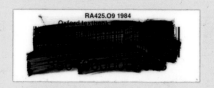
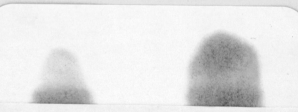

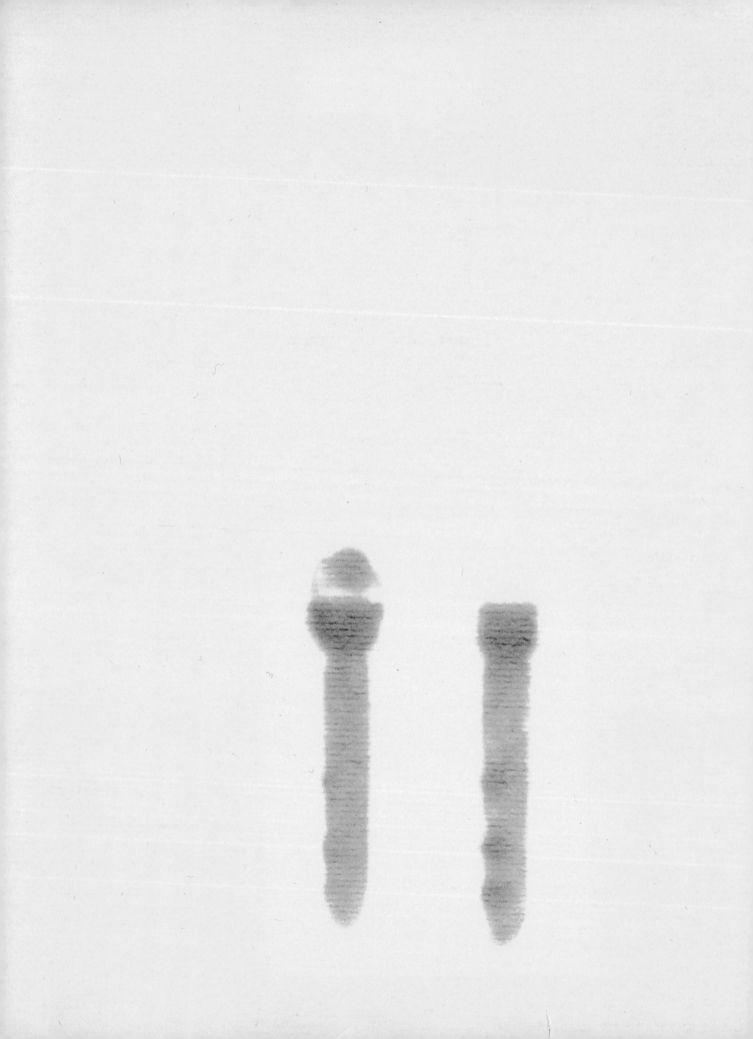

OXFORD MEDICAL PUBLICATIONS

Oxford textbook of public health

Editors

Walter W. Holland, MD, FRCGP, FRCP, FFCM

Professor of Clinical Epidemiology and Social Medicine,
Department of Community Medicine, and Honorary Director,
Social Medicine and Health Services Research Unit,
St. Thomas's Hospital Medical School (United Medical and Dental Schools),
London SE1 7EH, England.

Roger Detels, MD, MS

Professor of Epidemiology and Dean,
School of Public Health, Center for Health Sciences,
University of California, Los Angeles, CA 90024, USA.

George Knox, MD, BS, FRCP, FFCM

Professor of Social Medicine, Department of Social Medicine,
Health Services Research Centre,
University of Birmingham Medical School,
Edgbaston, Birmingham B15 2TG, England.

Ellie Breeze, MSc

Research Assistant, Department of Community Medicine,
St. Thomas's Hospital Medical School,
(United Medical and Dental Schools), London SE1 7EH, England.

Oxford textbook of public health

VOLUME 1

History, determinants, scope, and strategies

Edited by

Walter W. Holland, Roger Detels, and
George Knox
with the assistance of
Ellie Breeze

OXFORD NEW YORK TORONTO
OXFORD UNIVERSITY PRESS
1984

Oxford University Press, Walton Street, Oxford OX2 6DP

London New York Toronto
Delhi Bombay Calcutta Madras Karachi
Kuala Lumpur Singapore Hong Kong Tokyo
Nairobi Dar es Salaam Cape Town
Melbourne Auckland

and associated companies in
Beirut Berlin Mexico City Nicosia

Oxford is a trade mark of Oxford University Press

British Library Cataloguing in Publication Data

Oxford textbook of public health.
Vol. 1; History, determinants, scope and
strategies
1. Public health
I. Holland, Walter W.   II. Detels, Roger
III. Knox, George
614   RA425
ISBN 0-19-261369-3

Library of Congress Cataloging in Publication Data
Main entry under title:

Oxford textbook of public health.

(Oxford medical publications)
Bibliography: p.
Includes index.
Contents: v. 1. History, determinants, scope, and strategies.
1. Public health—Collected works.   I. Holland,
Walter W.   II. Series. [DNLM: 1. Public Health.
WA 100 O98]
RA422.5.O9 1984   362.1   84-14717
ISBN 0-19-261369-3

Typeset by Cotswold Typesetting, Cheltenham
Printed in Great Britain by Thomson Litho Ltd, East Kilbride, Scotland

Preface

It is not an easy task to follow in the footsteps of such a renowned editor as Professor Hobson. We were however very honoured when, on the retirement of Professor Hobson, the Oxford University Press approached us about taking up the challenge of revising Hobson's *Theory and practice of public health*. Since this work first appeared in February 1961, Professor Hobson was responsible for taking it through no less than five editions. Many eminent public health academics and practitioners have contributed to this book and it has been recognized as a standard textbook on the subject. Sadly, Professor Hobson died after a long illness at the end of November 1982. After an early training in public health starting as a medical officer of health and then as a specialist in hygiene and epidemiology in the army, he went on to be a lecturer in social medicine at Sheffield University, becoming professor in 1949. From 1957 until his retirement, he served in a variety of posts at the WHO, where his major responsibilities were always concerned with education and training. His interest in this and in the international aspects of health were well exemplified by the first edition of *Theory and practice of public health*. One of the major strengths of the book has been its international nature and its link to the WHO.

On accepting the daunting task of revising this major work our first step was to look dispassionately at its role within public health, a field which has evolved and changed greatly over the last 25 years. We decided that although this book is held in great esteem in the western world it was appropriate now to introduce major revisions and thus, increase its relevance to the problems facing us as we approach the twenty-first century. A particularly important advance has been the recognition in recent years that the problems in public health facing developing countries are quite different to those facing the developed world. The interests of WHO, quite correctly, have been focused on developing countries. We consider that this book should concentrate on presenting a comprehensive view of public health as it relates to developed countries. (Perhaps there is a place now for a comparable textbook concerned specifically with developing countries.) This is not to say, however, that the content will not prove relevant and of interest to the student of public health from a developing country.

The *Oxford textbook of public health* attempts to portray the philosophy and underlying principles of the practice of public health. The methods used for the investigation and the solution of public health problems are described and examples given of how these methods are applied in prac-tice. It is aimed primarily at postgraduate students and practitioners of public health but most clinicians and others concerned with public health issues will find some chapters relevant to their concerns. It is intended to be a comprehensive textbook present in the library of every institution concerned with the health sciences. The term 'public' is used quite deliberately to portray the field. Public health is concerned with defining the problems facing communities in the prevention of illness and thus studies of disease aetiology and promotion of health. It covers the investigation, promotion, and evaluation of optimal health services to communites and is concerned with the wider aspects of health within the general context of health and the environment. Other terms in common use, such as community medicine, preventive medicine, social medicine, and population medicine have acquired different meaning according to the country or setting. This gives rise to confusion and we have avoided their use since this book is directed to a worldwide audience. Public health, we believe, is more evocative of the basic philosophy which underlies this book.

The first volume aims to lead the reader through the historical determinants of health to the overall scope and strategies of public health. Through knowledge of historical aspects of the subject we may gain an understanding of what it is possible to achieve now and in the future. Only by grasping the underlying strategies of public health can we determine whether specific actions are feasible or not. In outlining the scope of public health we have emphasized that this covers not only the environment but also the social and genetic determinants of disease, which may ultimately enable us to identify those at greatest risk and thus to prevent the development and onset of disease and disability. The scope has now been broadened further by the growing concern with the provision and development of health services. This is clearly a function of public health. The approaches towards public health and the underlying political realities differ from country to country. However there are a few basic concepts common to every situation and these are outlined.

The major determinants of health and disease are dealt with in the second section of this volume, which paints, with a broad brush, the factors concerned with the development of disease, such as the physical environment, infectious agents, the social environment, war and social disorder. It is also important to have an understanding of the methods governments employ to control health hazards as well as their overall policies towards health. This we illustrate by describing the widely different approaches adopted on the two sides of the Atlantic. The strategies both for tackling modern hazards and for modifying behaviour through education are considered. To draw all these themes together into the same perspective, the final three chapters, prepared by three specialists with broad experience of public health in the context of the world as a whole, consider overall public health strategies relevant to the western as well as the developing world.

Volume 2 of this textbook is concerned with the process of public health promotion, Volume 3 with the investigative methods used in public health, and finally Volume 4 with a description of the specific applications of public health methods of controlling disease processes, and, with tackling the problems of disease in specific client groups.

The development of public health policy is dependent upon a series of scientific methods, and we do not attempt in this book to cover all the methods and their applications. However it is to be hoped that those examples that have been chosen will illustrate to the reader the way in which particular problems can be approached. Each chapter includes a comprehensive list of further reading which should equip the reader with the means of obtaining a deeper knowledge should he or she wish to pursue any theme further.

This is the first of what we hope will be many editions. As each chapter was submitted to the editors we have attempted to identify gaps and areas of overlap. There is no doubt however that some remain. It is only through feedback from readers that we will be able to adapt, modify, and improve further editions. If the book is successful it will be entirely due to the effort of the contributors who undertook with great patience a tremendous amount of work. They were bombarded with instructions, advice, reminders, and modifications and we would like to express our thanks and extend our apologies to all of them. Our gratitude also goes to our secretaries and assistants who coped so admirably with the enormous task of compiling this work. We hope that it will be widely read by all those concerned with the formulation and execution of public health policy and that it will provide a suitable framework for devising approaches to some of the problems challenging public health today.

W.W.H.
London   R.D.
August, 1984   G.K.

Contents

List of contributors

Anthony C. Allison, BM, DPhil (Oxon), FRCPath
Director, Institute of Biological Sciences, and Vice President for Research, Syntex Research Division of Syntex (USA) Inc., 3401 Hillview Avenue, P O Box 10850, Palo Alto, CA 94303, USA.

Joan Z. Bernstein, Esq.
Partner of Wald, Harkrader and Ross, 1300 Nineteenth Street, Northwest, Washington, DC 20036, USA.

Lester Breslow, MD, MPH
Professor of Public Health and Dean Emeritus, School of Public Health, Center for Health Sciences, University of California, Los Angeles, CA 90024, USA.

Central Directorate on Environmental Pollution
Department of the Environment, Romney House, 43 Marsham Street, London SW1P 3PY, England

Sidney P. Chave, PhD, FRSH
Emeritus Senior Lecturer in Community Health, London School of Hygiene and Tropical Medicine, London WC1E 7HT, England.

Roger Detels, MD, MS
Professor of Epidemiology and Dean, School of Public Health, Center for Health Sciences, University of California, Los Angeles, CA 90024, USA.

Virgil H. Freed
Head and Professor, Department of Agricultural Chemistry, Oregon State University, Corvallis, OR 97331, USA.

Michael Freedman, Esq.
Director of Issue Development at Common Cause, 2030 M Street, Northwest, Washington, DC 20036, USA.

J. Gallagher, MD (Public Health), MA (Education), FFCM
Consultant, World Health Organization, Copenhagen, Denmark.

Clifford Graham, LLB, Barrister-at-Law
Under Secretary, Department of Health and Social Security, Euston Tower, 286 Euston Road, London NW1 3ND, England.

Basil S. Hetzel, MD
Chief, Division of Human Nutrition, Commonwealth Scientific and Industrial Research Organization, Kintore Avenue, Adelaide 5000, Australia.

Gene I. Higashi, MD, ScD
Associate Professor, Department of Epidemiology, School of Public Health, University of Michigan, Ann Arbor, Michigan 48109, USA.

Richard E. Isaacson, PhD
Project Leader, Pfizer Central Research, Eastern Point Road, Groton, Connecticut 06340, USA.

Leo Kaprio MD, PhD, FAPHA, FFCM (Hon)
Regional Director for Europe, World Health Organization, Copenhagen, Denmark.

M.F. Lechat, MD, DTM, DrPH
Professor of Epidemiology and Head, Department of Epidemiology, Louvain's University School of Medicine, Brussels, Belgium.

Philip R. Lee, MD
Professor of Social Medicine and Director, Institute for Health Policy Studies, School of Medicine, University of California, San Francisco, 1326 Third Avenue, San Francisco, CA 94143, USA.

M.G. Marmot, MBBS, MPH, PhD
Senior Lecturer in Epidemiology, Department of Epidemiology, London School of Hygiene and Tropical Medicine, London WC1E 7HT, England.

Alan Maynard, BA(Hon), BPhil
Professor of Economics and Director of the Centre for Health Economics, University of York, Heslington, York YO1 5DD, England.

Arnold S. Monto, MD
Professor, Department of Epidemiology, School of Public Health, University of Michigan, Ann Arbor, Michigan 48109, USA.

J.N. Morris, MD(Hon), DSc(Hon), FRCP, FFCM
Professor and Senior Research Fellow, Department of Human Nutrition and Community Health, London School of Hygiene and Tropical Medicine, London WC1E 7HT, England.

K.W. Newell, MD, DPH, MCCM(NZ)
Professor of Tropical Community Health, Department of International Community Health, Liverpool School of Tropical Medicine, Pembroke Place, Liverpool L35 QA, England.

Joseph P. Newhouse, PhD
Head, Economics Department, The Rand Corporation, 1700 Main Street, Santa Monica, CA 90406, USA.

Ellie Scrivens, PhD
Lecturer in Social Sciences, Department of Community Medicine, St. Thomas's Hospital Medical School, (United Medical and Dental Schools), London SE1 7EH, England.

Arland T. Stein
Reed Smith Shaw McClay, Union Trust Building, P O Box 2009, Pittsburgh, PA 15230, USA.

S. Leonard Syme, PhD
Professor of Epidemiology, School of Public Health, University of California, Berkeley, CA 94720, USA.

Hugh H. Tilson, MD, DrPh
Director of Product Surveillance and Epidemiology, Burroughs Wellcome Co., Research Triangle Park, NC 27709, USA.

Abbreviations

AAV	Adeno-associated virus
ACGIH	American Conference of Governmental and Industrial Hygiene
ADP	Adenosine diphosphate
AEA	Atomic Energy Authority
AF	Attributable fraction
AHA	Area Health Authority
ALARA	As low as reasonably achievable (in environmental pollution control)
AMA	American Medical Association
ASTM	American Society for Testing of Materials
BPM	Best practicable means (in environmental pollution control)
CAT	Computed axial tomography
CDC	Centers for Disease Control
CDP	Community Development Project
CF	Complement fixation
CHC	Community Health Council
CHD	Coronary heart disease
CHESS	Community Health and Environmental Surveillance System
CMHC	Community Mental Health Center
CMV	Cytomegalovirus
CON	Certificate of Need
CPE	Cytopathic effect
DHA	District Health Authority
DHHS	Department of Health and Human Services
DHSS	Department of Health and Social Services
DNA	Deoxyribonucleic acid
DPH	Diploma in Public Health
EB virus	Epstein–Barr virus
ECG	Electrocardiogram
ECHO virus	Enteric cytopathic human orphan virus
ECT	Electroconvulsive therapy
EEC	European Economic Community
EF2	Elongation factor
ELISA	Enzyme-linked immunosorbent assay
EM	Electron microscopy
EPA	Environmental Protection Agency
EPEC	Enteropathic strains of *Escherichia coli*
EPSDT	Early periodic screening detection and treatment
EQO	Environmental quality objectives
EQS	Environmental quality standards

FA	Fluorescent antibody
FAO	Food and Agriculture Organization
FPC	Family Practitioner Committee
FTC	Federal Trade Commission
GDP	Guanosine diphosphate
GHS	General Household Survey
GNP	Gross national product
GP	General Practitioner
G6PD	Glucose 6-phosphate dehydrogenase
Hb	Haemoglobin
HbA	Adult haemoglobin
HbF	Fetal haemoglobin
HbS	Sickle-cell haemoglobin
HDFP	Hypertension Detection and Follow-up Program
HI	Haemoglutinin inhibition
HLA	Human lymphocyte antigen
HMO	Health Maintenance Organization
HSA	Health Systems Agencies
HSC	Health and Safety Commission
HSE	Health and Safety Executive
IAEA	International Atomic Energy Agency
IAPI	Industrial Air Pollution Inspectorate
IBRD	International Bank for Reconstruction and Development (UN)
ICAO	International Civil Aviation Organization
ICRCC	Interdepartmental Committee on the Redevelopment of Contaminated Land
IDDM	Insulin-dependent diabetes mellitus
IgA	Immunoglobulin A
IgE	Immunoglobulin E
IgG	Immunoglobulin G
IgM	Immunoglobulin M
IMCO	International Maritime Consultative Organization
IPI	Industrial Pollution Inspectorate
IQ	Intelligence quotient
Ir-genes	Immune response genes
Is-genes	Immune suppression genes
JOD	Juvenile onset diabetes
LD_{50}	Median lethal dose
LPS	Lypopolysaccharide
MHC	Major histocompatibility complex
MOH	Medical Officer of Health

MRC	Medical Research Council	RAWP	Resource Allocation Working Party
MRFIT	Multiple Risk Factor Intervention Trial	RCI	Radiochemical Inspectorate
mRNA	Messenger ribonucleic acid	RF	Rheumatoid factor
NDV	Newcastle disease virus	RHA	Regional Health Authority
NIH	National Institutes of Health	RIA	Radioimmunoassay
NII	Nuclear Installations Inspectorate	RNA	Ribonucleic acid
NHS	National Health Service	RS virus	Respiratory scyncytial virus
NPDES	National Pollutant Discharge Elimination System	RWMAC	Radioactive Waste Management Advisory Committee
OASDI	Old Age, Survivors, and Disability Insurance	SHPDA	State Health Planning and Development Agency
OECD	Organization for Economic Co-operation and Development	SIP	State Implementation Plan
OPCS	Office of Population Censuses and Surveys	SMMR	Standardized maternal mortality ratio
OSHA	Occupational Safety and Health Administration	SMR	Standardized mortality ratio
PA toxin	*Pseudomonas aeruginosa* toxin	TCDC	Technical co-operation between developing countries
PCB	Polychlorobiphenyls	UN	United Nations
PCA	Parliamentary Commissioner for Administration	UNDP	United Nations Development Programme
		UNICEF	United Nations Childrens Fund
PSRO	Professional Standards Review Organization	VD	Venereal disease
QUALS	Quality adjusted man years	WHO	World Health Organization

**The discipline of
health and disease**

1 The origins and development of public health

S.P.W. Chave

INTRODUCTION

Public health, as an organized system of health protection for the population, came into being in England in the nineteenth century. It began there because England was the first country to undergo the experience of the Industrial Revolution which transformed it from a land of small farms to one of smoking factories and 'dark satanic mills'.

Much of the knowledge on which the first measures to protect the public health were to be based had been acquired long before. In the Middle ages segregation and quarantine had been used in attempts to prevent the import and spread of leprosy and plague. Probably as a result of these actions leprosy died out in England in the fourteenth century. Plague, which entered the country in 1348, continued to erupt at intervals until 1665 after which, for reasons that are still not fully understood, it disappeared.

In 1720, when plague threatened to invade England again, the Government sought the advice of Richard Mead (1673–1754). He recommended the appointment of a Council of Health with wide powers to enforce a strict system of quarantine. In the event the threat did not materialize but the idea of the Council of Health was to be realized later on. For when in 1805 yellow fever threatened to enter the country from Gibraltar, a Board of Health was set up under the Privy Council to advise on the introduction of quarantine and other measures to meet the emergency. Once again the threatened invasion did not occur and the Board was dissolved in the following year.

Until the eighteenth century the control of the movement of people through segregation and quarantine was still the only method employed to prevent the outbreak and spread of infectious disease. Then, in that century new methods of prevention were developed. The first of these was environmental control. This came about through the pioneering work of three men, each working in a different environment, but all facing the common problems of 'fevers' and filth diseases in the populations with which they were concerned. John Pringle (1707–82) in the army, James Lind (1716–94) in the navy, and John Howard (1726–90) in the prisons, showed how improvements in environmental conditions could reduce the toll of disease, which in the fighting services caused a greater loss of lives than did warfare, and in the prisons, caused more deaths than all the public executions in the country put together. Lind was also responsible for another

important preventive measure, namely the use of citrus fruit to prevent the occurrence of scurvy among seafarers.

But the most important advance in prevention at this time came with the discovery of vaccination by Edward Jenner (1749–1823). This not only provided a safe and effective [against] smallpox, one of the great killing and [diseases] of the time, it also laid the foundations [of the] science of immunology.

Such was the knowledge already available and awaiting wider application when England came through the Napoleonic Wars.

INDUSTRIALIZATION AND REFORM

England emerged from the Napoleonic Wars victorious abroad only to face serious social, economic, and political problems at home. These problems arose in part from the effects of the long wars with France, but more particularly from the dislocations brought about by the rapid advances in industrial technology based on the harnessing of steam power. Rapid industrialization was accompanied by equally rapid urbanization. Extensive enclosures of farm land drove thousands of country people from their small holdings to the new industrial towns to become 'hands' to serve the new machines.

The industrial towns grew apace, many of them such as Manchester, Liverpool, Leeds, and Sheffield increased their populations by 50 per cent in a decade. The demand for housing far outpaced the available supply. Houses were hastily built with little thought for suitability of soil or site, for water supply or drainage. Dwellings were packed together back-to-back within easy reach of the factories, and the people were packed together inside them. Accumulations of refuse and soil-heaps, and unwholesome cess-pools were common features of the narrow courts and alleys. Dirt, disease, and malnourishment flourished. Chief among the diseases were typhoid and typhus, not by then distinguished, tuberculosis, smallpox, scarlet fever, and measles. Mortality was high, infant mortality particularly so, in many places as high as 200 per 1000 births.

England paid for the economic benefits of increased production with the social costs of unplanned urbanization.

At this time the country was without even the rudiments of a system of public health. There was on the Statute Book a

3

well intentioned, but futile, Act to establish a system of quarantine if epidemic disease threatened, and each year Parliament voted £2000 to the National Vaccine Establishment for the prevention of smallpox. Apart from this, neither the law nor the government had any concern for the public health. Furthermore, the people in the industrial towns had no voice in political affairs either centrally or locally, through which they could express their complaints. There was a need for reform, indeed there was clamour for it, and reform, when it came, came quickly and decisively. Within the space of five years a like number of enactments was made which were not only important advances in themselves, but also paved the way for further developments which were to follow over the next 50 years.

There was first, the great Reform Act of 1832, which radically re-shaped the House of Commons, the main seat of political power. It swept away the so-called 'rotten boroughs', the constituencies which had lain in the pockets of the great landowners for generations, and redistributed parliamentary seats having regard to the distribution of the population, thus enfranchizing the new industrial towns. The Act also extended the parliamentary vote to the urban middle class.

This was followed by the Factory Act of 1833. Working conditions in the factories, cotton mills, and coal mines were harsh in the extreme. Child labour was extensively employed and exploited. At the beginning of the century children began their working lives at the age of five years and toiled for up to 16 hours a day for a pittance of a wage. Between 1802 and 1825 several Acts of Parliament had been passed to raise the minimum age for employment, and to reduce hours of work. They had all failed because there were no means of enforcing them, and so parents and employers, each for their own financial reasons, had tacitly conspired to ignore them. The Act of 1833, which was drafted by Edwin Chadwick, of whom more will be heard, was important not only because it made it unlawful to employ children under the age of nine years in the factories, and limited their hours of work, but because it instituted a system of inspection to ensure that the law was being observed. Four inspectors were appointed with powers of entry who were required to report directly to Parliament. The practice of inspection and report once embodied by law into the administrative system was to be widely employed in the future. The Factory Act of 1833 was to be followed by further enactments made through the century which dealt with working conditions and with the safety, health, and welfare of industrial workers.

The year 1834 brought the Poor Law Amendment Act which reformed the system of administering relief to the poor. This had been established by the great Elizabethan Poor Law of 1601 which had made the parish responsible for caring for its own poor. For this purpose a poor rate was levied on the occupancy of land which was used to provide work for the workless and to relieve the needs of the sick, the impotent, and the aged. By the nineteenth century the old system was getting out of hand. It had become clear that the unit of administration, the parish, was too small. There were over 15 000 parishes in England and Wales, each of which was a law unto itself, so that benefits varied in different parts of the country. Across the south of England a system known

as 'Speenhamland' was spreading. Speenhamland was a small village in Berkshire, where in 1795 the local justices had ruled that poor relief should be tied to the cost of living, specifically to the price of a loaf of bread. Thus, when the price of bread rose, poor relief was raised accordingly. But not only relief, but also the wages of the lowest paid were subsidized out of the poor rate. Although the intention here was probably humanitarian, its results were pernicious. For there was now no inducement for employers to raise wages as prices rose, but to keep them down, knowing that they would be supplemented out of the poor rate. The effect of this was to pauperize and demoralize the honest working man. But more than that it placed an intolerable burden on the poor rate itself. The system was badly in need of overhauling. Accordingly, in 1832 a Royal Commission was set up to review the working of the Poor Law. It reported two years later and its recommendations were immediately embodied in the Amendment Act of 1834 which created the 'New Poor Law'. In the event this was to lead to the founding of the public health movement, as we shall see later.

Meanwhile, in 1835, the Municipal Corporations Act did for local government what the Reform Act had done for Parliament. It brought an end to the self-perpetuating oligarchies which had held power in the municipalities since the Middle Ages, and extended the local vote to all ratepayers. This was an important step not least because it was the local authorities which were, in time, to become the agents for sanitary administration and reform.

Finally, in this series of enactments came the Births, Marriages and Deaths Registration Act of 1836, which founded the system of civil registration. From 1538 every parish church had been required to keep a register of baptisms, marriages, and burials. From early in the seventeenth century, during visitations of plague, Bills of Mortality based on parish records, had been collated and published in the City of London. From 1660 these had been issued weekly. It was on these Bills that John Graunt (1620–72) had carried out his pioneering statistical studies which have earned him the title of 'father of medical statistics'. In 1801 the first national census was taken which showed that the population of England and Wales numbered about eight million. Since then a census has been taken every ten years with the exception of 1941. The Act of 1836 established the General Register Office in London, created the post of Registrar-General and required compulsory registration of births, marriages, and deaths. Through the initiative of Edwin Chadwick the cause of death was made registrable from the beginning. Chadwick was also instrumental in securing the appointment of William Farr (1807–83), a young mathematically-minded doctor, to the staff of the new Office. Farr remained there for 40 years and in that time he created the system of national vital statistics which is used to this day, and which has become a model for many other countries.

Appended to the First Report of the Registrar-General in 1841 was a letter addressed to him by William Farr. In this he discussed the causes of death and related them to various environmental and other factors. These letters, written by Farr over the next 40 years, created what was, in effect, a new branch of medical literature. It was the statistical information tabulated and interpreted by Farr, and published in the Annual Reports of the Registrar-General, which provided the information-base for the work of the public health service through the years that were to follow.

THE RISE OF THE PUBLIC HEALTH MOVEMENT IN ENGLAND: CHADWICK AND SIMON

We turn now to the beginnings of the public health movement. It began as a problem of the Poor Law and was first seen as a possible means of reducing expenditure on poor relief. The Poor Law Amendment Act of 1834 had created what came to be called the New Poor Law. This introduced a single scale of benefit across the country, with no local variations. The unit of administration became, not the parish, but the union of parishes. This reduced the number of poor law authorities from 15 000 to 660. In each Union, a Board of Guardians of the Poor was elected by the rate-payers to administer the scheme locally. A Poor Law Commission was set up in London which sent inspectors round the country to ensure that the rules were being observed. And the rules? In principle they were quite simple. There was to be no more outdoor relief for the able-bodied. There would be no more Speen-hamland.* An unemployed man could not receive relief unless he was prepared to enter the workhouse with his family, where husband would be separated from wife, to prevent them bringing more pauper children into the world, and where children would be separated from their parents. Further, the Act laid down the 'test of lesser eligibility' which meant that the workhouse should be the lowest paymaster and the hardest taskmaster of all.

It was a harsh system, a cruel system. Its purpose was to encourage industry, and discourage idleness through the deterrence of the workhouse test, for it was believed that if a man really wanted work, if he looked hard enough he would find it. This then was the New Poor Law and the man who was appointed to administer it was Edwin Chadwick (1800–90).

Chadwick began his career by training in the law, but before being called to the Bar he came under the influence of Jeremy Bentham (1748–1832), the ageing reformer and philosopher. Bentham was the leading proponent of the Utilitarian philosophy which held that the good of the community should take precedence over all other considerations. According to Bentham, the test of the 'utility' of any social institution was the extent to which it contributed to 'the greatest happiness of the greatest number'. He proposed that this principle should be embodied in far-reaching reforms of the law, government, and administration, and should also include the setting up of a ministry of health.

Chadwick became secretary to Bentham and was with him when he died. It was his close association with the old philosopher, and his acceptance of his ideas, which determined the future course of Chadwick's life. Instead of pursuing

a lucrative career in the law, he chose the hard and thorny path of the reformer. In 1832 he accepted an appointment on the Royal Commission on the Poor Law and with Nassau Senior (1790–1864) was the joint author of its Report. Following the passing of the Act in 1834 he became Secretary to the Commission and thus its chief executive officer.

As a young man Chadwick had already become aware of the close connection that exists between poverty and sickness, indeed he had already written about it. Now at the Poor Law Commission he came face to face with the facts of that association. He saw the way in which sickness would strike down the wage-earner, bringing him to an early grave, thus throwing his widow and orphans onto the Poor Law. What a waste this was, he said. Chadwick was no great humanitarian, no one has ever accused Chadwick of having a heart! But he loathed waste, and this was gross waste of life and resources. Moreover, it was preventable waste. Prevent the sickness and you would prevent the poverty and thus the drain on the resources of the Poor Law.

In 1838, at Chadwick's suggestion, the Commission employed three doctors to conduct an inquiry into the fevers prevalent in London, having regard to their prevention. Their reports described the grossly insanitary conditions which prevailed in the poorer districts of the metropolis and the diseases which were rife among the inhabitants. These findings made a profound impression on Parliament and, as a result, again on Chadwick's prompting, the Commissioners were asked to conduct a similar inquiry covering the whole country. Chadwick organized the inquiry himself and wrote the Report on it which was published in 1842. Entitled *'General Report on the Sanitary Conditions of the Labouring Population of Great Britain'* it was a damning and fully documented indictment of the appalling conditions in which masses of the working people were compelled to live, and die, in the industrial towns and rural areas of the Kingdom.

Chadwick claimed that the annual loss of life due to filth and bad ventilation was greater than that in any war in which the country had ever been engaged. The effect upon the population of such a shockingly insanitary environment was to make them 'short-lived, improvident, reckless, and intemperate' in conditions which fostered 'the most abject degradation'. In propounding the problem, Chadwick also propounded his remedy which came to be known as his 'Sanitary Idea'.

As fully developed the 'Sanitary Idea' consisted of three parts. The first was a theory of causation. Chadwick accepted the prevailing view that disease is caused by foul air arising from the putrefaction and the decomposition of organic matter and waste. In fact it can be said that Chadwick's inquiry confirmed the theory, because it was in the most insanitary and ill-ventilated quarters that mortality was at its greatest. Second, there was the remedy for the problem. This was simply a drainage system backed by a supply of running water to flush away the filth and so the foul air associated with it. The basis of Chadwick's drainage system was the glazed earthenware pipe which had recently been invented. Chadwick showed that a network of these pipes could effectively drain a district, and do so better, and more cheaply, than the brick-built sewers of disposal which had done duty

*The Speenhamland system, that is, relief in aid of wages, was abolished in 1834. It was revived in 1974 as the Family Income Supplement under which workers on low pay have their wages supplemented out of government funds.

for this purpose in the past. In essence this was an arterio-venous system which would replace the earth closet by the WC. Third, was Chadwick's proposal for implementing his scheme. He proposed that a local board of health should be set up in every district in the land charged with the task of sanitary improvement. However, Chadwick had little faith in local initiative especially where local money had to be spent. So he recommended that a central board of health should be set up which would send out inspectors to ensure that the local boards were carrying out their duties. Chadwick's proposal was a plan for a national public health service whose structure would parallel exactly that of the Poor Law which he was then administering and of which he was the author.

This was the 'Sanitary Idea', and it was while penning it that Chadwick put forward a further proposal which was to be of lasting importance. He wrote:

that for the general promotion of the means necessary to prevent disease it would be a good economy to appoint a district medical officer, independent of private practice, with the security of special qualifications, with responsibility to initiate sanitary measures and reclaim the execution of the law.

This was the moment of conception of the Medical Officer of Health – the MOH.

There had been a cadre of medical officers in the public service before this time, namely the medical officers of the Poor Law. However, their concern was mainly with *treatment*, the task of the new officer was to be essentially with *prevention*. And, as Chadwick said, it would be a good economy. The principal reason in Chadwick's mind in bringing the MOH to birth was not humanitarian, but economy, because it promised to be cost-effective.

Chadwick's report was a best-seller. Ten thousand copies were printed and sold and it was read and debated right across the country. As a result, Peel's Government was obliged to take action. In 1843, it appointed a Royal Commission on the Health of Towns to repeat Chadwick's inquiry, which it did, and confirmed his findings. This is not altogether surprising because Chadwick 'precognized' the witnesses and drafted the Commission's first Report and its final recommendations. A further outcome of Chadwick's work was the formation of the Health of Towns Association which, with the support of many important figures in public life, conducted a widespread campaign for sanitary reform throughout the country.

Thus it was that in 1848, on the basis of the Reports of the Royal Commission, backed by public pressure exerted through the Association, and with cholera in the land acting as a spur, the first Public Health Act in British history went on to the Statute Book. The Act represented a watered-down version of Chadwick's proposals, mainly because it was permissive in character rather than obligatory, as Chadwick would have had it.

It set up a General Board of Health, but gave it a life of only five years in the first instance. It did not require the establishment of local boards but allowed their formation if the people so desired, that is, on a petition of 10 per cent of the ratepayers. However, the General Board could compel the setting up of a local board in any district where the average death rate reached 23 per 1000 persons, as it did in many places. Further, the Act did not require the appointment of a MOH, but permitted a local board to make such an appointment if it wished.

In this respect, however, the provisions of the Act had already been anticipated in two places. It was in Liverpool, on 1 January 1847, that the MOH first saw the light of day. Under a private Act, the Liverpool Corporation, inspired by the 'Sanitary Idea', had secured Parliamentary sanction for the appointment of an MOH, and immediately used its newly won power to appoint William Henry Duncan (1805–63) to that post. Duncan was a local physician with a profound concern for the sanitary problems of his town – and they were legion. Following his appointment he took up his new task with energy and dedication.

But Duncan is more important for what he was than for what he did. Far more important in the long run was the appointment in 1848 of John Simon (1816–1904) as the first MOH of the City of London. For Simon (pronounced 'Simmone') was to win for the new office the seal of approval and acceptability that could never have been done by Chadwick. In his new post he set a high standard of informed and impartial comment on all matters affecting the public health which won respect and gained attention well beyond the confines of the City. His reports to the City authorities, couched in the rich flowing language of the educated Victorian gentleman he was, were published verbatim in the columns of *The Times* newspaper and read right across the country. Simon was already addressing himself to the nation. But now we must leave Simon in the City and turn our attention to the General Board of Health.

The Board was appointed in 1848 after the passing of the Public Health Act. It consisted of three persons; Lord Morpeth, a minister, representing the government; Viscount Ashley, afterwards as Earl of Shaftsbury to become well-known for his humanitarian work on behalf of children, who was the unpaid member; and Edwin Chadwick who was the full-time paid member. Two years later Dr Southwood Smith, a friend of Chadwick's, who had been prominent in the health of towns movement, was appointed as a part-time member to advise on burial matters. But Chadwick was, in effect, the Board and acted as such.

The beginning of the Board's career was marked by the second visitation of cholera in which 54 000 people perished. On the occasion of the first outbreak in 1831–32, when 30 000 people died, a Central Board of Health had been set up, along the lines which had been suggested long before by Richard Mead, but it had been allowed to lapse after the ending of the epidemic. The significance of the new machinery which was created in 1848 was that it was intended to be permanent.

The Board began by attempting to mobilize the nation's defences against the cholera epidemic. In this it was successful in securing the passage of the Nuisances Removal and Prevention Act which gave powers of compulsion on sanitary matters to local authorities. In the next four years 183 local boards were set up covering over two million people. Chadwick from his desk in Whitehall issued copious directions setting out in immense detail how they were to perform their functions.

In its early days the Board acquired some public esteem for its efforts to combat cholera and for its fight against apathetic boards of guardians who sought to obstruct its work. However, as time passed this goodwill was dissipated, largely through Chadwick himself. He claimed a wide scope for state intervention in an age when *laissez-faire* was the doctrine of the day. He took the view that professional civil servants knew better than elected representatives, and showed contempt for public opinion. Instead of persuasion he used the methods of the bully and before long he made himself the most detested man in the Kingdom. Chadwick succeeded in antagonizing almost every section of the community. He antagonized local interests by his flagrant use of 'centralizing' powers; he antagonized ratepayers because of the heavy costs of his sanitary schemes; he antagonized the doctors, for whom he had little time, because the 'Sanitary Idea' does not need doctors, it needs engineers; but he even antagonized the engineers by the partiality he showed to those who would do his bidding against those who critically maintained their professional independence. But more than this Chadwick antagonized *The Times* newspaper. On one occasion it wrote 'We would rather take our chance with the cholera than be bullied into health by Mr. Chadwick'. All this hostility came down on Chadwick's head in 1853 when the time came to renew the life of the Board. The Government introduced a short Bill to extend the life of the Board for a further five years but the House of Commons threw it out. The Government was defeated on the issue, the General Board of Health was dissolved and Chadwick was dismissed.

This first attempt to establish a central department with responsibility for the public health was broken on the personality of the man who had conceived it. Active to the end of his long life, Chadwick was never again entrusted with any public office. Yet the 'Sanitary Idea' of which he was the author remained the driving force behind the public health movement for another 50 years.

In the year following Chadwick's downfall the Government re-established the Board, but only as a shadow of its former self, for now it was shorn of any centralizing powers. One important step was taken, however, and that was to appoint John Simon as the full-time salaried medical officer to the Board. The life of the new Board was renewed annually for five years and then the Government decided to let it quietly disappear. However, on the representation of the Prince Consort this was not done, and in 1858, at his suggestion, the powers and duties of the Board were transferred to the Privy Council where a medical department was set up with Simon as its head. For the next ten years public health remained quiet under Simon's leadership. Where Chadwick had bullied Simon sought to persuade. Chadwick had aimed to extend the powers of the centre, whereas Simon accepted local feeling and attempted to work with it. Through his inspectors, his annual reports, and his personal initiatives he made steady but sound progress within a legal framework that was permissive rather than obligatory.

Simon used his limited resources to employ the best medical scientists of the day to investigate the entire range of infectious diseases, as well as the living and working conditions of the people. In this he was building up a fund of knowledge that would provide a scientific foundation for the development of sanitary law and administration for the future.

ENVIRONMENTAL HYGIENE AT ITS PEAK

When Gladstone took office in 1868 he found the sanitary scene in a state of near chaos. This had arisen largely because the rapid growth of towns had created the need for the extension of local administration to such matters as paving, lighting, drainage, and sewerage which had been met by the indiscriminate appointment, under private Acts, of *ad hoc* bodies to oversee these various services. By 1869 there were said to be at least 160 Acts of Parliament in force making sanitary provisions, but so mixed up as to their administration that even the lawyers could not unravel them. The time was ripe for reform. Gladstone immediately appointed the Royal Sanitary Commission to review the whole situation. In its report, published in 1871, the Commission made three important recommendations which were to determine the scope and pattern of the public health system in England for the next 50 years. They were that:

1. There should be one central department with responsibility for the public health.
2. The country should be divided into administrative districts, each of which should be responsible for sanitary action at the local level.
3. The mass of sanitary legislation should be consolidated into a single statute.

In brief, there should be one central department, one authority in each district, and one sanitary law applying to the whole country.

Thus it was that the Local Government Board Act of 1871 created the central department, the Public Health Act of 1872 created the local sanitary authorities, and the Public Health Act of 1875 codified the law. Each of these enactments had important implications for the future and they will therefore be briefly considered in turn.

First, the Local Government Board Act. Simon, in his evidence to the Royal Commission had advocated the creation of a strong central department of public health with a cabinet minister at its head, and that every local health officer should stand in an official relationship to the minister who would thus head the national public health service. In the event, the Government decided to bring together Public Health and the Poor Law into a single department, thus creating the nineteenth century equivalent of the Department of Health and Social Security of the present time. And so the Local Government Board came into being. This was undoubtedly the biggest setback that English public health ever suffered. For the arrangement within the department was such that public health was subordinated to the pinch-penny policies of the destitution authority, with its avowed policy of deterrence. The Board never showed any appreciation of the real health needs of the nation. Advances there were, important advances, but rarely indeed were they the result of leadership from the centre. Instead, they came about most often through local initiative and voluntary effort taken up and led by enterprising medical officers of health. When the Board was set up, Simon was appointed as its medical officer. However, he found the subordination of himself and the medical division so humiliating that after four years he resigned and took his retirement.

The Public Health Act of 1872 virtually created a national public health service. It not only established a sanitary authority in every district in the land, but it also required each one of them to appoint a medical officer of health. The Public Health Act of 1848 had allowed local authorities to appoint a MOH if they wished, but, in fact very few had done so. Most of them had looked on the past as an expensive luxury they could afford to do without, and by 1870 only 92 authorities outside London were employing the services of a MOH. Now there were to be more than a thousand of them! This really put the MOH on the map and right across the country.

The need to provide training for doctors entering the new specialty was quickly felt. It was first met in Dublin in 1870 where Trinity College established a post-graduate course leading to a Diploma in State Medicine, shortly after to be called the Diploma in Public Health, the DPH. Cambridge followed in 1875 and before long almost every University and medical school in the country was running a DPH course. In 1886 the qualification was put under the supervision of the General Medical Council and made registrable. Two years later Parliament set the seal of statutory approval on the qualification by requiring the medical officer of health of any district having a population of 50 000 to hold the DPH. In this way the MOH won his spurs as a specialist, and the DPH became the criterion of proficiency in public health, the hallmark of this specialty in the Faculty of Medicine. In the course of time the DPH also became a requirement for public health practice in many of the countries of the British Commonwealth as they adopted, and adapted, the British system of public health law and administration.

During the 1870s, and for some time after, the work of the MOH continued to be concerned primarily with the environment, especially with housing and sanitation, and with infectious diseases. It was carried out within the framework of the Public Health Act of 1875. This had codified the sanitary law and provided a charter for action by the public health service for the next 60 years. The conceptual basis of the Act was the 'Sanitary Idea'. It was scarcely influenced by the discoveries of the bacteriologists. Noxious effluvia from cesspools, sewer gas from drains, and obvious dirt and filth, rather than germs, were the enemies to be tackled through sensible, practical sanitary action. Thus, on the basis of a false hypothesis much public good was to be achieved.

The Public Health Act of 1875 signalled the high-water mark of environmental hygiene as a notionally complete system of health for the nation, and it continued under its own momentum for many years. However, towards the end of the century the 'Sanitary Idea' began to be overtaken by a new idea, the concept of the individual and his or her personal health needs.

The great feats of sanitary engineering had been accompanied by substantial improvements in the public health. Between 1840 and 1900 the crude death rate had fallen from 25 to 15 per 1000, while the expectation of life of a male at birth had increased from 40 years in 1840 to 50 years in 1900 – a massive improvement in health adding years to the life of the average man. But there were no grounds for complacency, because the infant mortality rate, perhaps our most sensitive index of social health, had remained obstinately high at about 150 per 1000 births, indicating that about 1 in 7 of all babies born under Queen Victoria did not live to see their first birthday, while each year some 4000 mothers were dying in childbirth.

It was becoming clear that environmental sanitation was not enough to secure an adequate standard of health for the great mass of the people, but that what were needed were services directed specifically towards the needs of vulnerable groups, of which the first were mothers and children. This swing of interest in the public health movement, away from a primary concern with the environment towards personal health coincided closely, as will be shown later, with the turn of the century. Moreover, it took place not only in Britain but also on the continent of Europe and in the US. It is to this development that we shall now turn briefly.

THE BEGINNINGS OF PUBLIC HEALTH IN FRANCE, GERMANY, AND THE UNITED STATES

Wherever, in Europe or North America, industrialization took place on a wide scale, the consequences were similar to those which had occurred in England, and called for similar remedies.

In France, following the Revolution in 1789, the Convention passed a series of laws which aimed to establish a system of medical care for the population. This was to include the appointment of three medical practitioners in every district of the country. However, the system remained one on paper only, for it was never implemented. In the years that followed, industrialization proceeded steadily and was accompanied by insanitary housing in unplanned towns, the exploitation of child labour in the factories, and by outbreaks of epidemic diseases, all of which called for government intervention. However, it was not until after the founding of the Second Republic in 1848 that action was taken. In that year two laws were passed, the first of which established a central public health council to advise the government, and the second created a network of such councils to advise local prefects on matters affecting the health of the people. These councils were mainly concerned with environmental sanitation and with conditions in the factories. The system proved to be of only limited effectiveness largely because the functions of the councils were purely advisory. However, nothing was done to improve the system until the end of the century, by which time problems of maternal and child health had come to the fore. The first steps in this direction consisted in the opening of milk stations in poor districts to provide cheap milk to nursing mothers, and centres to advise mothers on infant care.

In the German states, awareness of the need for governments to take action to protect the public health had emerged during the eighteenth century and had found expression in the concept of 'medical police' (or polity). By this was meant the establishment by government of an organized system of health protection for the people and its implementation through administrative regulation. The principal exponent of this idea was Johann Peter Frank (1748–1821) who embodied his proposals in his *Complete System of Medical Police* in six volumes published between 1779 and 1819. In this monumental work he traced the course of a person's life from the womb to the tomb laying down in great detail how his or her every action should be regulated to ensure total well-being. It was a system designed to produce a nation of fit people who could support the rule and ambitions of an autocratic ruler. Indeed, it is true to say that Frank was the public health representative of enlightened despotism. Frank's work influenced developments in some of the German states, but it was so closely associated with absolutist Government that after the fall of Napoleon interest in it steadily declined, although it was never forgotten. Thereafter, it was not until after 1848 that progress in sanitary reform began to be made, and even then, by reason of the autonomy of the states, it was uneven in quality.

Following the Franco-Prussian War, and the creation of the Second Reich in 1871, it became possible for the first time to establish a central department of public health to exercise surveillance and jurisdiction over the whole country. Again, as in other countries at that time, the principal concern was with the environment, and great strides were made to bring about improvements in general sanitary conditions in the towns and cities. One notable advance in the provision of medical care came in 1883, when Chancellor Bismarck introduced his system of social insurance. It was a compulsory contributory insurance scheme providing sick benefit and maternity benefit, compensation for industrial accidents and disability, widows and orphans, and old age pensions. It was paid for by deductions from the pay-packets of the workers, by payments by the employers, and supplemented by the State. Bismarck's system became a model for other European countries, including Britain.

At this time Germany began to give attention to the health of children and by the end of the century had established a system of routine medical inspection of children in the schools of the State.

In the US, the conditions which had brought the sanitary reform movement into being in England were to be repeated, somewhat later, and more slowly. Outbreaks of epidemic diseases brought quarantine measures and environmental control into play. As early as 1804, New York had appointed a City Inspector of Health who was responsible for environmental sanitation, health administration and the collection of vital statistics. Shortly after, a Board of Health was set up to advise the Common Council on public health matters. Large-scale immigration put pressure on housing accommodation in the towns, and standards of hygiene, which in the working class areas had never been high, steadily deteriorated.

Chadwick's inquiries in England acted as a stimulus to similar activities in the US. In 1848 John Griscom, a former City Inspector of Health, published a report on *The Sanitary Condition of the Labouring Population of New York*, which clearly showed the influence of Chadwick. It described the conditions in the urban slums, and pointed the way to measures of reform which were to be undertaken during the next 30 years. Central to the programme was the concept of 'preventable death'. Recurrent epidemics of yellow fever, cholera, smallpox, typhoid, and typhus, reinforced Griscom's recommendations for the creation of a proper system of public health administration.

From 1845 a number of voluntary associations grew up, similar to the Health of Towns Association in Britain, which acted as a stimulus to official action. The local sanitary survey, begun by Griscom, became a useful weapon with which to counter the vested interests which opposed any movement for local reform, as well as to encourage government action. The best known of these surveys was that conducted by Lemuel Shattuck (1793–1859) in Massachusetts, and published in 1850. Shattuck was a bookseller and publisher who had a profound concern for the health problems of his state. He had secured the passing of a state law introducing civil registration which became a model for other states. He was also responsible for the setting up of a Commission, with himself as chairman, to make a sanitary survey of the state. The Report, which he wrote himself, is as important a landmark in the US as is Chadwick's in England. It embodied proposals for the creation of a sound public health organization. But action on the Report was slow, and Shattuck died before his recommendations were implemented in his home state.

Meanwhile there was progress in New York State. In 1864 a Council of Hygiene and Public Health had been set up which immediately carried out a survey and revealed the insanitary conditions prevailing in some parts of the City. Public concern was aroused, and as a result, a bill was passed which led to the establishment of the Metropolitan Board of Health, with responsibility for sanitary administration in the metropolitan district of New York State. This was followed ten years later by the founding of the New York City Health Department, whose principal duties were to take practical steps to improve the general environment, and to control the spread of infectious diseases.

The creation of the Metropolitan Board of Health marked a turning point not only in New York but in the US as a whole. For it brought into being a system of public health organization and administration which became a model for other states. The development of state departments of health gave rise to the idea of a central health department for the nation. In 1878 Congress passed a bill creating the National Board of Health. Its duties were to advise the Federal Government, and the states, on matters affecting the health of the people. It continued until 1883 when it was brought to an end. It failed through the antagonism of the states, who felt that the Board posed a threat to their rights. Seventy years were to elapse before a central department of health was to be re-established in the US.

During the latter part of the nineteenth century the US was forging ahead with industrialization and as a result caught up with, and surpassed, Britain as an industrial nation. But, as in Britain, industrialization brought a welter of health and social problems. Rapid industrialization, unplanned urban growth, and a new flood of immigrants from Europe all combined to produce city slums where poverty, malnutrition, disease, and vice were endemic.

This prompted socially-minded people to combine together to form voluntary societies to tackle these problems, often in association with government agencies.

Among these problems infant and child mortality were especially prominent. Thus it was as the nineteenth century neared its end, that steps began to be taken in the US, as also in France, Germany, and Britain, representing the industrialized countries of western Europe, specifically to protect and promote the health of children.

THE SWING TO PERSONAL HEALTH IN BRITAIN

It can be said with some truth that for the British people the twentieth century began on 22 January 1901, the day on which Queen Victoria breathed her last. Certainly the passing of the old Queen marked the end of an era of the greatest importance in the social, political, and economic development of Britain and of its influence across the seas. But, for those whose concern is with public health, the Edwardian period which followed was a veritable seed-time, the harvest of which was to be reaped over the next 50 years.

It began in 1902 with the Midwives Act, which established the Roll of Midwives under the control of the Central Midwives Board. This marked the end of the career of 'Mrs Gamp', the untrained, unwashed handywoman who performed her lowly function for small fee, and replaced her with a trained professional midwife, at first under the surveillance of the medical officer of health, and later as a member of his staff. Improved care of mothers in childbirth was to contribute to the slow, but steady, decline in maternal mortality that took place in the years that followed.

Public concern over the fitness of the nation, particularly as a result of the disclosure that no less than 40 per cent of the men who had volunteered for service in the army in the Boer War (1899–1902) had been rejected because they were unfit, led to the setting up by Balfour's Conservative Government of the Committee on Physical Deterioration, to examine the problem. The Committee found little evidence of deterioration. Undeterred, however, they went on to make a series of bold, sensible, and practical recommendations which together amounted to a blue-print to protect and improve the health of the nation's children.

The immediate outcome of this Report was the provision of school meals in 1906 and the founding of the School Medical Service in 1907. The implementation of these two proposals was a tacit admission on the part of the nation that large numbers of the children who had been swept into school by the introduction of compulsory education could not benefit from the teaching provided, either because they were hungry or because they were sick. Despite opposition from those who feared that providing meals for hungry children would be an encouragement to parental irresponsibility, wiser counsels prevailed, and before long thousands of children were enjoying the bowl of soup and hunk of bread which made up the first school meals.

More important in the long run was the setting up of the School Medical Service, which instituted a system of routine medical inspection of all children in the local authority schools. This was similar to the schemes which were already in operation in France, Germany, Belgium, and Sweden. It is important to note that this, the first of the British personal health services, was not put under the control of the Local Government Board. Through the initiative of Robert Morant (1863–1920) the far-sighted Permanent Secretary of the Board of Education, a medical department was set up there under Dr George Newman (1870–1948). Morant and Newman devised a simple procedure for linking the new service for schoolchildren to the public health service as a whole. They encouraged the appointment of the MOH as the principal school medical officer for his district. So, from this time onwards, the MOH wore two hats, namely as the medical officer of health responsible to the Public Health Committee of his authority, and the principal school medical officer and so responsible to the Education Committee of the same authority. This was a happy arrangement that lasted until 1974.

The system of routine medical inspections soon yielded a wealth of information, never before available, about the poor physical condition of large numbers of children in schools, and highlighted the need for the provision of medical care.

Under the Act, the duty of inspection lay with the local education authorities; the responsibility for obtaining treatment lay with the parents. But the school doctors found themselves repeatedly inspecting children whose disorders and disabilities were going untreated, either through the unwillingness, or more often through the inability, of parents to obtain the necessary treatment, or to pay for it. Nor, if they could not pay, were they willing to take their children to the doctors of the Poor Law because of the stigma this incurred. So from 1912, on the advice of Newman and Morant, the Board of Education began to make grants to local authorities for the setting up of minor ailment clinics. These provided treatment for the common conditions of the skin, the ears, the nose, mouth, and throat; they also provided dental treatment and spectacles. These clinics were to make an important contribution to the health care of children until the coming of the National Health Service (NHS) in 1948.

By this time the Poor Law was once again giving rise to public disquiet. The old system was full of anomalies, and the stigma which surrounded it acted as a deterrent to many of those in genuine need. In 1905 the Conservative Government set up a Royal Commission to review the system. The Commission consisted of eighteen persons including Octavia Hill the housing reformer; Charles Booth the pioneer of social inquiry and author of *London Life and Labour*; George Lansbury later to become one of the leaders of the Labour Movement; and Beatrice Webb who, with her husband Sidney Webb, was responsible for many contributions to social science and social policy. The Commission worked hard for five years and in the end produced not one Report, but two – the Majority and Minority Reports on the Poor Law. On only one issue of substance did the two Reports agree; they both called for the abolition of the Boards of Guardians. Thereafter, they differed completely in their approaches. The Majority Report was palliative, i

commended that the powers and duties of the Guardians
ould be transferred to the local authorities. The Minority
eport, which was written by Beatrice Webb, was more
dical and analytic. It examined the causes of poverty and
w it not as a sin, or a personal failing, as was maintained by
e 'Majority', but as a social evil having social causes to be
et by social action. It called for the complete break-up of
e Poor Law system, and recommended that the problem of
overty be dealt with by a considerable expansion of the
owers of the local authorities, and by government interven-
on in the national economy to prevent the recurrent cycles
f boom and slump. It also proposed that a State medical
rvice be set up, with hospitals linked to the public health
rvice at the local level.

The two Reports were laid before the Liberal Government
1909, but despite the admitted urgency of the need for the
oor Law to be reformed, neither that government, nor any
her for the next 20 years, was prepared to take action. And,
in the end it was the Majority Report which was to be
plemented, it is also true to say that in the long run the
fluence of the Minority Report was to be the greater. For it
ontributed greatly to changing public opinion. There
adually grew up the idea, accepted today, but unfamiliar
en, that society has a responsibility to all its members, and
articularly the disadvantaged, which, in the end, was to be
alized in the establishment of the Welfare State.

The nineteenth century had left a legacy of the twin related
ils of poverty and sickness, those evils which had con-
onted Chadwick long before, and which still remained
bstinately undefeated. The Committee on Physical Deterior-
tion and the Royal Commission on the Poor Law had both
ighlighted the problem and suggested possible courses of
ction. It was Lloyd George's National Health Insurance
cheme which set out to tackle both evils simultaneously. It
as patterned closely on the insurance scheme which
ismarck had introduced in Germany and which Lloyd
George had studied at first hand. It was a compulsory contri-
utory scheme paid for by a weekly deduction from the
orker's pay packet supplemented by a contribution from
he employer and the Treasury. It provided the wage-earner
ith medical care from a general practitioner (GP) without
ayment, but, what was equally important, it also provided a
ash benefit to help to compensate for loss of earnings during
he period of sickness absence. Thus, it staved off the spectre
f financial disaster which had haunted every working class
amily since the coming of the factory system, and it did so
ithout recourse to the Poor Law.

The Act was passed in 1911 but, at first, the doctors
eclined to work with it, partly because they saw it as a threat
o their professional freedom but also for financial reasons. It
ook a year of patient negotiation by Robert Morant, whom
Lloyd George had taken from the Board of Education to
ecome the first chairman of the National Insurance Commission, to overcome the objections of the medical
profession. As a result the implementation of the Act was
delayed until January 1913.

Lloyd George's scheme had two serious deficiencies, it did
not provide hospital treatment for workers and, further, it
provided nothing at all for their dependants. Nevertheless it

was an affirmation of the principle that the health of the
worker is of national concern and that it is in the national
interest to prevent the waste of human resources and, not
least, that of poverty arising out of sickness. The National
Insurance Act of 1911, which embodied the National Health
Insurance scheme, was the first step along the path which was
to lead to the provision of medical care for all.

The Edwardian period really came to an end on 4 August
1914, the day when the lamps went out over Europe and the
Great War, 'the War to end Wars', broke out, and the price
was paid in the slaughter of a generation on the fields of
Flanders. The War saw the introduction of services for the
detection and treatment of tuberculosis on the one hand, and
of venereal diseases on the other. Tuberculosis had been
known through the nineteenth century as 'the captain of the
men of death' because, whereas cholera and the other
epidemic diseases came and went, tuberculosis was always
present. By now treatment was available; it was long-term in
sanatoria. These were built in country areas by the county
authorities and were backed by the setting-up of tuberculosis
dispensaries by the local authorities, for the detection of
cases, the follow-up of contacts, and the supervision and
after-care of patients. The venereal diseases (VD), and
especially syphilis, became a serious problem during the War.
Diagnosis through the Wasserman reaction, and treatment
through Ehrlich's 'magic bullet', Salvarsan, were now
available. The Local Government Board saw to the establishment of VD clinics by all the local authorities. These clinics,
like the tuberculosis dispensaries, came under the control of
the MOH.

It was during the War that the Maternity and Child Welfare
Service came into its own. This had been brought about
through three quite separate developments which had already
taken place in France. The first was the milk depot supplying
free milk to nursing mothers, of which the first had been
opened in St. Helen's in Lancashire in 1899. The second was
the school for nursing mothers to teach them about the care
and nurture of their babies – the first of these had been
founded in St. Pancras in London in 1907. The third was the
medical clinic for infants, of which the first had been set up in
Liverpool, also in 1907. Gradually these three elements came
together under one roof providing food supplements, health
education, and medical supervision of mother and baby, and
so the maternity and child welfare clinic came into being.
There was a considerable expansion of this service during the
War, for with the men away at the Front, young mothers
were left to fend for their families on their own. The local
public health departments rose to the occasion by setting up
these clinics in almost every district in the country.

The Local Government Board maintained oversight of this
development, and then, as the War was ending secured the
passing of the Maternity and Child Welfare Act, which
required local authorities to provide a service which most of
them had been giving for many years. This was the swan-song
of the Local Government Board, for it had long outlived its
usefulness. Although its duty was to provide for need, its
dead hand, and the stigma associated with it, had prompted
successive governments to provide health and welfare services
outside its ambit. Thus, school meals, school medical inspec-

tion and treatment, old age pensions which began in 1908, labour exchanges which were first opened in 1908, and the National Health Insurance scheme were all organized and administered outside the Board. In each case it had been a deliberate act of policy to separate these newer provisions from the socially unacceptable scope of the Poor Law and the Local Government Board.

Thus it was that in 1918 public pressure and political wisdom combined to sweep the Board away and in 1919 to found the Ministry of Health. Before dealing with the new Ministry, however, we will consider the development of child care services in the United States.

CHILD CARE IN THE UNITED STATES

The movement to protect infant and child health in the US really dates from the turn of the present century, although its beginnings can be traced back earlier. As in France and Great Britain it was composed of three elements – education of the mother and improved nutrition and medical care for the child.

The first steps were taken in the 1860s by private organizations who appointed suitable working class women as 'sanitary visitors' to give practical instruction to poor mothers on the management of their infants. In 1874, the New York City Health Department reinforced this activity with a leaflet on child care which was widely distributed for many years. The next step came in 1878 with the opening of a 'milk station', the first of many, to provide milk for nursing mothers. During the late 1890s there came a slow but steady expansion of facilities and programmes for child care in many states. In 1899 New York went a step further when one of the City's milk stations began to function as a consultation and advice centre for mothers on matters concerned with the health and welfare of their babies. Other centres were soon to follow this example.

In 1908 a Division of Child Hygiene was established in the New York City Health Department under Josephine Baker (1873–1945). She instituted a system of home visits by public health nurses to mothers on the day following the birth of their babies, which resulted in a substantial decline in infant mortality.

Meanwhile, services for schoolchildren had also been developing. In the 1870s the medical inspection of school-children was carried out sporadically in a number of states. At the outset, the main purpose of the inspection was to detect and exclude children suffering from infectious diseases. Once begun, however, the system was expanded to deal with minor infections and skin conditions. In 1902 Lina Rogers, who had been involved in this work for some years, was appointed as the first full-time school nurse in the US. In 1906 Massachusetts passed a law requiring every schoolchild to be examined annually. It is interesting to note that, as in England, this service was put under the control of the Education Department and not of the Health Department, on the grounds that a better standard of care would be provided. Some states followed suit, but others did not and, as a result, school health work became a somewhat uneven and patchy affair.

The discovery that large numbers of children attending school were obviously suffering from malnutrition gave rise to the 'school lunch' movement. New York gave the lead in 1908 by setting up a scheme for providing free lunches to needy children at school, and this example was soon followed elsewhere.

In 1912, special clinics began to be set up, similar to the minor ailment clinics in England, to provide treatment for schoolchildren suffering from the common conditions of the skin, ears, eyes, teeth, and tonsils.

Another very important development which took place in 1912 was the setting up, with federal funds, of the Children's Bureau. This was charged with the task of investigating and reporting on all matters pertaining to the health and welfare of children in all sections of the population. In the years that followed, the information collected by the Bureau provided the basis for federal and state action which was to be taken in the interests of the health of mothers and children.

During the First World War the Federal Government sponsored a programme for the health care of mothers and children. In 1921 Congress passed the Maternity and Infancy Act which came about directly as a result of the recommenda-tions of the Bureau. This Act initiated a programme of federal-state co-operation which continued until 1929 when it was allowed to lapse. In 1935 it was re-established on a more ambitious scale by the Social Security Act. This authorized the Children's Bureau to make annual grants to the states to enable them to extend and improve their services for mothers and children and also for handicapped children. The work of the Children's Bureau continued during the Second World War when it administered an emergency programme of maternal and child care for the wives of servicemen.

It will have been seen that since its inception 70 years ago, the Children's Bureau has played a leading part in the development of services for mothers and children at all administrative levels in the US. The close parallel between the US and Britain in the pattern and growth of these services is also noteworthy.

THE MINISTRY OF HEALTH AND THE PUBLIC HEALTH

The British Ministry of Health was founded in 1919 with Christopher Addison, a doctor, as its first minister. He took Robert Morant from the National Insurance Commission where he had been serving as Chairman since 1911, and made him Permanent Secretary, that is chief administrator, of the Ministry. Then he appointed Dr George Newman as the first Chief Medical Officer, a post which he held with great distinction for 16 years. The three men then set to work to determine the policy and programme of the new department. Its primary duty was 'to take all such steps as may be neces-sary to secure the health of the people', but to this were added two further heavy burdens – housing and the Poor Law.

Housing, or more particularly, the shortage of housing in towns, was a problem that had plagued the nation for half a century. The nub of the problem was that with rising public health standards, it was becoming increasingly difficult for private enterprise to build houses to let at rents which working people could afford to pay, and which would yield an adequate return on the capital investment, while the local authorities could not cope with the problem because they did not have the resources. The War had exacerbated the problem by bringing new building to a halt. Lloyd George had won the general election of 1918 on the slogan 'A Land fit for Heroes' but when they came back from the Front many of them were homeless heroes. The problem was laid on the shoulders of the Ministry of Health and there it remained until 1951. It was this problem which dominated the attention and energies of the department for the first ten years of its life.

The second charge laid upon it was the Poor Law, which despite, or perhaps because of, the two Reports of the Royal Commission still remained unreformed. It might then be asked, was the new Ministry just the old Local Government Board under a new name? Most certainly it was not. The difference was esentially one of attitude and objective. The orientation of the Ministry was to health, positive and constructive, and not to that deterrence which had characterized the Board. From then onwards the old Poor Law began to be administered with a new humanity; it was increasingly seen as a social service supporting health. Guardians were encouraged to ameliorate the harsh conditions prevailing in the workhouses, to bend the rules so long as they did not break the law, while the Ministry itself took steps to raise the standards of staffing and care in the infirmaries.

Quite early, the department began to make plans to bring the Poor Law to an end, but in the economic climate of the 1920s, and with its preoccupation with housing, it was ten years before action could be taken. Then, in 1929, Neville Chamberlain, the Minister of Health in Baldwin's Conservative Government, took the decision to implement the recommendations of the Majority Report of the Royal Commission. The Local Government Act which followed abolished the Boards of Guardians and transferred their powers and duties to the Local Authorities. These were required to set up committees to administer, not poor relief, but 'public assistance' as it was now called. Thus, the Poor Law lived on under a new name until 1948 when the National Assistance Act of that year declared, 'The existing Poor Law shall cease to have effect'. And that brought to an end a system of local responsibility for local poor which had lasted from 1601.

However, the Act of 1929 did more than this, for it transferred all the institutions of the Poor Law to the local authorities, including the infirmaries. In time, these were to become municipal hospitals under the executive control of the MOH.

By this time the MOH of the large towns was responsible for the traditional environmental services of water supply and sewage disposal, for the control of food and food hygiene, for the public health aspects of housing, for the control and prevention of infectious diseases, for the maternity and child welfare clinic with its attendant health visitors and midwives, for the tuberculosis dispensary, and the VD clinics. Then, in his other role, the MOH was responsible for the school medical service. To all this was now added the responsibility for the administration of the municipal hospital. Curative and preventive medicine had been brought together under the MOH, who was now at the height of his powers. This

was the position the MOH was to hold for almost 20 years until the coming of the NHS in 1948.

STEPS TO THE NATIONAL HEALTH SERVICE

In 1939 war came again and the MOH was immediately involved in the evacuation of children from the towns to the greater security of the countryside, and later in coping with the effects of the bombing of the cities. In this they were stretched as never before, for in addition to the management of local casualty services and co-ordination with the hospitals, the MOH still retained responsibility for providing the whole range of public health services for a population living and working under very difficult and abnormal conditions. Fears of large scale epidemics were met by a massive stepping-up of the immunization programme, and of mass X-ray, all of which bore fruit not only then but later. An additional wartime measure came with the setting up of a network of laboratories, covering the whole country, to provide diagnostic and other services to local public health departments. This proved to be so useful that, in due course, it became a permanent part of the public health establishment.

War can bring out the best as well as the worst in people, and so it was on that occasion. A new spirit of idealism was abroad, a feeling that the nation was fighting not to restore the conditions of the past but to create a more humane, a more caring society than had existed before. Thus it was that in the dark days of 1941, Winston Churchill's Coalition Government appointed a committee under William Beveridge (1879–1953) to plan a new system of social security that could be brought into being when the conflict was over. Beveridge produced his Report over his own hand in 1942. It embodied a scheme for a comprehensive system of social insurance which would provide benefits to meet the crises of birth and death, of unemployment, and injury, and for support in old age. In essence it was a plan to banish 'Want' from society. It breathed the spirit of the Minority Report, which is not to be wondered at, because as a young man Beveridge had been an assistant to the Webbs, and it fell to him to realize the aspirations of his mentors.

Beveridge said that his scheme would rest on three assumptions which must be met. They were first, that there should be a system of family allowances, financed outside the social security system, to give additional support to young families; second, that governments should through their policies maintain full employment, so that never again would the national insurance scheme be bankrupted by mass unemployment as it had been in 1931; and third, 'that a comprehensive national health service will ensure that for every citizen there is available whatever medical treatment he requires, in whatever form he requires it, domiciliary, institutional, general, specialist or consultant, and will ensure the provision of dental, ophthalmic and surgical appliances, nursing and midwifery, and rehabilitation after accidents, and that this be provided without payment at the time of need'.

This was Beveridge's prescription for a national health service. He incorporated this proposal as a basic assumption underlying his social security system because, like Lloyd

George and Chadwick before him, he believed that sickness is a major cause of poverty. He held that a national health service would raise the general level of health and fitness in the nation, that it would reduce the toll of sickness-absence from work, that it would increase national productivity and so national prosperity. Thus, a national health service could pay for itself.

His proposal for such a service was not a new one, it had a respectable history. In 1909, the Minority Report had recommended the creation of a state medical service. In 1920, the Dawson Committee appointed by Dr Addison, the first Minister of Health, had put forward a plan for a comprehensive health service based on a system of health centres providing both preventive and curative care. In 1926, a Royal Commission on the National Health Insurance Scheme had recommended its extension to include the worker's dependants, but doubted whether hospital care could be financed through contributory insurance. In 1937, Political and Economic Planning, an unofficial body, produced a detailed study of the health services and made equally detailed proposals for their development. Then, in 1938, the British Medical Association put forward its plan for a 'General Medical Service for the Nation'.

All these plans and proposals were on the table in 1944 when the Conservative Government came to produce its White Paper setting out its proposals for a national health service. However, the general election of 1945 swept all that away and brought in Clement Attlee's Labour Government committed to a programme of nationalization and to the creation of the 'Welfare State'. Aneuran Bevan became Minister of Health and immediately scrapped his predecessor's proposals and shortly after came forward with his own.

Bevan's plan for a national health service took the form of a tripartite structure. General practice would be organized through local executive councils, of which there were to be 120; the personal health services would be provided by the councils of the counties and county boroughs (the large towns and cities) now to be designated Local Health Authorities, of which there would be 160; and with a state take-over of all hospitals, voluntary and municipal, to be administered by 14 Regional Hospital Boards and by Boards of Governors for the teaching hospitals.

It was this scheme which went onto the Statute Book in the National Health Service Act of 1946. Then followed a year of difficult negotiations to deal with the objections to the scheme raised by the doctors, which in some ways paralleled those of 1912. This time the principal issues were the method of remunerating GPs, who were adamant in refusing to enter a State salaried service; the freedom of doctors from direction, and the right to continue private practice; and the right to buy and sell practices. The discussions were protracted, and at times bitter, but in the end the difficulties were resolved. GPs would not become employees of the State, but each would hold an individual contract with the local executive council, and remuneration would be based on a capitation fee. There would be no direction of doctors, private practice could continue, and hospital consultants would be able to treat private patients in paybeds in the hospitals. The buying and selling of practices would cease but the government provided

the sum of £66 million by way of compensation, and also created a pension scheme for retiring doctors.

So it was that after a year of conflict there was peace and harmony on 5 July 1948, the Appointed Day, when the NHS came into being. It provided comprehensive medical care for every man, woman, and child in the country without payment, and backed this with the positive provisions of the personal health and preventive services. This was its achievement. The expected rush of patients to the surgeries of the GPs to obtain free treatment did not happen. What did occur was an almost overwhelming rush to the dentists and opticians to obtain dentures and spectacles, thus indicating a hitherto massive unmet need.

But what happened to public health? The MOHs had expressed the hope that the new service would be provided through the local authorities. However, their colleagues, the GPs flatly refused to accept any arrangement that might put them under the control of locally elected councillors. So it was, that under the tripartite structure preventive and curative medicine went their separate ways and the MOHs lost their responsibility for hospitals.

PUBLIC HEALTH IN THE POST-WAR PERIOD

The 'Appointed Day' marked the end of the period in which the local municipal hospitals had been linked to the local public health services through the MOH. The transfer of that control to the Regional Hospital Boards brought something like dismay at first, but as the country moved into the post-war period it brought new opportunities, new challenges, and saw the development of what came to be called 'Modern Public Health'.

The opportunities came with the need to provide caring and supportive services to meet the needs of the increasing numbers of old people in the population, and for the physically and mentally handicapped. The challenges came with the changing pattern of disease, as the infectious diseases of the past gave way, through immunization and the use of antibiotics, to what may be called the 'behaviourally-based' conditions of the present. By these we understand lung cancer, coronary heart disease, death and disablement on the roads, the large, but mainly hidden, problem of alcoholism, the rising problem of drug addiction, the increasing incidence of venereal disease in young people, and, on another dimension, the large numbers of unwanted pregnancies. All this demanded new approaches, new methods of detection and prevention. It gave an impetus to the expansion of traditional prevention into what came to be called primary, secondary, and tertiary prevention. It also saw a new importance, and a new meaning, given to health education as a potentially valuable instrument of prevention and, indeed, of health promotion.

The same period also brought opportunities to make further improvements in the environment. The 'smog' episode in London in December 1952, as a result of which 4000 people died, led to the passing of the Clean Air Act in 1956. The provisions of the Act were enforced by the public health departments of the local authorities and effectively brought an end to serious air pollution in the urban areas of the country. This in turn made it worthwhile to clean the great public buildings of the cities by removing the layers of grime that had been deposited on them for more than a century. But more important still, the cleansing of the atmosphere in the towns was accompanied by a measureable decline in the prevalence of chronic respiratory disease. Another significant step to deal with a growing environmental problem was taken in 1960 with the Noise Abatement Act. This made excessive noise a statutory nuisance which could be dealt with under public health law. These two measures can be looked on as the tailpiece of the programme of sanitary reform carried out by the public health movement in the Victorian period.

It was in this way that the fifteen years following the 'Appointed Day' saw the expansion of the personal health services and the extension of environmental control under the MOH. However, disappointment lay ahead. In the 1960s came the 'revolt' of social workers. By this time almost every department of local government was employing social workers. They now claimed that they were professionals in their own right, and that they should no longer be regarded as hand-maidens to other professionals. Their arguments were accepted by the Seebohm Committee which was appointed to examine the issue in 1965. As a result, in 1970, social work was hived off to a new independence in the social services departments, which then came into being, and the MOH lost half his staff and incidentally, also half his budget.

However, the MOH was nothing if not resilient, and towards the end they were building bridges across to general practice, through the attachment of health visitors and nurses to GPs as they moved into group practice and into health centres. This was to be one of the last initiatives of the MOH, as we shall see, as we turn to developments in the NHS itself.

FROM PUBLIC HEALTH TO COMMUNITY MEDICINE

After 1948 the NHS proceeded somewhat unsteadily on its three legs for 20 years. By this time it was clear that there were serious defects in its structure which were hampering its effectiveness. With the three branches of the Service organized and administered separately, it was inevitable that there would be gaps between them. This was particularly true in the continuity of patient care which was almost entirely absent. Inevitably too, there were expensive overlaps, notably in the provision of maternity services. But worst of all there was no machinery through which to plan comprehensively to meet local needs at the local level.

Aneuran Bevan had intended that the three branches of the Service should be brought together in working relationships in health centres, as the Dawson Committee had proposed in 1920. But partly through lack of finance, but more particularly because of the unwillingness of GPs to enter them very few health centres had been built.

In 1962, the Porritt Committee put forward a well-argued case for the integration of the three branches of the Service. This was to be achieved through the formation of area health boards each to be responsible for the total health care of its local population. This began the debate, not so much on the principle of integration, for this was soon accepted by the medical profession, the politicians, and by the public, but on how the integration was to be achieved. Two Labour Secre-

taries of State, Kenneth Robinson and Richard Crossman, put forward their proposals in successive Green Papers. These were superseded by the Conservative Government's proposals which were embodied in Sir Keith Joseph's Consultative Document. This endorsed the principle of unification, and proposed that it should be achieved through a three-tier structure consisting of a central department, and regional and area health authorities, the latter to have a district level of management. The Consultative Document was particularly noteworthy for the emphasis that it gave to the need for effective management. It was this scheme which was passed into law in 1973 and which came into being on 1 April 1974.

The re-structuring of the NHS was to have profound effects upon the public health services. When integration began seriously to be mooted it became clear that there would be no place in a unified service for the MOH. This local health officer whom we had known since the time of Chadwick would become an anachronism, and therefore had to go. But it was equally clear that there must be a doctor, in each of the areas into which the country was to be divided for health service purposes, who would be informed on the health status and needs of the local population, and would advise the health authority on how best to use its available resources to meet those needs. Who should this be? Not the MOH, for this had never been his job, nor was he trained to do it. So to fill this role a new specialist was created – the 'community physician'. The community physician was conceived as the specialist in social, or community, medicine. By social medicine, as the subject was first called, is meant the application of medicine, not to the individual person or patient, which is clinical medicine, but to the population. Public health had always been population orientated in its programmes of prevention, but social medicine represents an extension of the public health idea. It is concerned with all the factors affecting the distribution of health and ill health in populations, including their use of health services.

The subject had achieved its first measure of academic respectability in England in 1943, when John Ryle (1889–1950) gave up the Regius Chair of Physik at Cambridge to take the new chair of social medicine that had been established at Oxford. The post-war period saw a considerable expansion of social medicine as an academic discipline, with the creation of new university departments and professorial chairs, the founding of a journal and a learned society devoted to the subject. During this period social medicine was busy defining its field, establishing epidemiology as its basic science and making use of statistical methods as the 'tools of the trade'.

The next step came in 1968 with the Report of the Royal Commission on Medical Education (Todd Report). For the first time, an official document referred not to *social* medicine but to *community* medicine, and defined it in terms which embraced social medicine, but went beyond it, by giving greater emphasis to the organizational and administrative aspects than had academic social medicine in the past. It was within the context of community medicine as defined by the Todd Commission that reference was now made to the community physician as the practitioner of community medicine. The job specification, as it would be in the re-structured Health Service, was spelled out in detail in 1970 by the Hunter Committee, by which time a training course for the new specialist had been started at the London School of Hygiene and Tropical Medicine under Professor J.N. Morris. In 1972, the Royal Colleges of Physicians of the UK collaborated in founding the Faculty of Community Medicine, thus signifying the formal recognition of the new specialty. Thereafter, Membership of the Faculty of Community Medicine (MFCM) was to become for the community physician of the future what the DPH had been to the MOH of the past.

So we come to the night of Sunday 31 March 1974. On that night, the medical officer of health, the local health officer whom we had had in England since 1847, passed into the pages of the history book. And on the following morning there arose out of the ashes, like the phoenix, the community physician. That day marked an end and a beginning. It marked the end of a system of public health that went back to the Royal Sanitary Commission and beyond that to the founding fathers, John Simon and Edwin Chadwick. It marked the beginning of a new system in which the community physician would occupy a key role within the structure of an integrated health service which offered comprehensive health care for all the people.

Over the 127 years of the MOH's life there had been profound social, economic, and demographic changes, changes which in their turn had influenced the health of the people the MOH served. For example, since Duncan had taken up his appointment in 1847, the population of the country had almost trebled, from 17 to 49 million; the birth rate had fallen by half, from 31.5 to 16 per 1000; the death rate had been cut by half, from 24.7 to 11.6 per 1000; the infant mortality rate had tumbled from 164 to 18 per 1000 live births; and the expectation of life of a male at birth had risen from 40 years in 1847 to nearly three score years and ten in 1974. These figures give some idea of the advances in the quality and quantity of life which had taken place during this period, and to which the public health movement had made its own contribution under the leadership of the MOH, whose career had now come to an end.

THE INTEGRATED HEALTH SERVICE

In the history of the NHS, Monday, 1 April 1974, the day of reorganization, ranks second in importance only to 5 July 1948, the day when the Service was born. The purpose of the reorganization was to enable the Service to attain to its objectives more effectively. But what were those objectives? They were well set out by the Royal Commission which was appointed in 1976 to review the Health Service.

The Commission said that it should:

1. encourage and assist individuals to remain healthy;
2. provide equality of entitlement to health services;
3. provide a broad range of services to a high standard;
4. provide equality of access to those services;
5. provide a service free at the time of use;
6. satisfy the reasonable expectations of its users;
7. remain a national service reponsive to local needs.

The unified structure was set up to establish an improved system of management for the Health Service which would enable a more effective use to be made of its available resources to subserve these ends.

Reorganization brought together the hospital and specialist services, the family practitioner services and the personal health services, into a single administrative structure. Within the new structure, the central department, under the Secretary of State, was responsible for the general oversight of the Service, for national policy and planning, for allocating resources to the 14 Regional Health Authorities and for monitoring their performance. The Regional Health Authority (RHA), was responsible for developing regional plans, for providing services needing a regional rather than an area approach, for allocating resources to the Area Health Authorities and for monitoring their performance. The Area Health Authority (AHA) was the key operational level. It was responsible for planning and developing services to meet local needs. Its boundaries were co-terminous with those of its local authority with which it was required to work closely. The day-to-day operation of local services was based on the health district. Two-thirds of the 90 AHAs were divided into two or more health districts. There were 170 of these, their size and number being determined by the size of the population considered suitable for the administration of local health services, usually between 150 000 and 250 000. Each district was planned to include a district general hospital. The district was not a separate level of administrative authority, it was part of the area administration, so organized as to enable the AHA to meet community needs most effectively.

This then was the new machinery. The principles on which it worked were delegation downwards and accountability upwards; and within management itself, decision-making was through consensus reached between responsible officers.

On the day of reorganization, the community physician (or community medicine specialist) came into being. Community physicians were appointed to key positions at every level of the Service, including the district. The broad functions of the community physician were first, as a *specialist,* to provide information to clinicians, and to advise them on possible approaches to care, having regard to the relation between health and local authority services, especially to the available social services. Second, as a *manager,* to be concerned with the planning of services, with the provision and interpretation of information, with the monitoring and evaluation of services and programmes, and with the development of measures for the prevention of disease and the promotion of health. Third, as an *adviser* to local authorities in matters affecting the public health. It is to the latter function that we must now turn.

The re-structuring of the Health Service brought about profound changes in the organization of public health. The public health departments of the local authorities vanished on 1 April 1974 along with the MOH. All the medical personnel who formerly worked for the local authorities moved across to the National Health Service. Likewise, the personal health services passed to the new health authorities. These included maternal and child care, health visiting, home nursing and midwifery, health centres, family planning, vaccination and immunization, community epidemiology, the ambulance service; and separately, the school health service.

However, environmental services remained with the local authorities and became the responsibility of the newly-formed environmental departments. Their duties were carried out by environmental health officers under the chief environmental health officer. These officers were formerly known as public health inspectors and before that as sanitary inspectors. Prior to 1974 they had formed part of the staff of the MOH. Now under the new arrangement there was to be no direct medical control or supervision of environmental health.

Nevertheless, the local authorities still retained their statutory duties in respect of communicable diseases and food poisoning and, for these purposes, they were required to appoint a 'proper officer'. They were also recommended to appoint a medical officer to advise on environmental health, on the health aspects of the social services, and on other relevant matters within their purview. The medical adviser, as also the proper officer, was to be in the employ of the Health Service and not of the authority. These appointments were held either by the district community physicians or by community physicians specializing in environmental health or in social services. It was in this way that an attempt was made to bridge the gap between personal and environmental health which had been brought about by the reorganization.

Despite the magnitude of the changes made by the integration of the Health Service, the transfer of responsibility to the new authorities took place remarkably smoothly. Inevitably it took time for new working relationships to be established, especially with the local authorities. Change is always made easier when it can bring with it extra resources. It was therefore unfortunate that reorganization took place only a few months after the oil crisis of 1973. This seriously affected the national economy and led to reductions in public expenditure. The years that followed were marked by increasing financial stringency, so that a plan which was intended to raise the standards of health care of the nation was hampered in its achievement by lack of resources.

The Health Service had, therefore, to adjust to a lower rate of growth which was scarcely more than enough to keep up with demographic changes, particularly with the increasing proportion of old people in the population. It therefore became all the more necessary to determine a set of priorities which should guide the distribution of the available resources within the Service. The plan which was produced proposed that greater weight should be given to preventive services and to community care at the expense of the acute services. Priority should also be given to the expansion of services for the mentally ill, for the mentally handicapped, for young children, and for the aged, while the rate of growth of the acute services should be kept below that of the service as a whole. In the years that followed some attempt was made by the AHAs to implement these proposals.

The unification of the Health Service made it possible for the first time to introduce a more rational basis for allocating resources across the country, so as to provide a greater measure of equality. In 1975 a Working Party was set up to recommend how this might best be done. In its Report, the Resource Allocation Working Party proposed that allocations should be made on the basis of a formula which took into account population size, with weightings for variations in the use of services by different age groups, and also mortality ratios. It was through the application of this formula that the most deprived regions received additional resources, allowing for modest expansion, while the allocations to the best provided regions sufficed for little more than the maintenance of the existing level of services.

One noteworthy development in this period was the new emphasis given to prevention. This started as a national campaign to encourage people to become more responsible for their own health. Its message was that the NHS could provide health services but it could not provide health. Many of the causes of ill health lay in the way people chose to live their lives, that is, in their life-styles. Improved health could depend upon people changing their life-styles, for example, by giving up cigarette smoking, by drinking alcohol only in moderation, by taking regular exercise, by improving diet and avoiding obesity, and eschewing resort to addictive drugs. In furtherance of this policy additional funds were allocated to the Health Educational Council to be used both for the 'Better Health' campaign and also for the training of health education officers to be employed by the area health authorities.

Within a few years of the reorganization it was becoming clear that the new arrangement had not brought all the benefits that had been hoped for. Unification had been achieved on paper but hardly in effect. The hospitals, general medical services and the personal health services still functioned to a large extent in isolation, not least because of the complexities of the communications system. It was apparent that there were too many levels of management, too many committees and too much paper passing between them. All this reflected on the community physicians appointed to several types of posts. The continuing demands upon them to deal with problems of immediacy left little time or opportunity to devote to wider issues of prevention and health promotion. There were uncertainties too about their role. The preoccupation with 'management' tended to diminish them, as medical specialists in the eyes of clinical colleagues.

Thus the new situation had thrown up problems that were general to the system and some that were specific to the practitioners of community medicine. Accordingly, the decision was taken to simplify the structure by eliminating one level of administration, namely, that of the area. This took effect on 1 April 1982, when the 90 AHAs were abolished and their functions were taken over by 192 District Health Authorities (DHAs). These are now responsible for assessing the health needs of their local communities, and for planning and providing services and programmes to meet those needs within the resource allocations made by the RHAs, to whom they are now directly responsible. And, as before, a key figure in the structure, with responsibilities that may now be performed with greater effect, is the district medical officer – the community physician.

PUBLIC HEALTH AND MEDICAL CARE IN WESTERN EUROPE AND THE UNITED STATES

In the countries of western Europe, organized public health has come a long way since it was primarily concerned with cleaning up the environment, providing sanitary services, and controlling epidemic diseases. Since the beginning of this century a wide range of personal services has been developed to protect the health of specific population groups of which mothers, infants, schoolchildren, industrial workers, and the elderly are among the most prominent. Although administrative systems providing environmental and personal health services vary from one country to another, the most common pattern takes the form of a three tier structure with a central controlling department delegating to and supervising, provincial, regional, or county authorities, and then down to the local, district, or municipal bodies which are responsible for services at the local level.

As public health services and standards have improved in these countries, so an increasing interest has been shown in the provision of medical care as a function of the state. The post-war period has seen the extension of government involvement in the provision of medical care in the home, in the clinic or health centre, and in the hospital, so as to provide a more or less comprehensive system of health cover for the whole population. These health systems are commonly financed through compulsory insurance schemes, with contributions from the employees, the employers, and the State. In some countries, for example, the Netherlands, Denmark, and West Germany, private insurance organizations, supervised by the State, but having a greater or lesser degree of autonomy, play an important part in the health care system. In other countries, such as France, Belgium, and Sweden, patients pay for their treatment by a medical practitioner on a prescribed scale, and then recover part of the costs through the insurance scheme.

The British system, which is financed out of general taxation has already been described. To complete this chapter we will briefly consider the development of medical care in the US. In the early years of the twentieth century advancements in medical science and practice caused hospital treatment to become increasingly expensive, and so beyond the reach of many working people. As a result, various proposals were put forward for insurance schemes to cover the costs of hospital care. In 1915 the American Medical Association appointed the Social Insurance Committee which immediately organized a national conference on the subject. The outcome was a draft bill which could be laid before state legislatures to establish a system of insurance. Sixteen states introduced the bill, but opposition arose to the principle of these schemes, and within a short time the movement collapsed. For the next ten years medical insurance was an unfashionable topic.

Meanwhile, between the two World Wars many states and local authorities began to open health centres to provide a wide range of services including maternal and child care, vaccination and immunization, and health education. Along with this development voluntary associations also grew rapidly in number and scope. Each of these took as its area of concern either a particular disease, for example, tuberculosis, or a disability such as blindness or deafness, or some section of the community, for example, the elderly. These associations served to arouse public interest, to mobilize local resources, and to supplement the work of the official agencies. This was valuable work, but on the debit side, this welter of well-intentioned activity was marked by the absence of co-ordination and the duplication of effort. This gave rise to some confusion in the mind of the public.

After 1925 the subject of the costs of medical treatment began to be raised again, and two years later the Committee on the Costs of Medical Care was set up to study the problem. Over the next five years the Committee issued 28 reports. On its main recommendations the Committee was divided between a majority and a minority group. The majority favoured a system of voluntary insurance to cover the costs of medical and hospital care, and also proposed that these services should be made available to the poor at the expense of the State. The minority completely rejected any system of prepayment for medical care. These issues continued to be the subject of public debate for some time to come.

In 1936 the National Health Survey confirmed yet again the close association between sickness and poverty, by showing that morbidity and mortality were highest among families in receipt of relief. This led to further proposals to establish a more equitable system of providing medical care. Some of the proponents of these schemes called for the state provision of medical services, but others argued in favour of systems based on private insurance. In the years that followed attempts to promote government action through the states all failed, but schemes of private insurance burgeoned. The largest of these was the Blue Cross Hospital Service Plan which by 1953 had 42 million subscribers. The piecemeal provision of these many schemes lacked co-ordination and central planning. They also left those on low incomes without any proper provision of medical care.

In 1953, seventy years after the demise of the Board of Health, Congress enacted legislation to create the Department of Health, Education and Welfare so that once again the US had a national health agency. Its main functions were to encourage the activities of the state and local health departments through grants-in-aid, to sponsor research and to be responsible for the international aspects of health. The fifty states retained, and still retain, their autonomy in matters concerning public health. Each state has its own board of health with two main departments concerned with health and welfare respectively. The state departments of health deal with public health and sanitation, including the control and prevention of infectious diseases, maternal and child health, dental care, and mental health. They also administer the state hospital services. The departments of welfare are responsible for the care of handicapped and deprived children, for the community care of the mentally ill, and for dealing with a wide range of social problems. They also administer financial relief to the indigent.

Since 1966 the involvement of the government in the provision of medical care has increased considerably, notably through the Medicare and Medicaid schemes. Medicare is concerned with the elderly, and provides for a proportion of the costs of medical and hospital care to be recovered out of public funds. Medicaid meets the cost of these services for the low income group, also out of government funds.

The principal characteristic of the American system is the emphasis that is placed on personal responsibility for health care within the context of a free enterprise system. However, the provision of care for those who cannot meet the costs of the private systems has now been accepted as a duty of government, and is made through the agencies which are responsible for the public health. The similarity in objectives and the differences in organization, between the US and the UK and other west European countries are patent. They are the result of the historical development not only of their health services but also of their social, political, and economic systems.

SELECT BIBLIOGRAPHY

General reading

Frazer, W. M. (1950). *A history of English public health, 1834–1939*. Baillière, Tindall and Cox, London.

Newman, G. (1939). *The building of a nation's health*. Macmillan, London.

Newsholme, A. (1927). *Evolution of preventive medicine*. Baillière, Tindall and Cox, London.

Rosen, G. (1958). *A history of public health*. MD Publications, New York.

Sand, R. (1952). *The advance to social medicine*. Staples Press, London.

Simon, J. (1890). *English sanitary institutions*. Cassell, London.

Trevelyan, G. M. (1937). *British history in the nineteenth century and after*, 2nd edn. Longmans, London.

Walker, M. E. M. (1930). *Pioneers of public health*. Oliver and Boyd, London.

Watkin, B. (1975). *Documents on health and social services, 1834 to the present day*. Methuen, London.

The nineteenth century

Checkland, S. G. and Checkland, E. D. A. (1974). *The Poor Law Report of 1834*. Penguin, Middlesex.

Commission for Inquiring into the State of the Large Towns and Populous Districts (1844). *Reports*. HMSO, London.

Farr, W. (1885). *Vital statistics, a memorial volume of selections from the writings of William Farr*. Facsimile of the 1885 edn. New York Academy of Medicine, New York (1975).

Flinn, M. W. (ed.) (1964). *Report on the Sanitary Condition of the Labouring Population of Great Britain, Chadwick, E. (1842)*. Edinburgh, University Press.

Fraser Brockington, C. (1965). *Public health in the nineteenth century*. Livingstone, London.

General Board of Health. (1854). *Report on the administration of the Public Health Act for 1848–1854*. HMSO, London.

Hanlon, J. J. (1950). The background and development of public health in the United States. In *Principles of public health administration*, p. 26. Mosey, St. Louis.

Lambert, R. (1963). *Sir John Simon, 1816–1904*. MacGibbon and Kee, London.

Lewis, R. A. (1952). *Edwin Chadwick and the public health movement 1832–1854*. Longmans, London.

Massachusetts Sanitary Survey Commission (1850). *Report by L. Shattuck and others*. Fascimile edn. Harvard University Press, Cambridge, Mass (1948).

Paterson, R. G. (1948). Health of Towns Associations in Great Britain. 1844–1849. *Bull. Hist. Med.* 22 (No. 4), 373.

Privy Council. *Annual reports of the Medical Officer (J. Simon) 1858–1870*. HMSO, London.

Royal Sanitary Commission (1871). *Report*. HMSO, London.

Simon, J. (1854). *Reports relating to the sanitary condition of the City of London*. J. W. Parker, London.

The twentieth century

Abel-Smith, B. (1978). *National Health Service, the first thirty years*. HMSO, London.

British Medical Association (1938). *A general medical service for the Nation*. BMA, London.

Chave, S. P. W. (1980). The rise and fall of the medical officer of health. *Community Med.* **2**, 36.

Crew, F. A. E. (1949). Social medicine as an academic discipline. In *Modern trends in public health* (ed. A. Massey) p. 46. Butterworth, London.

Department of Health and Social Security (1971). *National Health Service reorganization. Consultative document*. HMSO, London.

Department of Health and Social Security (1972). *Report of Working Party on Medical Administrators*. (Hunter Report.) HMSO, London.

Department of Health and Social Security (1976). *Prevention and health—everybody's business*. HMSO, London.

Department of Health and Social Security (1977). *Priorities in the health and social services; the way forward*. HMSO, London.

Department of Health and Social Security, Resource Allocation Working Party (1976). *Report: Sharing resources for health in England*. HMSO, London.

Eurohealth Handbook (1978). Robert, S. First, New York.

Interdepartmental Committee on Local Authority and Allied Personal Social Services (1968). *Report*. (Seebohm Report.) HMSO, London.

Interdepartmental Committee on Physical Deterioration (1904). *Report*. HMSO, London.

Interdepartmental Committee on Social Insurance and Allied Services (1942). *Report*. (Beveridge Report.) HMSO, London.

Jordan, W. S. (1978). *Community medicine in the United Kingdom*. Springer, New York.

Local Government Board (1918). *Forty-seventh annual report, 1917–1918, with review of events since 1871*. HMSO, London.

Mackintosh, J. M. (1953). *Trends of opinion about the public health, 1901–1951*. Oxford University Press, London.

Ministry of Health, Consultative Council on Medical and Allied Services (1920). *Interim report on the future provision of medical and allied services*. (Dawson Report.) HMSO, London.

Ministry of Health. *On the state of the public health. Annual reports of the Chief Medical Officer*, 1921 to present. HMSO, London.

Morris, J. N. (1969). Tomorrow's community physician. *Lancet* **ii**, 811.

Morris, J. N. (1975). *Uses of epidemiology*, 3rd edn. Churchill Livingstone, London.

Pater, J. E. (1981). *The making of the National Health Service*. King Edward's Hospital Fund, London.

Political and Economic Planning (1937). *Report on the British Health Services*. HMSO, London.

Read, D. (1972). *Edwardian England*. Harrap, London.

Royal College of Physicians of London (1962). *A review of the medical services in Great Britain* (Porritt Report). Social Assay, on behalf of Medical Services Review Committee, London.

Royal Commission on Medical Education (1968). *Report*. (Todd Report.) HMSO, London.

Royal Commission on the National Health Service (1979). *Report*. (Merrison Report.) HMSO, London.

Royal Commission on the Poor Laws and Relief of Distress (1909). *Report and Minority Report*. HMSO, London.

Ryle, J. A. (1948). *Changing disciplines*. Oxford University Press, London.

Warren, M. D. (1973). The concept of community medicine. *Community Health* **4**, 275.

World Health Organization, Regional Office for Europe (1965). *Health services in Europe*. WHO, Copenhagen.

2 Current scope

Roger Detels and Lester Breslow

INTRODUCTION

As indicated in the preceding chapter, public health is the organization of local, state, national, and international resources to address the major health problems affecting communities.

In the nineteenth and early twentieth centuries these health problems were primarily associated with aspects of early industrialization, that is, crowding, undernutrition, exhaustion, and faecal contamination of water supplies. These social conditions resulted in a high prevalence of tuberculosis, enteric infections, infant mortality, and acute respiratory diseases. Public health organizations emerged through which communities, states, and nations could deal with important health problems. From the outset public health embraced both social action and scientific knowledge. This partnership, for example, meant linking the anti-poverty (reform) movement with the findings of epidemiology and bacteriology to combat such diseases as tuberculosis and typhoid fever.

Now, at the end of the twentieth century many of the major health problems facing Britain, the US and other highly industrialized nations stem from advanced technology, a richer diet, and a lengthened life span. In this chapter we will present broadly the current scope and strategies of public health as well as issues which confront public health organizations in the developed countries. Subsequent chapters will present specific topics in greater detail.

The first part of this chapter will outline the major health problems facing these countries, including infectious diseases, chronic diseases, and mental health. The second part will discuss determinants of health such as nutritional problems, environmental hazards, and disorders resulting from life-style choices. The third part will deal with the scientific responses which public health uses to cope with these problems, including a discussion of strategies basic to public health, such as epidemiology, and those which are borrowed and modified from other disciplines such as the social, biological, and physical sciences. The programmatic scope of public health will then be outlined in relation to its activities directed toward influencing medical care, health-related behaviour and control of the environment. The fifth section will be devoted to the strategies for applying these scientific approaches to public health problems, and the final section will deal with the interaction of the various governmental and voluntary actions aimed at improving the health of the community.

The reader should be aware that public health is only one of the major determinants of a community's health. Of fundamental importance are the economic and social conditions which directly influence the level and mode of living, as well as the resources which can be specifically devoted to health promotion and disease intervention. The prevailing economic and social conditions determine more than the extent of poverty and concomitant inability to obtain the necessities of life. Such forces also influence, for example, decisions about the cigarette issue in so far as agriculture, trade, economy, and politics are involved in addition to health.

The magnitude and success of public health efforts will vary both in time and place within different areas in the world. None the less, the principles of public health remain the same. The actions which should be taken are determined by the nature and magnitude of the problems affecting the health of the community. What can be done will be determined by the scientific knowledge and resources available. What is done will be determined by the social and political situation existing at that time in that place.

HEALTH PROBLEMS

Infectious disease

Pandemics of infectious disease now rarely threaten developed nations even though they occurred with alarming frequency in the past. The decreasing danger from infectious disease agents has resulted largely from the provision of safe drinking water, better handling of sewage, improved personal hygiene and improved nutrition, especially in infancy.

Today the major infectious disease problems affecting people in developed countries are usually related to: (i) changing life-styles and technical advances which lead to changes in the characteristics and manifestations of known pathogens, and, possibly, the introduction of new pathogens; or (ii) the application of preventive measures including vaccination. For example, the increase in sexual freedom and the emergence of antibiotic-resistant agents have resulted in a rise in sexually transmitted diseases. Among homosexually active males and some other groups an outbreak of acquired immune deficiency and related conditions such as Kaposi's sarcoma is occurring which is probably a reflection of changes in life-style (Gottleib *et al.* 1981; CDC 1982). The widespread immuniza tion of children against certain infectious diseases such as rubella has increased the average age at which these diseases occur, resulting in the more frequent complications associated with infection at an older age (Robinson *et al.* 1982). Previously known pathogens are being identified as causing new clinical syndromes – for example, venereal disease in men and women due to *Chlamydia* which are better known for causing ocular and respiratory diseases (Grayston and Wang 1975) and herpes virus (Josey *et al.* 1972).

Although public health advances have eliminated the threat of major epidemics of the traditional infectious diseases, these still occur among groups which for various reasons, including poverty, have not benefitted fully from the public health practices that have led to control of these diseases in the majority of the population. Influenza and agents causing high morbidity, but relatively infrequent death such as those responsible for the 'common cold' remain major problems. Despite the availability of excellent vaccines, outbreaks of measles, rubella, and polio still occur. In addition, several diseases such as tuberculosis are constantly reintroduced into developed countries which receive refugees from developing countries. More effective vaccines for hepatitis, influenza, and pneumonia have been recently developed but the optimal strategy for their use is still being debated.

Individuals who survive disease because of improved medical technology are often susceptible to agents which usually do not cause disease in healthy individuals. Cyto-megalovirus, for example, affects primarily individuals whose immune systems have been compromised possibly due to treatment with drugs or to other factors. Conversely, exposure to infections may be involved in chronic disorders such as multiple sclerosis.

The public health professional in developed countries hence must be constantly alert to changing relationships between infectious disease agents, chronic disease, the susceptibility of members of the community, and the environment which may result in new clinical syndromes. Relatively few of these new clinical entities will be due to hitherto completely unknown agents. Frequently, they will be attributable to the dynamic epidemiology of infectious disease arising from the otherwise successful application of public health strategies, use of new technologies, rapid changes in life-styles, and the emergence of new population groups including individuals who survive because of advances in medical technology.

Chronic disease

Beginning in the nineteenth and continuing through the twentieth century, industrialization has vastly changed the way people live and, correspondingly, the nature of their health problems. This change is made particularly apparent by comparing the leading causes of death among the US population in 1900 and 1980 (Table 2.1).

Heart disease, cancer, stroke, and accidents now cause more than two-thirds of all deaths. A different pattern appears, however, when disability or illness rather than death is used as the measure of health. Tables 2.2 to 2.4, illustrate the functional impact of various kinds of acute and chronic conditions. More than half of all restricted-activity days occur because of acute conditions. Only after the age of 45 years do chronic conditions become a more important cause for restriction of activity (Table 2.2). Beyond age 65 years the average person suffers restriction of activity from one or several chronic conditions for the equivalent of almost one month a year, about one-third of that time confined to bed (Table 2.2). Upper respiratory conditions (mostly common colds) account for more than one-fourth of all acute conditions and influenza for almost as high a proportion

Table 2.1. *Age-adjusted death rates per 100 000, leading causes of death, United States, 1900 and 1980*

1900		1980	
Cause	Rate	Cause	Rate
Influenza and pneumonia	210	Heart disease	205.3
Tuberculosis	199	Cancer	134.2
Heart disease	167	Accidents	43.4
Stroke	134	Stroke	41.5
Diarrhoea and related diseases	113	Influenza and pneumonia	12.6
Cancer	81	Cirrhosis/chronic liver disease	12.6
Accidents	76	Suicide	12.2
Diabetes	13	Diabetes	10.1
Suicide	11	Homicide	11.4
Homicide	1	Tuberculosis	0.5
All other causes	775	Diarrhoea	0.7*
		All other causes	109.6
All causes	1779	All causes	594.1

*Figure is for 1978. Not available for 1980.
Source: McGinnis (1982). (From *Annual Summary of Births, Deaths, Marriages and Divorces: United States*, 1930; *Monthly Vital Statistics Report*, Vol. 29, No. 13, Sept. 17, 1981; and unpublished data, National Center for Health Statistics.)

Table 2.2. *Restricted-activity and bed-disability days due to acute and chronic conditions per person per year, United States, 1977*

	All conditions		Acute conditions		Chronic conditions	
	Restricted-activity days	Bed disability days	Restricted-activity days	Bed-disability days	Restricted-activity days	Bed-disability days
All ages	17.4	6.8	9.4	4.2	8.0	2.6
Under 17 years	11.2	5.2	10.0	4.8	1.2	0.4
17–44 years	14.2	5.4	9.1	3.9	5.1	1.5
45–64 years	24.4	8.2	8.6	3.7	15.8	4.5
65 years and over	36.5	14.5	10.1	4.5	26.4	10.0

Source: Department of Health, Education and Welfare (1980).

Table 2.3. *Annual incidence of acute conditions per 100 persons under 65 years of age, United States, 1976*

Condition	Incidence	
All acute conditions	231.9	
Total respiratory	126.9	
Upper respiratory		64.4
Influenza		56.1
Other		6.4
Injuries	33.4	
Infective and parasitic diseases	26.6	
Digestive system	11.0	
All other	34.0	

Source: Department of Health, Education and Welfare (1978).

(Table 2.3). Specific well-defined infective and parasitic diseases are responsible for only about one-tenth of them.

Heart disease is the major chronic condition resulting in limitation of activity (Table 2.4). Arthritis and rheumatism follow and impairments of the back, spine, hips, and lower extremities or other musculoskeletal disorders all result in a considerable amount of limited activity.

Significant success in the prevention of chronic disease has been achieved in the area of public health dentistry. The introduction of fluoride into municipal water supplies and dentifrices has dramatically reduced the incidence of dental caries over the last several decades. The major dental public health problem in developed countries is now periodontal disease. Reduction of this disease will depend on the ability of the dental community in motivating the public to practise better oral hygiene and to improve their nutritional habits. In this respect the strategies which must be used by public health dentistry are similar to those needed to reduce the incidence of the other major chronic diseases.

Health problems among the elderly are an increasing concern of public health, both because more people are living longer and because of the greater frequency of disabling illness among them. Until recently, the main factor extending the average duration of life, was the reduction in fatal

Table 2.4. *Percentage of persons with specific chronic conditions among persons with chronic limitations of activity, United States, 1974*

	All degrees of activity limitation (%)	Unable to carry on major activity (%)
Heart condition	16.2	24.1
Arthritis and rheumatism	15.0	15.8
Impairment of back or spine	7.0	4.2
Hypertension without heart involvement	6.7	6.6
Impairment of lower extremities and hips	6.4	5.4
Visual impairment	5.9	8.1
Other musculoskeletal disorders	5.9	4.3
Mental and nervous conditions	5.1	7.6
Diabetes	4.9	6.9
Asthma	4.9	2.5

Source: Department of Health, Education and Welfare (1977).

diseases in infancy and the early years of life. The average duration of life after age 45 years remained fairly steady until about 1970. Since then, the life expectancy of individuals of 45 years of age has increased by two years, compared with the five years gained during the entire period from 1900 to 1970. The major interest in preventing and controlling chronic disease is not just extending the duration of life but maintaining the quality of life as well.

Mental disorders

Mental disorders requiring some form of mental health services in the US have been estimated to affect 15 per cent of the population (Task Panel Report to President's Commission on Mental Health 1978). Thus, these disorders represent a significant portion of all health problems. In the US the cost of mental illness in 1978 was $17 billion annually, that is, 11 per cent of the nation's health care expenditures.

These disorders include psychoses, neuroses, mental retardation, alcoholism, dependency disorders, child abuse, and learning disabilities. Despite the considerable progress that has been made in the past few years in understanding the aetiology of mental illness and in treating a wide variety of mental disorders, public health efforts directed toward prevention and treatment have not been adequately implemented. Two out of every five persons with psychosis and one out of five with schizophrenia have never received treatment (Task Panel Report to President's Commission on Mental Health 1978).

Until the twentieth century the public health approach to individuals with mental illness or mental retardation was to place them in custodial institutions and thereby exclude them from society. In the US significant changes in this approach did not occur until after the Second World War when, for the first time, the problem of mental illness received national attention. In particular, a strong effort was made to reduce the number of patients in mental institutions and return these individuals to their local communities. Further impetus for this effort came in the early 1950s with the use of new psychoactive drugs which allowed many mentally ill persons to live normal lives in the community. In the US the number of persons in state mental hospitals declined from more than 550 000 in 1955 to less than 200 000 in 1975 (Task Panel Report to President's Commission on Mental Health 1978). Federal legislation in 1963 to establish Community Mental Health Centers (CMHC) was another significant effort to promote de-institutionalization and to reduce the role of state and county mental hospitals in caring for the mentally ill.

Largely as a result of insufficient resources, these Centers were unable to provide adequate care to the large number of persons requiring it. As many as 50 per cent of patients released from large mental institutions have had to be reinstitutionalized (Task Panel Report to President's Commission on Mental Health 1978).

Although there have been numerous efforts within the past 25 years to attribute a variety of different mental disorders to specific genetic, physical or psychosocial factors, most mental disorders have not, in fact, been associated with specific causes.

They seem to result from multiple determinants (Lieberman 1975). Never the less, in a few areas specific links have been made between certain biological factors and certain mental disorders. For example, mental retardation due to Down's syndrome results from a defect in one of the chromosomes (trisomy 21) which occurs at a much greater frequency in pregnancy among women over 35 years of age. This condition can now be diagnosed *in utero* by amniocentesis, allowing the termination of pregnancies which would result in children with Down's syndrome.

Paralleling the approach which acknowledges the need to deal with physical health problems within a broad social context, there has come recognition that mental illness cannot be understood or treated independently of socio-economic conditions. In mental health this approach reflects awareness that mental disorders are more frequent and the type of problem experienced more severe in the lowest socio-economic segment of the population. Yet, in the US, this segment of the population is least likely to seek or receive care. Other populations unlikely to receive adequate care are those with chronic mental illness, children, adolescents, and the elderly. In 1978, a Presidential Commission noted that the future organization, delivery, and financing of mental health services must be planned to address this lack (Task Panel Report to President's Commission on Mental Health 1978). This will require the creation of networks of high quality comprehensive mental health services that are adequately funded through public and private sources and are appropriately staffed by trained mental health personnel.

Other significant developments in the past two decades that are likely to result in improved methods of prevention and treatment of mental disorders are: (i) the increased number and types of mental health professionals and the increased range of services they provide in a variety of diverse settings; (ii) an increased understanding of the role of personal and community support systems in helping individuals with short-term as well as chronic mental or physical health problems; (iii) an increased awareness of the value of early detection and intervention in the early developmental stages of mental disorders; and (iv) the advances made in understanding the biochemical mechanisms of certain psychoses and other biologically based or genetically determined mental disorders.

Until recently, at least, the mentally ill have not shared fully in the rights and expectations taken for granted by the vast majority of people in the industrialized nations. The means to provide the mentally ill with these rights and privileges are now becoming available. It must be a part of the public health agenda to assure these rights to those suffering from mental illness.

DETERMINANTS OF HEALTH

Although public health and medicine have done much to prevent disease and improve health, there has been increasing recognition that individuals, themselves, can play a major role in determining their own health through nutritional, environmental, and life-style choices. The spectacular achievements of microbiology and related biomedical sciences which have

evoked wide, and deserved admiration have unfortunately tended to obscure the important influence of life-style which public health must now also emphasize.

Nutrition

Fifty years ago the major nutritional problems throughout the world were: the lack of adequate, safe, affordable supplies of food; inadequate knowledge of the dietary needs of humans; and wide-scale ignorance among the public concerning the relationship of nutrition to health and disease. Large segments of the population in industrialized nations were not aware of the need for a balanced diet including components from all the major food groups. Even if they had been aware of nutritional needs, essential foods were often not available due to poverty or because of transportation and distribution problems affecting a wide range of foods. For example, fresh fruits and other major sources of vitamin C were often almost unobtainable in northern climates for major portions of the year. Finally, provision of safe foods, uncontaminated by parasites, bacteria, and viruses, was difficult in the absence of refrigeration.

The high prevalence of infective and parasitic disease conditions led to undernutrition and, in turn, made individuals more susceptible to infectious disease agents because of their compromised nutritional status. For example, individuals with ascaris infection could be undernourished in the face of what appeared to be an adequate diet and would thus be more susceptible to infections with other disease agents.

Most of these nutritional problems of fifty years ago have been resolved in the developed countries. On the other hand, these problems persist in the developing countries and even among certain groups of people in developed countries, for example, among the poor and immigrants whose access to health care may be limited.

The major nutritional problem in the developed countries, however, appears now to be overnutrition, particularly an excessive consumption of fats, refined carbohydrates, and salt, which promote diseases such as coronary heart disease, diabetes, hypertension, and dental caries. The importance of these factors has been emphasized by various scientific bodies, such as the US National Academy of Sciences in a recent report, and health organizations, such as the American Heart Association (National Research Council 1982). On the other extreme are the food faddists, who out of a desire to lose weight or for other reasons, subject themselves to nutritionally unsound diets which adversely affect their health.

The resolution of several current health problems requires intensive, additional research into the relationships between nutritional factors, health, and disease. For example, diet varies in populations with high and low risks of cancer. Studies of such differences may lead to insight into how nutritional factors promote or inhibit cancer.

Nutritional surveys and surveillance such as those carried out by the US National Center for Health Statistics can identify problems of malnutrition using questionnaires and anthropometric measurements such as height-weight index, ponderal index, and skin-fold thickness. Education about properly balanced diets and diseases induced by poor nutrition should be expanded, especially among expectant mothers, children, and the elderly in whom nutritional problems are more likely to occur. Finally, opportunities for nutritional intervention through fortification and supplementation of common foods, such as the addition of vitamin D to milk, iodine to salt, vegetables to sausage, and vitamins to bread, need continuing examination.

Environmental conditions

In the early part of the twentieth century the public health professional was concerned largely with ensuring the provision of biologically safe water and food to the public, and the safe removal of sewage and garbage. The health consequences of ingestion of toxic substances such as lead and the use of radioactive substances to paint dials on watches were not recognized as important to public health.

Systems are now in place in most developed countries to assure the supply of biologically safe water and foods, and the proper removal of sewage and garbage. The environmental problems of importance in the developed countries now largely result from the explosion of technology over the last several decades. For example, the production of chemicals in the US has grown from 1.9 billion pounds in 1940 to over 375 billion pounds in 1980. This increase in the production of chemicals has also been accompanied by a tremendous expansion of the spectrum of chemicals to which the public is exposed.

The major current, environmental threats to health arise from chemical pollution of the air, water, and land. (See Volume 3, Chapters 18 and 19.) Unfortunately, health effects from such pollution may occur years after exposure and are thus difficult to document. These health effects may be the result of cumulative burdens of chemicals in tissues, or the deposition of chemicals in parts of the body which are not readily accessible for evaluation, for example, the brain. The registration of individuals in potentially hazardous occupations would help identify the specific health hazards associated with certain exposures.

Safeguarding the health of the public requires regulation of pollutants. Establishing and maintaining acceptable levels of pollutants is complicated by two factors: (i) the difficulty of ascertaining dose-response relationships, particularly for diseases with a long induction period; and (ii) the economic burden which may result from regulatory actions. Whereas intervention in infectious diseases has met with enthusiastic support from the public, control of toxic substances in the environment has, until very recently, not been vigorously supported by the public. Inadequate understanding of the relationships between chemical pollutants and resultant disease, and the expense related to surveillance, regulation, and control of toxic substances has deterred action. The application of stringent controls may cause other problems such as increased costs and unemployment. Thus, regulation often rests more with the courts and legal procedures than on scientific expertise and judgment.

Resolution of important issues confronting society may themselves introduce health hazards. Thus, the need to develop energy-efficient housing has increased the levels of indoor pollutants with heightened potential for occurrence of related disease. In addition, certain life-styles may promote the action of specific toxic substances. For example, the likelihood of developing lung cancer from exposure to asbestos is increased about sevenfold by smoking.

Protecting the public's health against environmental and occupational hazards in the future will depend upon research into the acute and long-term health effects of the myriad substances being released into the environment, and into techniques for neutralizing or eliminating them, as well as on surveillance and enforcement of regulations. Such efforts will be expensive and unpopular so that careful considerations should be given to implementing those which will have a high probability of yielding a positive effect on the health of the community.

Life-style

In addition to specific nutritional patterns and physical features of the environment, the way people live substantially influences health. Life-style can be subdivided into two sets of behaviours, those which are primarily personal, and those which are primarily social or collective in nature.

Most people in industrialized society have access to possibilities of consumption that, if followed to the extreme, can generate serious health problems. These include cigarettes, alcohol, excessive calories, and reduced physical demand. Their choices in these and similar matters exert a profound influence on whether an individual will suffer and die prematurely from lung cancer, coronary heart disease, cirrhosis, chronic lung disease, trauma, and other major causes of illness and death in the latter part of the twentieth century.

Analysis of Canadian experience, for example, indicates that 18 per cent of all deaths and 18 per cent of all premature years of life lost from 1 to 70 years of age are, conservatively, attributable just to cigarette smoking and excessive consumption of alcohol (Ouellet et al. 1977). Cigarette smoking alone has been judged responsible for more than 300 000 deaths annually in the US (Califano 1979). A 1965 general population survey in Alameda County, California, identified seven personal habits – exercising at least moderately; drinking alcohol moderately, if at all; eating moderately, that is, maintaining optimum weight; eating regularly; eating breakfast; not smoking cigarettes; and sleeping 7–8 hours regularly – to be strongly associated with health (Belloc and Breslow 1972). At every age, from 20 to 70 years, persons who followed all seven of these habits had better physical health status than those who followed six, six better than five, five better than four, four better than three, and three better than two or fewer. The same relationship held with respect to mortality rates expressed in longevity (Table 2.5).

These habits, of course, do not develop in a vacuum. The extent to which a person acquires them depends on circumstances such as, for example, the advertising, price, and peer support of cigarette smoking. Social policy affecting these matters hence becomes an important issue for public health. Also, there is a danger that public health practitioners will compromise their credibility by advocating unpleasant changes

Table 2.5. *Average remaining lifetime based on death rates of three health practice groups, and California life-table, 1959–61*

Age (years)	Number of health practices			California 1959–61
	0–3	4–5	6–7	
Men				
45	21.6	28.2	33.1	27.6
65	10.6	13.7	17.4	13.3
Women				
45	28.6	34.1	35.8	33.1
65	12.4	17.3	19.9	

Source: Belloc and Breslow (1973).

in life-style which are not supported by scientifically sound studies.

A second aspect of life-style significantly associated with health embraces peoples' relationships to their social networks. Considerable evidence now links health to marital status, degree of closeness to friends and relatives, and social group involvement. The Alameda County study assessed the role of the social network in health and mortality (Berkman and Syme 1979). Table 2.6 displays the extent to which social connections are associated with mortality. This association is largely independent of physical health status, health practices, use of health services, socio-economic status, age, sex, and race.

Population

Success in reducing death rates has increased population pressures. In developed countries the decline in mortality took place gradually with a commensurate decline in birth rates as survival of infants increased. In developing countries the drop in mortality has occurred over a shorter time period and without a commensurate drop in birth rates. This has resulted in rapidly expanding populations in those countries where food and other vital resources are limited.

Currently the less developed countries are expanding their populations four times as rapidly as the developed countries.

Table 2.6. *Age-adjusted mortality rates per 100, all causes, men and women aged 30–69, social network index and health practices index, Alameda County, 1965–74*

Social network index	Health practices			Total
	0–4	5	6–7	
Men				
I (fewest connections)	21.5	9.9	10.5	15.6
II	14.6	11.7	9.9	12.2
III	10.3	9.9	6.6	8.6
IV (most connections)	7.8	9.5	4.2	6.2
Total	12.3	10.2	6.7	9.5
Women				
I (fewest connections)	15.2	8.5	10.0	12.1
II	10.4	7.5	4.0	7.2
III	5.8	4.7	4.3	4.9
IV (most connections)	6.5	2.4	4.4	4.3
Total	9.3	5.6	4.7	6.4

Source: Berkman and Syme (1979).

Since the former countries also have a higher proportion of individuals of reproductive age or younger, the higher birth rates are likely to continue for at least the next several decades. Thus, it is estimated that by the year 2000 nearly 80 per cent of the world's population will be concentrated in developing countries (Volume 2, Chapter 4).

It is clear that unless efforts to control population growth are successful the population of the earth will outstrip its ability to sustain itself. Therefore, a major public health effort must be directed at controlling population growth. These efforts must include the continued development and implementation of more effective, safe contraceptive methods as well as education efforts, both in their use and the need for them.

In the more developed countries where population growth has declined to replacement levels the proportion of elderly has increased, introducing new problems. These shifts in age distributions should be anticipated as population growth is decreased in the rest of the world.

SCIENTIFIC RESPONSES

Public health is the application of the scientific disciplines to the resolution of the health problems outlined above. It is imperative that public health base itself on scientific evidence. The range of sciences used extends from those specific to public health, such as epidemiology, to those shared with other fields.

Epidemiological strategies

Epidemiology is the core science of public health and preventive medicine. The methodology is used to describe the distribution, dynamics, and determinants of disease and health in human populations. Although there are many definitions, the Greek root of the word *epidemiology* delineates well the scope of the discipline: 'The study of that which is upon the people'. The epidemiologist seeks to identify those characteristics of people, the agents of disease, and the environment which determine the occurrence of disease and health. In order to accomplish that objective, the epidemiologist describes: (i) disease occurrence (time characteristics); (ii) the population affected (person characteristics); and (iii) the nature of the environment in which the disease is occurring (place characteristics) which contribute to knowledge about the natural history of the disease and ways to control it. For example, epidemiologists have observed that coronary heart disease occurs primarily among men middle-aged and older in developed countries, who overeat, have high blood pressure, smoke cigarettes, do little exercise, and who have a family history of heart disease.

For studying these matters, epidemiologists must have good information on the occurrence of disease, and on the relevant characteristics of the population and the environment. The need for this information has stimulated the development of health information systems for co-ordinating existing sources of data and guiding the development of necessary new sources.

Epidemiologists depend to a considerable extent upon comparing disease frequencies in different populations. To make these comparisons it is necessary to estimate rates of disease occurrence. Information about populations is usually obtained through a census, or sometimes by sample survey. Rates which depend on census data are likely to be increasingly inaccurate with the number of years which have elapsed since the data were collected. In addition, detailed information on populations derived from a periodic census is often not available for one or more years following the actual collection of data. In some communities information on population characteristics may be obtained at more frequent intervals by examining an appropriately selected probability sample of the population. This information can be particularly useful at times distant from the date of census collection.

The potential of health information for documenting disease occurrence and developing hypotheses has expanded rapidly over the last decade. This advance is a result not only of the rapid development of computer technology but also because of the entry into the field of individuals whose major discipline is epidemiology. Prior to the last decade, the majority of epidemiologists in the US were physicians who took an additional year or more of training to supplement their biomedical education. Non-physicians in the UK, however, made several significant contributions to epidemiological methodology, for example, the great biostatistician, Bradford Hill. Both physician and non-physician epidemiologists are essential to the field. Many non-physician epidemiologists have concentrated primarily on methodological issues. For example, they have contributed greatly to the further development of techniques which distinguish factors which are truly related to disease from those factors which are related only indirectly to disease and, thus, may confound a true causal association.

The capacity of the epidemiologist for ascertaining the distribution, dynamics, and determinants of disease depends upon the availability of several other scientific disciplines. For example, laboratory procedures derived from chemistry, biochemistry, microbiology, and immunology can be used for obtaining information about the environment, the agents of disease, and the changes which occur in man. Epidemiology looks to statistics, on the other hand, for mathematical methodologies which describe the strength of correlations between the multiple factors which may promote the occurrence of disease. The balance of this section will be devoted to a description of the changing contributions of these various disciplines to the field of public health.

Biostatistics

Advances in epidemiological methodology have been accompanied by rapid progress in biostatistics, particularly the development of computer technology. Through its application, biostatisticians have developed multivariate techniques to determine the relationship of mutiple factors to disease occurrence while simultaneously observing the relationship of these variables to each other. Sophisticated techniques for the analysis of events in relation to time are enhancing the value of the cohort study design. Because the computer can process massive amounts of information rapidly, it has been possible to develop and test mathematical models that describe hypothetical relationships and disease

outcomes based on a variety of assumptions. The degree to which the actual occurrence of disease matches the models confirms or refutes these relationships.

These new statistical techniques using computer technology have been directed towards more sophisticated analytical approaches in epidemiology as well as to clinical trials. The potential of statistics to contribute to public health through further development of computer methodology is great.

Laboratory sciences

The laboratory sciences have long played an essential role in public health. Many of the advances against infectious diseases depended upon microbiology to provide isolation techniques and markers of prior infection or exposure. The rapid expansion of vaccines against viral diseases reflect new procedures for isolating viruses using cell cultivation techniques that were developed in the late 1930s. These cell culture techniques facilitated the manufacture of live vaccines using attenuated viruses, that is, viruses which have lost their virulence characteristics for man but not their capacity for stimulating immunity. Recently, microbiologists have fragmented disease agents into particular components and selected those which are responsible for the immune response. Vaccines are now also being developed which utilize genetic recombination.

Startling as these recent developments in microbiology and immunology have been, equally important contributions to public health are coming from the laboratory sciences of chemistry, biochemistry, and engineering. For example, the studies of the chemical interactions of primary pollutants in the atmosphere which lead to development of photochemical oxidants can suggest intervention strategies.

In summary, rapid advances in the field of epidemiology have resulted from new epidemiological methods as well as from the availability of new techniques in biostatistics and the laboratory sciences – microbiology, chemistry, and engineering. Epidemiology will continue to draw upon them to help provide the basic information needed for the development and application of effective public health strategies for disease control and health promotion.

Social sciences

Recent decades have brought recognition that individuals can control many of the determinants of disease through their choice of exercise, eating patterns, and alcohol consumption. Behavioural factors also determine the response to illness, particularly to subtle manifestations of disease, and thus affect the ability of the individual to function normally. The role of the behavioural sciences (including psychology, sociology, and anthropology) in public health is thus increasing.

Each of the behavioural sciences approaches behaviour from a different vantage point. Psychologists emphasize individual differences; sociologists draw inferences from analyses of how groups of people, whole communities or nations or sub-sets of them, behave *en masse*; and anthropologists stress the cultural patterns that influence behaviour from generation to generation.

Behavioural science techniques have proved valuable in understanding factors influencing health. For example, social survey methodology has greatly enhanced our capacity to understand relationships of behaviour to disease and to discern trends that are highly important to public health. Psychological investigation of peoples' knowledge and attitudes yields insight into the habitual and life-style practices that are related to health, and often suggests ways of promoting health. Sociological investigation of the group processes that determine a community's norms and values, and adherence to them, likewise leads to an understanding of how people behave and thus how they can be influenced to follow a healthy life-style. Anthropology elucidates the cultural traditions that influence what people do in everyday life and suggests approaches to health promotion specific for various cultural groups.

Within the field of public health, health education draws upon these disciplines to apply effective techniques to cultivate healthy behaviour.

In addition to this behavioural science approach to health, it is necessary also to note that the socio-economic milieu in large measure influences the choices that people make. Life-style does not consist of behaviour elements selected by an individual in a vacuum; it reflects the circumstances of life.

Demography and vital statistics

John Graunt is commonly considered the father of vital statistics because of his early studies of the Bills of Mortality in London and a parish town of Hampshire. He collected and examined the birth and death records maintained by parish clerks from 1603 to 1662. (His original report was reprinted in 1939 – see also Lilienfeld 1976.) From that epochal work he drew important inferences about the population and its health. For example, he analysed mortality, including infant mortality, seasonal variation of deaths, and longevity, as well as fertility and the excess of male births. His studies laid the groundwork for what has become vital statistics.

Over the past three centuries demography, the study of human populations, has been closely intertwined with public health. Vital statistics include delineation of: (i) births and the rates of their occurrence in various elements of the population; (ii) fertility – that is, the ratio of births to women aged 15–49 years; (iii) mortality, including deaths among infants and in subsequent ages as well as trends, specific causes, and determinants of deaths; and (iv) migration patterns. All of these are important to public health.

Information about the occurrence of disease may be obtained through aggregated data derived from death certificates, birth certificates, hospitals and clinics, surveys, and registries. Computer technology facilitates analysis of mortality in relation to the characteristics which are coded on each person's death certificate. In addition, information from birth certificates and other sources can be linked to the occurrence of death, thus providing additional information about the characteristics of persons or events that may cause death.

Data concerning non-lethal diseases are more difficult to obtain than the birth and death information which must be recorded by law. In the US, the Centers for Disease Control (CDC) publish a morbidity and mortality weekly report which contains information on certain diseases, obtained through reporting from local health departments. Hospital discharge abstracts and summaries provide further information. Special surveys may be carried out, in addition to ongoing national health surveys administered to a probability sample of the population. Disease-specific registries also provide information about changing trends in disease occurrence, mortality and duration of survival. Most well-known among these are cancer registries, but comparable data bases are also being developed for diabetes, coronary heart disease, and other chronic diseases.

Demography focuses on population trends such as growth – that is, the excess of births over deaths, and in-migration over out-migration, and age-distribution. Public health statistics are concerned with information about the health of populations. Both fields are devoted to satisfying social concerns about people. Mutual interest in factors determining fertility illustrates the continuing interrelationships of public health and demography.

PROGRAMMATIC SCOPE OF PUBLIC HEALTH

With the maturation of industrial society three approaches for the protection and improvement of health – behavioural, environmental, and medical – have become apparent. They comprise the programmatic scope of public health. Most current health problems are being tackled through a combination of these approaches, as illustrated in Table 2.7. From time to time, and in various circumstances, public health agencies may focus on one or another of the three types of approaches, but a comprehensive programme includes them all.

Table 2.7. *Approaches to current health problems*

Health problem	Preventive medical measures	Environmental measures	Influences on behaviour
Infant deaths	Pre-natal and paediatric care	Home hygiene; reduce exposure to toxic agents	Support healthy life-styles; parent education
High blood pressure	Detect hypertension and treat it vigorously	Reduce fat and salt in processed foods	Heighten public awareness of significance of overweight, salt
Loss of teeth	Repair caries; remove calculus	Fluoridation; reduce production and promotion of refined sugars	Encourage tooth brushing and flossing; prudent diet
Lung cancer	Detect and treat disease early	Curtail promotion of cigarettes; reduce occupational exposures to pulmonary carcinogens	Encourage no cigarette smoking

Source: Breslow (1983).

Medical care

Beginning with Bismarck, the western nations have generally provided medical care of varying kinds and degree as a social benefit to industrial workers. In most countries some care has also been extended to others, particularly to families of workers, the elderly, and the poor. For example, the British National Health Service covers virtually the whole population. On the other hand, the US relies almost entirely on private arrangements for employed persons and their families except for work injuries. Large-scale governmental assistance for health care services goes only to the elderly and the poor.

Medical care can be examined from several perspectives: medical and economic, for example, as well as from the standpoint of public health. The medical profession, reflecting both the centuries-old tradition of healing and recent advances in medical science, looks upon medical care as the main means to relieve suffering and restore health. Economists view medical care principally in terms of cost and, therefore, examine the increasingly large public, as well as private, expenditures with concern. Public health considers medical care to be one means of protecting and improving the health of people, but also is concerned with cost, especially in so far as it constitutes a barrier to health care for some groups. The public health focus on medical care emphasizes the potential for enhancing a community's health.

Provision of medical services is usually determined in a specific country by cultural and traditional patterns. Thus, in Britain the individual general practitioner and his or her panel of patients are the predominant care module, with referral to the hospital consultant as necessary. In the US, however, the former life-long, physician–patient relationship has now often been replaced by clinics where the patient sees no particular physician; by specialists such as paediatricians, general internists, and obstetricians, who see patients only during certain limited periods of their lives; and, most recently, to a growing extent by free-standing emergency medical services. Different medical service patterns are continuously evolving in both countries. For example, in Britain the trend is for general practitioners to work within a group practice, and group-practice prepayment plans are expanding in the US. The community medicine movement, as this has developed in the US, aims at adapting medical services more closely to community needs by directing attention to locale and by incorporating social workers, nutritionists, and other personnel into the services.

Public health, however, uses medical care primarily to achieve prevention. Thus, public health agencies have organized immunization activities and, especially in the US, maternal and child health services. Over the past few decades these efforts have contributed to spectacular achievements in control of communicable disease and infant mortality and, thus, have provided a strong rationale for integrating preventive and curative services. In the past, curative services have generally received priority over preventive services on grounds of urgency.

Most physicians and medical care agencies generally follow what may be termed the complaint–response system of medicine – patients are taught to recognize and bring their health complaints to the doctor whose response is to diagnose and treat any illness that may be present. Prevention, if advocated at all, is usually a minor consideration.

A new system of medical care, which gives priority to promoting health and preventing disease, has been slowly emerging in the US. Individuals' health is monitored through periodic appraisal geared to age and other factors that determine both current and future prospects of health. Thus, infant care concentrates on growth, appearance of defects, immunization status, and any necessary corrective action to assure the healthiest possible development. When a person has reached 50 years of age, the focus shifts to blood pressure, weight/height ratio, blood-sugar, blood-cholesterol, cancer detection, cigarette and alcohol consumption, and other physical and behavioural characteristics. This approach, emphasizing the maintenance of health through systematic, early diagnosis and prevention, must yet be fully evaluated.

In addition to the relative emphasis that should be accorded preventive versus curative efforts, several other issues currently affect the public health approach to medical care. In past years many procedures and drugs have been put into widespread use without sufficient consideration of their effectiveness. Initiatives are now underway, for example, by the Medical Research Council and the Department of Health and Social Security in Britain, and the Congressional Office of Technology Assessment in the US, to establish a better system for evaluating the effectiveness of drug regimens and medical technologies.

These initiatives, in part, express concern about the rapidly rising cost of medical care in the western nations which make it especially unwise to devote resources to items of questionable, and in some instances even negative, value to health. Another issue raised by the cost factor is the efficiency of medical service, that is, how can the best possible quality of medical care be provided with a given amount of resources? The organization of medical personnel, for example, into groups, as well as the provision of incentives to personnel, offer possibilities for raising the productivity of medical services. A third cost-related problem that must be considered is the extent to which medical resources should be used for highly expensive procedures and devices such as kidney or heart replacement which benefit only a few at great expense. Expanding technology and limited resources together are forcing consideration of the ethical as well as the health and economic consequences of medical care.

Thus a major programmatic thrust of public health in the immediate future will be renewed emphasis on medical care as a means of improving health. However, the balance of the various components of medical care will shift from primarily curative or complaint oriented to preventive and promotive services.

Influencing behaviour

As noted earlier in this chapter the way people live largely determines their health. Thus, a prime responsibility for public health is to develop effective strategies to promote healthy life-styles.

Several approaches are being tested. One is to convert the national and even international milieu so that it favours healthy behaviour – for example, the various national and WHO campaigns against cigarette smoking. Such activities, however, often result in confrontation with powerful, entrenched economic interests. Tactics in the struggle to turn public policy explicitly towards the side of health must be high on the public health agenda.

A second approach is the so-called medical model, that is, using the doctor–patient relationship, or analogues of it, to influence health-related behaviour. The tactic is a one-to-one, or sometimes a small group, effort in a health-oriented environment to guide individuals toward healthy behaviour. It offers promise particularly when people have, or can be induced to have, concern about particular health problems such as coronary heart disease, and then are willing to undertake the indicated change of their habits.

Several nation-wide studies have evaluated this general strategy. In the US the Hypertension Detection and Follow-up Program and the Multiple Risk Factor Intervention Trial exemplify efforts at evaluation of interventions (HDFP 1979; MRFIT 1982). In Europe the WHO has sponsored a cardiovascular disease intervention trial, based on paired factories in several countries (WHO 1982).

Community-wide intervention constitutes a third approach to influencing behaviour in the interest of health. The focus in this case is to identify and enhance positive trends towards health such as smoking cessation in a geographically-defined population. This technique which uses sample surveys to determine baseline levels followed by a broad effort utilizing broadcast and news media, community organizations, and the health professionals is being formally tested in several places in the world.

Environmental control

Attempts to control pollution of the environment including the occupational setting are complicated by the problem of identifying those pollutants which pose health hazards to humans. Pollutants such as radiation which have no apparent immediate effect on humans can cause disease after many years of chronic and persistent exposure. Some pollutants may cause disease by accumulating in the body. However, the accumulation of these substances may occur in parts of the body such as bone, in which it is difficult to measure levels.

A highly desirable approach to control is to obtain the voluntary co-operation of industry. However, control mechanisms which are often expensive have seldom been voluntarily adopted by industry.

In the middle decades of the twentieth century the western nations became increasingly aware of threats to health occurring through contamination of the environment. This concern led in the US, for example, to implementation of the National Environmental Act in 1969 which directed the federal government to plan policies in the light of the effect that these policies would have on the environment. The National Environmental Act was followed in the next decade by a series of legislative actions creating regulatory agencies directed at

protection of the environment, and especially reduction of pollutants. These are discussed further in Chapter 9.

During the first part of the 1980s the governments in the US, as well as the UK and Europe, have faced increased challenges to their regulatory activities. The deteriorating fiscal situation of federal and local governments has caused legislatures to question the advisability of handicapping industrial operations at a time when these are deemed necessary for economic recovery. The 1980s will present serious difficulties in maintaining and improving the quality of the environment. Innovative approaches, such as combining the control of wastes and the development of new energy sources and techniques for recycling waste products, will be needed.

In summary, the programmatic scope of public health embraces medical, behavioural, and environmental measures designed to improve health at the community level. Although particular agencies and personnel address specific aspects of community health, public health embraces the whole range of activities.

PUBLIC HEALTH STRATEGIES

As outlined above, public health strategies include the maintenance of effective surveillance of threats to community health, implementation of sound intervention measures, and continuing evaluation of their effectiveness.

Surveillance

Effective intervention into factors affecting community health depends upon reliable knowledge concerning the occurrence and distribution of these factors in the community. Thus, the backbone of public health strategy is the development and maintenance of an accurate, reliable health information system upon which actions can be based. Such surveillance systems should include information on the occurrence of infectious and chronic diseases, environmental, including occupational exposures, behavioural characteristics, and medical services. Information must be collected on a regular basis and reported rapidly, particularly for the infectious diseases and hazardous environmental exposures. Tardy reporting of information about disease outbreaks or sudden radiation hazards, for example, might slow down the implementation of effective intervention procedures. Currently, the surveillance systems used by public health agencies, in general, do not fully meet these criteria for reporting.

The most extensive experience in surveillance work has concerned the communicable diseases. There are fewer reporting mechanisms for chronic diseases.

Currently, surveillance for environmental hazards and occupational exposures is less satisfactory than surveillance for either infectious or chronic diseases. Most urban areas have systems for monitoring quality of air and quality of water for human consumption although provisions for monitoring new contaminants such as cadmium and magnesium are inadequate. Considerable attention also needs to be directed to surveillance of recreational waters, toxic dump sites and radiation exposures. In addition, workers continue to be exposed to unsafe working conditions, particularly workers in small industries which are more difficult to monitor and regulate. Details of the current surveillance systems are discussed in subsequent chapters.

Until information systems provide accurate, reliable, rapid reporting on all principal factors affecting community health, effective programmes cannot be fully realized.

Intervention

Public health efforts to protect communities from health hazards include reducing the number of susceptible individuals, medical intervention, modification of the environment, and promoting healthy behaviour of both communities and individuals.

Although we have achieved remarkable success in the development of biological approaches to disease control, we have not yet achieved comparable success in nutritional intervention, promotion of healthy environments and life-styles, insuring safe workplaces, or behavioural intervention strategies. These should clearly have priority in public health for the immediate future.

Evaluation

An important component of public health strategies is evaluation, both of the quality of surveillance information and the effectiveness of intervention procedures. This should be part of the surveillance or intervention procedures but it can also be the subject of separate studies. Ideally, such evaluations should be continuous. For example, the effectiveness of pertussis (whooping cough) vaccine in preventing disease has been well established and has not changed appreciably over time. The ratio of risk of adverse outcome from vaccination to risk of acquiring disease, however, may be changing in part because of the success in reducing the incidence of whooping cough so that in developed countries the risk of vaccine-related encephalitis may be greater than the risk of acquiring whooping cough. Thus, re-evaluation of current vaccine strategies may be called for.

The effectiveness of community strategies for promotion of healthy life-styles can also be evaluated. The Stanford three-city study, for example, evaluated different strategies for reducing behavioural risk factors for disease (Farquhar *et al.* 1977).

Evaluation of environmental intervention may be more easily accomplished if the appropriate technology for measuring levels is available. If it is not available more indirect measures of effectiveness may be necessary.

In summary, surveillance, intervention, and evaluation are the backbone of public health strategies to prevent disease, eliminate health hazards and promote health.

ORGANIZATION OF PUBLIC HEALTH

Government structure

Organization of health services, both public and private, tends to be conditioned by the cultural, political, and organi-

zational patterns of the countries in which they are located. Thus, in Britain there is a national health service covering preventive, community, and clinical health. On the other hand, in the US the tendency has been to follow the tradition of state and local governmental autonomy in community health services; but individual, clinical services have been left largely in the private sector with governmental payment for certain segments of the population.

United States

The basic concept of government in the US has been for the states to relinquish only those rights of jurisdiction which are essential to maintain the union. Public health has followed this political pattern with strong state and local jurisdiction. Most public health programmes have been conducted at the local level, under state regulation, with only broad directions or incentives provided by the federal government. Thus, the local jurisdictions – the country, city, or township – through authority delegated from the states, typically assume primary responsibility for communicable disease surveillance and control, maternal and child health services, environmental surveillance and control, and other public health activities.

The role of the federal government in public health has evolved for the most part on a piecemeal basis. Usually it has assumed responsibility for meeting needs which were not otherwise met by private, local, or state agencies. These initiatives have generally been categorical in nature, directed primarily at specific disease problems or segments of the population such as the poor. Exceptions to this approach have been the creation of the National Institutes of Health, the major research funding source in the US; certain regulatory agencies such as the Environmental Protection Agency and the Food and Drug Administration; and the agencies and programmes stemming from the 1935 Social Security Act, the basic social security legislation for the nation.

The US Department of Health, Education and Welfare has published *Healthy People* (Surgeon General 1979) and *Promoting health and preventing disease; objectives for the Nation* (Centers for Disease Control 1979), and other documents indicating a broad approach to prevention of disease and promotion of health in the US. Such documents, however, do not have the force of legislation and have served mainly as guidelines and encouragement for local health agencies. The role of the federal government remains largely to suggest and encourage (sometimes with specific subsidies) actions that are implemented (or ignored) at the local level. These are discussed further in Volume 2, Chapter 13 and Volume 3, Chapter 25.

Europe

In the European nations the philosophy of central control of public health has predominated, perhaps because of their smaller size and more homogeneous populations. The majority of the European nations have a national health scheme of one type or another which is administered federally. Thus, to a larger degree than in the US, public health activities can be implemented centrally through an organized system. In some countries such as those in Scandinavia, federal registration of individuals further facilitates public health actions.

The presence of a national health scheme, however, has not guaranteed a more effective public health programme. Often the agencies within these federal governments do not command the respect and resources accorded the clinical components and, therefore, are not as effective as they could be (Evans 1982).

For example, many of the European countries lack schools of public health or their equivalents which prepare professionals to lead public health programmes. None the less, access to medical care and equity have often been greater in these systems than in the US.

Whatever the governmental structure for public health, the need for good management is increasingly recognized. The responsibility for handling budgets that are often substantial, complex organizations involving many different categories of people, and maintaining effective relationships with a wide array of health as well as other bodies, requires great managerial skill. In fact, the inadequate preparation in management skills of many health professionals who have occupied public health administrative posts in the past, has induced some governing authorities to call upon 'managers' rather than public health experts for the key positions in public health. Too often, then, the task of public health administration has been reduced to budget control or complying with already adopted laws and regulations. As a result, little attention is given to health problems or their solution. The ideal, of course, is to combine the talent for leadership in public health with managerial skill.

In conclusion, the organization of public health appears to be determined at every level – local, state, and national – largely by cultural and historic factors resulting in a wide array of, often complex, organizational arrangements.

Non-governmental public health agencies

Voluntary health agencies have flourished in the US and to a somewhat lesser extent in Europe. They tend to be organized around specific disease entities; for example, the American Cancer Society, the American Heart Association, and the American Lung Association. Their success has encouraged the development of many more such groups, devoted to practically all the major diseases and several lesser ones.

They are typically organized at the national level with state divisions and local chapters. These voluntary health agencies bring together physicians who are leaders in the particular fields and interested members of the public. They involve millions of people in fund-raising for, and operation of disease control activities. In this way they have contributed much to the level of enlightenment and activity concerning health, particularly in the US. Their programmes usually include support of health research, professional education, public education, and demonstration services devoted to the particular category of disease with which the organization is concerned.

These voluntary health agencies have become a considerable force in American public health. They are able to operate with fewer constraints than governmental departments and thus, have often broken new ground in the field. For example, the American Heart Association and the American Cancer Society have been particularly active in bringing the concepts of risk factors and healthy life-styles before the American public.

SUMMARY

The scope of public health in the last part of the twentieth century has greatly expanded. Not only have the number of recognized health hazards to the public increased, the strategies available to resolve them have grown commensurately. Public health has borrowed and adapted knowledge from the physiological, biological, medical, physical, behavioural, and mathematical sciences, and has been quick to recognize the potential of new fields such as the computer sciences for improving, safeguarding, maintaining, and promoting the health of the community.

As the major communicable diseases have been brought under control through public health measures, more effort has been directed at chronic disease control, mental health, a safe environment, reduction of accidents, violence and homicide, and promotion of healthy life-styles. Although the biological sciences remain an important underpinning of public health, the contribution of the physical and behavioural sciences is increasingly recognized. As in the past many public efforts will need to be implemented through legislation and development of public awareness and consensus, as well as through service.

The effectiveness of such efforts in the past and the realization of the cost-effectiveness of preventive strategies for promoting and maintaining health have brought renewed attention to public health and have set the stage for a new public health revolution.

REFERENCES

Belloc, N.B. and Breslow, L. (1972). Relationship of physical health status and health practices. *Prev. Med.* **1**, 141.

Berkman, L.F. and Syme, S.L. (1979). Social networks, host resistance and mortality: a nine-year follow-up study of Alameda County residents. *Am. J. Epidemiol.* **109**, 186.

Breslow, L. (1983). The potential of health promotion. In *Handbook of health, health care and the health profession* (ed. D. Mechanic) p. 50. Free Press, New York.

Califano, J.A. (1979). Forward to smoking and health. A report of the Surgeon General. US Department of Health, Education and Welfare Publication No. (PHS) 79-55066. Washington, DC.

Centers for Disease Control (1980). *Promoting health, preventing disease: Objectives for the Nation.* US Government Printing Office, Washington, DC.

Centers for Disease Control (1982). Update on acquired immune deficiency syndrome (AIDS) – United States. *Morbidity and Mortality Weekly Report* **31**, 507.

Department of Health, Education and Welfare (1977). *Health, United States, 1976-1977.* DHEW Publication No. (HRA) 77-1232. Washington, DC.

Department of Health, Education and Welfare (1978). *Health, United States—1978.* DHEW Publication No. (PHS) 78-1232. Washington, DC.

Department of Health, Education and Welfare (1980). *Health, United States—1979.* DHEW Publication No. (PHS) 80-1239. Washington, DC.

Evans, J.R. (1982). Measurement and management in medicine and health services. In *Population-based medicine* (ed. M. Lipkin and W.A. Lybrand). Praeger Scientific Publishers, New York.

Farquhar, J.W., Maccoby, N., Wood, P.D. *et al.* (1977). Community education for cardiovascular health. *Lancet* i, 1192.

Gottlieb, M.S., Schoff, R., Schanker, H.M., Weisman, J.D., Fan, P.T., Wolf, R.A., and Saxon, A. (1981). *Pneumocystis carinii* pneumonia and mucosal candidiasis in previously healthy homosexual men. *N. Engl. J. Med.* **305**, 1425.

Graunt, J. (1939). *National and political observations metnioned in a following index, and made upon the bills of mortality.* Printed by Tho. Roycroft for John Martin, James Allestry and Tho. Dicas, London, 1662. W.F. Willcox (ed.). Johns Hopkins Press, Baltimore. Cited by Lilienfeld, A.M. in *Foundations of epidemiology* (1976). Oxford University Press, New York.

Grayston, J.T. and Wang, S.P. (1975). New knowledge of chlamydiae and the diseases they cause. *J. Infect. Dis.* **132**, 87.

Hypertension Detection and Follow-up Program (HDFP) Co-operative Group (1979). Five-year findings of the Hypertension Detection & Follow-up Program. II. Mortality by race-sex and age. *JAMA* **242**, 2572.

Josey, W.E., Nahmias, A.J., and Naib, Z.M. (1972). The epidemiology of Type 2 (genital) herpes simplex virus infection. *Obstet. Gynecol. Surg.* Suppl. **27**, 295.

Lieberman, E.J. (ed.) (1975). *Mental health: the public health challenge.* American Public Health Association, Washington, DC.

McGinnis, J.M. (1982). Targeting progress in health. *Public Health Report,* **97**, 295.

Multiple Risk Factor Intervention Trial (MRFIT) Research Group (1982). Multiple Risk Factor Intervention Trial – risk factor changes and mortality results. *JAMA* **248**, 1465.

National Research Council, Committee on Diet, Nutrition and Cancer Assembly of Life Sciences (1982). *Diet, nutrition and cancer.* National Academy Press, Washington, DC.

Ouellet, B.L., Romeder, J.M., and Lance, J.M. (1977). *Premature mortality attributable to smoking and hazardous drinking in Canada,* Vol. 1. Department of Health and Welfare, Canada.

Robinson, R., Duenhoeffer, F.E., Holroyd, J.J., Blake, L.R., Bernstein, D., and Cheery, D. (1982). Rubella immunity in older children, teenagers and young adults: a comparison of immunity in older children, teenagers and young adults: a comparison of immunity in those previously immunized with those unimmunized. *J. Pediatrics.* **101**, 188.

Smith, R.J. (1982). Hawaiian milk contamination creates alarm. *Science* **217**, 137.

Surgeon General (1979). *Healthy People: The Surgeon General's report on health promotion and disease prevention.* DHEW Publication No. (PHS) 79:55071. Washington, DC.

Task Panel (1978). *Report to President's Commission on Mental Health,* Volume II Appendix, pp. 4, 5, 16. US Government Printing Office, Washington, DC.

WHO European Collaborative Group (1982). Multifactorial trial in the prevention of coronary heart disease: 2. risk factor changes at two and four years. *Eur. Heart J.* **3**, 184.

Determinants of health and disease

Origins of disease

3 Genetic evolution and adaptation

Anthony C. Allison

INTRODUCTION

An important determinant of health and disease is inherited predisposition. Sometimes the pattern of inheritance of a disease conforms with expectations for dominant genes with the relatively high penetrance, recessive genes, or sex-linked recessive genes (McCusick 1978). Although most of these genes are uncommon, there are so many of them that their cumulative effects are substantial from the public health point of view. Often the primary gene products are known: usually they are enzymes, but they may be other proteins such as haemoglobins, immunoglobulins, or receptors for lipoproteins or other ligands. This molecular biological information clarifies the pathogenesis of the diseases in question, and the straightforward pattern of inheritance simplifies population genetic analysis. Selection of varying intensity operates against the abnormal phenotype, in the sense that survival to and through reproductive age is reduced or there is a reproductive disadvantage for other reasons. Hence there is in principle an equilibrium between the rate of elimination of these genes by selection and the rate of their replacement by recurrent mutation. However, improved medical care has relaxed selection against some of these genes, as discussed below, so that such an equilibrium will not be attained for a long time.

Other genes affecting susceptibility to disease are polymorphic, in other words the gene frequency reached in the past, when selection was intense, exceeds that attributable to recurrent mutation (see glossary on p. 49). Such genes are of special interest from the point of view of genetic evolution and adaptation. They show that diseases can themselves act as selective agents, thereby influencing the genetic composition of populations. Three examples will be considered in some detail in this chapter because they illustrate different general points: abnormal haemoglobins, glucose 6-phosphate dehydrogenase deficiency, and genes of the major histocompatability complex (MHC). Linkage of MHC genes with a number of diseases, or in some cases with subsets of patients having particular diseases, has been firmly established, and possible explanations for such associations will be discussed.

For a long time confusion has been generated by attempts to fit complex and difficult human pedigree analyses into simple Mendelian ratios, on the assumption that diabetes mellitus, for example, is a single disease. However, analyses of linkage with MHC genes make it clear that there are several types of diabetes mellitus with different genetic associations and different environmental factors facilitating their expression. The same is true of hepatitis and many other common diseases. A few examples are discussed to illustrate theoretical points such as selective interactions of genes at different loci and practical points such as difficulties of determining the prevalence of diseases and identifying genetically predisposed individuals.

A final point considered in the chapter is the changing intensity and nature of selection. Formerly, infectious diseases killed many persons before reproductive age was complete; in some cases at least, such effects acted differentially on different genotypes, thereby producing selection. During the past century there has been a major demographic transition in the more industrialized countries from a period of high birth and death rates to a period of low birth and death rates. The opportunity for selection has been correspondingly reduced, although not eliminated altogether. There has been a much smaller reduction in selection through infectious diseases in the developing world.

As a result of improved medical care, selection against diseases with well-defined genetic causation, such as galactosaemia and phenylketonuria, and those with clear but less well-defined inherited predispositions, such as diabetes mellitus, has been relaxed. This has led to concern about the accumulation of genes for inherited disorders in advanced societies. The maximum rates at which such genes can accumulate in populations can be calculated, and this has some bearing on related ethical problems.

ABNORMAL HAEMOGLOBINS

The prototype abnormal human haemoglobin is sickle-cell haemoglobin (HbS). Several human populations are polymorphic for this variant. Each molecule of normal adult human haemoglobin (HbA) is a tetramer composed of two α-chains and two β-chains. In HbS the sixth amino-acid residue from the N-terminus of the β-chain is replaced by a point mutation, presumably resulting from a single nucleic acid base substitution (GAA to GUA). In HbA the glutamic acid residue in this site provides a negative surface charge to the whole tetramer, whereas in HbS the neutral amino acid, valine, in this position provides a combining site allowing polymerization of deoxygenated Hb molecules, which form rigid helical aggregates able to distort the red cell from a discoid to a sickle shape. Moreover, HbS more readily associates with the red cell membrane than does HbA, with consequences discussed below.

Individuals heterozygous for the sickle-cell gene have both HbA and HbS, usually 25–40 per cent of the latter. Each red cell contains a mixture of the haemoglobins, and the transformation to the sickle shape takes place only when the partial pressure of O_2 is lower than usually encountered in the circulation. The heterozygotes are therefore healthy except under extreme anoxic conditions, such as high-altitude flights in unpressurized aircraft. In sickle-cell homozygotes no HbA is formed; the majority of the Hb is HbS, although a small amount of fetal haemoglobin (HbF) is also present. These cells assume the sickle shape at partial pressures of oxygen encountered *in vivo*, so the SS homozygotes are prone to develop sickle-cell disease, a haemolytic and painful vaso-occlusive condition aggravated by infections which produce sickle-cell crises.

Another polymorphic variant is HbC, in which the same glutamic acid residue in the normal molecule, residue 6 of the β-chain, is replaced by lysine. Persons homozygous for HbC have a haemolytic disease, and CS heterozygotes suffer from a variety of sickle-cell disease usually milder than that manifested by SS homozygotes.

A third abnormality is β-thalassaemia, in which the β-polypeptide chain is deficient owing to a structural or regulatory mutation leading to a relative deficit in the formation of β-chain messenger RNA. As a result there is excessive production of α-chains, which are unstable in the absence of β-chains, precipitate, and bind to the erythrocyte membrane. Individuals homozygous for the β-thalassaemia gene (an allele of HbA, HbS, and HbC) have a severe haemolytic disorder, thalassaemia major, and seldom survive to adulthood and to reproduce. Heterozygotes having both HbS and β-thalassaemia suffer from another variant of sickle-cell disease, often of moderate severity.

Although with good medical care some individuals with sickle-cell disease can survive to adulthood and even reproduce (though pregnant women often experience difficulty), there is no doubt that under the conditions prevailing in Africa for centuries very few sickle-cell homozygotes could have reproduced. Hence, the fitness of SS homozygotes has been close to zero and the loss of S genes from populations through death of homozygotes has been much greater than could be replaced by recurrent mutation.

Despite the loss of S genes in this way, the mutation became polymorphic in several populations. Over a large part of Africa south of Sahara and north of Zambia, the frequency of HbS heterozygotes in many tribes is 20 per cent or higher, rising to 40 per cent in some populations. Allison (1954*a*) suggested that the sickle-cell polymorphism might be maintained because HbS heterozygotes are relatively resistant to falciparum malaria and have a greater chance of surviving through the dangerous years of first exposure to the disease before immunity is acquired.

In support of this hypothesis, high frequencies of HbS were found in East African populations living in regions where falciparum malaria was endemic but not in populations living in non-malarious areas (Allison 1954*a*). This was true of populations with different linguistic affinities and blood groups, suggesting a strong selective effect of a local environmental factor such as malaria. In young Ugandan children, four months to four years of age, who had not yet acquired strong immunity to falciparum malaria, lower parasite counts were found in those with HbAS than in those with HbA (Allison 1954*b*). These observations were confirmed by several other groups investigating African children, and potentially lethal infections such as cerebral malaria were observed much less frequently in children with HbAS than in those with HbA (reviewed by Allison 1964).

An important advance was the development by Trager and Jensen (1976) of a method for continuous propagation of *Plasmodium falciparum* in cultures of human erythrocytes. It was then possible to compare under controlled conditions the multiplication of the parasite in normal erythrocytes and in those with abnormal haemoglobins. In two laboratories *P. falciparum* was found to grow less well in erythrocytes bearing HbS than those bearing HbA under low partial pressures of O_2 (Friedman 1978; Pasvol *et al.* 1978). Such relatively anoxic conditions would be expected where *P. falciparum* completes its asexual bloodstream cycle of replication attached to endothelial cells of post-capillary venules. Hence the findings with cultured cells nicely complement the observed protection provided by HbS *in vivo*. *Plasmodium falciparum* also grows poorly in erythrocytes bearing HbC and HbE (Friedman *et al.* 1979). The growth of the parasite in thalassaemic cells is strongly inhibited under conditions of oxidant stress (Friedman 1979). Oxidant stress could be produced by effector cells of the immune system bound to parasitized erythrocytes (Allison 1983). Thus acquired cell-mediated immunity, elicited by frequent attacks of falciparum malaria, would be expected to have synergistic effects with abnormal haemoglobins in protecting hosts against infections with this parasite. Sensitivity of erythrocytes to oxidant stress is increased in β-thalassaemia because the excess α-chains oxidize membrane lipids and thereby consume antioxidants such as reduced glutathione (Allison 1983).

The implications for population genetics of the abnormal haemoglobins were pointed out by Allison (1954*c*). Natural selection is expressed by the concept of fitness, which is the contribution of a genotype to the next generation and hence a measure of its capacity to survive and reproduce. For an autosomal locus with two alleles, when the heterozygote has an increased fitness over both homozygotes a stable equilibrium with both alleles can exist (Fisher 1930). It is termed a balanced polymorphism. Among the adult Baamba of Uganda, who have a frequency of about 40 per cent S heterozygotes, no S homozygotes have been observed, confirming the lethality of that condition in the African bush. If these alleles are close to equilibrium, the heterozygotes must have a fitness of about 1.25, which is the highest known fitness for any human genotype. The results suggest a mortality through direct or indirect effects of falciparum malaria of at least 25 per cent of children, in other words a powerful selective effect of the disease. Among the Baamba, 4 per cent of children born are S homozygotes liable to sickle-cell disease. Over vast areas of central Africa the frequency of S heterozygotes is about 20 per cent, implying that 1 per cent of the millions of children born are S homozygotes, creating a substantial public health problem. The S gene is also polymorphic in some non-African populations, including people living in formerly malarious parts of Greece, Turkey, southern Arabia, and India (see Livingstone 1967).

In the absence of selection in favour of the heterozygote (for example when Africans were moved to the US), the frequency of the S gene would be expected to fall exponentially (Allison 1954c), representing a transient polymorphism. The HbS frequency in different populations of US Blacks now varies from about 5 to 17 per cent (Livingstone 1967). Taking into consideration genetic variants, the incidence of sickle-cell disease in this population is about 1 in 300 births, an unfortunate genetic legacy of past selection.

The existence of natural selection can be demonstrated by comparing the observed phenotype and expected genotype frequencies in representative samples of young children, before selection has taken place, and samples of adults from the same community (Allison 1956). Where the frequency of S is high and thalassaemia is rare, as in certain East African populations, haemoglobin phenotypes can be equated with genotypes. From the frequency of the S gene in the adult population ($p=$ in effect $0.5 \times$ the heterozygote frequency) and the Hardy–Weinberg equilibrium, the expected frequencies of S homozygotes, heterozygotes, and normal homozygotes are p^2, $2p(1-p)$, and $(1-p)^2$, respectively. The observed distribution in young children showed insignificant departure from this expectation whereas in the adult population there was a significant excess of S heterozygotes and deficiency of S homozygotes (Allison 1956).

Similar considerations apply to β-thalassaemia, which is polymorphic in some Mediterranean and other countries. In Sardinia, Greece, New Guinea, and several other countries β-thalassaemia is common in lowland areas, which were formerly malarious, and rare in montane regions which remained free of that disease. This distribution, along with the poor growth of *P. falciparum* in cultured thalassaemic erythrocytes, provides strong evidence that malaria was the major selective factor accounting for the polymorphism of this gene. The consequence is a high frequency of heterozygotes (up to 20 per cent) and a correspondingly high incidence of homozygotes with thalassaemia major (up to 1 per cent) in parts of Italy, Greece, Turkey, and some other countries, as well as in migrants from these countries to North and South America and north-western Europe.

In some populations the co-existence of two or more abnormal haemoglobins complicates the population genetics. For example, over a large part of West Africa HbS and HbC co-exist, and in parts of Greece and Turkey HbS and β-thalassaemia co-exist. Because S-β-thalassaemia and SC heterozygotes have decreased fitness, Allison (1956) postulated that these genes must be mutually exclusive in populations; in other words, where the frequency of C or β-thalassaemia is high that of S must be low. Subsequent observations have confirmed that prediction. It is not known whether there is an equilibrium involving three alleles (which is theoretically possible) or whether in West Africa the C gene is being replaced by the S gene, as suggested by Livingstone (1967).

The relationship between the abnormal haemoglobins and malaria provided the first, and still the most direct and convincing, evidence that disease can act as an agent of natural selection, producing a change in gene frequencies, in other words evolution, in human populations.

MALARIA AND GLUCOSE 6-PHOSPHATE DEHYDROGENASE (G6PD) DEFICIENCY

The existence of this sex-linked genetic trait in Americans of African origin was revealed by the correlation of G6PD deficiency with their sensitivity to the antimalarial drug primaquine (Carson et al. 1956). Later it became apparent that there are two polymorphic varieties of G6PD deficiency (the African A- and the Mediterranean B- forms), a non-deficient form polymorphic in Africans (B+) as well as several rare deficient variants. Furthermore, G6PD$^-$ individuals show haemolysis when exposed to several different drugs or dietary constituents, such as fava beans, which exert oxidant stress on erythrocytes.

As soon as an assay that could be used under field conditions became available, the distribution of G6PD deficiency was studied in East and West Africa (Allison 1960; Allison and Clyde 1961). The essential findings, which have been repeatedly confirmed, were that G6PD deficiency is common in malarious areas of East Africa (15–20 per cent of males affected) and in West Africa from Nigeria to the Gambia. It is absent from non-malarious parts of East Africa. Many studies (reviewed by Livingstone 1967) have supported the view that high frequencies of both the African and Mediterranean varieties of G6PD deficiency occur only where malaria has been endemic.

Allison and Clyde (1961) found significantly lower *P. falciparum* rates and counts in the G6PD$^-$ children. Bienzle et al. (1972) reported that Nigerian female children heterozygous for the deficiency (Gd^{A-}/Gd^A) showed significantly lower *P. falciparum* counts than other children, and other observations are discussed by Allison (1983).

Roth et al. (1983) have shown that *P. falciparum* grows poorly in erythrocytes from persons hemizygous or heterozygous for the Mediterranean variety of G6PD deficiency in the presence of 17 per cent O_2. Presumably the protection would be even greater under conditions of oxidant stress (Friedman 1979), so that synergistic effects with cell-mediated immunity are likely. These observations, together with the distribution of G6PD deficiency and the observed protection against malaria, leave little doubt that malaria has been the major selective factor accounting for this polymorphism. Provided that female heterozygotes have a selective advantage, equilibrium can be maintained. Females heterozygous for G6PD deficiency show mosaicism of their erythrocytes (some having a normal content of G6PD, others full enzyme deficiency), which may be sufficient to provide some protection against malaria while rarely increasing susceptibility to haemolysis from dietary or other factors, which are haemolytic in enzyme-deficient male hemizygotes.

The best known manifestation of this susceptibility to haemolysis is favism following ingestion by enzyme-deficient persons of fava beans (*Vicia fava*), which is common in

Mediterranean and Middle Eastern countries. The susceptibility of G6PD-persons to haemolysis following exposure to drugs can pose public health problems. For example, in the region of Adana in Turkey *Plasmodium vivax* infection still occurs. The exoerythrocytic cycle of infection with this parasite, which allows recurrence, can only be terminated by the use of primaquine, but some 20 per cent of persons in the area are G6PD deficient and liable to severe haemolysis following treatment with the drug.

Since both G6PD deficiency and abnormal haemoglobins protect against malaria, and individuals with both traits are not at a disadvantage, a positive correlation of their frequency in populations would be expected, and is observed (Allison 1964).

THE MAJOR HISTOCOMPATIBILITY COMPLEX

The HLA and H-2 complexes of man and the mouse respectively are the prototype MHC systems which have been analysed in detail, although comparable systems exist in all vertebrates so far examined. First studied with the intention of finding genetic markers for transplantation, the MHC emerged as a remarkable cluster of linked genes controlling cell surface determinants, which produce a great deal of genetic diversity in natural populations. The MHC determinants influence a variety of cellular interactions, including immune responses.

There are three classes of HLA factors: class 1 – comprising HLA-ABC antigens, class 2 – comprising D/DR and related antigens, and class 3 – comprising certain complement factors (for example C2, C4a, C4b, Bf). The ABC antigens are controlled by genes at three closely linked loci (Fig. 3.1). The D antigens are detectable by mixed leucocyte culture using homozygous typing cells, and the DR (D-related) antigens by serological methods using B-lymphocytes. Typing for D-antigens with homozygous typing cells probably reveals grouped combinations of lymphocyte-activating determinants rather than single determinants. The D/DR region refers to a chromosome region controlling all antigens resembling DR. Both the α- and β-polypeptide chains of these class 2 molecules are encoded by genes within the D/DR region, which probably contains a number of different α- and β-genes (Shackelford *et al.* 1982). In general the β-chains seem to be more polymorphic than the α-chains. The MT, MB, DC, and LB antigens are thought to be present on β-chains different from those of the DR molecules, encoded by genes at closely linked loci. The primed lymphocyte typing technique has proved useful in studying D/DR antigens, including a new series of lymphocyte-stimulating antigens, termed SB, encoded by genes located on the centromeric side of the DR locus (Shaw *et al.* 1981).

Linked genes code for three classes or families of molecules denoted I, II, and III (Hood *et al.* 1982). The association of these genes over the 500 million years of vertebrate divergence suggests that selection constraints have maintained linkage among these gene families. The most remarkable feature of the MHC in the mouse and man is the extensive genetic polymorphism presented by certain class I and class II genes, but not all of them, suggesting functional requirements for diversity in some of the gene products and uniformity in others.

Class I molecules comprise a 45 000 daltons class I polypeptide, an integral membrane protein, noncovalently associated with β2-microglobulin, a 12 000 dalton polypeptide encoded by a gene on another chromosome. These are expressed on most cell types. Class II antigens are encoded by genes of the I region in mice and DC, DR, and SB regions in man. Each class II molecule has an α-chain (30 000–33 000 daltons)· and a β-chain (27 000–29 000 daltons). Class II molecules are expressed selectively on certain cell types, such as macrophages and B-lymphocytes, and it is known that antigens have to be presented to lymphocytes in association with class II molecules to elicit immune responses. The capacity of mice to respond well to defined antigens depends on their I-region (immune-response-associated) genes, which code for class II molecules. By analogy human DC, DR, and SB genes are likely to control capacity to respond to particular antigenic determinants, and therefore function as immune response genes. In this way they could influence susceptibility to a variety of diseases.

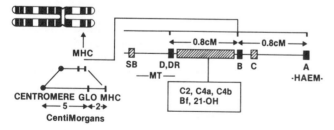

Fig. 3.1. Map showing the location of the MHC complex. The MHC complex is located on the short arm of human chromosome 6, approximately 7 centiMorgans from the centromere and 2 centiMorgans distal to the *Glo* locus which codes for the enzyme glyoxylase. Genes for SB are on the centromeric side of the D/DR region and for MT are in the DR region. The precise order of loci for complement components and 21-OH between DR and B is unknown. The recessive gene *haem* producing haemochromatosis is closely linked to A but its precise location is unknown.

HLA haplotypes and linkage disequilibrium

The term haplotype is used to describe a chromosomal segment inherited *en bloc* from one parent. In a family such a segment is manifested by a particular combination of HLA-A, -B, and -DR phenotypes, from which probable genotypes can be derived. Within a family it can be assumed that the entire segment is identical unless there is evidence of recombination. When different families in a population are compared, combinations of phenotypes vary, but not in a random fashion. There is a tendency for certain genes at different loci to occur together on the same chromosome or haplotype more often than expected by chance. The existence of population associations between products of linked genes, such as antigens of the HLA loci, is termed linkage disequilibrium, which is important when considering associations of HLA with disease.

A well-known example is the A1, B8 haplotype. In north Europeans the frequency of allele A1 is 0.17 and that of B8 is 0.11, so that if they were not associated the expected frequency of the A1, B8 haplotype would be $0.17 \times 0.11 = 0.019$, which is less than one-fourth of the observed frequency, 0.088 (Bodmer and Bodmer 1978). The extent of linkage disequilibrium (Δ or D) can be defined as the difference between the observed and expected haplotype frequencies:

$$\Delta = 0.088 - 0.019 = 0.069$$

In this case the contribution of linkage disequilibrium to the total haplotype frequency is 0.069/0.088, or nearly 80 per cent. Less than 10 of the nearly 300 possible pairwise combinations of HLA-A and -B locus alleles show significant linkage disequilibrium in western European and North American populations.

Theoretical analysis (see Bodmer and Bodmer 1978) shows that in a random mating population in the absence of selection, Δ should be 0 at equilibrium. If Δ is at any time not 0 it should approach 0 at a rate $(1-r)$ per generation, where r is the recombination fraction between the two loci. The more tight the linkage between two genes, the longer it will take linkage disequilibrium to reach zero. Hence one explanation for observed linkage disequilibrium is that there has not yet been time for populations to reach equilibrium with respect to the two relevant alleles. For HLA-A and -B alleles, given a recombination fraction of 0.8 per cent, linkage disequilibrium would in the absence of selection be expected to decrease by a factor of 5 in 200 generations, or some 5000 years. Thus failure to reach equilibrium is unlikely to explain persistent HLA-A and -B combinations found throughout Caucasoid populations which were separated more than 5000 years ago. Likewise, non-random mating, migration and population admixture are unlikely explanations for observed linkage disequilibrium (Bodmer and Bodmer 1978). It is therefore probable that the persistent linkage disequilibrium observed for some pairs of alleles at the HLA loci is due to the effects of natural selection. This does not necessarily imply interactive selection between the alleles, since linkage disequilibrium can persist for considerable lengths of time as a result of selection affecting alleles at one or more loci closely linked with those under consideration. Nevertheless, as Fisher (1930) showed, natural selection favouring pairwise combinations of alleles at different loci can produce persistent linkage disequilibrium. Such a model is consistent with recent observations on the associations of HLA phenotypes with disease and with the molecular biology of the antigens, as discussed below.

RELATIVE RISK

The strength of an association between a genetic marker and a disease is defined by the relative risk, a term originally suggested by Woolf (1955). The relative risk indicates how many times more frequently a disease develops in individuals carrying an antigen or other genetic marker than in individuals lacking it. Traditionally, relative risk is calculated from the 2×2 table shown in Table 3.1, and is the cross-product ratio or odds ratio for alleles at the loci being considered.

Table 3.1. *Estimates of the strength of an association between a genetic marker and a disease*

(1) The 2×2 Table:

	Percentage of individuals	
	Genetic marker present	Genetic marker absent
Patients	a	b
Controls	c	d

Frequency of marker in patients: $h_p = \dfrac{a}{a+b}$

(2) Relative risk (RR) $= \dfrac{a \times d}{b \times c}$

(3) Attributable fraction (AF) $= (\dfrac{RR-1}{RR})(\dfrac{a}{a+b}) = (\dfrac{RR-1}{RR})\,h_p$

(Positive associations: RR > 1)

(4) Preventive fraction (PF) $= \dfrac{(1-RR)\,h_p}{RR(1-h_p) + h_p}$

(Negative associations: RR < 1)

Adapted from Svejgaard *et al.* (1983).

Although this is a useful term, its limitations should be recognized. For example, the ascertainment of patients is a limiting factor, particularly when a disease is heterogeneous and/or is expressed only in ageing subjects; the prevalence of the disease in the population in question must be known if a true relative risk is to be calculated (see Svejgaard *et al.* 1983). Especially when different races are compared, control frequencies of genetic markers and the prevalence of the disease in question may vary greatly and can make a major contribution to cross-product ratios (see Dawkins *et al.* 1983). Thus the whole 2×2 table and derivations from it should be presented and not just cross-product ratios. The 2×2 table should be adjusted so that the terms $(a+b)$ and $(c+d)$ are equal (for example, by using percentages). If it is intended to estimate the likelihood of development of a disease in a random member of the population, it is essential that $(a+b)/(a+b+c+d)$ is approximately equal to the known prevalence of the disease.

Definition of diseases can be difficult for many reasons. Taking the examples discussed more fully below, diabetes mellitus is the end result of several different disease processes, each of which has a distinct set of genetic associations. Ankylosing spondylitis has a component of sacroiliitis but the latter may not be accompanied by ankylosis of vertebrae (Dawkins *et al.* 1983). The disease group should have unequivocal disease, using if possible internationally standardized criteria; the control group should have no sign of disease. If different races are being compared, it should be established that the diseases under study are truly comparable, no easy task.

Another estimate of the strength of an association between HLA and disease is the so-called attributable fraction (AF) calculated as shown in Table 3.1. The attributable fraction provides an estimate of the extent to which a disease is due to a disease-associated factor, and is well known from epidemiology (Miettinen 1976). When the relative risk exceeds unity, the attributable fraction can under certain conditions provide information about the degree of linkage disequilibrium between an HLA gene and a hypothetical disease-susceptibility gene (Bengtsson and Thomson 1981). When the relative risk is less than unity, the so-called preventive fraction (PF) can be calculated.

The difference between relative risk and attributable fraction can be illustrated by the increased frequencies of the complement factor BfF1 and of DR3 in insulin-dependent diabetes mellitus (Svejgaard *et al.* 1983). BfF1 confers a higher relative risk for the disease (15.0) than does DR3 (2.9). However, BfF1 has a much lower frequency in the healthy population than DR3, so the attributable fraction for BfF1 is only 0.21 whereas that of DR3 is 0.35. The presence of BfF1 in an individual is a better predictor of insulin-dependent diabetes mellitus than is the presence of DR3. At the population level BfF1 contributes less to the development of the disease than does DR3.

Another approach designed to overcome problems of varying age of onset and incomplete penetrance is sib-pair analysis (Day and Simons 1976; Thomson and Bodmer 1977). Analysis of HLA haplotype sharing in affected sib pairs eliminates both of the above problems. If HLA and/or genes closely linked to HLA have no influence on the development of a disease, affected sib-pairs will share haplotypes as expected: 25 per cent will share both, 50 per cent will share one and 25 per cent will share no haplotypes. By investigating whether the observed distribution of haplotype sharing differs from that expected, the null hypothesis can be tested. Parents of affected sibs should be HLA typed to establish the expected haplotype sharing.

ASSOCIATION OF IMMUNE RESPONSE AND IMMUNE SUPPRESSION GENES WITH THE MAJOR HISTO-COMPATABILITY COMPLEX

McDevitt and Benacerraf (1969) showed that some strains of mice and guinea pigs are able to respond well, while others respond poorly, to particular synthetic peptide antigens, which present a limited number of antigenic determinants. The immune response (*Ir*) genes controlling such differences were found to map in the I-region of the mouse MHC. Immune suppression (*Is*) genes map in the same region (Benacerraf and Germain 1978; Dorf 1981). Defined products of the I region in the mouse are I-A (immune-response-associated) or class 2 antigens, the composition of which has been described above.

Three major findings have helped to define the role of MHC products in immune responses. The first is the phenomenon of genetic restriction. Rosenthal and Shevach (1973) found that guinea pig T-lymphocytes respond well to antigens only when they are on the surface of histocompatible antigen-presenting cells. Zinkernagel and Doherty (1974) found that sensitized T-lymphocytes kill virus-infected target cells only when the latter are histocompatible. Later analyses of these phenomena showed that the helper subset of T-lymphocytes requires exposure to both foreign antigens and self class 2 MHC products to respond with the production of interleukin-2, a growth factor for other subsets of lymphocytes. The cytolytic subset of T-lymphocytes, which is generated by exposure to antigen in the presence of interleukin-2, releases interferon-γ and other mediators, and kills target cells bearing virus or other antigens on their surfaces, only when these antigens are associated with class 1 MHC products. In other words, the class 1 and class 2 MHC products are recognition units required for cellular co-operation in the elicitation of immune responses and the effector phase of immune responses, respectively. Evidence that class 2 antigens of the MHC complex restrict *Ir*-gene controlled proliferation of T-lymphocytes has been reviewed by Nagy *et al.* (1981), who conclude that certain genotypes lack the capacity to respond to particular antigenic determinants because of gaps in the MHC product repertoire. Such failures to respond might on the one hand increase susceptibility to infectious diseases and on the other hand prevent autoimmune diseases.

For many years it was believed, following Burnet (1949), that clones of antibody-producing B-lymphocytes reacting with autoantigens are eliminated or inactivated during ontogeny. However, normal persons were found to have B-lymphocytes with receptors for autoantigens (Bankhurst *et al.* 1973), so that self-tolerance is not due to deletion of auto-antibody-forming clones but to immunoregulation: the absence of T-lymphocyte help for autoantigens and the presence of a subset of T-lymphocytes suppressing auto-immune responses (Allison *et al.* 1971). Abundant experimental evidence in support of this interpretation has accumulated (reviewed by Allison 1977). Hence definition of *Is*-genes linked to the human MHC, and analysis of their role in controlling alloimmune and autoimmune responses, is of special interest. These two processes are not unrelated: growth and differentiation factors produced as a result of immune responses to alloantigens can stimulate proliferation and differentiation of clones of lymphocytes with receptors for autoantigens, with resulting autoantibody formation. Thus the requirements for antigen-presenting cells with class 2 structures reacting functionally with autoantigens, and of helper T-lymphocytes with receptors for autoantigens, can be by-passed (Allison 1977). An example is the formation of autoantibodies during graft-versus-host reactions (Fialkow *et al.* 1973; Grebe and Streilein 1976).

Attempts have been made to define *Ir*- and *Is*-genes linked to human MHC complex markers. Hsu *et al.* (1981) studied HLA-associated genetic control of human lymphocyte proliferative responses to several synthetic polypeptides. On the basis of stimulation indices, individuals could be classified as high, intermediate, or low responders. Family studies suggested that high responses to these antigens are inherited as HLA-linked dominant traits. A strong association of Dw2 with IgE and IgG antibody responses to the ragweed allergen Ra5 has been reported (Marsh *et al.* 1982). Analyses of killing of virus-infected and allogeneic cells by human T-lymphocytes (McMichael *et al.* 1977; Dickmeiss *et al.* 1977) indicate that some MHC products are superior to others in the presentation of foreign antigens to immunocompetent cells. Although all these findings are preliminary, they are consistent with the presence in humans of *Ir*-genes linked to defined MHC antigens.

Evidence for genetic control of T-lymphocyte-mediated suppression in humans has been published by Sasazuki *et al.* (1983). Proliferative responses of peripheral blood cells to streptococcal cell wall antigen were found to be inherited in a manner suggesting that a high response is recessive and a low response is dominant; suppression in culture was mediated by the generation of antigen-specific Leu-2a$^+$, 3a$^-$ lymphocytes, not monocytes. Sasazuki and his colleagues postulate the existence of an *Is*-gene in linkage disequilibrium with HLA-MT1. The same authors described an analogous antigen-specific suppressor cell under the control of an *Is*-gene in linkage disequilibrium with HLA-Bw52, Dw12, in the presence of which the response of lymphocytes to schistosomal antigen is low. Absence of this *Is*-gene in homozygous individuals, who show a strong immune response in the antigen, predisposes them to post-schistosomal cirrhosis.

Sasazuki *et al.* (1983) also analysed 104 families with allergy to cedar pollen allergen, and obtained evidence for another HLA-linked *Is*-gene suppressing IgE responses to the allergen through antigen-specific Leu-2a$^+$, 3a$^-$ lymphocytes. Absence of this *Is*-gene in the homozygous state predisposed individuals to cedar pollinosis because of their high IgE responses to the allergen. This *Is*-gene was found to be in linkage disequilibrium with HLA-Dw44, DEn-MT1, 2-MB3. Sasazuki and his colleagues suggest that the statistical associations of many diseases with MHC products might be explained by the presence of *Is*-genes in strong linkage disequilibrium with particular alleles at loci in the HLA-D region such as D, DR, MT, and MB.

This is an attractive hypothesis which requires rigorous testing through international co-operative studies. The tests will not be easy, since correlations of *in vitro* suppression tests using human peripheral blood lymphocytes with *in vivo* immune responses, including autoimmune responses, are not straightforward. Nevertheless, let us suppose that several dominant *Is*-genes linked with DR genes exist, and that there are two recessive alleles, one linked with DR3, and concomitantly with B8 through linkage disequilibrium, and the other linked with DR4. When the recessive *Is* alleles are both expressed in homozygous form, in some DR3/4 heterozygotes, major suppressor mechanisms will not be operative: immune responses to both alloantigens and autoantigens will be high and prolonged. Let us postulate, further, that one of the dominant *Is* alleles is linked with DR2 and concomitantly with B7; in the presence of this allele immune responses to alloantigens and autoantigens will be suppressed.

This example can be compared with what is actually found. Eddlestone and Williams (1978) pointed out that several diseases in which immune responses to alloantigens and autoantigens are believed to play a pathogenic role are associated with B8: gluten-sensitive enteropathy, Graves' disease, Addison's disease, chronic active hepatitis, and insulin-dependent diabetes mellitus. Subjects with B8 showed high levels not only of autoantibodies but also of antibodies against exogenous bacterial and virus antigens. Diabetics with B8 likewise had higher titres of antibodies against Coxsackie viruses than those with other genotypes. In insulin-dependent diabetes mellitus B8 is associated not so much with the presence of autoantibodies reacting with pancreatic islet cells

as with their persistence for years after the onset of the disease (see below). B8 is associated with a high relapse rate in thyrotoxic patients after a full course of medical treatment. Insulin-dependent diabetes mellitus, Graves' disease, and Addison's disease are now known to be more strongly associated with DR3 than with B8 (Svejgaard *et al.* 1983). Two other organ-specific autoimmune diseases (the Sicca syndrome and myasthenia gravis) and a generalized autoimmune disease, lupus erythematosus, have also been associated with DR3 (Table 3.2).

Two rare but instructive types of isoimmunization in pregnancy are associated with DR3. One is immunization against the platelet-specific antigen, Zw^a, in mothers lacking this antigen who give birth to children with isoimmune neonatal thrombocytopenia; this condition is strongly associated with B8 and more strongly with DR3 (Svejgaard *et al.* 1983). The second is herpes gestationis, a vesiculo-bullous eruption of the skin of pregnant women associated with autoantibody and complement deposition along the dermo-epidermal junction. Stasny *et al.* (1983) have found herpes gestationis to be strongly associated with DR3, and even more strongly with DR3/4 heterozygotes (relative risk 23.5). In women with herpes gestationis, Stasny and his colleagues found a high frequency of antibodies against foreign (often paternal) HLA antigens, suggesting that maternal immune responses against alloantigens may have been accompanied by the formation of autoantibodies against dermal antigens, perhaps by the mechanism discussed above for graft-versus-host disease.

DR3/4 heterozygotes also show increased susceptibility to insulin-dependent diabetes mellitus (see below). In contrast frequencies of DR2, and concomitantly B7, are decreased in coeliac disease and juvenile diabetes mellitus (Scholz and Albert 1983). All these findings are consistent with the model presented: that in some DR3/4 heterozygotes 'switch off' signals of immune responses are deficient. The particular disorder manifested would depend on which powerful 'switch on' signals for immune responses operate in that individual, determined by exposure to antigens in the presence of a complex of *Ir*-genes.

These observations do not, of course, confirm the model, and alternative explanations should be considered. For example, the increased susceptibility of DR3/4 heterozygotes to several diseases could result from the presence on antigen-presenting cells of unique class 2 molecules which allow them to interact efficiently with a range of alloantigens and auto-antigens. Interactions of two *Ir*-genes based on hybrid I-region antigens have been reported (Fathman 1980). In the example quoted, heterozygotes could have unique antigens produced by combination of α- and β-chains of DR3 and DR4, namely $\alpha_3\beta_4$ and $\alpha_4\beta_3$; if more than one locus is involved, the heterogeneity of products would be greater. A clone of human T-lymphocytes has been obtained selectively recognizing restriction elements encoded by interacting D regions of two different haplotypes (Hansen *et al.* 1982).

The DR3, B8 combination appears again in a remarkable association with IgA deficiency (Oen *et al.* 1982; Hammarstrom and Smith 1982). IgA deficiency may be accompanied by increased susceptibility to pulmonary and/or gastrointestinal infections, but it is also observed in about 1 in

Table 3.2 *Associations between HLA and some diseases*

Condition	HLA	Frequency (%)		Relative risk	Attributable fraction
		Patients	Controls		
Hodgkin's disease	A1	40	32.0	1.4	0.12
Idiopathic haemochromatosis	A3	76	28.2	8.2	0.67
Behcet's disease	B5	41	10.1	6.3	0.34
Congenital adrenal hyperplasia	B47	9	0.6	15.4	0.08
Ankylosing spondylitis	B27	90	9.4	87.4	0.89
Reiter's disease	B27	79	9.4	37.0	0.77
Acute anterior uveitis	B27	52	9.4	10.4	0.47
Subacute thyroiditis	B35	70	14.6	13.7	0.65
Psoriasis vulgaris	Cw6	87	33.1	13.3	0.81
Dermatitis herpetiformis	D/DR3	85	26.3	15.4	0.80
Coeliac disease	D/DR3	79	26.3	10.8	0.72
	D/DR7 also increased				
Sicca syndrome	D/DR3	78	26.3	9.7	0.70
Idiopathic Addison's disease	D/DR3	69	26.3	6.3	0.58
Graves' disease	D/DR3	56	26.3	3.7	0.42
Insulin-dependent diabetes	D/DR3	56	28.2	3.3	0.39
	D/DR4	75	32.2	6.4	0.63
	D/DR2	10	30.5	0.2	–
Myasthenia gravis	D/DR3	50	28.2	2.5	0.30
	B8	47	24.6	2.7	0.30
SLE	D/DR3	70	28.2	5.8	0.58
Idiopathic membraneous nephropathy	D/DR3	75	20.0	12.0	0.69
IgA deficiency in blood donors	B8	49	24.3	3.0	0.33
	DR3	81	24.6	13.0	0.75
Zw^a-immunized mothers	B8	73	24.6	8.4	0.64
Multiple sclerosis	D/DR2	59	25.8	4.1	0.45
Optic neuritis	D/DR2	46	25.8	2.4	0.27
C2 deficiency	D/DR2				
	B18				
Goodpasture's syndrome	D/DR2	88	32.0	15.9	0.82
Rheumatic arthritis	D/DR4	50	19.4	4.2	0.38
Pemphigus (Jews)	D/DR4	87	32.1	14.4	0.81
IgA nephropathy	D/DR4	49	19.5	4.0	0.37
Hydralazine-induced SLE	D/DR4	73	32.7	5.6	0.60
Hashimoto's thyroiditis	D/DR5	19	6.9	3.2	0.13
Pernicious anaemia	D/DR5	25	5.8	5.4	0.20
Juvenile rheumatoid arthritis:					
pauciarticular	D/DR5	50	16.2	5.2	0.40
All cases	D/DRw8	23	7.5	3.6	0.17

The above information has been extracted from the HLA and Disease Registry (Svejgaard *et al.* 1983). Relative risks and attributable fractions are explained in Table 3.1.

700 apparently healthy blood donors. In groups of the latter strong associations with B8 and DR3 were found. Thus failure to secrete an entire class of immunoglobulins is HLA related. This again appears to be a disorder of regulation rather than an absence of the structural genes for IgA, since the subjects have B-lymphocytes with surface membrane IgA.

ASSOCIATIONS OF HLA AND DISEASE

An international HLA and Disease Registry has been established in Copenhagen. This registry provides a comprehensive compilation of HLA and disease associations, based on published reports and information made available to the registry. The *Third Report of the HLA and Disease Registry* (Ryder *et al.* 1979) compiled information up to 1979, and the list has been updated to 1982 by Svejgaard *et al.* (1983), see Table 3.2. In this table the principal known associations of HLA-A, -B, -C, and DR are summarized. Ankylosing spondylitis is more strongly associated with B27 than DR, suggesting that the former association is primary while the latter follows secondarily from linkage disequilibrium. Likewise the association of psoriasis with Cw6 appears to be primary. However, in many cases the association with D/DR is closer than with HLA-A, -B, or -C. Since *Ir*- and *Is*-genes are presumed to be located in the D/DR region, it is not suprising that most of the D/DR-associated diseases are believed to have an immune component in their pathogenesis.

However, linkage with HLA or DR does not necessarily have that implication. An example is congenital adrenal hyperplasia due to 21-OH hydroxylase deficiency, which is an autosomal recessive trait. Studies of families with intra-HLA recombinants show that the locus concerned maps between HLA-B and D/DR genes (Dupont *et al.* 1980). Thus the locus controlling congenital adrenal hyperplasia, which may well code for the 21-OH hydroxylase enzyme, is probably associated with HLA-B47 through linkage disequilibrium rather than because the B47 antigen plays any role in the pathogenesis of congenital adrenal hyperplasia. The complete penetrance of 21-OH hydroxylase deficiency and its expression at birth greatly facilitates genetic analysis.

Other HLA-associated disorders have varying ages of onset, and presumably, penetrance of the genes in question. In the case of idiopathic haemochromatosis these difficulties have been to some extent overcome by affected sib-pair analysis (Simon *et al.* 1977) and by linkage analysis of HLA with serum transferrin saturation as marker (Kravitz *et al.* 1979). Both groups of investigators concluded that idiopathic haemochromatasis is an autosomal recessive disorder closely linked to HLA. The locus concerned and the biochemical mechanism controlled by it have not yet been defined, but may not involve HLA antigens directly. Nevertheless, the linkage with HLA allows the probable identification of siblings with haemochromatosis, and iron depletion can be commenced before organ damage develops.

In this chapter there is space to discuss only a few associations of HLA with diseases, to illustrate general points about the analysis of such relationships. One of the principal points to emerge is that many diseases are heterogeneous in their aetiology and genetic associations, for example diabetes mellitus. The heterogeneity of genetic and environmental interactions giving rise to diseases, and of their responses to therapy, is a major lesson for social medicine. Two other examples will be mentioned to underline the point. Stasny *et al.* (1983) report that classical rheumatoid arthritis, with rheumatoid factor (RF) in adults, is associated with DR4 whereas in patients with clinical arthritis indistinguishable from rheumatoid arthritis, but who do not produce RF, the frequency of DR4 is the same as in controls. Only the minority of children with polyarthritis, who produce RF, show an increase in DR4. DR3 is more strongly associated with subacute cutaneous lupus erythematosus than with systemic lupus erythematosus.

Although the association of DR3/4 heterozygotes with several diseases is striking, it is not the only combination predisposing to disease. Coeliac disease is more prevalent in DR3/7 heterozygotes, perhaps because an *Ir*-gene for a sensitizing response to gluten is linked with DR7. Drug-induced diseases have genetic associations different from those of the naturally-occurring diseases which they mimic: hydralazine-induced systemic lupus erythematosus is not associated with DR3 (Svejgaard *et al.* 1983) and penicillamine-induced myasthenia gravis is associated with B235 and concomitantly DR1, in contrast to B8 and concomitantly DR3 in the naturally-occurring disease (Dawkins *et al.* 1983).

Ankylosing spondylitis

The finding by Brewerton *et al.* (1973) and Schlosstein *et al.* (1973) that antigen B27 is present in 85–95 per cent of patients with ankylosing spondylitis, as compared with about 9 per cent of controls, provided convincing evidence for a genetic basis of susceptibility to the disease. With a relative risk of 87 in Caucasoids and 192 in Japanese, it remains the strongest known association of an HLA or D/DR antigen with a disease. An increase in frequency of B27 is found in anky-losing spondylitis associated with two other chronic rheumatic disorders, acute uveitis and Reiter's disease (see Sachs and Brewerton 1978). Even in the absence of sacroili-itis, 15 of 38 patients with acute uveitis and 29 of 84 patients with Reiter's disease were also B27-positive. However, the distribiution of B27 in non-specific urethritis was similar to that in healthy controls, suggesting that B27 is related to joint involvement rather than urethritis itself. Patients with reactive anthritides following other acute infections (such as those caused by *Salmonella* spp, *Yersinia enterocolitica*, and *Klebsiella pneumoniae*) also have a highly significant increase in B27 in the absence of features of ankylosing spondylitis. Patients with Cronin's disease and ulcerative colitis show an increased frequency of B27 only when they also have spondy-litis. Hence the frequency of B27 is increased not only in patients with ankylosing spondylitis, which may be accompanied by Crohn's disease or ulcerative colitis, but also in patients with Reiter's disease, acute uveitis, and reactive arthritides in the absence of ankylosing spondylitis. Although the association of this group of chronic rheumatic disorders with B27 has been recognized for a decade, the underlying aetiological factors are still unknown and illustrate the diffi-culty of providing a precise genetical and biochemical explanation of HLA associations with diseases.

Genetic analyses of population and family data suggest that susceptibility to ankylosing spondylitis is due to a domi-nant gene with incomplete penetrance. Kidd *et al.* (1977) esti-mate that the frequency of the ankylosing spondylitis suscept-ibility gene in Caucasoids is 0.022 and that it is nearly always (93 per cent of times) together with B27; the penetrance was estimated to be 38 per cent.

Dawkins *et al.* (1983) reported that in a Caucasoid popula-tion of Western Australia, sacroiliitis was essentially restricted to individuals with B27. The sacroiliitis was usually unaccom-panied by ankylosing spondylitis and was found in about 18 per cent of B27 subjects of either sex above 50 years of age. Some patients with psoriasis, ulcerative colitis, and other diseases have sacroiliitis in the absence of B27, but even in these diseases, which are not themselves associated with B27, the presence of B27 is associated with sacroiliitis. More than 20 per cent of patients with these diseases develop sacroiliitis. They conclude that B27 confers susceptibility to sacroiliitis but is not sufficient. It seems likely that a gene present in 10–20 per cent of the population interacts with B27 to produce sacroiliitis. In diseases such as ulcerative colitis and psoriasis the second gene is common. A third gene is required for expression of ankylosing spondylitis, which is commoner in males than females, suggesting sex linkage or sex limitation.

Studies of various populations indicate the need for caution before B27 itself is identified as the principal predis-posing factor to sacroiliitis and ankylosing spondylitis (Sachs and Brewerton 1978). In Japanese, a mixed Israeli population, and people indigenous to north India, the frequency of B27 in ankylosing spondylitis was as high as in Caucasoids. In Haida Indians of North America, with a 50 per cent frequency of B27, sacroiliitis was found in 10 per cent of males and B27 in all 27 ankylosing spondylitis cases tested. However, 38 per cent of 193 Pima Indians had evidence of sacroiliitis and of these only 26 per cent were B27 positive, which is similar to the frequency observed in the control population. The frequency of both ankylosing spondylitis and B27 is low in American Blacks and only 49 per cent of these patients have B27. In summary, the close association of ankylosing spondylitis with B27 in Caucasoid and Japanese populations suggests a disease susceptibility gene closely linked to B27; the lesser association in Blacks and Pima Indians may have resulted from recombination within the HLA region.

The genetic data therefore cast doubt on the identity of the B27 gene and the gene for susceptibility to sacroiliitis and ankylosing spondylitis. Nevertheless, the striking correlation between this HLA specificity and seronegative arthropathies has encouraged attempts to provide an immunochemical explanation for such associations (see Geczy et al. 1983). A serological relationship between the B27 antigen and certain membrane antigens of *Klebsiella pneumoniae* has been found. Antigens in the outer membrane of the organism can modify B27, or a closely related cell surface structure. The authors suggest that modified B27 elicits immune responses able to injure specific target tissues bearing altered self-determinants (for example, synovium and cartilage). The destruction of appropriate target cells may trigger a complex chain of events culminating in the development of ankylosing spondylitis. In addition to the modification of B27 to provide the target antigen, an immune response gene (perhaps located in the D/DR region) may control the magnitude of the immune response which is elicited. Thus, despite the strong association of B27 with AS and seronegative arthropathies, which has long been known, the chemical and immunological basis of the association remains speculative.

Diabetes mellitus

Diabetes mellitus is a clinical syndrome characterized by an increase in blood glucose and an absolute or relative deficiency of insulin. It is a complex of diseases rather than a single entity, with several distinct genetic and environmental factors interacting to produce the end point of diabetes. It is usual to classify diabetics according to whether their disease can be controlled by oral hypoglycaemic drugs or requires insulin therapy, and whether the disease is of juvenile or adult onset. Some limitations of this classification will be mentioned below. More recently the role of viruses in pancreatic islet cell damage (Notkins 1977; Yoon et al. 1979), the existence of autoantibodies against islet cells (Doniach and Botazzo 1977; Irvine 1980), and the finding that some types of diabetes are associated with HLA antigens have provided further insight into the pathogenesis of the disease.

In insulin-dependent diabetes mellitus (IDDM) DR4 is increased in all ethnic groups, DR3 is increased in Caucasoids and DR8 in Japanese (Svejgaard et al. 1983). Analyses in Caucasoids showed the increases of B8 and B15 to be secon-

dary to those of DR3 and DR4, respectively, with which they are in linkage disequilibrium. About 58.6 per cent of affected sib-pairs share both, 36.9 per cent share one and only 4.6 per cent share no parental haplotypes; this difference from the distribution expected on the assumption of no linkage is highly significant. The relative risk of developing IDDM is much greater in DR3/DR4 heterozygotes than in persons with other genotypes (Contu et al. 1982; Svejgaard et al. 1983). Juvenile-onset diabetes (JOD) is also highly significantly associated with the heterozygote type DR3/DR4 in all populations tested, including Basques who are classified as non-Caucasoids (Scholz and Albert 1983). The frequency of the DR2 antigen is decreased in JOD in all populations, suggesting linkage of DR2 with a gene protecting against this disease (Scholz and Albert 1983).

Autoantibodies reacting with the cytoplasm of human pancreatic islet cells (ICAb) are much commoner in patients with IDDM than in those with diabetes that can be controlled by oral hypoglycaemic agents (Doniach and Botazzo 1977; Irvine 1980). The prevalence of ICAb is some 60–80 per cent at the time of diagnosis of IDDM but only 20 per cent 2–5 years after diagnosis. ICAb are rare in diabetics whose disease can be controlled by diet and in persons without diabetes. Persistent ICAb are often associated with evidence of other signs of organ-specific autoimmunity, together with an increase in thyroid and gastric parietal cell antibodies in the first-degree relatives of patients. The increased frequency of DR3 again appears in patients with idiopathic Addison's disease (most of whom have adrenocortical autoantibodies – Irvine 1980) and in Graves' disease (who have thyroid-stimulating autoantibodies), suggesting relaxed suppression of autoantibody formation in this group as a whole, as discussed above.

All these observations provide strong evidence for inherited predisposition to diabetes mellitus, although attempts to analyse the human data in terms of simple genetic models have failed (Svejgaard et al. 1983). Experimental animal models provide clues to the complexity of the situation. There has been interest in the role of viruses and toxic chemicals in the pathogenesis of diabetes mellitus. A variant of Coxsackie B4 virus isolated from the pancreatic islet cells of a boy dying acutely of diabetes was found to be more diabetogenic in experimental animals than most strains of Coxsackie B4 virus (Yoon et al. 1979). The pancreatic islet cells of different strains of mice vary in susceptibility to infection with certain viruses (Notkins 1977). Viruses not only damage infected cells; they can elicit autoimmune responses (Allison 1977). The inherited predisposition of certain strains of mice, rats, and chickens to autoimmune diseases is well known (see Allison 1977). Toniolo et al. (1980) reported that sub-diabetogenic doses of streptozoticin can condition mice so that they are more prone to develop diabetes following infection with Coxsackie virus. Moreover, strains of mice resistant to encephalomyocarditis virus-induced diabetes can be rendered susceptible by pretreatment with sub-diabetogenic doses of streptozoticin (Toniolo et al. 1980). The association of diabetes with obesity is well known. Thus, in human diabetes mellitus, inherited susceptibility factors are likely to interact with infectious agents, toxic chemicals, immune, metabolic, and other factors in a complex manner. Nevertheless, attempts should be made to identify major pathogenic factors operating in groups of patients.

The limitations of existing classifications of diabetes mellitus have been emphasized by Irvine (1980). In some centres patients are treated with insulin before systematic attempts are made to control the disease by oral hypoglycaemic agents; such patients may be classified as insulin-dependent when they are not. ICAb are found in IDDM of both juvenile and adult onset, and their presence may be a more reliable guide to pathogenesis than age of onset or insulin requirement, since either could follow from a non-immunological cause such as a virus infection or particular sensitivity to a chemical agent. Most studies of a relationship between ICAb and HLA have concerned the association with B8 (Irvine 1980), whereas in IDDM and JOD linkage with DR3 and DR4 is tighter and deserves further analysis in relation to ICAb. Identification of individuals with ICAb who are likely to develop insulitis and consequent diabetes is an important practical consideration. Rats genetically predisposed to diabetes treated with the immunosuppressive drug cyclosporin A do not develop the disease (Laupacis et al. 1983), and preliminary evidence from the same group of investigators suggests that cyclosporin A treatment may also be beneficial in some human patients with diabetes mellitus.

Coeliac disease

Coeliac disease is an enteropathy associated with sensitivity to ingested gluten. Dissecting microscopical and routine histological examination show a flat or nearly flat jejunal mucosa, and gluten withdrawal is followed by clinical, haematological, and morphological improvement. An immune response conferring sensitivity to gluten is believed to be involved in the pathogenesis of the disease, although this is difficult to establish unambiguously. The observed linkage with HLA antigens is consistent with an immunological interpretation but does not prove it.

The association of B8 with coeliac disease was reported in the US by Falchuk et al. (1972) and in England by Stokes et al. (1972), and has been repeatedly confirmed in children and adults. In populations where the frequency of B8 is high, such as that of the west of Ireland, where it reaches 87 per cent, the prevalence of coeliac disease is also high (Mackintosh and Asquith 1978). Later, DR3 and DR7 were found to be significantly increased in groups of patients with coeliac disease (Scholz and Albert 1983). The primary association with DR3 leads to secondary associations with B8 and A1 through linkage disequilibrium. There is a decrease in the frequency of DR2, and concomitantly that of B7, in coeliac disease, suggesting that DR2 and B7 are associated with a protective gene. A remarkably constant feature in different populations is the high frequency of DR3/DR7 heterozygotes in the different patient populations (Scholz and Albert 1983). The number of DR3/7 heterozygotes in the group of patients exceeded the sum of the two types of homozygotes, DR3/3 and DR7/7. This suggests the simultaneous presence of two susceptibility genes, one associated with DR3 and the other with DR7, rather than a recessive susceptibility gene associated with both DR3 and DR7.

Analysis of affected sib-pairs showed 56 per cent sharing two parental HLA haplotypes, 40 per cent one haplotype, and only 4 per cent sharing no haplotypes, confirming the linkage between HLA and coeliac disease. Combining the population and sib-pair data, Scholz and Albert (1983) conclude that at least three different HLA-linked genes influence susceptibility to coeliac disease: one gene associated with DR3 and another with DR7 increase susceptibility while a third associated with DR2 provides resistance.

From the practical point of view, typing could be useful for identifying patients, but only when the clinical picture and/or the results of other screening tests make the diagnosis of coeliac disease possible (Mackintosh and Asquith 1978). Even susceptible DR3/DR7 heterozygotes should not have jejunal biopsies unless there is a strong indication. In coeliac families typing could be useful to identify individuals at risk before weaning on to gluten-containing foods.

CHANGING OPPORTUNITIES FOR SELECTION

In any population natural selection occurs because different genotypes produce different numbers of offspring and because different proportions of their offspring survive to the age of reproduction. Differential reproduction and survival provide the opportunity for selection. The demographic transition from a period of high birth and death rates to the lower birth and death rates in the more advanced countries has obviously reduced the opportunity for selection, but has not eliminated it altogether. In these countries both birth and death rates are largely controlled. In 1800 the average American woman passing through reproductive life had seven children; today she has three or less (Kirk 1968).

Nevertheless about 1 in 10 married women remains childless, with infertility resulting from infectious diseases of the reproductive tract or other causes, so that some opportunity for selection still occurs. Mortality is to a large extent postponed beyond the age of reproduction, which implies that the opportunity for selection in this way is greatly reduced. In 1840 about 50 per cent of American women died before the end of the reproductive years whereas the figure is now only about 4 per cent. For males the present figure is a little higher, about 6 per cent.

Crow (1966) has proposed an 'Index of Opportunity for Selection' that tells how much potential genetic selection is inherent in the pattern of births and deaths. Of course these differences may not be heritable – hence the term opportunity for selection. If a trait is completely heritable and perfectly correlated with fitness, the index tells its rate of increase. Otherwise, and this is the situation in practice, it provides only an upper limit.

The Index, I, is defined as V/x^2, where V is the variance and x the mean number of progeny per parent. This can be separated into components due to mortality and to fertility differences. Table 3.3 shows the trends in the fertility component of the Index in the US. The pattern has changed from uniform high fertility (x small, I_f small) through low fertility with considerable variability from family to family (x small, I_f large) to the most recent situation where the family size is more uniform and I_f is again small. Meanwhile, the index due

Table 3.3. *Changes in mean number of children and the fertility component of the index of opportunity for selection, I_f, in the United States*

Date of mother's birth	Mean no. children	I_f
1839	5.5	0.23
1861–65	3.9	0.78
1901–05	2.3	1.14
1911–15	2.2	0.97
1921–25	2.5	0.63

Note: This includes both white and non-white and both married and unmarried. Data from US Census (Crow 1966).

to mortality has dropped from about 1 for those born a century ago to less than 0.1 for current death rates.

These values quantify what has already been pointed out, that the opportunity for selection from differential postnatal mortality is greatly reduced. Prenatal mortality has changed much less, and probably contributes at least 0.3 to the total index. The opportunity for selection from fertility differences first increased and then decreased.

If all the differential viability and fertility were genetic, the total index would still be large enough to produce a considerable amount of selection. But the more important question of how much genetically effective selection is still occurring cannot be answered in general terms: specific examples must be considered.

Some trends are clear: infectious diseases have been drastically reduced in many parts of the world. A few decades ago a gene producing a decreased susceptibility to smallpox would have had a selective advantage; now that smallpox is eliminated the advantage has disappeared. Genes for resistance to tuberculosis and other bacterial infections would have had great selective advantages a century ago, whereas in Europe and the US the advantage would now be slight. Nevertheless, malaria and bacterial diseases still exert considerable selection in developing countries.

The greater mobility of contemporary populations will also have genetic consequences; there is certain to be less inbreeding as persons tend to find mates away from their home environs. This should decrease the incidence of rare recessive diseases and cause some increase in general health and vigour –although the latter may not be measurable directly. A second consequence of mobility may be an enhanced degree of assortative marriage. The greater participation in higher education, the stratification of students by aptitude, and the growth of communities with similar interests and attainments all can lead to increased correlations between husband and wife. Added to this is the greater range of choice created by affluence and mobility so that any inherent preferences for assortative marriage are more easily realized. The effect of assortative marriage is to increase the population variability. There is already a high correlation in IQ between husband and wife, and this may well increase. To the extent that this trait is heritable there will be greater variability in the next generation than would otherwise be the case: more geniuses as well as more at the other end of the scale.

The population always carried a number of deleterious genes. Many of them are recessive, or nearly so, and owe their incidence to mutation and opposing selective forces. They may or may not be at equilibrium; probably many are not, for the conditions determining the equilibrium may change faster than the time necessary for equilibrium to be reached. In any case, an environmental change that makes a gene less likely to cause death or sterility will cause that gene to be more frequent in later generations than it would otherwise be. How great is this effect?

Consider first a rare recessive gene causing a disease that can now be treated. Let p be the relative frequency of this gene. Then, with random mating, the proportion of persons homozygous for this gene will be p^2. Let the probability of death or infertility in untreated cases (relative to the normal population) be s and in treated cases t. Then, as a result of the treatment, a fraction $(s-t)p^2$ recessive genes will be transmitted to the next generation that, in the absence of the treatment, would be eliminated by death or failure to reproduce. If p' is the proportion of recessive genes that would otherwise be present in the next generation, the proportion of harmful genes in the next generation is $p' + (s-t)p^2$. The incidence of the disease is the square of this.

Ordinarily p and p' are very similar, for the gene frequency is likely to be near equilibrium. Letting $p' = p$, the incidence in the next generation is $p^2 (1 + ip)^2$, where $i = s - t$ is the improvement produced by the treatment, measured in terms of survival and reproduction.

The proportion by which the incidence is increased is

$$\frac{p^2 (1 + ip)^2}{p^2} = 2ip,$$

approximately, where p is small.

A familiar example is phenylketonuria, which can now be treated with considerable success by a low phenylalanine diet. If untreated persons hardly ever reproduce, s is nearly 1. If the treatment is fully successful, $t = 0$; so $i = 1$. The gene frequency, p, in this case is about 0.01; thus the proportion of increase is $2ip = 0.02$. An increased incidence of 2 per cent per generation would mean about 40 generations for the incidence to double. Even allowing for a geometric, not an arithmetic increase, it would take close to 1000 years for this to occur.

The situation is quite different with a rare dominant gene. In this case, if p is the frequency of the gene in this generation, and p' the frequency in the next generation in the absence of treatment, the fraction of deleterious genes added as a consequence of the treatment is ip. Thus, the proportion in the next generation is $p' + ip$, or if p and p' are approximately equal the proportion by which the incidence is increased is simply i.

If the mutant has a constant but reduced penetrance, P, the proportion of increase is approximately iP. In summary, the proportion increase in incidence in the next generation for simple inheritance is approximately:

Recessive	$2pi$
Dominant	i
Dominant with penetrance P	Pi

In practice, the relatively rapid increase in frequency of dominant genes due to improved medical care may not be important because of genetic counselling. If the disease severe or painful, the person with it will not wish to inflict it on his or her children. If the disease is mild or treatment is effective, the parents may not hesitate to expose their children to a risk of up to 50 per cent of developing the disease.

In more complex cases involving interactions of several genes and environmental factors, such as diabetes mellitus, only broad generalizations can be offered. If the condition depends on recessive genes (for example, recessive alleles of *Is*-genes in the example discussed above), the rate of increase will still be slow.

Whether conditions have been so stable in the past that most genes were near equilibrium frequencies, it is evident that environmental factors relevant to the selective value of many genes are changing rapidly – far more rapidly than the gene frequencies can change. Although improved medical care is certainly increasing the frequency of disease-producing genes in human populations, the rate of increase does not justify the alarmist predictions that some distinguished geneticists have made. The benefits clearly outweigh the disadvantages, although the latter must be recognized and dealt with if possible, for example by genetic counselling and prenatal detection of abnormalities.

REFERENCES

Allison, A.C. (1954*a*). The distribution of the sickle-cell trait in East Africa and elsewhere, and its apparent relationship to the incidence of subtertian malaria. *Trans. R. Soc. Trop. Med. Hyg.* **48**, 312.

Allison, A.C. (1954*b*). Protection by the sickle-cell trait against subtertian malarial infection. *Br. Med. J.* **i**, 290.

Allison, A.C. (1954*c*). Notes on sickle-cell polymorphism. *Ann. Hum. Genet.* **13**, 39.

Allison, A.C. (1956). The sickle-cell and haemoglobin C-genes in some African populations. *Ann. Hum. Genet.* **21**, 67.

Allison, A.C. (1960). Glucose-6-phosphate dehydrogenase deficiency in red blood cells of East Africans. *Nature* **185**, 531.

Allison, A.C. (1964). Polymorphism and natural selection in human populations. *Cold Spring Harbor Symp. Quant. Biol.* **29**, 137.

Allison, A.C. (1977). Autoimmune diseases: concepts of pathogenesis and control. In *Autoimmunity, genetic, immunologic, virologic and clinical aspects* (ed. N. Talal) p. 91. Academic Press, New York.

Allison, A.C. (1983). Cellular immunity to malaria and babesia parasites: a personal viewpoint. In *Progress in immunobiology* (ed. J. Marchalonis). Raven Press, New York.

Allison, A.C. and Clyde, D.F. (1961). Malaria in African children with deficient erythrocyte glucose-6-phosphate dehydrogenase. *Br. Med. J.* **i**, 1345.

Allison, A.C., Denman, A.M., and Barnes, R.D. (1971). Co-operating and controlling functions of thymus-derived lymphocytes in relation to autoimmunity. *Lancet* **ii**, 135.

Bankhurst, A.D., Torrigiani, G., and Allison, A.C. (1973). Lymphocytes binding human thyroglobulin in healthy people and its relevance to tolerance for autoantigens. *Lancet* **i**, 115.

Benacerraf, B. and Germain, R.N. (1978). The immune response genes of the major histocompatibility complex. *Immunol. Rev.* **38**, 70.

Bengtsson, B.O. and Thomson, G. (1981). Measuring the strength of associations between HLA antigens and diseases. *Tissue Antigens* **17**, 356.

Bienzle, V., Ayent, O., Lucas, A.O., and Luzzatto, L. (1972). Glucose-6-phosphate dehydrogenase and malaria. Greater resistance of females heterozygous for enzyme deficiency and of males with a nondeficient variant. *Lancet* **i**, 107.

Bodmer, W.F. and Bodmer, J.G. (1978). Evolution and function of the HLA system. *Br. Med. Bull.* **34**, 309.

Brewerton, D.A., Caffrey, M., Hart, F.D., James, D.C.O., Nicholls, A., and Sturrock, R.D. (1973). Ankylosing spondylitis and HLA-27. *Lancet* **i**, 904.

Burnet, F.M. (1949). *The clonal theory of acquired immunity.* Cambridge University Press, London.

Carson, P.E., Flanagan, C.L., Ickes, C.E., and Alving, A.S. (1956). Enzymatic deficiency in primoquine-sensitive erythrocytes *Science* **124**, 484.

Cavalli-Sforza, L.L. and Bodmer, W.F. (1978). *The genetics of human populations.* Freeman, San Francisco.

Crow, J. (1966). The quality of people: human evolutionary changes. *Bioscience* **16**, 863.

Contu, L., Deschamps, I., Estradet, H. *et al.* (1982). HLA haplotype study of 53 juvenile insulin-dependent diabetic (I.D.D.) families. *Tissue Antigens* **20**, 123.

Dawkins, R.L., Christiansen, F.T., Kay, P.H. *et al.* (1983). Disease associations with complotypes, supratypes and haplotypes. *Immunol. Rev.* **70**, 5.

Day, N.E. and Simons, M.J. (1976). Disease susceptibility genes. Their identification by multiple case family studies. *Tissue Antigens* **8**, 109.

Dickmeiss, E., Soberg, B., and Svejgaard, A. (1977). Human cell-mediated cytotoxicity against modified target cells is restricted by HLA. *Nature* **270**, 526.

Doniach, D. and Bottazzo, G.F. (1977). Autoimmunity and the endocrine pancreas. *Pathobiol. Annu.* **7**, 327.

Dorf. M.E. (1981). Genetic control of immune responsiveness. In *The role of the major histocompatibility complex in immunobiology* (ed. M.E. Dorf) p. 221. Garland, New York.

Dupont, B., Pollack, M.S., Levine, L.S., O'Neill, G.J., Hawkins, B.R., and New, M.I. (1980). Congenital adrenal hyperplasia. *Joint report in histocompatibility testing 1980* (ed. P.I. Teraski) p. 693. UCLA Tissue Typing Laboratory, Los Angeles, California.

Eddlestone, A.L.W.F. and Williams, R. (1978). HLA and liver disease. *Br. Med. Bull.* **34**, 295.

Falchuk, Z.M., Rogentine, G.N., and Strober, W. (1972). Predominance of histocompatibility antigen HL-A8 in patients with gluten-sensitivity enteropathy. *J. Clin. Invest.* **51**, 1602.

Fathman, C.G. (1980). Hybrid I region antigens. *Transplantation* **30**, 1.

Fialkow, P.J., Gilchrist, C., and Allison, A.C. (1973). Autoimmunity in chronic graft-versus-host disease. *Clin. Exp. Immunol.* **13**, 479.

Fisher, R.A. (1930). *The genetical theory of natural selection.* Oxford University Press, London.

Friedman, M.J. (1978). Erythrocytic mechanism of sickle-cell resistance to malaria. *Proc. Natl. Acad. Sci. USA* **75**, 1994.

Friedman, M.J. (1979). Oxidant damage mediates variant red-cell resistance to malaria. *Nature* **280**, 245.

Friedman, M.J., Roth, E.F., Nagel, R.L., and Trager, W. (1979). The role of hemoglobins C, S, and N_{BALT} in the inhibition of malaria parasite development *in vitro*. *Am. J. Trop. Med. Hyg.* **28**, 777.

Geczy, A.F., Alexander, K., Bashir, H., Edmonds, J.P., Upfold, L., and Sullivan, J. (1983). HLA-B27, *Klebsiella* and ankylosing spondylitis: biological and chemical studies. *Immunol. Rev.* **70**, 23.

Grebe, S.C. and Streilein, J.W. (1976). Graft-versus-host reactions: a review. *Adv. Immunol.* **23**, 120.

Hammarstrom, L. and Smith, C.I.E. (1982). T cell clones restricted to 'hybrid' HLA-D antigens? *J. Immunol.* **128**, 2497.

Hansen, G., Sönderstrup, G., Svejgaard, A., and Claesson, M.H. (1982). T cell clones restricted "to hybrid" HLA-D antigens? *J. Immunol.* **128**, 2497.

Hood, L., Steinmetz, M., and Malissen, B. (1983). Genes of the major histocompatibility complex of the mouse. *Annu. Rev. Immunol.* **1**, 529.

Hsu. S.H., Chan, M.M., and Bias, W.B. (1981). Genetic control of major histocompatibility complex-linked immune responses to synthetic polypeptides in man. *Proc. Natl. Acad. Sci. USA* **78**, 440.

Irvine, J. (1980). Immunological aspects of diabetes mellitus: a review (including the salient points of the NDDG report on the classification of diabetes). In *Immunology of diabetes* (ed. J. Irvine) p. 000. Teviot Scientific Publications, Edinburgh.

Kidd, K.K., Bernocco, D., Carbonara, A.O., Daneo, V., Steiger, U., and Ceppellini, R. (1977). Genetic analysis of HLA associated diseases: the 'illness susceptible' gene frequency and sex ratios in ankylosing spondylitis. In *HLA and disease* (ed. J. Dausset and A. Svejgaard) p. 72. Munksgaard, Copenhagen.

Kirk, D. (1968). Patterns of survival and reproduction in the United States: implications for selection. *Proc. Natl. Acad. Sci. USA* **59**, 662.

Kravitz, K., Skolnick, M., Cannings, C. *et al.* (1979). Genetic linkage between hereditary haemochromatosis and HLA. *Am. J. Hum. Genet.* **31**, 601.

Laupacis, A., Gardell, C., Dupre, J., Stiller, C.R., Keown, P., and Wallace, A.C. (1983). Cyclosporin prevents diabetes in BB Wistar rats. *Lancet* **i**, 10.

Livingstone, F.B. (1967). *Abnormal hemoglobins in human populations,* p. 470. Aldine Press, Chicago.

McDevitt, H.O. and Benacerraf, B. (1969). Genetic control of specific immune responses. *Adv. Immunol.* **11**, 31.

Mackintosh, P. and Asquith, P. (1978). HLA and coeliac disease. *Br. Med. Bull.* **34**, 291.

McKusick, V.A. (ed.) (1978). *Mendelian inheritance in man,* p. 533. Johns Hopkins University Press, Baltimore.

McMichael, A.J., Ting, A., Zweerink, H.J., and Askonas, B.A. (1977). HLA restriction of cell-mediated lysis of influenza virus-infected human cells. *Nature* **270**, 520.

Marsh, D.G., Hsu, S.H., Roebber, M. *et al.* (1982). HLA-Dw2: a genetic marker for human immune response to short ragweed pollen allergen Ra5. I. Response resulting primarily from natural antigenic exposure. *J. Exp. Med.* **155**, 1439.

Miettinen, O.S. (1976). Estimability and estimation in case-referent studies. *Am. J. Epidemiol.* **103**, 226.

Nagy, Z.A., Baxevanis, C.N., Ishii, N., and Klein, J. (1981). Ia antigens as restriction molecules in Ir-gene controlled T-cell proliferations. *Immunol. Rev.* **60**, 59.

Notkins, A.L. (1977). Virus-induced diabetes mellitus: brief review. *Arch. Virol.* **54**, 1.

Oen, K., Petty, R.E., and Schroeder, M.L. (1982). Immunoglobulin A deficiency: genetic studies. *Tissue Antigens* **19**, 183.

Pasvol, G., Weatherall, D.J., and Wilson, R.J.M. (1978). Cellular mechanism for the protective effect of haemoglobin S against *P. falciparum* malaria. *Nature* **274**, 702.

Rosenthal, A.S. and Shevach, E.H. (1973). The function of marcrophages in antigen recognition by guinea pig T lymphocytes. *J. Exp. Med.* **138**, 1194.

Roth, E.F., Raventos-Suarez, C., Rinaldi, A., and Nagel, R.L. (1983). Glucose-6-phosphate dehydrogenase deficiency inhibits *in vitro* growth of *Plasmodium falciparum. Proc. Natl. Acad. Sci. USA* **80**, 298.

Ryder, I.P., Anderson, E., and Svejgaard, A. (eds.) (1979). *HLA and disease registry. Third report.* Munksgaard, Copenhagen.

Sachs, J.A. and Brewerton, D.A. (1978). HLA, ankylosing spondylitis and rheumatoid arthritis. *Br. Med. Bull.* **34**, 275.

Sasazuki, T., Nishimura, Y., Muto, M., and Ohta, N. (1983). HLA-linked genes controlling immune response and disease susceptibility. *Immunol. Rev.* **70**, 51.

Schackelford, D.A., Kaufman, J.F., Korman, A.J., and Strominger, J.L. (1982). HLA-DR antigens: structure, separation of subpopulations, gene cloning and function. *Immunol. Rev.* **66**, 134.

Schlosstein, L., Terasaki, P.I., Bluestone, R., and Pearson, C.M. (1973). High association of an HL-A antigen, W27, with ankylosing spondylitis. *N. Engl. J. Med.* **288**, 704.

Scholz, S. and Albert, E. (1983). HLA and diseases: involvement of more than one HLA-linked determinant of disease susceptibility. *Immunol. Rev.* **70**, 77.

Shaw, S., Kavathas, P., Pollack, M.S., Charmot, D., and Mawas, C. (1981). Family studies define a new histocompatibility locus, SB, between HLA-DR and GLO. *Nature* **293**, 745.

Simon, M., Bourel, M., Genetet, B., and Fauchet, R. (1977). Idiopathic hemochromatosis. Demonstration of recessive transmission and early detection by family HLA typing. *N. Engl. J. Med.* **297**, 1017.

Stasny, P., Ball, E.J., Dry, P.J., and Nunez, G. (1983). The human immune response region (HLA-D) and disease susceptibility. *Immunol. Rev.* **70**, 113.

Stokes, P.L., Asquith, P., Holmes, G.K.T., Mackintosh, P., and Brooke, W.T. (1972). Histocompatibility antigens associated with adult coeliac disease. *Lancet* **ii**, 162.

Svejgaard, A., Platz, P., and Ryder, L.P. (1983). HLA and disease 1982 – a survey. *Immunol. Rev.* **70**, 193.

Thomson, G. and Bodmer, W.F. (1977). The genetic analysis of HLA and disease associations. In *HLA and disease* (ed. J. Dausset and A. Svejgaard) p. 84. Munksgaard, Copenhagen.

Toniolo, A., Onodera, T., Yoon, J.-W., and Notkins, A.L. (1980). Induction of diabetes by cumulative environmental insults from viruses and chemicals. *Nature* **288**, 383.

Trager, W. and Jensen, J.B. (1976). Human malaria parasites in continuous culture. *Science* **193**, 673.

Woolf, B. (1955). On estimating the relation between blood groups and disease. *Ann. Hum. Genet.* **19**, 251.

Yoon, J.-W., Austin, M., Onodera, R., and Notkins, A.L. (1979). Virus-induced diabetes mellitus. Isolation of a virus from the pancreas of a child with diabetic ketoacidosis. *N. Engl. J. Med.* **300**, 1173.

Zinkernagel, R.M. and Doherty, P.C. (1974). Restriction of *in vitro* T-cell-mediated cytotoxicity in lymphocytic choriomeningitis within a syngeneic or semi-allogeneic system. *Nature* **248**, 701.

GLOSSARY

Attributable fraction: The extent to which a disease is due to a genetic or other disease-associated factor (see pp. 39–40 and Table 3.1)

Fitness: The contribution of a genotype to the next generation. It is the product of the probability of survival (to and through reproductive age) and fertility, and is expressed by comparison with other genotypes.

Haplotype: This term (from haploid genotype) describes a combination of genetic determinants that leads to a set of antigenic specificities (or other gene products) which is controlled by one chromosome and so inherited together from one or other parent.

Linkage disequilibrium: This is the existence in populations of associations between products of linked genes such as HLA antigens, for example A1, B8, and DR 3 (see pp. 38–39).

Opportunity for selection: The amount of potential genetic selection that is inherent in the pattern of births and deaths in a population. This can be estimated from the index described on p. 45.

Polymorphism: The presence of two or more allelic genes in a population in frequencies higher than expected from recurrent mutation. Polymorphism can be transient or balanced. When it is balanced, opposing selection forces tend to stabilize gene frequencies, for example, when a heterozygote is at a selective advantage over either homozygote (Fisher 1930). In the case of sex-linked genes, if female heterozygotes have an advantage over other genotypes, balanced polymorphism can be attained (Cavalli-Sforza and Bodmer 1978).

Relative risk: The prevalence of a disease in persons carrying a genetic marker as compared with its prevalence in persons from the same population lacking the marker (the latter expressed as unity) (see pp. 39–40 and Table 3.1).

Selection: Unequal survival and reproduction of several genotypes resulting from differences in fitness.

4 Population and nutrition

Basil S. Hetzel

INTRODUCTION

Food intake is essential for the maintenance of the living processes of the human organism. Food is taken by man in the form of a diet which is duly digested, absorbed, and metabolized by complicated transformations which enable it to be used by cells. Waste products are excreted through the kidneys, lungs, skin, and bowels. Excess intake above metabolic requirements is stored in the form of fat – to provide stores for times of scarcity of food. But in the twentieth century, the excess of food intake over requirements in the western world has been so great, that overnutrition is widespread and a major risk to the health of people living in industrialized countries.

In the developing countries, there is a shortage of food and therefore energy for metabolism which affects approximately one-third of their populations as estimated by the available food supply and the energy needs of the estimated population (FAO 1977). This shortage of food leads to loss of weight and eventually wasting of the body as seen in the clinical condition of marasmus in children.

There are other criteria for estimating the shortage of food. These include food intake necessary for survival (used by FAO), a minimum of food intake necessary for normal growth of children (used by WHO) or that necessary for improvement of health and well-being (maximum) (used by World Bank). Energy intake for survival can be calculated as 1.2 times basal metabolic rate. This is used by FAO and is a minimum level. There are only limited relevant data generally available. Hence the aggregate actual food supply and the estimate of population need is used to indicate the extent of deficiency of food in the absence of evidence of significant storage of food. (Discussion at 8th Session of the ACC/Subcommittee on Nutrition, Bangkok, Thailand, February 1982.)

In this chapter we shall begin by considering the general relation between food and population and then proceed to examine in detail the relation of food to health and disease. The three major human ecosystems will be considered with special reference to their patterns of food supply and different patterns of health and disease. These are (i) the hunter-gatherer; (ii) the peasant agriculturalist; and (iii) the affluent industrial ecosystems. The dietary transition will also be considered because most dietary patterns are changing all over the world with important impacts on health and disease. Finally, the causes of hunger and overnutrition will be reviewed with reference to the factors determining food production, food transport, and food consumption including social, economic, and political considerations.

In Volume 4, devoted to the 'Application of Public Health Methods to Control of Disease Processes', Chapter 2 reviews the subject of assessment of nutrition status, the prevention and control of nutritional disorders in developing countries, and the role of nutrition in the prevention and control of the major health problems of developed countries.

FOOD AND POPULATION

There is an intimate relationship between food supply and the size of human populations. In the hunter–gatherer societies such as that of the Australian Aborigines the size of nomadic groups is kept small (up to 30) because of the uncertainty of the food supply. It was necessary for infanticide to be practised while the weak or frail were inevitably left behind to die. These measures drastically limited the size of populations. The Australian Aborigines also continue suckling for 3–5 years after birth which is an important mechanism for control of reproduction.

The maintenance of such small groups resulted in a relative lack of infectious diseases particularly those that are airborne. However, food supply was always precarious and starvation must have been a major cause of death, although there is little evidence available.

A greatly improved food supply followed the adoption of the raising of crops in the First Agricultural Revolution about 10 000 years ago. Continuity of food supplies could be ensured with much more confidence, subject of course to the risk of drought, pests or other natural hazards. Improvement in the supply of food leads to better nutritional status, better resistance to infection, and lowered mortality in infancy and childhood. Then, as numbers increase so does the pressure on the food supply, and this may eventually lead to undernutrition and a rise in mortality from infection. Larger groups living in settled agricultural communities are much more at risk from infectious disease, particularly airborne infections and this would limit the rise in population.

This general argument, developed in recent years particularly by McKeown (1976), has become widely accepted in the light of modern experience in developing countries. Malnutrition is a major factor in deaths from infectious disease especially in infancy and childhood (Bengoa 1971). In a recent report Behar (1974) concluded: 'One half to three quarters

50

all statistically recorded deaths of infants and young children are attributed to a combination of malnutrition and infection'. The predominant importance of nutrition in resistance against infection is demonstrated by the much higher death rate from measles and diarrhoea in the poorer countries than in the richer ones. The reason for this is not that the virus is more virulent, nor a lack of medical care, but a lack of resistance in poorly nourished children. Similar factors operate with respiratory infections and tuberculosis. In a recent study of mortality in infancy in Latin America it was concluded that malnutrition was an associated cause in 57 per cent of all deaths among children aged under five years (Behar 1974). Thus an adequate diet is very important in reducing mortality from infection.

The Second Agricultural Revolution dating from the mid-eighteenth century in Europe led to a greater abundance of food than ever before. This revolution followed the establishment of peace due to exhaustion by the wars of religion and the realization of the need for religious toleration. Law and order was established with the rise of national states with greatly improved communications. Improvement in agriculture could now occur – assisted by the introduction of the potato from North America. Maize was also introduced into southern Europe. The potato provided a much greater return in energy for a unit of land. Other new crops included clover and other legumes. Crop rotation, mixed farming with winter feeding with clover and root crops, and finally farm implements were also very significant developments. In Britain these improvements were sufficient to feed a population that trebled in size between the end of the seventeenth century and the mid-nineteenth century without significant import of food.

Once again as in the case of the First Agricultural Revolution, increase in population occurred due to fall in mortality from respiratory and intestinal infections particularly in younger age groups, with improved nutritional status. This led to an excess of population in rural areas and the migration to the cities which provided the manpower for the industrial revolution. This created a new pressure on food supplies which now had to be provided to increasing numbers of city dwellers away from the site of production. So the transport and preservation of food became as important as production. Food supplies were at risk due to such factors leading to higher costs apart from the vagaries of nature. In such circumstances the urban epidemics of tuberculosis developed in a setting of undernutrition and confined living conditions in many European cities (such as Glasgow) which sprang up with the industrial revolution.

Subsequently, in the second half of the nineteenth century, the Sanitary Revolution dating in Britain from the passing of the Public Health Act in 1848, led to effective control of the water- and food-borne diseases – typhoid, dysentery, and less specific diarrhoeal diseases. The effect of all these factors on death rates in England and Wales is shown by a fall in crude death rate from 24 to 17 per 1000 between 1850 and 1900 (crude death rate is the death rate uncorrected for the age structure of the population).

Detailed analysis revealed that nearly half this fall was attributable to reduction of mortality from tuberculosis – the result mainly of improved nutrition and housing. Most of the rest of the fall was due to reduction in mortality from

typhus and other filth-related fevers (23 per cent), diarrhoea, dysentery, and cholera (9 per cent); small pox (6 per cent); and scarlet fever (2 per cent) in which improved nutrition would also have played a significant role (McKeown 1976).

These measures continued to be of major importance in reducing death rate until after 1950 when the antibiotic era arrived. The striking fall in the standardized death rate in England and Wales from 1841 to 1971 is matched by the fall in death rate from respiratory tuberculosis. The marked decreases evident in both rates before 1941 indicate the importance of environmental improvement and better nutrition.

The developing world

In Asia and Africa, the establishment of colonial rule by the European powers during the nineteenth century led eventually to similar improvements in law and order, transport and communications. Food supply gradually improved with fall in death rate from infection in the twentieth century. However, this decline in mortality has greatly accelerated since 1950 and is associated with other public health measures such as a safer water supply through improved sanitation, and the introduction of drugs and insecticides such as DDT for the anopheline mosquito, vector of malaria. These measures are thought to have been responsible for half the fall in mortality in the Third World – an effect additional from that to be expected due to improvement in agriculture and food supplies (Gwatkin and Brandel 1982).

However, this post-war decline in mortality has led not just to an increase but a 'population explosion' in countries such as India, Pakistan, Indonesia, and China – together now providing two billion people or over one-half of the world's total population (Table 4.1).

This 'explosion' is due to the different age distribution of deaths in developing countries compared to developed countries. In developing countries 45 per cent of all deaths occur in children under the age of five. The saving of children's lives has a much greater effect on population as they are now able to grow up to procreate. Hence the 'explosive effect' on population.

Decline in mortality with consequent rise in population is the first stage of the demographic transition which is generally considered to be the central event in the recent history of the human population. During the transition a population evolves from a balance of high mortality and high fertility to a balance of low fertility and low mortality (Fig. 4.1).

In western Europe the death rate began to fall in the seventeenth and eighteenth centuries, but fertility remained high for

Table 4.1. *Estimated population of selected countries (in millions) (From Clark and Turner 1971)*

	1965	1970	1975	1980	1985
India	487	555	633	717	808
Indonesia	105	121	140	161	184
Pakistan*	116	137	162	191	224
China	695	760	826	894	965

*Includes Bangladesh.
Source: UN Population Study No. 49. September, 1971.

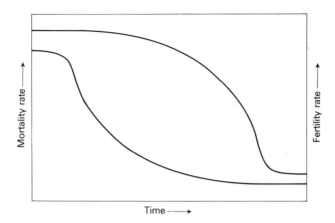

Fig. 4.1. The demographic transition. Before the transition a high birth rate is approximately balanced by a high death rate. When the transition is complete a low birth rate is balanced by a low death rate. The decrease in mortality precedes the decrease in fertility so that over this period the population grows rapidly – this is characteristic of developing countries since the Second World War.

several decades leading to a rapid growth of population (Fig. 4.1). The annual increase was between 0.5 and 1 per cent. Eventually the birth rate began to fall in the course of industrialization so that the growth of the population has slowed as the birth rate approached the death rate. Similar transitions to low mortality and low fertility have taken place in the US, Australia, Canada, and Japan. Demographic transitions are also well under way in countries with fairly advanced economic development such as Argentina, Cuba, and Singapore.

However, in most developing countries, the demographic transition has not proceeded so far. Although death rates have been falling for 75 years, fertility has only just begun to fall (20 per cent less in the late 1970s than 15 years before) and this disparity has produced the rapid population increase or explosion with increases of more than 2 per cent, which leads to a doubling of the population every 33 years. In some regions the growth rate is high enough to lead to a doubling of the population in less than 20 years.

It follows that control of this population increase can only be achieved by further reduction of fertility – further reductions in mortality are proving more difficult to achieve but will not be significant. The major question of population control is discussed further in Volume 2 (Chapter 4).

THREE MAJOR ECOSYSTEMS

The word ecosystem refers to the dynamic relationship that exists between man and his fellow men, the plants and the animals, and the physical environment on which all living beings depend. The concept includes an active interchange in which the various components are interdependent. The food system is one basic feature of the ecosystem which has in turn shaped social and cultural mores and been a major determinant of health and survival.

Let us now consider in some detail three major human

ecosystems representing three different patterns of food production associated with three greatly different patterns of health and disease. These are:
1. The hunter-gatherer ecosystem.
2. The peasant agricultural ecosystem.
3. The affluent industrial ecosystem.

The hunter–gatherer ecosystem

Man and his predecessors were primarily vegetarians. Hunting has developed gradually over the past one million years as man developed tools and formed small groups. However, the great mass of mankind remained primarily vegetarian until the last century. This suggests that man's body has indeed evolved in relation to such a diet. The hunter-gatherer life-style has been in existence for 30 000–50 000 years. The men do the hunting, but the supply of meat is intermittent, while the women collect plant foods. There are a number of these groups remaining in the world today in whom dietary studies have been made and their nutritional status studied. These include the Australian Aborigine and the Kung Bushmen in Africa (N.W. Botswana).

Nutritional status

Data on the Australian Aborigine are available from Arnhem Land (McArthur 1960) and Central Australia (Elphinstone 1971). In Arnhem Land, daily caloric intake was found to vary between 1170 and 2160 with animal protein intake varying between 16 and 300 g per person. Observations of Aboriginal people living out of contact with Europeans in the Great Sandy Desert of Western Australia (Elphinstone 1971) provided data on the chemical analyses of various edible seeds – protein content ranged from 12–44 per cent, fat 2–28 per cent, and fibre 4–20 per cent. A detailed catalogue of the plant foods is available. Snakes, lizards, and mice were described as reasonably plentiful (Hetzel and Frith 1978).

More information is available regarding the diet of the Kung Bushmen of South Africa (Bronte-Stewart et al. 1960; Wehmeyer et al. 1969) largely composed of the Mongonga (or Mangetti) fruit which can be cooked into a porridge or soup. In addition ants are an important source of food – 150 ants a day would provide 60 g protein, 118 mg calcium, 48 mg iron, 142 mg copper, and 220 mg phosphorus as well as providing a source of thiamine and riboflavin. Bushmen are reported to eat 100–300 ants per day.

In the Kung there is evidence that growth is normal during the first year of life with a fall-off later – which may be due to caloric undernutrition (Hansen et al. 1969). Another study shows good nutrition (Bronte-Stewart et al. 1960). Breast feeding is prolonged with the introduction of animal protein in the second six months of life in the form of bone marrow and pre-chewed meat. In the Kung, menarche usually occurred at the age of 15 years, the first baby was born at the age of 19 years and was usually breast-fed for four years. There is little evidence of malnutrition in the African Bushmen.

Simple observations indicate that aborigines have a lighter lean body frame more like a well-trained athlete than a typical sedentary white Australian (Elphinstone 1971). Mature height is within the normal European range, 151–181 cm, with mean of 167.1 cm in the Pintubi in Central Australia (Abbie 1957

52) and 147–185 cm, mean 167.1 in 22 Aborigines in the Great Sandy Desert (Elphinstone 1971). Earlier reports (White 1915; Basedow 1932) indicate good nutrition of Central Australian Aborigines. Biochemical data indicate normal serum iron, calcium, vitamin, and folate levels in Aborigines living in Arnhem Land. There was no evidence of anaemia and vitamin C levels were also normal. In Central Australia there was evidence of low serum cholesterol (Casley-Smith 1958–59). In The Great Sandy Desert of Western Australia there was no evidence of mineral or vitamin B_{12} deficiencies. Haemoglobin levels were normal in 51 of 57 examined.

Health and disease

The order of precedence of food distribution – old men, hunting men, children, dogs, and women suggest females are the most likely to develop malnutrition and two cases of scurvy in adolescent females were found in the Great Sandy Desert by Elphinstone (1971). Abdominal distention is frequent in children without other evidence of impaired health. In general the limited size of the Aboriginal communities makes it difficult to gather substantial epidemiological data. However, the data available do indicate the good health status of the nomadic Central Australian Aboriginal people. Studies of the blood pressure in Central Australian Aboriginals indicate low levels as late as 1975 (Edwards et al. 1976). Little or no evidence of atheroma or arteriosclerotic heart disease was found in a series of 44 autopsies (Schwartz and Casley Smith 1958a,b).

Careful restriction of numbers in relation to the food supply was obviously essential for survival but those that survived certainly impressed the first European observers. The deterioration of health following contact with the white man and destruction of the ecosystem with the establishment of the Reserves has been reviewed elsewhere (Hetzel and Frith 1978).

The peasant agricultural ecosystem

The growing of crops and domestication of animals appeared first in the Mesopotamian region from 8–9000 BC. Agriculture provided the base for the great ancient civilizations of China, Egypt, Maya, and classical Greece.

The growing of crops and complete dependence on them presents the ever present danger of crop failure. The classical European example of this is the Irish potato famine of 1845–46, but famines have occurred frequently in recent years in the developing world – e.g. India, Ethiopia, and the Sahel countries.

Dependence on a single crop such as a cereal or a root vegetable also leads to the liability to specific deficiency diseases. These are more likely to occur in children because of the extra nutrients required for growth. Examples of such deficiency diseases are keratomalacia (due to vitamin A deficiency) which may lead to complete blindness due to softening and scarring of the cornea, beri beri due to vitamin B_1 (thiamine) deficiency produced by milling and removal of the husk of rice – formerly a very common disease in Asia, pellagra in maize eaters due to lack of nicotinic acid and its

precursor tryptophane. Other examples are endemic goitre and endemic cretinism (brain damage) due to dietary iodine deficiency, and iron deficiency causing anaemia. Deficiency of protein is associated with kwashiorkor. These conditions are reviewed in general terms by Bengoa (1971) and will be discussed in detail in Volume 4, Chapter 2.

Papua New Guinea

An example of a primitive stone age peasant agricultural ecosystem is the New Guinea village. The initial migration of hunter-gatherers to New Guinea is thought to have occurred 20 000–50 000 years ago. Gradually this system was replaced by a seminomadic 'slash-and-burn' agriculture using a stone age technology in the tropical forest. Groups varying in size from 20 to 200 lived in the hills or on the plains surrounded by their gardens established after clearing the jungle by fire. Their food was almost entirely vegetable – taro, bananas, yams, and sugar cane which restricted the population to elevations not greater than 2135 metres. Subsequently about 350 years ago the sweet potato was introduced which made possible the development of larger settled communities in altitudes up to 2700 metres. The greater occupation of altitudes above 2000 metres presumably reflected population pressure and led to heavy dependence on the sweet potato. This provided only a marginal intake of protein due to its low content and its susceptibility to frosts (Sinnett 1977; Sinnett and Whyte 1981).

Nutritional status

A dietary survey among the people of Murapin in the western Highlands was undertaken in which all food consumed by each of 90 subjects was weighed over seven consecutive days (Sinnett 1977; Sinnett and Whyte 1981). Sweet potato supplied over 90 per cent of the food, intake of meat was negligible and non-tuberous vegetables accounted for less than 5 per cent of food intake. Similar dependence on a single vegetable staple has been reported from other Highland communities in Papua New Guinea. The daily energy intake was 9.6 MJ (2300 kcal) for males and 7.4 MJ (1770 kcal) for females; 94.6 per cent of the energy was derived from carbohydrate, 3 per cent from protein, and only 2.4 per cent from fat. Males consumed 25 g and females 20 g of protein per day (Australians consume 42 per cent of their energy from fat and eat approximately 100 g of protein per day). Intake of fibre was very high (34 g per day in males and 27 g per day for females compared with Australian and European figures of 15–20 g per day).

On this diet there was a progressive increase in body weight reaching a maximum between 20 and 29 years compared to European populations in which weight increases into middle age and even after the age of 70 years. By contrast in New Guinea there is a progressive loss of weight between the third and seventh decades (23 per cent in males and 25 per cent in females).

Growth in height was not completed until the age of 18 years in females and 24 years in the case of males. Values at all ages were lower than in Australians (British schoolchildren reach full adult stature by 15 years in females and 17 years in males –Tanner et al. 1966). This delayed growth is associated with delayed onset of puberty which is generally true of the people of

Table 4.2. *Indices of mineral nutrition in New Guinea. (From Hetzel 1974)*

Area	Urinary nitrogen (g/24 h)	Urine sodium (mEq/24 h)	Urine potassium (mEq/24 h)	Urinary iodine (μg/24 h)
Highland	2.7 ± 1.7 (74)	32 ± 35 (131)	149 ± 80 (131)	11.5 ± 12.4 (91)
Coastal	6.8 ± 5.5 (30)	77 ± 56 (30)	41 ± 39 (30)	49.0 ± 55.0 (31)
Australian population	10–15	100–150	50–100	80–150

The number of subjects appear in parentheses.

Papua New Guinea. Extensive studies by Malcolm (1970) in the Bundi people have indicated the importance of lowered protein intake to this delayed growth although genetic factors also play a part. It is suggested that genes for more rapid growth and taller stature may have been selectively removed by a high death rate for infants and toddlers from malnutrition and infection. An advantage for survival in conditions of sub-optimal nutrition is therefore conferred on slow-growing, short-statured populations.

An indication of the mineral nutritional status of New Guineans is provided by the data in Table 4.2 which compares urinary excretion of nitrogen, sodium, potassium, and iodine in a group of New Guinea subjects in Highland areas with those living near the coast (hospital orderlies receiving some European dietary supplements). There were lower levels of sodium and nitrogen excretion and higher levels of potassium excretion in the Highlands reflecting the higher vegetable intake. The data indicate very low levels of iodine excretion in the Highlands with higher levels at the coast. Normal 24 hour excretion levels of an urban Caucasian diet would be 10–15 g nitrogen, 100–150 mEq sodium, 50–100 mEq of potassium, 80--150 μg iodine. The lower levels of iodine excretion indicate severe iodine deficiency which is associated with high rates of endemic goitre and endemic cretinism among these Highland peoples (Hetzel 1974). The low level of sodium excretion indicates a very low salt intake and the low level of nitrogen excretion a very low protein intake.

Health status

In New Guinea, infection is the major cause of death: pneumonia and gastroenteritis in the Highlands, and malaria and dysentry in the Lowlands. Tuberculosis, leprosy, and parasitic infections are also common.

Limited autopsy studies reveal little atherosclerosis in Papua New Guineans, although there is some evidence of a recent increase – seven cases of atherosclerotic heart disease were seen (all in males) in a series of 146 autopsies carried out at the Port Moresby General Hospital between January 1973 and April 1974. The average period of urban contact was sixteen years for these subjects.

Blood pressure reaches a maximum in the third decade in Murapin (130 mm Hg systolic and 84 mm Hg diastolic in males and 121 mm Hg and 78 mm Hg respectively in females) in contrast to Europeans in whom a progressive increase occurs with age. These findings are relevant to the low salt intake in New Guinea (usually less than 1 g per day compared to 10 g per day in Europeans).

There was no clinical or electrocardiographic evidence of coronary heart disease (780 subjects). Obesity and diabetes mellitus were also uncommon in these people as were bowel cancer and varicose veins. There is, however, evidence of a recent increase in obesity, serum cholesterol, diabetes, and coronary artery disease in urban areas (Maddocks 1978; Sinnett and Whyte 1981).

Thailand

Thailand is a tropical country with a population of 48 million (1981) which has more than trebled since 1946. Most of the land is flat alluvial plain except some parts in the north and north-east. Forested and mountainous areas exist in about 30 per cent of the total land. The other 70 per cent is under cultivation. Rice is the main produce from the cultivation each year. Among the crops of secondary agricultural importance are maize, cassava, rubber, beans, fruits, and vegetables. Fish ranks second to agriculture in the nation's economy. Rice provides 80 per cent of total energy, protein (10 per cent energy) derived mainly (60–70 per cent) from vegetable sources, and fat, 3–5 per cent of energy.

The spectrum of nutritional disorders reported recently by the Ministry of Public Health in Thailand is shown in Table 4.3. Comprehensive programmes designed to correct these deficiencies are now under way in Thailand. Priority is being given to improvement in the local village food production by increasing the nutritional value of the rice diet for children by adding mung beans and sesame oil to increase (fat) energy content, protein, and vitamin intake. Emphasis is being laid on retaining the whole husk in the milling of rice but it is difficult to alter the milling practices of many centuries. These questions will be considered further in Volume 4, Chapter 2.

The affluent industrial ecosystem

Industrialization dating from the eighteenth century in Europe, and moving with an accelerated pace through the nineteenth

Table 4.3. *Nutritional disorders in Thailand*

Type of malnutrition	Severity	Affected groups
1. Protein-energy malnutrition (PEM)	40–60% (of varying severity)	Children aged 6 months especially in the north-east.
2. Thiamine deficiency	Not available	Among infants and lactating women
3. Riboflavin deficiency	10–30%	Among growing population, pregnant and lactating women
4. Vitamin A deficiency	17% in preschool children	Among children with PEM and inadequate fat ingestion
5. Iodine deficiency	20–50%	Among adults in the north and the north-east, especially highlanders
6. Iron deficiency	43% in female 29% in male	Among adults and pregnant women, especially those living in the endemic area of hookworm infection

Source: Ministry of Public Health (Nutrition Division) Thailand, 1981.

Table 4.4. *Per caput consumption in the UK of various foodstuffs over the last three centuries. (From Burkitt and Trowell, 1975)*

g/day per head	1770	1870	1970
Fat	25	75	145
Sugar	10	80	150
Potatoes	120	400	240
Wheat flour	500	375	200
Cereal crude fibre	5	1	0.2

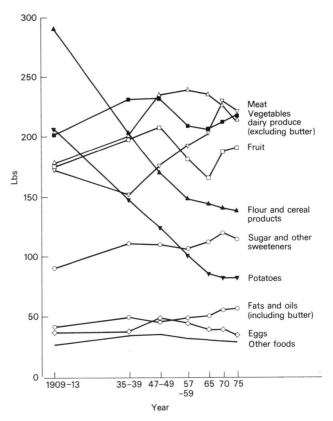

Fig. 4.2. Changes in consumption of foods in the US 1909–13 to 1975. Dairy produce consumption measured in quarts. (From Friend *et al.* 1979).

century has led to an unprecedented degree of affluence in the western world in the twentieth century. A striking feature of this increasing affluence has been the greater availability and increased consumption of foods containing sugar and fat. More efficient agriculture and the development of the food processing industry has led to this unprecedented situation.

Some information on the British diet over the last two centuries is summarized in Table 4.4 which indicates that there has been a very great increase in fat consumption (from 25 g per head per day in 1770 to 145 g per head per day in 1970). Sugar consumption has increased from 10 g per head per day to 150 g per head per day over the same period. A fall in wheat flour consumption from 500 g to 200 g since 1770 has been accompanied by a fall in crude cereal fibre due to a lower extraction rate of flour. Before 1770 the wheat flour was usually stone ground, lightly sifted wholemeal with a high crude fibre content. By 1870 the flour was still stone ground but moderately sifted and white in colour. By 1970 flour was roller milled white with only 70–72 per cent extraction. This fall in fibre from cereal intake is partly compensated for by the rise in potato consumption.

These changes, particularly the increase in fat and sugar intake, result in an increase in total energy (calorie) intake. A diet high in fat and refined sugar does not produce the feeling of satiety associated with high fibre intake. This is a significant factor in overconsumption of food of high sugar content. The absorption of refined sugar is much more rapid than the absorption from fibre which requires digestion so that an excessive insulin response is produced by the more rapid rise in blood sugar. This leads to the deposition of more fat in the tissues – and this is the reason that obesity is so likely to develop under these circumstances. A switch of diet from complex carbohydrate (fibre) to refined sugar is a major factor in a higher prevalence of obesity (defined as ≥ 20 per cent of desirable weight for height) in the twentieth century. Increased inactivity associated with labour-saving machinery and more recently the watching of television is the other major cause.

It is only in the twentieth century, and particularly since the Second World War, that meat has become so generally available in the western world. Even today meat is usually eaten only twice per week by most people in southern European countries. In Australia, New Zealand, the USA and Canada, and parts of South America, meat production has been much less costly and so meat has been consumed much more frequently than in Europe and surpluses have been available for export to Europe.

The changing trends in food consumption in the USA since 1903 are shown in Fig. 4.2. Notable decreases in the consump-

tion of flour, cereals, and potatoes have been associated with a rise in the consumption of meat, sugar, fats, and oils. The differences in daily supply of total fat by major regions of the world are shown in Fig. 4.3 for the two years 1965 and 1974. The relation of fat availability to income is clearly indicated.

Recent information on the nutrient content of the diet in the USA and Australia as representative western industrialized countries is shown in Table 4.5. The differences between the USA and Australia are relatively minor.

Such data are derived from dietary surveys in which the consumption of foods is determined by interview and/or questionnaire supported by actual measurements wherever possible. In fact, in spite of the difficulties of recall (which are considerable) there is a remarkable consistency in the data derived from such surveys. A limited number of national surveys have been carried out – as in the case of the HANES Survey in the USA (US Department of Health, Education and Welfare 1979). But the cost of such studies is great and the necessary resources have not usually been available. More limited studies, carried out with smaller groups, have provided the detailed data shown in Table 4.5 which is derived from a series of Australian surveys. Tables of food composition (Paul *et al.* 1978) provide the nutrient content of foods. These tables have to be constantly updated because of the changing patterns of food production including for example 'convenience' foods. The nutrient intake per day can be calculated from the

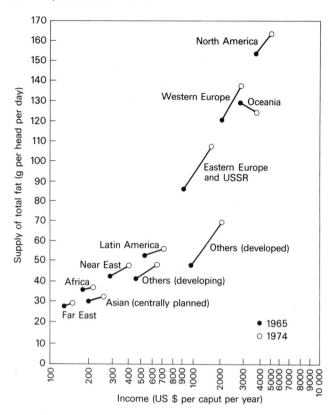

Fig. 4.3. Changes in daily per caput supply of total fat by regions in relation to income between 1965 and 1974. (From FAO 1978.)

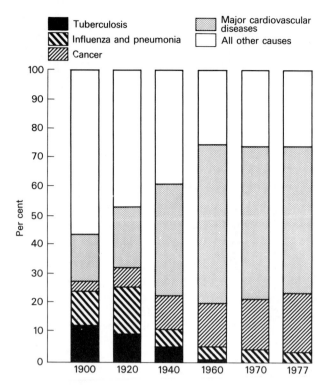

Fig. 4.4. Deaths for selected causes as a per cent of all deaths: US selected years (1900–77). (From Surgeon General's Report on Health Promotion and Disease Prevention 1979.)

frequency of use of each dietary item, the size of serving consumed (which can be identified by matching visually or actually weighing) and the nutrient content per 100 g.

The contrast between these data and those already cited for New Guinea and Thailand is very great (Table 4.5). Particularly striking differences are evident in fat and carbohydrate consumption. A notable change towards the western diet is apparent in Bangkok.

Health status

The major health problems causing mortality are coronary heart disease, responsible for approximately 30 per cent of

deaths, cancer, responsible for 20 per cent, and cerebrovascular disease, 13 per cent of deaths (Hetzel 1980). The changing trend in the USA away from the infectious diseases of tuberculosis and pneumonia towards cardiovascular diseases and cancer since the beginning of the twentieth century, is clearly shown in Fig. 4.4.

Coronary heart disease

The extensive epidemiological data relating diet and coronary heart disease were recently reviewed (Blackburn 1979). Reviews of clinical evidence and experimental studies have also been published (Lewis 1979; Wissler 1979).

The relationship between serum cholesterol levels and energy derived from saturated fat is now well established. Large differences in coronary heart disease mortality can be correlated with low (less than 10 per cent) saturated fat kilojoules as in Japan, Greece, Italy, and Yugoslavia, and high (more than 15 per cent) saturated fat kilojoules, as in all English-speaking countries with a high standard of living. These differences in intake are reflected in mean cholesterol levels of 151–158 mg/dl in the Greek islands and the Orient, compared to a level of 224 mg/dl in English-speaking countries. Mean cholesterol levels in children are approximately 50 mg/dl less than in the adult in each of these populations, so that levels in children predict the eventual level in middle age. There is evidence that strict vegetarians have approximately a 40 per cent lower rate of coronary heart disease mortality associated with much lower serum cholesterol levels. However, there has been considerable difficulty in correlating dietary differences with blood lipid

Table 4.5. *Dietary intake of major nutrients*

| | Per cent of energy (calories) | | | | |
| | USA* | Australia* | New Guinea† | Thailand‡ | |
				Rural	Bangkok
Carbohydrate	46	44	94.6	78	56
Simple	24	27			
Complex	22	17			
Fat	42	40	2.4	8	30
Saturated	16	19			
Mono- and					
polyunsaturated	26	21			
Protein	12	16	3	14	14

*Excluding alcohol – Baghurst and Record (1983).
†Data from the Murapin peoples – Sinnett and Whyte (1981).
‡Data kindly supplied by Dr Aree Valyasevi, Bangkok.

levels within populations (as opposed to between populations). This is attributed to the lack of precision of dietary assessment, and the relative homogeneity of the diet consumed in western countries (apart from the extreme of strict vegetarianism).

A recent switch from animal to vegetable fats in the last 15 years is thought to be relevant to the striking decline of coronary heart disease which has occurred in a number of western countries such as the USA, Australia, Canada, Belgium, Norway, and Finland (Walker 1977; Dwyer and Hetzel 1980; Hetzel and Dwyer 1981). Recent dietary intervention trials in Helsinki, Oslo, and Los Angeles indicate a fall in non-fatal coronary disease in men under 55 years of age associated with a fall in serum cholesterol levels. Evidence is also provided by the demonstration of the lesion in primates after a high fat intake; this lesion can be reversed, at least partially, by reduction in fat intake (Wissler 1979).

However, the relationship between diet and coronary heart disease indicates only one of several known risk factors. These also include genetic predisposition, high blood pressure, and cigarette smoking, which are well substantiated; stress and lack of exercise are less substantiated risk factors.

Cancer

International comparisons (Doll 1979) suggest that saturated fat predisposes to colonic cancer, the commonest single form of cancer (sexes combined) in affluent societies. Burkitt and Trowell (1975) suggest that cereal fibre protects against it and there is much evidence to support this. There is also evidence of the protective effect of green and yellow vegetables (Doll 1979) as well as a possible predisposing effect of alcohol (particularly beer) intake. It is likely that a balance of factors is involved that affect the bacterial flora of the bowel to produce carcinogens or pro-carcinogens from bile salts and other precursors (McMichael et al. 1979).

There is suggestive evidence of the importance of dietary fat intake as a predisposing factor in breast cancer, for example, a rise in incidence in Japanese moving to the US (see below). Other evidence relates earlier puberty and a diminished oestriol/oestradiol ratio with an increase in fat intake (McMahon et al. 1973). This leads to a longer exposure to an apparently unfavourable oestrogen profile until the first pregnancy. Fat intake may also be a factor in other endocrine-related cancers such as endometrial cancer. Dietary fat increases both prolactin and oestrogen production (Armstrong 1979).

Other conditions

Overnutrition, with sugar, fat, and alcohol, and the less active life-style characteristic of industrialized countries is associated with increasing rates of obesity. Obesity (with salt and alcohol intake) is a major factor in hypertension (itself a significant factor in cerebrovascular diseases) and in the development of diabetes mellitus in middle-age (hypertension affects 20 per cent of the population of industrialized countries, while diabetes affects at least 2 per cent of the population and 90 per cent of this associated with overweight) (Weinsier 1976; Howard 1975).

Increasing alcohol consumption is associated with increasing deaths from cirrhosis of the liver and alcoholic brain disease,

oesophageal and other upper gastro-intestinal cancer (Bruun et al. 1975; Hetzel 1978). It is also clearly related to deaths from road crashes (Hetzel 1979) and fetal damage, as in the fetal alcohol syndrome, characterized by a variable number of developmental defects including growth retardation, microcephaly and mental retardation, typical facial anomalies, congenital heart disease, and skeletal anomalies (Clarren and Smith 1978).

DIETARY TRANSITIONS AND HEALTH

There are a number of examples, now well documented, of dietary transitions associated with new health and disease effects. These have usually arisen as the result of western influence and more particularly through the introduction of such nutrients as refined sugar, saturated fat, salt, and alcohol. Current examples of transition in the hunter-gatherer eco-system are the Australian Aborigines, the Pima Indians, and the Eskimos, and from the peasant agricultural ecosystem, Papua New Guinea and the Pacific Islanders. Of these, the Pacific Islanders will be considered in detail. In addition, a notable dietary transition has been recorded in Japan with great improvement in nutritional status since the Second World War. Similar changes have occurred in China but unfortunately only limited data are available so far.

Further examples of dietary transition will be reviewed from studies of immigrant groups – notably the Japanese immigrants to Hawaii and California and the southern European immigrants to Australia.

The Pacific Islanders

Rapid social change is occurring in the small Pacific Island nations, many of which have only recently achieved independence. Many of these peoples have recently switched from a subsistence to a cash economy with a resulting drastic change in diet and life-style. A significant impact on nutrition and health status has occurred in this setting.

Extensive observations in several Pacific Island peoples have been made in recent years (Zimmett and Whitehouse 1981; Prior and Tasman-Jones 1981). Studies include Tuvaluans and Western Samoans who are both Polynesian and the Nauruans who are Micronesian (Zimmett and Whitehouse 1981).

Tuvalu (formerly the Ellice Islands) consists of eight islands (atolls) in the Central Pacific. The soil is poor and the main natural crops are coconut and pandanas. The main island is Funafuti with a population of 2000 only half of which are indigenous. A subsistence economy provides a diet of fish, coconut, bread fruit, and pulaka. A naval base was established in 1943 – which marked the beginning of a cash economy. Since 1943 there has been growing dependence on western goods so that 85 per cent of the food requirements are now imported. Motor cycles, motor cars, and motor boats have replaced the traditional means of transport.

Western Samoa is composed of 150 000 Polynesian people living on a group of islands in the Central Pacific. The islands are mountainous and covered by dense forest. The diet of the people in the main city of Apia includes canned goods, flour, sugar, and beer. Many of these people are in sedentary clerical positions. By contrast, in the rural areas there is less impact from imported foods. The staples continue to be consumed and the males work in plantations which involves heavy labour.

Nauru is the site of phosphate deposits which have made it the world's richest nation – the 4000 Micronesian inhabitants have an annual average per caput income of $US34 000 which they have received since the attainment of independence in 1968! In the ten years following independence the Nauruans became totally westernized. All food is imported – most of the heavy manual labour in the phosphate mine is performed by indentured Chinese labourers from Taiwan and by other Pacific islanders.

There is a progressive gradient in Western acculturation from the people of Funafuti and rural Western Samoans to the partially urbanized West Samoans and the fully urbanized Nauruans. A comparison of the diet of the least affected people in Funafuti and the most affected in Nauru and the Caucasion population is shown in Table 4.6. The distribution of nutrients

Table 4.6. *Mean nutrient intakes in Funafuti and Nauru islanders in comparison to American Caucasians*

| Nutrient | Funafuti | | Nauru | | Caucasian |
	Male	Female	Male	Female	General population
Energy (MJ)	13.1	11.0	30.0	22.0	13.2
(kcal)	3130	2620	7190	5220	3160
% carbohydrate	49	49	46	51	47
% fat	34	36	32	34	41
% protein	15	14	14	15	12

Source: Zimmet and Whitehouse, 1981.

is similar in all three groups and contrasts with traditional diets where there is a much higher contribution from complex carbohydrates.

The age standardized prevalence rates of diabetes mellitus in the four groups are shown in Table 4.7 which indicates that a

Table 4.7. *Prevalence of vascular diseases in Pacific Island populations (per cent)**

| | Funafuti | Western Samoa | | Nauru |
		Rural	Urban	
Diabetes mellitus †				
male %	5.3	2.8	12.6	41.9
female %	15.4	6.2	12.2	42.3
Hypertension ‡				
male %	11.6	20.1	35.7	47.5
female %	20.2	18.1	27.0	27.3
Coronary risk factors§ one or more (aged 20 years or more)				
male %	37	40	60	91
female %	56	46	70	86

*Retabulated from Zimmet and Whitehouse, 1981.

†Diagnosis – documented evidence of diabetes on a two-hour postloading plasma glucose of 8.9 nmol/l (160 mg/dl) or more after 75 g oral carbohydrate.

‡WHO criteria BP ≥ 160 mm Hg systolic and ≥ 95 mm Hg diastolic.

§Risk factors: 1. Body mass index ≥ 30; 2. Diastolic BP ≥ 95 mm Hg or systolic BP ≥ 160 mm Hg; 3. Serum cholesterol ≥ 6.8 mmol/l (260 mg/dl); 4. Serum triglycerides ≥ 1.8 mmol/l (160 mg/dl); 5. Smoking ≥ 20 cigarettes/day; 6. Diabetes mellitus.

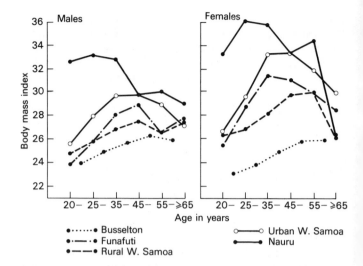

Fig. 4.5. Mean body mass index (weight/height²) by age group for males and females in Funafuti, Western Samoa, and Nauru compared with the Australian Busselton Caucasian Sample. (Reproduced with permission from Zimmet and Whitehouse 1981).

big rise has occurred with the acculturation gradient. Significant factors are genotype, as indicated by familial occurrence, and obesity which is of high prevalence. Mean body mass index, taking into account height and weight (Fig. 4.5), is higher for Nauru and Western Samoa compared to the Australian population (Busselton, Western Australia).

Observations of the age-standardized prevalence of hypertension in the four populations are also shown in Table 4.7 and Fig. 4.6. A similar gradient is shown to that already observed

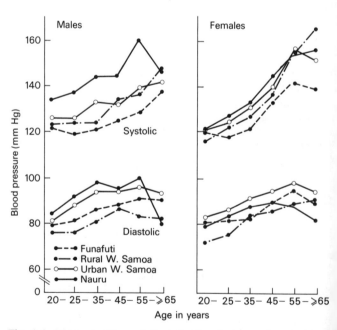

Fig. 4.6. Mean systolic and diastolic blood pressure by age group for males and females in Funafuti, Western Samoa, and Nauru (Reproduced with permission from Zimmet and Whitehouse 1981.)

for diabetes mellitus. The prevalence of coronary heart disease risk factors in the different populations also reveals the same gradation (Table 4.7). Overt coronary heart disease is still rare in these people, but as pointed out by Burkitt and Trowell (1975), the condition usually appears later than dietary transition.

These data indicate clearly the emergence of chronic non-infectious diseases following recent changes in diet and life-style in these Pacific islanders. The role of genetic factors is strongly suggested by the variation in occurrence of diabetes mellitus (rare after urbanization in Melanesians in contrast to Polynesians and Micronesians). The high susceptibility of the latter two groups is also shown by the Pima Indians (Bennett *et al.* 1976) and the Australian Aborigines after adoption of the western affluent diet (Wise *et al.* 1976).

The high prevalence of diabetes may be explained by the 'thrifty gene' hypothesis of Neel (1962). All these peoples have been periodically subjected to long periods of deprivation of food. In the Pacific, famines associated with hurricanes and tidal waves, were frequent. Those with a predisposition to diabetes may have been better able to survive such periods due to better maintenance of blood sugar levels. A similar mechanism has been suggested for the Australian Aboriginal (Wise *et al.* 1976).

The occurrence of these chronic diseases in such high prevalence represents a major loss to the work force and a heavy burden on costly medical care services. Their control, possibly through return to a more traditional type of diet, is an urgent priority to improve the health of these Pacific islanders.

The Japanese

The Japanese people underwent a dramatic change in nutritional status following the Second World War (1939–45). During the war food shortages were severe in many parts of Japan – the average daily consumption per adult was below 8.5 MJ (2000 kcal) from 1945 until about 1950. During this period there was an increase in tuberculosis but a fall in the prevalence of diabetes mellitus and also in the crude mortality from stroke (the yearly rate of 178 per 100 000 in the four years 1939–42 fell to 128 per 100 000 in the four years 1947–50). After 1950, with the Allied occupation, a dramatic change occurred with the adoption of a western life-style including diet. Large quantities of foods were imported including bread, wheat flour, cornflour, maize, and powdered milk. By 1967 the average Japanese male was eating 10.5 MJ (2500 kcal) and the average Japanese woman 9.4 MJ (2250 kcal) per day (Oiso 1971).

The changes in nutrient intake over the period 1950–75 are summarized in Table 4.8. The change to higher protein and fat content and reduced carbohydrate intake is clearly demonstrated. There has been a big increase in the proportion of saturated to unsaturated fats, increased consumption of milk and eggs, and a fall in consumption of rice, cereals, and potatoes. This changing dietary pattern was associated with the appearance for the first time of obese children in cities, and with an increase in coronary heart disease and diabetes mellitus, but rates are still low compared to western countries (Yamamoto 1981). A striking change from pigment to

Table 4.8. *Changes in adult nutrient intakes in Japan 1950–75*

		\multicolumn{4}{c}{Averages per caput per day}
		1950	1960	1972	1975
Energy (MJ)		8.7	8.7	9.5	9.1
(kcal)		2100	2100	2280	2190
Protein, total	(g)	68	70	83	80
Protein, animal	(g)	17	25	40	39
Lipids	(g)	18	25	50	52
Carbohydrate	(g)	420	400	360	340
Cereal energy	(g)	78	75	52	50

Source: Kagawa, 1978.

cholesterol gallstones has been reported, also indicating the effect of the dietary change (Yamamoto 1981).

In 1965, studies were initiated in a cohort of Japanese male immigrants to Honolulu, Hawaii, and to the San Francisco Bay area of California, and comparison made with a group of Japanese of similar age (45–69 years) living in Hiroshima and Nagasaki, Japan. Dietary surveys revealed striking differences although energy intakes were similar (Table 4.9). The main difference was in the starchy foods – 63.0 per cent of total energy in Japan compared to 46.4 per cent in Hawaii and 44.2 per cent in California. Fat intake was 15 per cent in Japan but 33 per cent in Hawaii (largely due to a fourfold increase in animal fats) and 37.5 per cent in California. Cholesterol intakes were similar. Sugar intake provided 11 per cent of calories in Japan, 16 per cent in Hawaii, and 17 per cent in California. Daily salt intake was assessed at 12–13 g in Japan and 8–9 g in Hawaii and California. The Japanese in California were slightly heavier than the Japanese Hawaiian men, who were an average 8 kg heavier than those living in Japan. Skin-fold

Table 4.9. *Diet and coronary heart disease rates in Japanese in Japan, Hawaii, and California. (Derived from Blackburn, 1979, and Marmot et al., 1975.)*

	Japan	Hawaii	California
Age	56.9 ± 5.8	54.4 ± 5.6	52.4 ± 6.1
Weight	55.2 ± 9.0	63.4 ± 9.0	65.9 ± 9.2
DIET/Total energy*	2164 ± 619	2275 ± 736	2262 ± 695
Carbohydrate (% cal)	63.0 ± 11.2	46.4 ± 11.0	44.2 ± 9.4
Simple %	11.3	16.1	17.0
Complex %	51.4	29.7	27.4
Fat (% cal)	15.1 ± 6.9	33.3 ± 9.4	37.5 ± 6.1
Saturated	6.7	23.4	26.4
Unsaturated	8.6	10.3	11.3
Serum			
Total cholesterol mg/dl	181.1 ± 38.5	218.3 ± 38.2	228.2 ± 42.2
Serum cholesterol			
(≥ 260 mg/dl per 1000)	31.6	124.0	162.5
CORONARY HEART DISEASE			
Age-adjusted prevalence rates per 1000. Definite and possible CHD by ECG	25.4	34.7	44.6
Deaths from coronary heart disease per 1000 per year men aged 45–64	1.3	2.2	3.7

*% energy (calories) except where stated otherwise.

measurements showed similar changes. Blood pressure levels were higher in California in all age groups. Serum cholesterol was lower in all age groups in Japan (4.7 mmol/l or 180 g/dl) compared to the levels in Hawaii and California (Table 4.9). Serum glucose levels at one hour after oral glucose (50 g) were lower in all age groups in Japan than in the same age groups in California. In Hawaii the levels were intermediate. Blood uric acid showed similar levels.

There was a higher mortality from coronary heart disease in the Japanese immigrants compared to the Japanese in Japan (Table 4.9). Cancer incidence rates have also been studied in Japanese migrants in comparison to rates in Japan. Data from a group of Hawaiian Japanese immigrants are shown in Table 4.10. It is apparent that there are falls in the rates of oesophageal and stomach cancers but rises in all the others with the exception of cervix uteri. Dietary changes are considered to be highly significant in these differences.

Southern Europeans in Australia

Between 1947 and 1969, large groups of immigrants came to Australia from southern Europe. These include, 278 000 Italians, 164 000 Greeks, 100 000 Yugoslavians, and 60 000 Maltese. The great majority of these immigrants came from rural villages in southern Italy, northern Greece, or Yugoslavia. As already indicated, their rates of coronary heart disease are low, associated with the simpler life-style of a peasant community.

There is evidence now available of increasing rates of coronary heart disease, and certain forms of cancer in relation

Table 4.10. *Comparison of cancer incidence rates* in Japan and for Japanese and Caucasians in Hawaii†*

Primary site of Cancer	Sex	Annual incidence/million people‡		
			Hawaii, 1968–72	
		Japan§	Japanese	Caucasians
Oesophagus	Male	150	46	75
		112		
Stomach	Male	1331	397	217
		1291		
Colon	Male	78	371	368
		87		
Rectum	Male	95	297	204
		90		
Lung	Male	237	379	962
		299		
Prostate	Male	14	154	343
		13		
Breast	Female	335	1221	1869
		295		
Cervix uteri	Female	329	149	243
		398		
Corpus uteri	Female	32	407	714
		20		
Ovary	Female	51	160	274
		55		

*From IARC, 1976.

†From Doll and Peto, 1981.

‡Ages 35–64 years, standardized for age as in IARC, 1976.

§For each type of cancer, upper entry shows incidence in Miyagi prefecture, 1968–71; lower entry shows incidence in Osaka prefecture, 1970–71.

Table 4.11. *Comparison of Australian death rates from coronary heart disease for Italian migrants and Australian-born per 100 000 men at risk. (From Stenhouse and McCall, 1970)*

Country of birth	Period of residence in Australia (years)	Age of men		
		40–49 years	50–59 years	60–69 years
Australia		169	592	1472
Italy (WHO 1963)		70	228	655
	0–6	16	123	260
	7–19	51	170	376
	20 +	130	344	758

to the period of residence in Australia. The longer the southern European immigrant resides in Australia the greater is his likelihood of contracting these diseases and contracting them more often than if he had remained in his native country (Table 4.11) (Stenhouse and McCall 1970; McMichael *et al.* 1980). Examination of deaths due to colorectal cancer reveals similar trends in migrants from Greece, Italy, and Yugoslavia. The risk is increased by 2–3 times after 15 years residence in Australia (Table 4.12). While many factors may operate there is no doubt that one important factor in these trends is diet.

A comparison of the diet available for consumption per person per day in Australia and Italy, and in Japan is shown in Table 4.13. This reveals the much higher intake of food derived from carbohydrate in the Italian population and the lower intake of fat particularly from saturated fat. Animal

Table 4.12. *Age–sex standardized relative risk of death (SRR), during 1962–76, from cancers of the colon and rectum in migrants to Australia, aged 30-plus, by duration of residence. (Australian-born population = 1.0; numbers of migrant deaths shown in parentheses)*

Country of origin	Cancer of			
	Colon		Rectum	
	≤ 16 years	>16 years	≤ 16 years	> 16 years
England	0.99 (497)	1.04 (2327)	1.23 (215)	1.04 (800)
Scotland	1.47 (126)	1.24 (675)	1.05 (33)	1.08 (216)
Ireland	0.62 (26)	1.06* (218)	1.17 (13)	1.18 (90)
Poland	1.02 (33)	1.14 (106)	0.43 (15)	1.34* (40)
Yugoslavia	0.47 (21)	0.66 (37)	0.46 (14)	1.34* (22)
Greece	0.36 (24)	0.69* (58)	0.34 (11)	0.70* (24)
Italy	0.37 (65)	0.70* (183)	0.48 (31)	0.80* (80)

*Differs from mortality ratio for ≤ 16 years, $p < 0.05$.

Source: McMichael *et al.*, 1980.

Table 4.13. *Nutrients available for consumption per person per day, USA, Italy, Japan, 1954–65 and Australia, 1962–65*

	USA	Australia	Italy	Japan
Total protein (g)	94	91	79	68
Animal protein (g)	68	60	27	16
Total carbohydrate (g)	372	411	423	425
Total fat (g)	135	130	77	25
Saturated fat (g)	49	(48)*	21	5
Polyunsaturated fat (g)	16	(16)*	13	7
Cholesterol (mg)	586	(397)*	246	129

*Actual consumption for an Australian group consuming 128 g total fat/day (Baghurst and Record 1983).

protein is also lower in the Italian population although total protein is not different, indicating a greater plant protein intake derived from cereal. These differences have been confirmed in a recent study of the diet of Italian migrants carried out in Perth (Hopkins *et al.* 1980). Current research suggests very strongly the importance of these differences in relation to the different rates of coronary heart disease and cancer in the two populations.

CAUSES OF NUTRITIONAL DISORDERS

As has been pointed out in the preceding two sections, there are in the broad sense, two major categories of nutritional disorders – those of undernutrition (due to deficit of protein, essential minerals or vitamins), and those due to overnutrition (due to excessive intake of energy (calories), fat, sugar, and alcohol).

Clearly in undernutrition we are dealing with a deficient intake of various essential nutrients. We can then ask what conditions in the environment led to such diets being available. This raises questions regarding the food supply, such as, availability of food, food products and distribution, imports and exports of food, marketing and the choice of food, dependent on income, education, and cultural factors. Finally there are social and economic structures that determine the nature of the food supply – the structures of food production in agriculture and the food processing industry, socio-economic structures in the distribution of wealth both within a nation and internationally. These social and economic structures have political implications which are also therefore relevant to nutritional disorders.

These various levels of causation of nutritional disorders can be grouped into three major categories (Jonsson 1981):

1. Immediate causes.
2. Underlying causes.
3. Basic causes.

We shall consider in detail these three categories of causation separately for undernutrition and overnutrition, and briefly discuss ways in which these causes can be eliminated or reduced with consequent improvement in nutrition and health.

Undernutrition

Immediate causes

Apart from dietary deficiency, immediate causes include excessive requirements due to coincident infection, and rapid growth during pregnancy, in infancy, and in adolescence. Undernutrition is being prevented or reduced by the provision of primary health care at village level in developing countries as a result of the major initiative by the WHO dating from the World Health Conference held at Alma Ata, Russia, in 1978. Primary health care includes health education, simple medical care by a volunteer trainee, preservation of a safe water supply through sanitation, vaccination, breast feeding, and improved food supply at village level.

Underlying causes

These include inadequate food supply due to failure of agricultural production or the distribution of food.

Failure of agricultural production to meet the need for food

Since the Second World War inadequate food supplies for larger or smaller groups of people have become very familiar. There were inevitably serious disruptions during the war and food rationing was necessary in many countries for survival. After the war, famine was widespread, but by 1955 food supplies in Europe had reached a level at least as good as before the war. However, in many developing countries inadequacies persist, and continue up to the present time.

The major factor in the persistence of nutrition problems is the increase in population size which has been discussed already. The FAO publishes annually an index based on estimates of national food production in relation to population. If the mean value for 1961–65 was taken as 100, indices for 1975 averaged 100 for countries in Africa, the Near East, the Far East, and Latin America, and 114 for countries in western Europe, North America, and Oceania (FAO 1977). It is clear that in the former group of developing countries agriculture is only just keeping up with the increase in population.

The solution of this problem through reduction in fertility has been briefly considered earlier in this chapter and will be further discussed in Volume 2, Chapter 4. Other possibilities to be considered are improvements in agricultural production through increase in land use for agriculture of many unused areas, or more efficient farming.

Agricultural production is subject to natural and man-made hazards. Natural hazards include the climate – the vagaries of which are still essentially uncontrollable. Drought is occurring somewhere in the world all the time – this applies particularly to India, China, parts of Africa, the Americas, and Australia. In India and China, years in which only 20 per cent of the average rainfall occurs may alternate with years of floods which burst the banks of rivers and so destroy the crops. Flood control through water engineering has been a high priority in the programme of the People's Republic of China since the Revolution in 1949 and the partial harnessing of the Yangtze and the Yellow Rivers was a great achievement. The provision of suitable dams with or without the development of hydroelectric power is a feature of modern development programmes in the Third World.

The major man-made hazard to agricultural production is soil erosion. The immediate factors are wind and water after removal of forest for agricultural purposes leads to loss of the permanent holding structure for the soil. This effect is compounded by the grazing of animals, particularly goats, who eat the roots of plants (unlike cattle or sheep) and also consume the bark and the leaves of trees and so destroy them. This leads to further loosening of the soil which is then washed away by rain or wind leaving an arid area. This process occurred in the production of the deserts of North Africa – formerly the pride of the Roman Empire providing a major source for grain and olive oil. After the fall of Rome, the Berber and Arab tribes grazed their flocks of goats, sheep, and camels without restriction over this area. Dams and reservoirs were neglected and so the stage was set for the formation of deserts. Similar changes occurred in Iraq and Iran where huge irrigation schemes involving the Tigris and Euphrates Rivers formerly supported large and flourishing populations.

Inefficient farming practices are characteristic of the Third World where patterns of farming have remained unchanged for many thousands of years. For example in Thailand and China the threshing floor for grain, the water buffalo, and the single farmer ploughing the paddy fields are still to be seen everywhere. Agriculture can be made more efficient as in Europe, but the problems of change including rural unemployment are very great.

In India, inefficient farming practices are reinforced by the religious (Hindu) taboo on the slaughter of cattle and the consumption of beef. The pressure on the land by these animals is very great when added to that of the human population. It has been estimated that half of India's enormous number of cattle have no economic value. In China by contrast, animals are much less frequent due to greater human pressure on the land and the absence of religious taboos.

A comparison of wheat and rice yields from various countries is shown in Table 4.14. The variations in

Table 4.14. *Yields of cereals in various countries in 100 kg per hectare. (From FAO, 1971)*

Wheat		Rice	
Netherlands	46.0	Spain	60.2
UK	42.1	Japan	54.8
United Arab Republic	26.5	USA	50.4
USA	21.4	Italy	49.8
Canada	18.2	Malaysia	27.9
USSR	13.8	Sri Lanka	26.3
India	12.3	Indonesia	20.9
Pakistan	11.1	Thailand	19.6
Iraq	5.6	India and Pakistan	17.0
Libya	2.3	Uganda	8.0

productivity are very great. They reflect the use of modern farming techniques in the developed countries which theoretically are available to developing countries. However, heavy inputs of energy in the form of fossil fuels are required which impose heavy constraints on most developing countries.

The Green Revolution, resulting from the development of high yield wheat and rice seeds by the International Maize and Wheat Improvement Center in Mexico, and the International Rice Research Institute in the Philippines respectively, has been a highly significant development. The new durable varieties of wheat (Sonora 64 and Lenna Reja 64) commonly yield 4 tons (even sometimes 5–8 tons) per hectare in comparison to 1–3 tons by the standard varieties. The same applies to IR8 rice where yields can be increased up to four times.

These new strains were first used on a large scale in 1967. In 1970–71 the harvest of food grain in India was adequate to meet national needs for the first time for many years. However, by 1974 India was importing cereals again to meet famine conditions in large areas of Maharastra. The new varieties require heavy fertilizer supplies so that they really require a heavier

outlay than a subsistence farmer can provide. The social inequalities and differences between rich and poor tend to be reinforced by the Green Revolution as the benefits have gone to large farmers, capitalists, and multinational corporations.

Increase in cereal production can be deviated for use for fuel as in the case of Brazil where sugar production is being used for the generation of alcohol to meet the shortage of fuel. Large areas of land have been set aside for this purpose rather than the production of food. Finally, increase in agricultural products can be used to produce cash crops for export rather than local food consumption. This applies to the production of soya beans by developing countries for the USA and the production of cheap meat by developing countries for developed countries.

Failure of food distribution

Poverty is the major reason for failure of food distribution – both in the Third World and in the West. In a celebrated and influential analysis Boyd Orr in 1936 published his book *Food, Health and Income*. It contained the results of a survey of 1152 families in each of which the food consumption was weighed for one week and a correlation made between the food consumption per head and the available income in each family. Orr found that 10 per cent failed to reach acceptable standards for energy, protein, vitamins A and C, and the minerals iron and calcium. In the next 40 per cent intakes of minerals and vitamins were below standard. This important study in a developed community is complemented by extensive similar data from developing countries.

In a recent review Reutlinger (1982) of the World Bank emphasizes that the most important determinants of hunger in developing countries are personal levels of income and the prices they must pay for food. Accelerated food production will alleviate hunger only to the extent that the scarce resources used in the process reduce poverty and food prices more than they would if used in other ways.

Basic causes

The basic causes of undernutrition are in the social, economic, and cultural structures that nations have developed over many centuries. There is also a network of international structures, particularly the relations between the developed world and the developing Third World.

It is now recognized more clearly that political and socio-economic factors are all important in the establishment and maintenance of undernutrition. Within a country there are social factors determining the distribution of wealth so that a minority is underprivileged – e.g. in the UK 10 per cent of the population in 1936 did not have enough money to buy the basic food required to maintain life. This situation has been greatly improved in Britain since the Second World War following the establishment of the National Health Service and the modern Social Security System.

Political initiatives on a much larger scale have led to the twentieth century revolutions in Russia and China with great improvement in food supplies for the whole populations of these countries. In China in 1981 there was no protein energy malnutrition – which is a remarkable achievement for a population of one billion. Less than 20 per cent of the land mass of China is arable compared with more than 50 per cent of the USA which has only a slightly smaller land mass (Chen Xue cun, Public Health Institute, Peking, personal communication) and supports less than one-quarter of the population of China.

Overnutrition

Immediate causes

As we have seen, excessive intake of energy due to over consumption of fat, sugar, salt, and alcohol is a major factor in the common diseases of the developed industrial world. This diet which is characteristic of the twentieth century, differs from previous diets in that there is much higher energy density and low content of fibre and other complex carbohydrates. The characteristic of this diet is an excessive intake of energy before satiety is achieved.

The evidence relating this affluent diet to the chronic non-infectious diseases has already been reviewed.

Underlying causes

The underlying cause of overnutrition resides in the nature of the food supply that has developed in the twentieth century. As already pointed out, a highly efficient agriculture has developed in the UK and elsewhere in Europe so that there are now surpluses, particularly the 'butter mountain'. The presence of such a butter mountain leads to attempts to promote the consumption of butter in EEC countries in direct conflict with the interests of good health and the reduction of premature death due to coronary heart disease.

In the USA, there are continuing attempts by primary industry particularly the meat industry, the dairy industry, the egg industry, and the liquor industry to promote their products in accordance with the practices of a free enterprise capitalist society. Similar considerations apply in other industrialized countries. The period of post-war affluence 1950–75 has been associated with heavier consumption of food, alcohol, and non-alcoholic beverages than ever before because all these items have been relatively cheap for the great majority.

There has until recently been a lack of awareness among the people of western nations of these relationships between diet and health. Indeed much of the research has been relatively recent and public controversies continue among scientists much to the confusion of the public. None the less there is evidence of a fall in consumption of dairy products and meat in some countries such as the USA and Australia which reflects greater awareness of health considerations (Walker 1977; Dwyer and Hetzel 1980). Lower fat meats such as chicken, pork, and fish are being consumed by increasing numbers. Consumer pressure for lower sugar content in fruit juices and soft drinks has led to production of increased quantities of these products (Hetzel 1980).

These recent developments indicate the operation of market forces in favour of better nutrition.

Basic causes

Food policy has until recently been determined by food producers – farmer organizations, farm and food companies (which have their political following), and government departments of agriculture. Effort goes not only into improving production with increased efficiency but also to the control of production and the maintenance of income with price supports and subsidies. The conflicts in this situation are well summarized in the statement by Jean Mayer following the White House Conference on Food, Nutrition and Health in 1969.

'Thus, we end up with the Department that simultaneously subsidizes farmers to increased production (through agricultural research, various direct aids to production), pays them not to produce and fixes prices or subsidies to save them from the consequences of over-production (of wheat, corn, cotton, and so forth), which would not have occurred had the government-subsidized programs not existed.'

The Inquiry of the US Senate Select Committee on Nutrition and Human Needs carried out an extensive examination of these issues as recorded in its reports *Nutrition and health* (1975) and *Dietary goals for the United States* (1977). These reports recommended National Food Policy Guidelines similar to those adopted in Scandinavian countries in 1968. These guidelines were the following:

1. Eat a variety of foods.
2. Maintain weight.
3. Avoid too much fat, saturated fat, and cholesterol.
4. Eat foods with adequate starch and fibre content.
5. Avoid too much sugar.
6. Avoid too much sodium.
7. If you drink alcohol do so in moderation.

Subsequent to these reports it is of great interest that in 1980 the US Department of Agriculture was involved in a programme of nutrition education along with the Department of Health, Education and Welfare designed to reduce the consumption of fat and sugar, and increase the consumption of complex carbohydrates.

Similar debates to these in the USA are proceeding in other developed countries in western Europe and in the British Commonwealth countries – Australia, Canada, and New Zealand.

The questions are considered at greater length in Volume 4, Chapter 2, when the question of prevention and the subject of national dietary guidelines is reviewed in detail.

SUMMARY

This chapter has explored the relationship between the nature of the food supply, states of health and disease, and the size of population. Food supplies either through scarcity or abundance have been a major determinant of the size of populations. The increase in food supply in the first and second agricultural revolutions has led to improvements in nutrition which in turn has led to increased resistance to infectious disease, particularly in younger age groups, and so to rises in population numbers. In developing countries, improvements in food supply have been unable to keep pace with the 'explosive' increase in population size due to falls in infant and child mortality. Very large numbers are still suffering from undernutrition with inadequate energy, mineral, or less commonly, vitamin intake. In the twentieth century, in developed countries, a mass excess of food intake (particularly fats and sugar) over requirement has occurred with the unprecedented occurrence of coronary heart disease as the major public health problem.

Communities differ greatly in their dietary patterns depending on differences in agriculture and food production. In the hunter-gatherer ecosystem the diet is mainly vegetarian which is associated with low fat intake and low rates of coronary heart disease – population numbers are carefully limited in view of the uncertainty of food supplies and good nutrition is usually maintained. In the peasant agricultural ecosystem the food supply tends to be of fixed pattern dependent on a staple cereal. Mineral and vitamin deficiencies are likely to occur and some form of supplementation is usually required to prevent these. In the affluent industrial ecosystem an unprecedented abundance of food, with high refined carbohydrate and fat content, and high intake of alcohol, together with a sedentary life-style has led to overnutrition with high rates of obesity, diabetes, hypertension, and coronary heart disease. Recent evidence suggests that certain common forms of cancer (e.g. breast, bowel) are also related to such a diet.

Dietary transitions due to changes in the pattern of food supply further indicate the close relation of food with health. In the Pacific Island populations a drastic change has occurred from a predominantly cereal and fish diet to a western diet with the appearance of diabetes mellitus, hypertension, and coronary heart disease. Similar changes have occurred in the Japanese with emigration to the USA and in the predominantly peasant southern European populations who have emigrated to Australia.

The immediate dietary causes of undernutrition and overnutrition arise from underlying factors in the pattern of agriculture and food production. The need to produce crops for cash or fuel in developing countries and the maintenance of existing patterns of agriculture ('the butter mountain') in the West are significant structural factors affecting food supply and public health. Such economic structures have major national and international political implications which require attention before major changes can come about that would improve nutrition and public health.

The adoption of dietary guidelines by many western countries designed to modify the western diet has encountered much opposition, but changes in food preference are occurring, dependent on nutrition education arising from recent research on the connections between food and health.

REFERENCES

Abbie, A.A. (1951–52). The Australian Aborigine. *Oceania* **22**, 91.

Armstrong, B.K. (1979). Diet and hormones in the epidemiology of breast and endometrial cancers. *Nutr. Cancer* **1**, 90.

Baghurst, K.I. and Record, S (1983). Intake and sources in selected Australian Sub-populations of dietary constituents implicated in the aetiology of chronic diseases *J. Food Nutr.* **40**, 1.

Basedow, H. (1932). Diseases of Australian Aborigines. *J. Trop. Med. Hyg.* **35**, 177.

Behar, M. (1974). A deadly combination. *World Health* Feb/March, 29.

Bengoa, J.M. (1971). The state of world nutrition. In *Man, food and nutrition* (ed. M. Rechigl, Jr) p. 1. CRC Press, Cleveland.

Bennett, P.H., Rushfort, N.B., Miller, M., Le Compte, P.M. (1976). Epidemiologic studies in diabetes in the Pima Indians. *Recent Prog. Horm. Res.* **32**, 333.

Blackburn, H. (1979). Conference on health effects of blood lipids: optimal distributions for populations, workshop report: epidemiological section. *Prev. Med.* **8**, 612.

Bronte-Stewart, B., Budtz-Olsen, O.E., Hickley, J.M., and Brock, J.F. (1960). The health and nutritional status of the Kung Bushmen of South-West Africa. *J. Lab. Clin. Med.* **56**, 187.

Bruun, K., Edwards, G., Lumio, M. *et al.* (1975). *Alcohol control policies in public health perspective,* Finnish Foundation for Alcohol Studies, Vol. 25. FORSSA, Finland.

Burkitt, D.P. and Trowell, H.C. (eds.) (1975). *Refined carbohydrate foods and disease: some implications of dietary fibre.* Academic Press, New York.

Casley-Smith, J.R. (1958–59). The haematology of the Central Australian Aborigines. Parts 1 and 2. *Aust. J. Exp. Biol. Med. Sci.* **36**, 23, 37, 451.

Clark, C. and Turner, J.B. (1971). World population growth and future food trends. In *Man, food and nutrition* (ed. M. Rechigl, Jr) p. 55. CRC Press, Cleveland.

Clarren, S.K. and Smith, D.W. (1978). The fetal alcohol syndrome. *N. Engl. J. Med.* **298**, 1063.

Doll, R. (1979). Nutrition and cancer: a review. *Nutr. Cancer* **1**, 35.

Doll, R. and Peto, R. (1981). Avoidable risks of cancer in the U.S. *J. Nat. Cancer. Inst.* **66**, 1161.

Dwyer, T. and Hetzel, B.S. (1980). A comparison of trends of coronary heart disease mortality in Australia, USA and England and Wales with reference to three major risk factors – hypertension, cigarette smoking and diet. *Int. J. Epidemiol.* **9**, 65.

Elphinstone, J.J. (1971). The health of Australian Aborigines with no previous associations with Europeans. *Med. J. Aust.* **2**, 293.

Edwards, F.M., Wise, P.H., Thomas, D.W., Murchland, J.B., and Craig, R.J. (1976). Blood pressure and electrocardiographic findings on the South Australian Aborigines. *Aust. N.Z. J. Med.* **6**, 167.

Food and Agriculture Organization (1971). *The state of food and agriculture.* FAO, Rome.

Food and Agriculture Organization (1977). *The state of food and agriculture.* FAO, Rome.

Food and Agriculture Organization (1978). *Dietary fats and oils in human nutrition. Report of an expert consultation jointly organized by the FAO and WHO, Rome, Sept. 1977.* FAO, Rome.

Friend, G., Page, L., and Marston, R. (1979). Food consumption patterns in the United States: 1909–13 to 1976. In *Nutrition, lipids and coronary heart disease* (ed. R. Levy, B. Rifkind, B. Dennis, and N. Ernst) p. 489. Raven Press, New York.

Gwatkin, D.R. and Brandel, S.K. (1982). Life expectancy and population growth in the Third World. *Scient. Am.* **246**, 33.

Hansen, J.D.L., Truswell, A.S., and MacHutchon, B. (1969). The children of hunting and gathering bushmen. *S. Afr. Med. J.* **43**, 1158.

Hetzel, B.S. (1974). The epidemiology, pathogenesis and control of endemic goitre and endemic cretinism in New Guinea. *N.Z. Med. J.* **80**, 482.

Hetzel, B.S. (1978). The implications of increasing alcohol consumption in Australia today. *Community Health Studies* **2**, 81.

Hetzel, B.S. (1979). A review of Australian research and action on alcohol and traffic safety. In *Proceedings 7th International Conference on Alcohol. Drugs and Traffic Safety, Melbourne, Victoria,* p. 354. Aust. Govt. Publishing Service, Canberra.

Hetzel, B.S. (1980). *Health and Australian society,* 3rd ed. Penguin, Melbourne.

Hetzel, B.S. and Dwyer, T. (1981). Soft fats: harder evidence. *Lancet* i, 1104.

Hetzel, B.S. and Frith, H.J. (eds.) (1978). *The nutrition of Aborigines in relation to the eco-system of Central Australia.* CSIRO, Melbourne.

Hopkins, S., Margetts, B.M., Cohen, J., and Armstrong, B.K. (1980). Dietary change among Italians and Australians in Perth. *Community Health Studies* 2, 67.

Howard, A. (ed.) (1975). *Recent advances in obesity research. Proceedings of the 1st International Conference on Obesity.* Newman Publishing, London.

International Agency for Research on Cancer (1976). *Cancer incidence in five continents,* Vol. III (Eds. J. Waterhouse, C. Muir, P. Correa *et al.*) p. 584. IARC Sci. Publ. 3, Lyon.

Jonsson, U. (1981). The causes of hunger. *Food Nutr. Bull.* 3, 1.

Kagawa, Y. (1978). Impact of Westernization on the nutrition of Japanese. *Prev. Med.* 7, 205.

Lewis, B. (1979). Conference on health effects of blood lipids: optimal distribution for populations, workshop report: clinical pathology section. *Prev. Med.* 8, 679.

McArthur, M. (1960). Report of the nutrition unit. In *Records of the American–Australian Scientific Expedition to Arnhem Land* (ed. C.P. Mounford). Melbourne University Press.

McKeown, T. (1976). *The modern rise of population.* Academic Press, New York.

McMahon, B., Cole, P., and Brown, J.B. (1973). Etiology of human breast cancer. *J. Natl. Cancer Inst.* 50, 21.

McMichael, A.J., Potter, J.D., and Hetzel, B.S. (1979). Time trends in colo-rectal cancer mortality in relation to food and alcohol consumption: United States, United Kingdom, Australia and New Zealand. *Int. J. Epidemiol.* 8, 295.

McMichael, A.J., McCall, M.G., Hartshorne, J.M., and Woodings, T.L. (1980). Patterns of gastrointestinal cancer in European migrants to Australia: the role of dietary changes. *Int. J. Cancer* 25, 431.

Maddocks, I. (1978). Papua New Guinea: Pari Village. In *Basic health care in developing countries: an epidemiological perspective* (ed. B.S. Hetzel) p. 11. Oxford University Press.

Malcolm, K. (1970). *Growth and development in New Guinea: a study of the Bundi People of the Madang Subdistrict.* Institute of Human Biology Monograph Series No. 1. Madang, New Guinea.

Marmot, M.G., Syme, S.L., Kats, H., Cohen, J.B., and Bolsky, J. (1975). Epidemiologic studies of coronary heart disease and stroke in Japanese men living in Japan, Hawaii and California. Prevalence of coronary heart disease and hypertensive heart disease and associated risk factors. *Am. J. Epidemiol.* 102, 514.

Mayer, J. (ed.) (1973). *U.S. nutrition policies in the seventies.* Freeman Press, San Francisco.

Ministry of Public Health, Thailand (1981). *Country report.* Nutrition Division, Bangkok.

Neel, J.V. (1969). Current concepts of the genetic basis of diabetes mellitus and the biological significance of the diabetic predisposition. In *Diabetes* (ed. J. Ostman and R.D.G. Milner) p. 68. Excerpta Medica, Amsterdam.

Oiso, T. (1971). Recent annual changes in nutrition in Japan. In *Diabetes mellitus in Asia 1970* (ed. S. Tsuji and M. Wada). Excerpta Medica, Amsterdam.

Orr-Boyd, J. (1936). *Food, health and income.* Macmillan, London.

Paul, A., Southgate, D., McCance, R.A., and Widdowson, E., (eds.) (1978). *The composition of food.* HMSO, London.

Prior, I. and Tasman-Jones, C. (1981). New Zealand Maori and Pacific. In *Western Diseases: their emergence and prevention (eds. H.C. Trowell and D.P. Burkitt)* p. 227. Arnold, London.

Reutlinger, S. (1982). *World Bank research on the hunger dimension* of the food problem. *Research News World Bank.* Winter 1981/82.

Schwartz, C.J. and Caseley-Smith, J.R. (1958a). Serum cholesterol levels in atherosclerotic subjects and in the Australian Aborigines. *Med. J. Aust.* 2, 84.

Schwartz, C.J. and Caseley-Smith, J.R. (1958b). Atherosclerosis and the serum mucoprotein levels of the Australian Aborigine. *Aust. J. Exp. Biol. Med. Sci.* 36, 117.

Sinnett, P.F. (1977). *The people of Murapin.* Institute of Medical Research, Papua New Guinea. E.W. Classey, Faringdon, Oxon.

Sinnett, P.F. and Whyte, H.M. (1981). Papua New Guinea. In *Western diseases: their emergence and prevention* (ed. H.C. Trowell and D.P. Burkitt) p. 171. Arnold, London.

Stenhouse, N.S. and McCall, M.G. (1970). Differential mortality from cardiovascular disease in migrants from England and Wales, Scotland and Italy, and native-born Australians. *J. Chronic Dis.* 23, 423.

Surgeon General's Report on Health Promotion and Disease Prevention (1979). *Healthy people.* Department of Health, Education and Welfare, Washington.

Tanner, J.M., Whitehouse, R.H., and Takaishi, M. (1966). Standards from birth to maturity for height, weight, height velocity and weight velocity for British children 1965. *Arch. Dis. Child.* 41, 454.

US Department of Health, Education and Welfare (1979). Fats, cholesterol and sodium intakes in the diets of persons 1–74 years. United States, In *Vital and health statistics of the National Center for Health Statistics* No. 54. DHEW, Hyattsville, Md.

US Senate Select Committee on Nutrition and Human Needs (1975). *Nutrition and health,* U.S. GPO, Washington, DC.

US Senate Select Committee on Nutrition and Human Needs (1977). *Dietary goals for the United States.* U.S. GPO, Washington, DC.

Walker, W.J. (1977). Changing United States life style and declining vascular mortality: cause or coincidence. *N. Engl. J. Med.* 297, 163.

Weinsier, R.L. (1976). Overview: salt and the development of hypertension. *Prev. Med.* 5, 7–14.

Wehmeyer, A.S., Lee, R.B., and Whiting, M. (1969). The nutrient composition and dietary importance of some vegetable foods eaten by the Kung Bushmen. *S. Afr. Med. J.* 43, 1529.

White, S.A. (1915). Aborigines of the Everard Range. *Trans. R. Soc. S. Aust.* 39, 725.

Wise, P.H., Edwards, F.M., Craig, R.J., Evans, B., Murchland J.B., Sutherland, B., and Thomas, D.W. (1976). Diabetes and associated variables in the South Australian Aboriginal. *Aust. N.Z. J. Med.* 6, 191.

Wissler, R.W. (1979). Conference on the health effects of blood lipids: optimal distribution for populations, workshop report: laboratory–experimental section. *Prev. Med.* 8, 715.

World Health Organization (1978). Declaration of Alma Ata. *WHO Chronicle* 32, 428.

Yamamoto, S. (1981). Japan. In *Western diseases: their emergence and prevention* (ed. H.C. Trowell and D.P. Burkitt) p. 337. Arnold, London.

Zimmet, P. and Whitehouse, S. (1981). Pacific Islands of Nauru, Tuvalu and Western Samoa. In *Western diseases, their emergence and prevention* (ed. H.D. Trowell and D.P. Burkitt) p. 204. Arnold, London.

FURTHER READING

Boyd-Orr, J. (1936). *Food, Health and Income*. Macmillan, London.

Davidson, S., Passmore, R., Brock, J.F., and Truswell, A.S. (1979). *Human nutrition and dietetics.*, 7th edn. Churchill Livingstone, Edinburgh.

Gwatkin, D.R. and Brandel, S.K. (1982). Life expectancy and population growth in the Third World. *Scient. Am.* **246, 33**.

Tanahill, R. (1975). *Food in history*. Paladin, St. Albans, Herts.

Trowell, H.C. and Burkitt, D.P. (eds.) (1981). *Western diseases: their emergence and prevention*. Arnold, London.

McKeown, T. (1976). *The modern rise of population*. Academic Press, New York.

5 Hazards in the physical environment

Virgil H. Freed

INTRODUCTION

Potential hazards in the physical environment can be categorized as either biological or physical. Biological hazards range from viruses and microorganisms through to higher organisms such as poisonous plants. The physical agents include such things as various types of radiation, noise, and chemicals. Biological agents are dealt with in other chapters as are such physical hazards as noise and radiation. Here I will concentrate on chemical hazards.

Some of these agents are indigenous to the environment while others arise as products or by-products of man's activities. The latter probably are of greater concern in public health but are also the most accessible to mitigation.

Chemical hazards in the physical environment, have received more attention in recent years than any other agents. In particular, concern has been focused on the anthropogenic chemicals such as vinyl chloride (Environmental Health Perspectives 1977b), halomethanes, PCBs (polychlorobiphenyls) (National Research Council 1979), and dioxins (Tucker et al. 1983), each of which has been implicated as a public health hazard.

Agents in the physical environment must be regarded as constituting not only an objective physical hazard, but also as a hazard to mental and emotional well-being. The depth of concern of residents in the vicinity of hazardous waste disposal sites or environmental exposure to chemicals, exacts its emotional toll as well (Slovic et al. 1979; Hay 1982; Levine 1983). It is incumbent on the public health practitioner, therefore, to keep both of these aspects in mind when addressing hazards within the physical environment.

It is as important when dealing with chemical hazards, as it is with biological hazards, to identify the source – whether point or non-point – and beyond this to have a firm grasp of how these agents move and behave in the environment to bring about the inadvertent exposure. It is to these topics that the following sections of this chapter are addressed.

SOURCES AND TYPES OF AGENTS

The sources of agents in the physical environment are many and varied. There are natural sources such as geological formation, vulcanism, decomposition of biological material, and water. The anthropogenic sources are as varied as human activity itself and include recovery of renewable and non-renewable resources, manufacturing, fabrication, agriculture, generation of energy, disposal of waste products, and so on. Sources rising out of man's activity may be categorized to either point, that is fixed sources, or non-point, that is sources that may be mobile or widespread. The agents themselves are sometimes categorized by the medium in which they are found, (for example, soil, food, water, air), by their physical state, and by class or composition (Lippmann and Schlesinger 1978).

Natural sources in some instances give rise to as much or more of a given agent than anthropogenic sources. For example, the sea is a source of a number of volatile halogen and sulphur substituted alkanes in amounts of $50–100 \times 10^6$ tons per year (Lovelock et al. 1972; Andreae and Raemdonck 1983). Similarly, volcanic activity annually results in the release of hundreds of millions of tons of sulphur dioxide and to a lesser extent hydrogen sulphide (Horne 1978). Anthropogenic sources give rise not only to a complex array of inorganic and organic agents but also to very substantial quantities of some of them. Combustion of fossil fuel for different purposes contributes annually almost 150 million tons of sulphur dioxide and in excess of 50 million tons of nitrogen dioxide (Lippmann and Schlesinger 1978). Similarly, combustion results in the release of polyaromatic hydrocarbons and a variety of other organic compounds (Bumb et al. 1980).

Mining and smelting of minerals results in the release of substantial quantities of mineral elements such as arsenic, beryllium, cadmium, chromium, lead, nickel, and other metals. In addition, mineral fibres, for example asbestos associated with the mineral or for use itself, escape into the environment in these operations. Utilization or manufacture of organic chemicals is a source of many millions of tons of waste and by-products of a great complexity. Whereas the polymers of the plastic industry are much less of a hazard, the monomers may comprise a significant public health hazard in a local region (Environmental Health Perspectives 1977b).

The biologically-based industries, specifically agriculture and forestry, contribute significant amounts of agents to the physical environment either through direct use or as waste products. Pesticides have received the most attention, but in addition, the industries must contend with crop and animal waste, and fertilizer contamination of water and air. Sediments arising from agriculture and forestry are a substantial concern for water systems (National Research Council 1977).

Table 5.1 provides examples of sources and types of agents in the physical environment.

Table 5.1. *Examples of sources and types of agents*

Source	Type of agent	Commonly encountered in
Natural		
Geological formation	As, Se, other metals	Water, plant
	Inorganic anions and cations	
Water	Halomethanes	Air
	Dibromoethane	
	salt aerosols	
Volcanoes	SO_2, dusts, organics	Air
Biota	Hydrocarbons, pollen	Air
	Mycotoxins	Food
Anthropogenic		
Point sources		
Mining and smelting	As, Cd, Pb, Hg	Air, water
	Asbestos	
	SO_2	
Manufacture fabrication	Metals (As, Cd, Hg, Pb, Cr, etc.), asbestos	Air, water
	Organics (phenols, hydrocarbons, chloroorganics, heterocycles)	
Combustion fossil fuels	Hg, SO_2, NO_x, CO	Air
(power generation, heating)	Hydrocarbons, other organics (e.g. PAH)	
Disposal	Complex mixtures of solids, metals	Water, air
	Organics	Soil
Non-point		
Cars/transportation	Hydrocarbons, CO, Pb, organics, NO_x	Air, roadside soil
Agriculture	NO_3, crop and animal wastes, pesticides	Water, air, some crops
Urban and rural runoff	PAHs, metals	Water
	Sediment, various organics	

DYNAMICS OF AGENTS IN THE ENVIRONMENT

Physical aspects

The pathway of a chemical through the environment following release from a source may be circuitous and have many feedback loops (Freed *et al.* 1977). On a large, even global scale, the pathways are dependent upon major factors of the ecological and climatic systems. These factors include solar energy flux and gravitational fields as well as atmospheric and aquatic gradients. The interaction of the physico-chemical properties of a substance plays a significant role in its transport and in its availability for transport even on the global scale. At lower levels of environmental resolution, it is probable that physical properties such as vapour pressure, water solubility, and partition coefficient are of major importance (Kenaga 1975; Chiou *et al.* 1977; Brown 1978). Wide differences in the environmental behaviour of chemicals and minerals are attributable, in large measure, to their physical properties. Table 5.2 lists several organic chemical substances and illustrates these differences in their physical properties.

Tracing a contaminant through the environment to ultimate exposure of man requires some understanding of the nature of the environment itself. The environment has been classified into five fundamental phases: the lithosphere, the hydrosphere, the atmosphere, and the biota (represented by plants and animals). The estimated relative masses of the different phases are as follows:

Animals	2×10^{13} kg
Plants	1.1×10^{15} kg
Atmosphere	5.3×10^{18} kg
Lithosphere	1.1×10^{17} kg
Hydrosphere	1.3×10^{21} kg

When released to the environment, a chemical will become distributed among different components of the environment depending on the properties of the chemical and the properties of the different components of the environment. Through interaction of these properties, the chemical will exhibit a greater affinity for and hence higher concentration in one or more compartments despite the cyclic and reversible nature of transport processes (Freed *et al.* 1977). A simplistic view of the chemical's distribution indicates a relationship similar to the Boltzmann equation shown below:

$$N_{ij} = N_0 e - \frac{\varepsilon\, ij}{\varkappa T}$$

If we assume that: $N_{ij} = n_{ij}$ and $N_{ij} = 0$
when: $i = j$ and $N_0 = N_1 + N_2 + N_3 + N_4 + N_5$

N_0 is the number of molecules of the chemical initially introduced and $N_1 \ldots N_5$ are the number of molecules in respective components of the environment. In the above equation ε represents the energy barrier between two components, $\varkappa$ represents the Boltzmann constant, and T represents the absolute temperature. To understand the behaviour of the chemical in environmental components, a knowledge of the physical and chemical properties of the chemical is needed. Table 5.3 summarizes the role of different physical properties in chemical transport and distribution. Chemicals experience a number of physical subprocesses in the environment including sorption, vaporization, dissolution, and micro-scale movement. The chemical's behaviour in any one of these subprocesses is related to its physical properties and also to its reactivity.

Table 5.2. *Properties of some commonly used chemicals*

Compound	Molecular weight	m.p. (°C)	b.p. (°C)	Solubility in H_2O p.p.m. (temp, °C)	Vapour pressure	Partition coefficient octanol/H_2O
DDT	354.5	108.5		0.0034 (25)	1.9×10^{-7} (20)	1.55×10^6
Dieldrin	381	175–176		0.25 (25)	1.9×10^{-6} (20)	
					2.6×10^{-6} (20)	
					2.0×10^{-6} (20)	
1,2-dibromoethane (EDB)	187.872	9.97	131.65	3520 (20)	7.69 (20)	98.8
					10.83 (25.1)	
1,2-dichloroethane	98.960	−35.4	83.483	8450 (20)	62.1 (20.21)	25.0
2,4-D (acid)	221	140.5		522 (25)	0.4 (160)	6.4×10^2
Malathion	330	2.85		145 (20)	0.55×10^{-5} (20)	781
				300 (30)		
Parathion	291	6.1		11.9 (20)	3.78×10^{-5} (20)	6.4×10^3
				11 (40)	1.96×10^{-5} (20)	
					4.39×10^{-6} (20)	
					5.7×10^{-6} (20)	
Leptophos	412	70.2–70.6		0.0047 (20)		2.0×10^6
		71.5–72.0		0.03 (25)		
Chlorpyrifos	350.5	42–43.4		0.4 (23)	1.87×10^{-5} (25)	1.29×10^5
Phosalone	368	48		10		2.0×10^4
				2.15 (20)		
Carbaryl (Sevin)	201	142		114 (24)	<0.005 (26)	
Propoxur (Baygon)	209	91.5		~2000 (20)	3×10^{-6} (20)	
Chlorpropham (CIPC)	213.7	41.4	247	102.3 (25)		
EPTC (Eptam)	189		235	375 (25)	1.55×10^{-1} (25)	
					1.62×10^{-2} (23)	
					1.97×10^{-2} (24)	

Table 5.3. *Role of physical properties in transport and distribution of chemicals in the environment*

Physical property	Related to
1. Solubility in water	Leaching, partitioning, mobility in environment
2. Partition coefficient	Bioaccumulation potential, sorption by organic matter
3. Vapour pressure	Atmosphere mobility, rate of vaporization
4. Reactivity	
Hyrolysis	Persistence in environment or biota
Ionization	Route and mechanism of adsorption or uptake, persistence, interaction with other molecular species

Sorption

Upon its release into the environment, a chemical is likely to encounter solid surfaces. Due to the dipole of the molecule (and other molecular forces) and the surface forces of the encountered solid, an interaction will occur that is important to the ultimate fate of the chemical and dictates its transport, bio-availability, and persistence. While the nature of the surface is important, the properties of the chemical often determine the degree of interaction (Hamaker 1975). The interaction for non-ionic compounds involves Van der Waals' forces and molecular dipoles. Ionic forms may react or interact through ion exchange. The overall interaction of a chemical with a surface may be written as follows:

Chemical + surface $\rightleftharpoons$ (chemical · surface) + (surface*) + (chemical*)

where asterisks represent unreacted chemical absorption at equilibrium.

The soil matrix represents a heterogeneous mixture of constituents such as organic matter, sand, clays, and inorganic salts. These constituents present a large surface area with many sites on which sorption can occur. While the bulk of the adsorption may be from solution, adsorption also occurs from chemicals present in the vapour state. Equilibrium in a chemical–soil system may be presented as follows:

$$P(H_2O)x = S(H_2O)_y \rightleftharpoons P(H_2O)_z S$$

where P and S represent the compound and soil matrix, respectively. With sufficient water present, the chemical molecule and the soil matrix will both be in the hydrated form. The symbols x, y, and z, in the equation denote the hydration number of the chemical, of the soil, and of the chemical–soil complex respectively. The equilibrium constant K_E for the reaction is:

$$K_E = \frac{[P(H_2O)_z S]}{[P(H_2O)x] \, [S(H_2O)y]}.$$

Here, the quantities in brackets represent the activity of the compound. An exact determination of K_E is difficult since it is very hard to obtain the exact volume occupied by the adsorbed chemical. Usually, adsorption data for a chemical–soil system are represented with a Freundlich isotherm:

$$x/m = KC^n$$

where x/m is the amount of chemical adsorbed per weight of the adsorbant, C is the equilibrium concentration of the chemical, and K and n are constants. For dilute solutions of many chemicals, the value of n approaches unity. Sorption also depends upon the specific chemical under investigation (Helling and Dragun 1981). Inorganic salts and organic cations may adsorb to clay portions of soil through exchange reactions. Most neutral organic molecules follow a physical type of sorption and the amount of chemical sorbed is in many cases inversely related to its solubility in water (Hamaker and Thompson 1972).

Sorption of chemicals from aqueous solution is in most cases an exothermic process. Usually a lowering of temperature leads to an increased heat of adsorption. For most non-ionized compounds the adsorption ranges only a few kcal/mole indicating a physical type of sorption; or, in some cases, weak hydrogen bonding between the adsorbate and the surface (Chiou *et al.* 1979; Chiou and Schmedding 1981). For most neutral organic molecules, sorption is of the physical type wherein a monolayer of the chemical is formed on the surface upon which many layers are built up. By analogy to the adsorption of gases on solids, the heat of adsorption for aqueous solutions of a chemical should be in the range of the heat of solution. The low energy involved in the adsorption of non-polar molecules by a soil has suggested to some investigators that this may be a partitioning process. This view gains credibility due to the close correlation between sorption of such molecules and soil organic matter.

Transport in soil

Another important process that controls the transport of a chemical in a soil matrix is the chemical's movement with water, a process termed leaching (Helling and Dragun 1981). Leaching may take place in three directions: downward (the usual direction of water movement), lateral, and upward. Upward movement, a result of upward mass transfer of water resulting from surface evaporation, may concentrate a chemical at the soil surface. There is a close correlation between sorption on soil organic matter and leaching as reflected by a chemical's partition coefficient (K_{oc}).

The movement of water downward in soil is thought to be in the form of a film and is produced by combined effects of capillary and gravitational forces. Chemicals are usually applied to the soil surface. Water also arriving at the surface may dissolve and carry the chemical with it as the water percolates through the soil. The displacement of the chemical under rapid percolation of water is predominantly with the bulk of the water solution. Counteracting this downward movement is the tendency for isodiametric (multidirectional) diffusion of the chemical in solution. Where water percolation is rapid, the movement of the chemical will be in the direction of water flow; but, as water percolation becomes slower, diffusion becomes a greater factor in determining the chemical's distribution. There is a dynamic equilibrium between the free chemical and the chemical in the sorbed phase as the chemical is carried through the soil profile. As a consequence, a chemical that is tightly sorbed to soil should be leached slowly and vice versa. In practice, the important factors controlling leaching are: (i) water solubility of chemical; (ii) extent of chemical adsorption; (iii) soil type; and (iv) amount and intensity of water percolation. A highly soluble chemical (having a low enthalpy of absorption) will be leached rapidly due to its tendency to go into solution. As a consequence, the amount of chemical carried in the soil will be proportional to the amount of water available to dissolve the chemical. Temperature plays an important role in the leaching of chemicals in soil since it also affects solubility.

Vaporization in transport

The vapour pressure of organic chemicals varies over a wide range from highly volatile substances such as fluorocarbons, chloroform, and vinyl chloride to moderately volatile compounds like parathion to slightly volatile materials such as DDT, PCBs, and polymers. An expression relating vapour pressure to quantity of chemical evaporating is found in the Langmuir equation (Freed *et al.* 1977):

$$Q = \beta P \sqrt{\left(\frac{M}{2\pi RT}\right)}$$

where β is the evaporation constant of a chemical under a given atmospheric condition, M is the molecular weight, T is the absolute temperature, and P is the vapour pressure in mm Hg.

The presence of suspended dust or aerosol particles may result in sorption of some of the vapours and will increase the partition function of the chemical between the atmospheric phase and other components of the environment. The sorbed chemical may then be transported some distance with the particulate. This partially explains why pesticides have been found in places where they have never been used (Haque *et al.* 1976; Machta 1978). Since the vaporization of a chemical from a surface is related to its diffusion into the air mass, air currents can increase the rate of vaporization.

Many chemicals in water will evaporate simultaneously with water. Vapour loss of a pesticide from a soil system is accelerated by the presence of moisture in the soil. This has been shown with such diverse materials as 2,4-D esters, thiol-carbamates, N-phenyl carbamates, triazines, and the organo-chlorine PCBs (Haque *et al.* 1974; Spencer and Cliath 1975, 1981; Miller 1978).

Although the vapour pressure of a chemical to a great extent determines the entry of that chemical into the atmosphere, caution must be exercised in interpreting vapour pressure data. The vapour pressure of a chemical can give a good estimate of air transport as long as the chemical is in the pure state or is evaporating from an inert surface. However when the chemical is bound to a surface, its vapour pressure cannot be used as an index for vapour transport. It should also be pointed out that while studying the vapour loss of a chemical from a soil surface, other factors controlling the release of the chemical may include: ambient temperature, the initial concentration of the chemical, moisture, and pH.

Solution behaviour

Major factors contributing to the partitioning of a chemical into the aquatic environment are its water solubility and it latent heat of solution. Many organic compounds in use today are hydrophobic, having water solubilities in parts-per-million (p.p.m.) or parts-per-billion (p.p.b.) range. This makes exact determinations of their solubilities quite difficult. This hydrophobic character also makes such compounds good candidates for biological accumulation.

Alkalinity or acidity may influence the stability and the solubility of many chemicals. For example, the solubility of the triazines usually increases with lowering pH and this is attributed to protonation of nitrogen with the ultimate formation of cationic species. The presence of salts in an aqueous solution may cause ion-association or ion-pair formation and directly affect chemical solubility.

As would be expected, temperature significantly influences the behaviour of organic chemicals in aqueous solutions. Though the exact mechanisms for solubilization of sparingly soluble chemicals is not known, solubility usually increases with temperature. The question still remains whether or not they form ideal solutions. However, an enthalpy of solution value can be obtained by using the Van't Hoff equation ΔH. This value may then be used as an index of the tendency of a chemical to dissolve. For some of the thiolcarbamate herbicides, temperature has the opposite effect on solubility (their solubility decreases with an increase in temperature). This may be due to hydrogen-bond formation between water and thiolcarbamates.

Other factors that may contribute to the transport and the persistence of chemicals in an aquatic environment are: (i) the presence of sediments and organic material; (ii) the presence of proteins and lipids (of the aquatic biota); (iii) effects of UV and other high-energy radiations that may cause decomposition of molecules.

The presence in water of soil particles of any type (soil, clay, sand, or biocolloid) will reduce the concentration of dissolved chemical by the process of adsorption. The extent of adsorption will depend on the nature of the suspended particles and the temperature.

Bioaccumulation

The accumulation of certain compounds in living organisms (bioaccumulation) has led to problems for populations of organisms (Blau et al. 1975; Kenaga 1975, Brown 1978). Most compounds that tend to bioaccumulate have a low water solubility and a high solubility in non-polar (lipophilic) solvents. The relation between water solubility and partition coefficient for a number of compounds is shown in Table 5.4. The partition coefficient of such compounds provides a good measure of their tendency to accumulate in living organisms. This, coupled with a refractoriness toward reaction, gives an indication not only of accumulation but transmission from one trophic level to another. The determination of the partitioning between an aqueous phase and a solvent phase can utilize a variety of organic solvents. The most desirable solvent, however, is one that more nearly resembles the adipose tissue of the living organism. While solvents such as olive oil and corn oil have been used, a more convenient and representative solvent is n-octanol.

Table 5.4. *Solubilities and partition coefficients of various compounds*

Compound	Solubility in water (p.p.m.)	Log (n-octanol H$_2$O partition coefficient)
Benzene	820 (22 ‡)[a]	2.13[d]
Toluene	470 (16)[a]	2.69[d]
Fluorobenzene	1540 (30)[a]	2.27[d]
Chlorobenzene	448 (30)[a]	2.84[d]
Bromobenzene	446 (30)[a]	2.99[d]
Iodobenzene	340 (30)[a]	3.25[e]
p-Dichlorobenzene	79 (25)[a]	3.38[b]
Naphthalene	30[a]	3.37[c]
Diphenyl ether	21 (25)[b]	4.20[b]
Tetrachloroethylene	400 (25)[b]	2.60[b]
Chloroform	7950 (25)[b]	1.97[f]
Carbon tetrachloride	800[a]	2.64[g]
p,p'-DDT	0.0031[i]–0.0034[j]	6.19[h]
p,p'-DDE	0.040 (20)	5.69[h]
Benzoic acid	2700 (18)[a]	1.87[d]
Salicylic acid	1800 (20)[a]	2.26[f]
Phenylacetic acid	16600 (20)[a]	1.41[d]
Phenoxyacetic acid	12000 (10)[a]	1.26[d]
2,4-D	890 (25)[b]	2.81[d]
2,4,5,2',5'-PCB	0.010 (24)	6.11
2,4,5,2',4',5'-PCB	0.00095 (24)	6.72
4,4'-PCB	0.062 (20)	5.58
Phosalone	2.12 (20)	4.30
Methyl chlorpyrifos	4.76 (20)	4.31

‡ Temperature in degrees centigrade.
Sources: (a) *Handbook of chemistry and physics* (1952); (b) Kenaga (1975); (c) Hansch and Fujita (1964); (d) Fujita *et al.* (1964); (e) Leo *et al.* (1971); (f) Hansch and Anderson (1967); (g) Macy (1948); (h) O'Brien (1975); (i) Bowman *et al.* (1960); (j) Biggar *et al.* (1967).

Chemical reaction

Such things as elemental composition, structure, and formula weight are required as identification of the compound. In some instances, this is sufficient to indicate to the chemist the more common reactions the substances may undergo. On the other hand, with new structures or new classes of compounds, the general knowledge of their chemistry may be restricted such that another chemist would not necessarily be in a position to predict characteristic reactions of the group.

There are certain reactions commonly encountered, particularly in biological systems, that might well be evaluated for each new compound. Among these reactions are oxidation, reduction, hydrolysis, alkylation, and dealkylation of oxygen and nitrogen or certain metallic atoms of molecules, esterification, and several types of conjugation with naturally occurring metabolites (Brink 1981). Many of these reactions are readily explored in the laboratory and would be recommended for consideration for study of compounds having a probable wide distribution in the environment.

It is not sufficient, however, to know just what reactions may occur, but in certain instances a knowledge of the rate and extent of those reactions is highly desirable (Brink 1981; Onishi and Brown 1981). For example, in analyses of environmental samples for chlorinated hydrocarbons, one takes advantage of the fact that DDT will undergo dehydrohalogenation with base, while PCBs do not. Or, again, one may take advantage of the relative rates of hydrolysis between certain organophosphate esters and carbamate acid esters in an analytical procedure. Beyond the utility of kinetic data in development of analytical procedures, this same information is useful in assessing the probable persistence of a compound in certain compartments of the environment.

A type of reaction particularly important for a number of compounds is the photochemical reaction (Zabic and Ruzo 1981). This may occur at exposed surfaces or, perhaps more often, when the compound by one mechanism or another finds its way into the atmosphere. For some compounds, the photochemical reaction results in rapid dismutation, but in others, for example dieldrin, a photochemical product of even greater activity may be formed. Though a vapour phase study of photochemical reactions requires elaborate instrumentation, the photochemistry of many compounds can be studied on thin-layer chromatographic plates by exposure to sunlight or artificial light sources.

EXPOSURE

There are several routes of human exposure to a chemical. The primary ones are dermal repiratory, and oral. These may be inadvertent routes of exposure whereas intravenous, subcutaneous, or intraperitoneal infection are advertent or intended routes of exposure (Hayes 1975).

In the case of a chemical in the environment, the predominant route of exposure will vary as to the nature of the activity, whether the compound is undergoing transport or is resident in a particular compartment of the environment, for example, water or food, and on the physico-chemical properties of the materials. Thus, with a compound of high vapour pressure, the probability of respiratory exposure is much greater than dermal or oral exposure. On the other hand, a compound of low vapour pressure and poor solubility might more frequently be encountered as a residue in food or water.

The route of exposure is important, both as to the amount absorbed and the rapidity of the response. This is due to the nature of the barrier, that is, skin, intestinal mucosa, alveolar cells, and the blood supply to the particular barrier or organ. The structure and chemistry of the absorbing organ is important as to whether it is preferential to partitioning lipid-soluble materials or whether hydrophilic substances pass with more ease across the barrier (Dugard 1977). As shown below, in general, the toxicity and rapidity of absorption decreases as the exposure occurs through intravenous, respiratory, oral, or dermal routes. The route of exposure is also a factor in toxicity in that it can influence the dosage producing toxicity in 50 per cent of a sample population. This is indicated in Table 5.5 for toxaphene, an organochlorine insecticide.

The difference in toxicity based on route of exposure is probably due in part to how rapidly the concentration of the chemical builds up in the susceptible organ or sites. Thus, one would expect for most substances that the skin, because of its corneum stratum, would reduce the rate of entry. Indeed, one finds a difference in dermal penetration depending upon the portion of the body that is exposed. This is illustrated by the penetration of parathion on skin of different regions of the body (Table 5.6).

Table 5.5. *Influence of route of exposure on median lethal dose of toxaphene*

Toxaphene Route of administration	Toxicity to rat LD_{50} mg/kg	Carrier
Intravenous	13	Peanut oil
Oral	90	Peanut oil
Dermal	930	Xylene
LC_{50} inhal.	3.4 mg/l (40% dust)	

Table 5.6. *Dermal absorption of an organophosphate, parathion*

Body area	Relative absorption (%)
Hands	12
Forearm	8
Upperarm	28
Feet	13
Cheek	46
Forehead	36
Scrotum	100

With many environmental chemicals, one route of exposure predominates. However, in an instance such as the waste chemical dump known as Love Canal, exposure is probably via all three routes – dermal, oral, and respiratory. Once the barrier seal of the dump was broken by construction, migration of the chemical was possible. Consequently, many of these substances would evaporate, even though of relatively low vapour pressure, to afford respiratory exposure. Some would be transported, adsorbed on dust particles, affording dermal exposure and others getting into water, possibly resulting in oral exposure.

It is thus apparent that physico-chemical factors play an important role, both in whether or not exposure will occur as well as whether or not the chemical will find access to the organism. The partition coefficient between lipids and water as indicated by the octanol–water partition coefficient is a factor in dermal absorption (Dugard 1977). There are upper and lower bounds to the partition coefficient favourable for absorption and these have been defined for a number of different substances (Hansch 1972; Kenaga 1972; Taylor 1978). The utility of the partition coefficient as an indicator of ease of internal exposure, that is passage into the organism, was first propounded by Overton and Meyer in the nineteenth century. Though not the full answer in every situation, it has none the less proved a fairly good predictor, not only for dermal absorption, but also for uptake of a variety of chemicals in a number of different species.

The vapour pressure of a compound is also important for exposure. While it has long been appreciated that the low boiling, high vapour pressure compounds, for example chloroform, vinyl chloride, ethylene dibromide, and sulphur dioxide, when released would result in respiratory exposure, the extent of respiratory exposure accruing from low vapour pressure compounds spread over large areas has only recently been appreciated. This has become increasingly apparent i cases of pesticide use or industrial waste disposal on soil surfaces. Thus, compounds having a vapour pressure in the order of 10^{-5} to 10^{-7} torr at 25°C will show substantial evaporative losses from a surface in a matter of a few days. The process, of course, is dependent, in part, on water providing competitive adsorption so as to prevent the organic molecule from becoming 'fixed' or adsorbed on colloidal particles.

It is apparent from the foregoing examples that the properties of the chemical are indeed important as factors in human exposure to environmental chemicals. Not only are the physical properties, but also the chemical reactivity are involved in the route and rate of exposure that are likely to be received, but the same factors interact with the environmental processes in a predictable manner to result in either increased or decreased probability of exposure (Hartung 1975; Freed *et al.* 1977). Thus, the movement, distribution, and persistence of the chemical, all of which relate to the possibility of exposure whether in an occupational or general environment is a function of chemical properties and environmental processes (Spencer and Cliath 1975; Freed *et al.* 1977; Maltoni 1977).

PUBLIC HEALTH CONCERNS

The presence of an agent in the physical environment may pose an objective physical hazard, a mental/emotional problem if perceived as a hazard, or remain only as a potential hazard (Slovic *et al.* 1979). In any event, the presence of such an agent (or agents) is the proper concern of public health. The extent to which a given agent will constitute an objective physical hazard is dependent upon the concentration in the environment and the characteristics of the material. A distinction is made between the intrinsic toxicity of a given material and the hazard, that is, the likelihood of harm, that it may pose (Davies *et al.* 1982). Several factors influence the hazard of a material, namely: (i) The innate danger or toxicity of the agent; (ii) The spectrum or range of species affected; (iii) The resident time or persistence of the material; (iv) The mobility of the agent in the environment; (v) The manner of handling and use.

The innate toxicity of an agent is a characteristic of the compound. It may be related to the reactivity, the molecular geometry, or atomic composition of the material but is only an indication of the chemical's potential for harm. Obviously if no exposure occurs there can be little hazard even though the chemical may be highly toxic. A common method of expressing the toxicity of compounds is that of the dose required to bring about an effect (usually death) within 50 per cent of a treated population, ED_{50}. However, as pointed out by Craig (1983), this is not an exact measurement but can be used for interchemical comparison.

There is wide variation in the susceptibility of different species to many agents in the environment. Thus one group may respond to very low levels of a given chemical where other species are tolerant of a much higher level. Kociba and Schwetz (1982), for example, found that the guinea pig is sensitive to small amounts of 2,3,7,8-tetrachlorodibenzo-*p*-dioxin but the hamster is tolerant of many-fold larger amounts. Such a pattern has been found for many other materials (Doull *et al.* 1980).

An agent may be very toxic and equally so to all species but if its residence in the environment is transitory, the hazard it poses may be small since it will not exist in sufficiently high concentration to cause a biologically significant exposure. Tetraethylpyrophosphate is an example of such an agent. On the other hand, an agent of somewhat lower toxicity but of far longer persistence becomes most worrisome, for example, PCBs (National Research Council 1979).

In evaluating whether an agent in the physical environment will be a hazard, one must consider the manner of handling and use. If directly released into the environment, whether from a point or non-point source, the distribution in the environment will occur as described in the earlier section. If the quantities are large in relation to the intrinsic toxicity, the hazard then will be multiplied (National Academy of Science 1975; National Research Council 1980; Environmental Protection Agency 1981).

Reference has been made to the role of concentration in determining the hazard of a specific chemical. Such a role is implicit in the dose–response relationship (Doull *et al.* 1980; Hayes 1982). As pointed out by Gehring (1979), even with many carcinogens there is a relationship between a dose and the length of time from exposure to response. Thus the lower the dose, the longer the time to appearance of the neoplasm.

As mentioned earlier, there are many agents, both organic and inorganic, to be found in the environment. They arise from both anthropogenic and geological activity from both point and non-point sources. Of the almost six million chemicals known, only about 60 000 are of significant use to man. And only a fraction of these escape into the environment in a sufficient quantity to be of significance biologically. However, even to enumerate all of these and assess the hazard afforded would be a formidable undertaking. The following serve as an example of the types of hazards found in the physical environment that are a source for concern.

Asbestos

Asbestos fibres escape into the environment during mining and manufacturing processes as well as in construction. It may be found in water and air to which humans will be exposed. It has also been demonstrated that there may be a familial exposure. Asbestos is a source of concern because of its production of neoplasms and particularly mesothelioma (Selikoff and Hammond 1979).

Arsenic

Arsenic is to be found in geological formations from whence it may be leached into water supplies. It also finds its way into the environment through activities such as mining, smelting, and, to a lesser extent in recent years, through the use of inorganic arsenic. It is both toxic and carcinogenic and for these reasons arsenic is a continuing public health concern (Environmental Health Perspectives 1977*a*).

Cadmium

Cadmium, a metal for which there are a number of uses, has been implicated in environmental poisoning incidents over the years. It has serious renal and neuromuscular effects (Environmental Health Perspectives 1979).

Mercury

The metal, mercury, held a fascination for the ancient alchemist but its worth was found in economic enterprises over the years. It has been used in medicine, agriculture, and industry for a wide variety of purposes. Its use as a catalyst in the plastic industry as well as numerous incidents of poisoning have served to focus on the hazard it represents in the physical environment. A finding of particular interest in the Minimata poisoning incident in Japan was that this metal, like some others, may be methylated in the environment to pose an even greater hazard through bioaccumulation and intrinsic toxicity (Goldwater and Stopford 1977).

Lead

Lead, both as a metal and salt, has long enjoyed wide use. It is reputed to have been used as drinking vessels in ancient times, as an alloy in more recent times, and as an organic derivative and additive to gasoline for the internal combustion engine. Both from these sources and from mining operations, lead has become widely distributed in the environment. Plumbism is a condition in children arising from the consumption of paints with a lead base (Environmental Health Perspectives 1977a).

Nitrogen

Nitrogen compounds, primarily the oxides, arise principally from high-temperature combustion in the form of nitrous oxide and nitrogen dioxide. These gases, demonstrated to cause respiratory problems, are of particular concern in closed spaces. Another oxide of nitrogen, nitrate, may arise from fertilizer, sewage waste, and to a lesser extent, conversion of nitrogen dioxide to nitrate by atmospheric electrical activity. Nitrate most frequently appears in water though it may, when occurring in large amounts in soils, be present in certain plants. Nitrate, even at moderate levels, is a particular hazard to the infant.

Sulphur

Like nitrogen, sulphur is encountered most frequently as one of its oxides. Sulphur dioxide or the sulphate as sulphuric acid are produced in large quantities in the combustion of fossil fuels. Again, its primary effect is on the respiratory tract (Lipmann and Schlesinger 1979).

Hydrocarbons

Hydrocarbons are compounds composed exclusively of carbon and hydrogen. This group includes such compounds as methane through to highly complex molecular structures such as the polyaromatic hydrocarbons. Some of the straight-chain compounds are of concern due to their effect on the peripheral nerves whereas the more aromatic compounds of concern are carcinogens. The polyaromatic hydrocarbons are to be found in many of the fossil fuels but also are formed in the combustion of these fuels. They have been shown to be widely distributed in the environment.

Halogenated hydrocarbons

This class has a wider distribution in the environment and includes a large number of industrially useful compounds, than any other group of organic compounds. The halomethanes, such as methylchloride, methylene dichloride, and chloroform find wide industrial use and for that reason are manufactured in substantial quantities. Halogenated methanes and ethylene dibromide are also formed in large quantities, presumably from biological action, in the sea. In fact, it has been estimated that the natural output of methyl chloride may equal or exceed that of the anthropogenic sources.

The halogenated hydrocarbons include not only the methane and ethane derivatives but also unsaturated hydrocarbons such as vinyl chloride, which causes angiosarcoma, chlorinated paraffins, polychlorobiphenols, polybromobiphenols, and a number of chlorinated products used as pesticides.

A distinctive feature of many of the halogenated hydrocarbons is their persistence in the environment. The halogen-carbon bond in many instances is quite refractory to being broken. On the other hand, there are certain of these, particularly the chain compounds, where there is sufficient activity to alkylate biopolymers. This class of compounds show a high degree of biological activity whether reactive or not, and cause a variety of diseases (DeBruin 1976).

Phenols and contaminants

Phenol, or carbolic acid, has long been recognized for its biological activity which arises primarily from the hydroxyl group on the benzene ring. The biological activity is shared by all members of the class to a varying degree. Nitrophenols have been employed as germicides, fungicides, and herbicides as well as an explosive (picric acid). Halogenated phenols are excellent biocides and have been used as antiseptics (methylene bistrichlorophenol), fungicides (orthochlorophenylphenol), and wood preservatives (pentachlorophenol). Pentachlorophenol has become widely distributed in the environment as a result of use (and possibly from chlorination of phenolic contaminated water) with the result that it shows up in human monitoring.

In the production of the chlorophenols, particularly trichlorophenol and pentachlorophenol, a number of contaminants are found. These include the chlorophenoxyphenols (pre-dioxins), dioxins, and benzofurans. These latter compounds, a frequent source of chloracne in manufacturing plants, are highly toxic and 2,3,7,8-dibenzodioxin, known as

TCDD, is reputed to be one of the most toxic synthetic organics known. TCDD is formed in the manufacture of certain chlorophenols and arises in combustion of chlorinated materials in municipal waste and, possibly, in the combustion of fossil fuels (Bumb *et al.* 1980).

Organic acids and esters

A diverse group of organic acids find utility but probably it is the esters of many of these acids used as plasticizers that have received greatest attention as an environmental hazard. Hundreds of millions of pounds of plasticizers are used annually to condition various plastics. In the manufacturing process, use, and disposal of the plastics, these plasticizers, such as the various alkyl phthalates, have escaped into the environment. Phthalates have been found in fresh and sea water as well as elsewhere. Exposure also comes through the use of these plasticizers.

Bipyridils

Bipyridils, primarily those used as herbicides, have received attention of late because of their unique toxic properties. The target organ of these compounds is the lungs and lesions produced by even moderate doses are always fatal once the compound has been absorbed (Summers 1980).

Pesticides

The chemicals used in the bioindustries and for vector control in health encompass many different classes of inorganic and organic chemicals. The hazard posed by halogenated hydrocarbons was first recognized because of their use as pesticides. Subsequently, however, there was added the cholinesterase inhibiting organophosphates and carbamates. Most classes of organic compounds are represented among the agents used as insecticides, fungicides, herbicides, and rodenticides. The very nature of the use of these chemicals insures their distribution in the environment; moreover, when used on food crops, small residues remain. The identifiable hazards which have arisen from the use of chemicals as pesticides can almost always be attributed to either overuse or abuse of the material proving once again the old adage that any chemical may be handled and used safely, and conversely that even relatively innocuous chemicals can be dangerous if misused (Hayes 1982).

CONSIDERATIONS ON HAZARDS

The multitude of hazards in the physical environment arising from either natural or anthropogenic sources is receiving increasing attention globally. Attempts to control or ameliorate these hazards take the form of new scientific and technical approaches as well as a more customary regulatory approach. It is important to reduce the hazards in the physical environment but at the same time to keep a perspective on the relative magnitude of the hazard. Very often, the course of action advocated to eliminate the hazard from a particular agent

may entail introduction of equal, or even more serious, consequence. Thus, to mitigate the likelihood of exposure to a chemical used in vector control, may result in a greater exposure to the diseased organism.

REFERENCES

Andreae, M.O. and Raemdonck, H. (1983). Dimethyl sulfide in the surface ocean and the marine atmosphere: a global view. *Science* **221**, 744.

Blau, G.E., Neely, W.B., and Branson, D.R. (1975). Ecokinetics: a study of the fate and distribution of chemicals in laboratory ecosystems. *AIChE J.* **21**, 854.

Biggar, J.W., Dutt, G.R., and Riggs, R.L. (1967). *Bull. Environ. Contam. Toxicol.* **2**, 90.

Bownan, M.C., Acree, M.K., Jr., and Corbett, J. (1960). *J. Agr. Food Chem.* **8**, 406.

Brink, R.H. (1981). Biodegradation of organic chemicals in the environment. In *Environmental health chemistry—a chemistry of environmental agents as potential human hazards* (ed. J.D. McKinney) p. 75. Ann Arbor Science Publishers, Ann Arbor.

Brown, A.W.A. (1978). *Ecology of pesticides.* Wiley, New York.

Bumb, R.R., Crummett, W.B., Cutie, S.S. *et al.* (1980). Trace chemistry of fires: a source of chlorinated dioxin. *Science* **210**, 385.

Chiou, C.T., Freed, V.H., Schmedding, D.W., and Kohnert, R.L. (1977). Partition coefficient and bioaccumulation of selected organic chemicals. *Environ. Sci. Tech.* **11**, 475.

Chiou, C.T., Peters, L.J., and Freed, V.H. (1979). A physical concept of soil-water equilibria for nonionic organic compounds. *Science* **206**, 831.

Chiou, C.T. and Schmedding, D.W. (1981). Measurement and inter-relations of octanol water partition coefficient and water solubility of organic chemicals. In *Test protocols for environmental fate and movement of toxicants*, p. 28. Association of Official Analytical Chemists, Arlington, Virginia.

Craig, P.N. (1983). Mathematical models for toxicity evaluation. *Ann. Rep. Med. Chem.* **18**, 303.

Davies, J.E., Freed, V.H., and Whittmore, F.W. (1982). *An agromedical approach to pesticide management: some health and environmental considerations.* University of Miami Medical School, Miami, Florida.

DeBruin, S. (1976). *Biochemical toxicology of environmental agents.* Elsevier, Amsterdam.

DHEW (1977a). *Arsenic and lead. Environmental health perspectives, Vol. 19.* DHEW publication No. (NIH) 77-218). Washington, DC.

DHEW (1977b). *Vinyl chloride related compounds. Environmental health perspectives. Vol. 21.* DHEW publication No. (NIH) 78-218). Washington, DC.

DHEW (1979). *Cadmium. Environmental health perspectives, Vol. 28.* DHEW publication No. (NIH) 79-218. Washington, DC.

Doull, J., Klassen, C.D., and Andur, M.O. (1980). *Toxicology: the basic science of poisons,* 2nd ed. Macmillan, New York.

Dugard, T.H. (1977). Skin permeability theory in relation to measurement of percutaneous absorption in toxicology. In *Dermatotoxicology and pharmacology* (ed. F.N. Marzulli and H.I. Maibach) p. 525. Hemisphere, Washington.

Environmental Protection Agency (1981). *Proceedings of the workshop on transport and fate of toxic chemicals in the environment.* US Environmental Protection Agency. Washington, DC.

Freed, V.H., Chiou, C.T., and Haque, R. (1977). Chemodynamics: transport and behaviour of chemicals in the environment – a problem in environmental health. *Environ. Health Perspect.* **20**, 55.

Fujita, R., Iwasa, J., and Hansch, C. (1964). A new substituent constant, π, derived from partition coefficients. *J. Am. Chem. Soc.* **86**, 5175.

Gehring, B.J., Watanabe, T.G., and Blau, G.E. (1979). Risk assessment of environmental carcinogens using pharmacokinetic parameters. *Ann. NY Acad. Sci.* **329**, 137.

Goldwater, L.J. and Stopford, W. (1977). Mercury. In *The chemical environment.* Vol. 6 (ed. J. Linehow and W.W. Fletcher) p. 38. Academic Press, New York.

Hamaker, J.W. (1975). The interpretation of soil leaching experiments. In *Environmental dynamics of pesticides* (ed. R. Haque and V.H. Freed) p. 115. Plenum Press, New York.

Hamaker, J.W. and Thompson, J.M. (1972). Adsorption. In *Organic chemicals in the soil environment.* Vol. 1 (ed. C.A.I. Goring and J.W. Hamaker) p. 49. Marcel Dekker, New York.

Handbook of chemistry and physics, 34th ed. (1952). Chemical Rubber Pub. Co.

Hansch, C. (1972). A computerized approach to quantitative biochemical structure–activity relationships. In *Biological correlation—the Hansch approach. Advances in Chemistry Series 114,* p. 20. American Chemical Society, Washington, DC.

Hansch, C. and Anderson, S.M. (1967). The effect of intramolecular hydrophobic bonding on partition coefficients. *J. Org. Chem.* **32**, 2583.

Hansch, C. and Fujita, T. (1966). *p-σ-π* Analysis. A method for the correlation of biological activity and chemical structure. *J. Am. Chem. Soc.* **86**, 1616.

Haque, R., Schmedding, D.W., and Freed, V.H. (1974). Aqueous solubility, adsorption, and vapor behavior of polychlorinated biphenyl arochlor 1254. *Environ. Sci. Technol.* **8**, 139.

Haque, R., Kearney, P.C., and Freed, V.H. (1976). Dynamics of pesticides in aquatic environments. In *Pesticides in aquatic environments* (ed. M.A.Q. Khan) p. 39. Plenum Press, New York.

Hartung, R. (1975). Accumulation of chemicals in the hydrosphere. In *Environmental dynamics of pesticides* (ed. R. Haque and V.H. Freed) p. 185. Plenum Press, New York.

Hay, A. (1982). *The chemical scythe.* Plenum Press, New York.

Hayes, W.J., Jr. (1982). *Pesticides studied in man.* Williams and Wilkins, Baltimore.

Hayes, W.J. Jr. (1975). *Toxicology of pesticides.* Williams and Wilkins, Baltimore.

Helling, C.S. and Dragun, J. (1981). Soil leaching tests for toxic organic chemicals. In *Test protocols for environmental fate and movement of toxicants,* p. 43. Proceedings of Symposium. Association of Official Analytical Chemists, Arlington, Virginia.

Horne, R.A. (1978). *The chemistry of our environment.* Wiley, New York.

Kenaga, E.E. (1972). Guidelines for environmental study of pesticides: determination of bioconcentration of potential. *Residue Rev.* **44**, 73.

Kenaga, E.E. (1975). Partitioning and uptake of pesticides in biological systems. In *Environmental dynamics of pesticides* (ed. R. Haque and V.H. Freed) p. 217. Plenum Press, New York.

Kociba, R.J. and Schwetz, B.A. (1982). A review of the toxicity of 2,3,7,8-tetrachlorodibenzo-p-dioxin (TCDD) with comparison to the toxicity of other chlorinated dioxin isomers. *Assoc. Food Drug Officials Q. Bull.* **46**, 168.

Leo, A., Hansch, C., and Elkins, D. (1971). Partition coefficients and their use. *Chem. Rev.* **71**, 525.

Levine, A. (1983). Psychosocial impact of toxic chemical waste dumps. *Environ. Health Perspect.* **48**, 15.

Lippmann, M. and Schlesinger, R.B. (1978). *Chemical contamination in the human environment.* Oxford University Press, New York.

Lovelock, J.E., Maggs, R.J., and Rasmussen, R.A. (1972). Atmospheric dimethyl sulphide and the natural sulphur cycle. *Nature* **237**, 452.

Machta, L. (1978). *Air concentration and deposition rates from uniform area sources.* MARC Report No. 10. Monitoring and Assessment Research Centre (International Council of Scientific Unions), University of London, London.

Macy, R. (1948). Partition coefficients of 50 compounds between olive oil and water at 20°C. *J. Ind. Hyg. Toxicol.* **30**, 140.

Maltoni, C. (1977). Recent findings on the carcinogenicity of chlorinated olefins. *Environ. Health Perspect.* **21**, 1.

Miller, D.L. (1978). Models for total transport. In *Principles of ecotoxicology* (ed. G.C. Butler) p. 71. John Wiley, New York.

National Academy of Sciences (1975). *Principles for evaluating chemicals in the environment.* National Academy of Sciences, Washington, DC.

National Research Council (1980). *Committee on prototype explicit analyses for pesticides. Regulating pesticides.* National Academy of Sciences, Washington, DC.

National Research Council (1979). *Polychlorinated biphenyls.* National Academy of Sciences, Washington, DC.

National Research Council (1977). *Environmental monitoring, Vol. IV.* National Academy of Sciences, Washington, DC.

O'Brien, R.D. (1975). Nonenzymic effects of pesticides on membranes. In *Environmental dynamics of pesticides* (ed. R. Haque and V.H. Freed) p. 331. Plenum Press, New York.

Onishi, Y. and Brown, S.M. (1981). Role of mathematical models for environmental assessment of toxicants. In *Test protocols for environmental fate and movement of toxicants.* p. 251. Proceedings of Symposium, Association of Official Analytical Chemists, Arlington, Virginia.

Selikoff, T.J. and Hammond, E.C. (1979). Health hazards of asbestos exposure. *Ann. NY Acad. Sci.* **330**, 1.

Slovic, P., Fischhoff, B., and Lichtenstein, S. (1979). Rating the risks. *Chem. Technol.* **9**, 738.

Spencer, W.F. and Cliath, M.M. (1975). Vaporization of chemicals. In *Environmental dynamics of pesticides* (ed. R. Haque and V.H. Freed) p. 61. Plenum Press, New York.

Spencer, W.F. and Cliath, M.M. (1981). Evaluating volatility of toxicants in soil and water. In *Test protocols for environmental fate and movement of toxicants,* p. 110. Proceedings of Symposium, Association of Official Analytical Chemists, Arlington, Virginia.

Summers, L.A. (1980). *The bipyridinium herbicides.* Academic Press, London.

Taylor, A.W. (1978). Post application volatilization of pesticides under field conditions. *J. Air Pollution Control Assoc.* **28**, 922.

Tucker, R.E., Young, A.L., and Gray, A.P. (1983). *Human and environmental risks of chlorinated dioxins and related compounds.* Plenum Press, New York.

Zabik, M.J. and Ruzo, L.O. (1981). Factors effecting pesticide photodecomposition studies. In *Test protocols for environmental fate and movement of toxicants,* p. 28. Proceedings of Symposium, Association of Official Analytical Chemists, Arlington, Virginia.

6 Infectious agents

Gene I. Higashi, Richard E. Isaacson, and Arnold S. Monto

INTRODUCTION

The concept that transmissible agents might be responsible for the production of at least certain diseases surfaced periodically during the early history of medicine, mainly based on empirical observations. The concept of contagion itself first appeared in the work, *De Res Contagiosa*, of Hieronymus Fracastorius in the sixteenth century. Progress was not made until much later, in the nineteenth century with the work of notable epidemiologists such as Snow and Budd, and microbiologists such as Pasteur and Koch. Only in the twentieth century did rapid advances in microbiology and parasitology with identification and description of many new agents allow precise characterization of infectious diseases and mechanisms of transmission. Certain general principles were developed, such as the idea that asymptomatic infection was frequent, and that the proportion of infections resulting in symptomatic illness or pathogenicity, varied with the agent and status of the host. It also became clear that the ability of an agent to survive in the environment determined its transmissibility, which in turn was usually related to its physicochemical characteristics. In this chapter, the features of the agents of infectious disease of public health importance will be discussed. It will be divided into discussion of viruses, bacteria, fungi, and parasites including protozoa and helminths. For more detailed descriptions of these agents, the reader is directed to standard texts on the particular subject.

VIRUSES

Mechanisms of viral infection

Viruses are infectious agents containing only one type of nucleic acid (RNA or DNA) enclosed in a protein covering of varied type. They are obligate intracellular parasites and cannot replicate without cells or survive for long outside the host body (Dulbecco and Ginsberg 1980). Thus transmission is the most hazardous part of the cycle of infection. Within the host, the virus replicates by making use of the metabolic processes of the infected cell. The replication process follows a series of sequential steps common to most animal viruses, and antiviral agents generally can be identified as operating on one or more of these steps (Bachrach 1978; Koch-Weser *et al.* 1980). A summary of these steps is given in Table 6.1.

The virus first attaches to specific receptor sites on the cell membrane; lack of such receptors is an explanation for the

Table 6.1. *Major steps in viral replication*

Early	Attachment of virus to cell
	Penetration and uncoating
Middle	Messenger RNA synthesis
	Protein synthesis
	Genomic nucleic acid synthesis
Late	Maturation and assembly of virion
	Release from cell

insensitivity of certain cells to a particular virus. Penetration occurs by mechanisms which differ among viruses. Thereafter, in the uncoating process, the viral nucleic acid is freed from the covering coat. Again, the site of this event will vary, as will its completeness. The replication itself begins with the transcription process. For DNA-containing viruses, the genome is transcribed to messenger RNA (mRNA) using either enzymes brought into the cells as with the poxviruses or using cellular RNA polymerases. The nucleic acid in certain single-stranded RNA viruses is already infectious (so called positive stranded) and no new mRNA is needed to initiate the process; with the negative-stranded viruses mRNA is transcribed using a viral transcriptase (Raghow and Kingsbury 1976). The oncogenic retroviruses represent a special case, possessing a reverse transcriptase for the production of DNA. Transcription is followed by translation, in which the mRNA is finally translated into viral proteins. Some of these proteins aid in producing new viral genomic RNA or DNA. Often the viral products are produced in excess of what is required for final assembly and release of the completed new virus. Assembly takes place in the cytoplasm and/or in the nucleus and, with more complex viruses, layers are laid down in a stepwise fashion. Release marks the end of the latent period of viral replication, and in the process of leaving the cells viruses may acquire a glycoprotein envelope as they bud through the cellular membrane.

As mentioned above, the lack of appropriate receptors is a common cause of resistance. However, resistance can also occur as a result of intrinsic inability of the cell to support the growth of a particular virus. If infection does take place, it can have a number of effects on the cells of the host. Most important in terms of production of acute disease is cytocidal infection. Cell destruction results when the viral proteins produced early in infection shut down cellular RNA and protein synthesis. Transformation may result if susceptible cells are infected with oncogenic viruses (Vogt and Dulbecco 1960). Certain viruses which do not produce either of these effects cause a steady-state infection, a situation in which virus is produced without destruction of the infected cells (Choppin 1964). Latency, another type of persistent infection, can result following acute infection by a number of processes, including integration of viral RNA in the host genome. When an acute infection does not resolve, and virus continues to be produced by cells, the situation is described as a chronic infection.

Cell damage is the most important element in the pathogenesis of viral infection. It can be produced by the action of the virus itself, or by immunological response to the products of viral infection. In the intact host, specific, predictable organ systems demonstrate the effects of viral replication pathologically. The poxviruses are recognized by their growth in the skin but other internal organs can also be involved, since virus is initially disseminated via the bloodstream. Viraemia is not present in other localized skin infections, while infections of the respiratory or enteric tract generally involve only the surface and do not disseminate. Infections of the nervous system may be produced by direct extension, as in rabies, or they may follow more generalized infection and viraemia as in poliomyelitis.

Exact mechanisms of recovery from viral infection are largely unknown although many of the elements are recognized. At one time, it was thought that depletion of the susceptible cells was responsible, but this is now known not to be the case. Circulating antibody is produced in response to viral infection, and, for diseases which last for several weeks, appears at a time when it could temporally be involved. However, most viral infections last for too short a period and have largely resolved before antibody is detected. Interferon has been proposed as a likely factor in recovery since it is produced by cells early in response to infection. Cell-mediated immune responses may also be involved; thus with the herpesvirus family, which typically persist as latent infections, depression of cell-mediated immunity, either naturally or as a result of therapy, often results in clinical recurrences. Indeed the immunodeficient patient in whom viral infection can sometimes not be contained gives important clues as to the role of various types of immunity with specific viruses (Koprowski and Koprowski 1975).

The same factors involved in recovery are involved in prevention, and here the situation is much better defined. Humoral antibody is clearly involved in prevention of a number of infections. Passive administration of antibodies has long been known to prevent measles and hepatitis A, and more recently hepatitis B (Maynard 1978); with influenza, levels of circulating antibody measured in individuals after vaccination or natural infection correlate well with protection (Bell *et al.* 1957). In the surface infections of the respiratory and presumably the enteric tract, secretory antibody is likely to be involved in the process (Rossen *et al.* 1971). The precise role of cell-mediated immunity in protection is not as well defined, but is undoubtedly of importance sometimes independently and sometimes in association with humoral antibody.

Recognition of viral infection

This is based on detection of the virus by isolation or identification of its antigens, and/or on detection of a significant antibody response. In Table 6.2 are listed common ways viruses are isolated (Lennette and Schmidt 1979). Embryonated or fertile hens' eggs have been employed for many years to isolate influenza viruses by amniotic or allantoic inoculation. This method is still used for vaccine production. The arthropod-borne viruses and other agents have been cultivated in the past by yolk-sac inoculation or by inoculation of suckling mice, although this has largely been supplanted by use of cell culture. Inoculation of suckling mice has been used for isolation of certain coxsackie viruses.

Cell cultures are the principal means for identifying viruses today in laboratories worldwide and especially in more developed countries. They may be of several varieties. Primary cell cultures result when organs or tissues taken from animals are treated to release individual cells and are placed into culture; these cells are capable of only limited further growth, and thus additional subcultivation is rarely practised. Examples are monkey and human embryo kidney or chick embryo cultures. These cultures are generally composed of a number of cell types, which would be expected considering their origin, and they may contain adventitious agents, persistent viruses which had infected the animal from which they were derived. In contrast to these cells, which cannot be propagated well, are the continuous cell lines. These lines are immortal, that is, they can be propagated indefinitely and are mainly derived from tumours (Rafferty 1975). They generally are of a single cell type, and grow readily under proper conditions. Because of their origin, their use for production of vaccines is unacceptable. Finally there are the diploid or semicontinuous cell lines, derived from normal cells, often embryonic, which maintain normal chromosome number. They can be propagated in the laboratory but have a finite number of divisions through which they can be carried. They are of one cell type, do not contain adventitious agents and are acceptable substrates for vaccine production. An example is the human embryo lung line, WI-38 (Hayflick 1965).

Growth of cytocidal viruses in cell culture is mainly recognized by its cytopathic effect, or CPE. Many viruses produce characteristic CPE specific to that type, while others simply destroy cells without producing a typical microscopic effect. In still other situations, little visible damage to cells occurs,

Table 6.2. *Isolation techniques for viruses of public health importance*

Substrate	Method
Embryonated eggs	Inoculation in amniotic, allantoic cavity, or yolk sac
Suckling mice	Intracerebral or intramuscular inoculation
Cell culture	Detection of viral growth by cytopathic effect, haemadsorption, etc.
Organ culture	Detection by measuring or visualizing virus produced

and other means for detecting the presence of virus must be employed. In the haemadsorption technique, red cells are added, which adsorb to certain viruses which bud from the viral membrane. These include influenza and parainfluenza viruses as well as the coronaviruses. Other methods used to identify the presence of virus include identification of viral components with antibodies tagged with fluorescent, radioactive, or similar compounds, and visualizing virus by electron microscopy (EM). The interference method has occasionally been used, that is inoculation of a cytocidal virus into a tube already possibly infected with an unknown specimen; the known virus will produce a cytopathogenic effect if the cell culture is not truly infected. Organ cultures, such as explants of human embryo trachea are used ordinarily for those agents which do not replicate in cell culture (Hoorn and Tyrrell 1969). Virus is identified by visualizing it in EM or by detecting the antigen by immunological procedures.

When it is difficult to cultivate viruses, or when rapid diagnosis is desired, techniques are employed for direct detection of the agent that use antibody which reacts with the viral antigen. This antibody is either itself tagged with a recognizable compound, or a tagged antibody, directed against the first antibody is used (Lennette and Schmidt 1979). The tag may be a fluorescent substance, a radioisotope or a compound which, when a substrate is added, produces a colour in the enzyme-linked immunosorbent assay (ELISA) (Herrman et al. 1979). A limiting factor in these assays is the quantity of virus contained in a particular specimen. Small amounts of virus may be detected by cell culture, since replication takes place, but in the methods just described only if more than a specific amount of virus is contained in the original specimen can it be recognized.

Serological techniques which may be used to identify viral infection by detecting rises in antibody are shown in Table 6.3 (Lennette and Schmidt 1979). In neutralization tests, infectious virus is exposed to antibody and then the mixture is inoculated into cell culture or other susceptible systems. Reduction in infectivity is measured in that system by several methods (Fujita et al. 1979). The test is sensitive and specific but is time consuming. For viruses which haemagglutinate, the haemag-

glutination inhibition test can be performed. Here the haemagglutinating potential of the virus is blocked by antibody. The test is relatively simple, and is specific and sensitive, although somewhat less than neutralization; non-specific inhibitors may be present in serum, which must be removed for accurate interpretation of the test. Complement fixation (CF) is a well-known generally available procedure suitable for most viruses. Complement-fixing antibody tends to be short lived, and is often directed against whole groups of viruses, rather than a specific type. This may make the test more valuable as a screening procedure. However, CF also tends to be less sensitive, especially in infants and young children.

Fluorescent antibody (FA), radioimmunoassay (RIA), and ELISA may all be considered together. They are carried out in a manner similar to that described above for detection of antigen, with the exception that for detecting antibody, known virus is used as antigen. Sensitivity and specificity of FA is often similar to that seen with CF. However, for RIA and ELISA sensitivity is high and, depending on the type of antigen used, the test can be made more specific (Murphy et al. 1981). The ELISA test is of potential importance in public health, since no radioactive reagents are needed. All of these tests can be specific as to isotype, so that IgG, IgM, and IgA antibodies can be separately identified. Such an ability is of value, for example, in the serodiagnosis of rubella or hepatitis when only a blood specimen after infection is available (Osterholm et al. 1980) and the presence of IgM antibody would indicate recent infection.

Diffusion techniques in agar gels are used to detect antibody to a number of viruses. This may involve precipitation based on single radial or double diffusion, or specialized techniques involving incorporation of red cells and complement into the agar, in which the principles of complement fixation apply. Such tests are of moderate sensitivity, and can be made more specific if subunit rather than whole virus antigens are employed.

Specific viruses involved in human infections

The viruses of concern in public health are numerous, and will be reviewed briefly in terms of their characteristics in the laboratory. In Table 6.4 are listed families of DNA-containing viruses of public health importance, with information on their structure. Terminology of viruses is in constant flux, and the nomenclature given may change over time (Melnick 1980).

Parvoviruses are the smallest viruses of vertebrates and are not of established significance in human disease. The adeno-associated viruses (AAV) are satellite viruses which can only multiply in the presence of helper adenoviruses. There is at present no evidence that they play a role in human disease independent of the adenoviruses with which they must grow (Yates et al. 1981). Norwalk and similar viruses of gastroenteritis have been called parvovirus on the basis of their appearance, but there is little evidence that they truly belong to this family (Greenberg et al. 1979). The papovaviridae family includes the papilloma virus of benign human warts and the polyomaviruses. These in turn include the polyomavirus itself, which when inoculated into mice and other laboratory animals produces a solid tumour, and the simian

Table 6.3. *Methods used to detect rise in antibody titre*

Method	Comment
Neutralization test	Neutralization of infectivity – specific and sensitive
Haemagglutination-inhibition	Suitable for only certain viruses – must remove non-specific serum inhibitors
Complement fixation	Antibody short-lived – may detect cross-reactive, antibody
Immunofluorescence	Moderately sensitive – requires appropriate microscope
Radioimmunoassay	Sensitive – requires use of radioisotopes
Enzyme-linked immunosorbent assay (ELISA)	Sensitive – special equipment not necessary
Antibody diffusion in agar	Variable sensitivity – requires little specialized equipment

Table 6.4. *DNA viruses of public health importance*

Family	Size (nm)	Structure	DNA	Envelope	Members
Parvoviridae	18–26	Icosahedral symmetry	Single stranded	No	Adeno-associated viruses,?Norwalk
Papovaviridae	45–55	Icosahedral symmetry	Double stranded	No	Papilloma (wart) virus, polyoma, simian virus (SV)$_{40}$
Adenoviridae	70–90	Icosahedral symmetry	Double stranded	No	Adenoviruses of most animals
Herpesviridae	100–200	Envelope around icosahedral capsid	Double stranded	Yes	Herpes, varicella-zoster, EB, cytomegalovirus
Poxviridae	230–300	Brick-shaped, complex	Double stranded	Yes	Vaccinia, smallpox, cowpox, monkeypox

virus SV$_{40}$. The latter agent was present as a contaminant in early batches of inactivated poliovaccines produced in monkey kidney. Because it is a polyomavirus with oncogenic potential, frequency of tumours in recipients has been evaluated but no clear effect has been found.

The adenoviruses are a large group of viruses mainly involved in respiratory infections of man, as well as other infections such as keratoconjunctivitis, cystitis, and most recently gastroenteritis (Jacobsson *et al.* 1979). The behaviour of the virus in man is dependent on its type, of which there are at least 34. Type specificity is related to the 'fibre protein' of the virus while the cross-reactive antigen is associated with the base protein. The CF test, as well as others, such as ELISA, detects the cross-reactive antigen while haemagglutination-inhibition (HI) or neutralization is more type specific. Growth of the viruses in permissive cell culture is slow with production of a typical cytopathogenic effect. In addition, the penton protein of the virus is toxic, and causes detachment of cells from the surface on which they are growing. Human adenoviruses produce tumours when injected into laboratory animals, and this potential is also dependent on their type; there is no clear evidence that this oncogenicity occurs in natural infection, although it has obvious implications in terms of vaccine development. As is true of certain other DNA viruses, adenoviruses can produce latent infections and prolonged shedding is characteristic.

The viruses thus far described have been non-enveloped and, since the viral envelope usually contains lipid, the non-enveloped viruses are generally resistant to lipid solvents such as ether or chloroform. Members of the herpesviridae are sensitive to these solvents. These agents in general are similar in that they all cause latent or recurrent infections. They are quite different in many other characteristics; the herpesviruses themselves are related to each other antigenically but not to other members of the family (Nahmias and Roisman 1973). They are readily grown in cell cultures of many types and produce typical CPE. Serodiagnosis is only rarely useful because of the recurrent nature of the infection. The varicella-zoster virus, in contrast, is much more difficult to grow in cell culture. The same virus is involved in chicken pox and in herpes zoster, its recurrent form. In addition to culture techniques, the agent may be detected around vesicles or in the vesicular fluid by identifying the typical giant cells or visualizing the virus by electron microscopy. Antibody determinations may be of use in identifying susceptibility, especially in immunocompromised children. Cytomegalovirus (CMV)

infections are widespread and again latency is characteristic. While there are cytomegaloviruses of various species, infection with a particular virus seems to be species specific. Congenital infection is the principal reason for public health importance of the agent, and can be identified serologically in the newborn by FA or other techniques which distinguish mother's IgG from children's IgM antibody. The virus replicates relatively slowly in cell cultures; thus isolation is not as simple a procedure as with many other viruses. It is also possible to detect inclusions in cells in the urine, which have characteristic appearance. Epstein Barr (EB) virus was first identified by Epstein and Barr in Burkitt lymphoma cells cultured *in vivo* (Epstein *et al.* 1965). This virus has proven difficult to cultivate and its identification by direct isolation is limited to the specialized laboratory. A number of serological procedures are available to confirm its aetiologic role in cases of suspected infectious mononucleosis.

Vaccinia is the best studied of the poxviruses while smallpox is the one which previously had the greatest impact on the human population. Although they do contain lipid, they are relatively insensitive to inactivation by lipid solvents, by disinfectants, or by drying, and thus the smallpox virus was well known to survive in crusts from infected individuals. The poxviruses can easily be isolated on the chorio-allantoic membrane of chick embryos on which it produces typical pox-like lesions. The isolates of variola virus can be distinguished from those of vaccinia or poxviruses of animals by antigenic characteristics. Virus can also be identified as to family in vesicular fluids by electron microscopy.

The families of RNA viruses are similarly listed in Table 6.5. The picornaviruses are a large family of relatively stable, non-lipid-containing viruses causing many different diseases in man. The term picornavirus itself indicates that they are small RNA-containing viruses. Table 6.6 lists prominent members of the family. The enterovirus and rhinovirus genera are of greatest importance in human infection and are distinguished in the laboratory by the fact that the former are acid stable and the latter acid labile (Hughes *et al.* 1973). This enables enteroviruses to pass through the stomach and infect the lower enteric tract. The polioviruses, three in type, can be cultivated in cell culture easily and quickly. Infection can also be identified serologically. At present, a recurring public health problem is distinguishing between revertent live attenuated vaccine strains causing paralysis and wild strains. This is accomplished in the laboratory by sensitive neutralization tests. Recent application of monoclonal antibody tech

Table 6.5. *RNA viruses of public health importance*

Family	Size (nm)	Structure	RNA	Envelope	Members
Picornaviridae	24–30	Icosahedral symmetry	Single stranded	No	See Table 6.6
Togaviridae	40–70	Icosahedral capsid – within envelope	Single stranded	Yes	Formerly portion of arbovirus. See Table 6.7
Reoviridae	60–80	Icosahedral double capsid	Double stranded Segmented	No	Reovirus, rotavirus, orbivirus
Coronaviridae	80–130	Spherical – club-shaped projections	Single stranded	Yes	Coronaviruses of man – Animal gastroenteritis, mouse hepatitis
Orthomyxoviridae	80–120	Spherical or filamentous-spikes on envelope	Single stranded Segmented	Yes	Influenza types A, B, and C
Paramyxoviridae	150–300	Spherical – envelope with spikes	Single stranded	Yes	See Table 6.8
Arenaviridae	85–120	Surface projections on envelope contain granules	Single stranded Segmented	Yes	Lymphocytic choriomeningitis, Lassa fever; Tacaribe group
Bunyaviridae	90–100	Spherical – envelope with spikes	Single stranded Segmented	Yes	Formerly portion of arboviruses – California group
Rhabdoviridae	175×70	Bullet shaped	Single stranded	Yes	Rabies, vesicular stomatitis virus
Retroviridae	100	Various	Single stranded	Yes	Oncogenic viruses

Table 6.6. *Members of family Picornaviridae*

Genus	Common member
Enterovirus	Poliovirus, coxsackie virus A and B, echoviruses, other enteroviruses
Rhinovirus	Rhinoviruses of humans and cattle
Cardiovirus	Encephalomyocarditis (EMC)
Aphthovirus	Foot and mouth disease

niques has increased the ability to differentiate between different wild strains, so that subtypes can be identified and separated for epidemiological purposes.

Most of the type A and B coxsackie viruses can now be isolated in cell culture. However, use of suckling mice is still necessary to identify each one of the 23 types. The group A viruses produce myositis and necrosis in voluntary muscles, while group B produce focal areas of degeneration in the brain plus other more distant changes. The list of diseases caused by these viruses is much longer than the classic herpangina by group A and pleurodynia by group B. As is the situation in suckling mice, they generally involve the muscles or central nervous system and are characteristically related to specific types. The name ECHO virus is an acronym for enteric cytopathic human orphan virus, orphan because they were isolated from stools of individuals without disease. However, most have been associated with illnesses, such as aseptic meningitis, febrile illness with rash, and, occasionally in institutional epidemics, enteritis. Cytopathic effects are observed on culture in primary monkey kidney, or in other commonly available cell systems. Specific serological diagnosis is difficult with the ECHO viruses, as with the coxsackie viruses, since cross-reactions are common in the tests generally available.

It was decided, after 23 coxsackie and 31 ECHO viruses had been identified, that any future enteroviruses that were not polioviruses would simply be termed enteroviruses and

numbered from 68 onward. This was done because of the overlapping characteristics of the genera. Enterovirus 70 is an example of these types, and is the cause of acute haemorrhagic conjunctivitis (Mirkovic *et al.* 1973). Rhinoviruses, made up of at least 115 types, are the most frequent cause of the common cold. They can be easily isolated in a limited number of cell systems, such as WI-38 (Monto and Cavallaro 1972). Diagnosis is usually carried out by virus isolation since the antibody response is mainly type-specific and without knowing the type of the infecting strain, selection of the proper virus to use is impossible.

The togaviruses are enveloped and relatively unstable when maintained without added protein. The family is mainly composed of agents which were formerly called arboviruses. They were defined as being transmitted biologically by an arthropod vector and exhibiting sensitivity to lipid solvents. The genera listed in Table 6.7 are classified by their cross-reactions in HI tests; the haemagglutinin is associated with spikes on the surface of the viral envelope. Viraemia typically occurs and allows the arthropod to become infected when it feeds. The agents multiply in the arthropod, and in some instances exhibit transovarian transmission. Isolation was previously carried out by intracerebral inoculation of suckling mice, which has largely been replaced by cell culture in many laboratories. Domestic fowl are also susceptible, and have been used as sentinel animals. The rubella virus shares

Table 6.7. *Members of family Togaviridae*

Genus	Members
Alphavirus (Group A arboviruses)	Easter equine, Venezuelan, western equine, encephalitis, sindbis, and others
Flavivirus (Group B arboviruses)	Yellow fever, dengue, Japanese B, St. Louis encephalitis, Murray Valley, West Nile fever, etc.
Rubivirus	Rubella
Pestivirus	Hog cholera

structural characteristics with these agents, and thus has been placed in the togavirus family although arthropods are never involved in transmission. The virus does possess a haemagglutinin in common with other togaviruses.

Of the reoviruses, only the rotaviruses are common pathogens for man. The term derives from respiratory enteric orphan virus and orphans the reoviruses themselves have remained. The double-stranded, segmental genome is the most characteristic feature of the family. The genera are somewhat different in EM and do not cross-react immunologically. The human rotaviruses are involved in enteric illnesses, especially of young children. It is difficult to isolate these viruses in cell culture and detection by ELISA is the method of choice, replacing direct visualization by EM (Yolken *et al.* 1977). The arbo-virus genus contains members which multiply in arthropods, including the agent of Colorado tick fever.

Coronaviruses were named because of their appearance; projections give the virion the appearance of a solar corona. The viruses in man cause common respiratory illnesses and are difficult to isolate. Organ culture of human embryo trachea has been required for isolation. Much of the information on their behaviour in man has come from serologic studies using CF, HI, and, more recently, ELISA methods (Monto and Lim 1974). The viruses in animals cause a variety of illnesses, including gastroenteritis. In man, the latter association has yet to be clearly documented. The influenza viruses, classic agents of respiratory infection of man, are the principal members of the orthomyxovirus family. The types are distinguished from each other on the basis of a common nucleoprotein antigen. The subtypes of type A and B are divided on the basis of their haemagglutinin and neuraminidase located separately on the spikes projecting from the virion. The shifts and drifts characteristic of these glycoproteins are related to the segmented genome of the virus, which has also allowed creation of live vaccine candidates by reassortment-recombination (Odagiri *et al.* 1982). The viruses are easily isolated in embryonated eggs and cell culture, and haemagglutination inhibition is the most commonly used serological procedure.

The paramyxoviruses are larger than the orthomyxoviruses, and their genome is not segmented. As shown in Table 6.8, these viruses are varied in their makeup. The parainfluenzaviruses are of four types, cause respiratory infection, and along with mumps and Newcastle disease virus (NDV) possess haemagglutinin and neuraminidase. The haemagglutinin and neuraminidase are located together on single spikes surrounding the virion, and the F protein responsible for cell fusion and haemolysis is located on other spikes. They

can be grown readily in cell culture and identification is facilitated by the haemadsorption technique (Shelokov *et al.* 1958). Complement fixation, HI, and neutralization tests can be used for serodiagnosis, with specificity greatest for the last technique and least for the first. The measles virus haemagglutinates but does not have a demonstrable neuraminidase. Like the parainfluenzaviruses, it haemolyses susceptible erythrocytes and on growth of cell cultures can be detected by haemadsorption. Viremia is associated with infection and antibody can be detected by a number of commonly available techniques. Respiratory syncytial (RS) virus is so named because of the typical CPE produced in susceptible cell culture. It is quite unstable and cultures containing it must not be subjected to freeze-thaw cycles before inoculation. No haemagglutination has been demonstrated for this agent, which is the most important cause of bronchiolitis in children, but which also produces common respiratory infections in adults. Secretory antibody appears to be of importance in preventing reinfection or modifying symptoms.

The arenaviruses and bunyaviruses are similar in certain characteristics but, as indicated by their being placed in separate families, are different in others. On EM, the arenaviruses have dense granules in the centre of the virion (arena = sand) and many of the agents infect rodent hosts, who shed virus for long periods. The bunyaviruses on the other hand are a large group of arthropod-borne viruses, of worldwide distribution. Like the togaviruses, they can be cultivated in the laboratory in suckling mice or cell culture. The principal member of the rhabdovirus family is rabies. The virus has a unique morphology and is enveloped, rendering it susceptible to lipid solvents. Glycoprotein projections cause haemagglutination of susceptible red cells. The virus can be cultured in laboratory animals and in embryonated eggs, but for public health purposes, the FA test is relied on for detection of viral antigen in animal brain or human cells. There are several related viruses, but since they do not infect man, the test can be considered specific. The retroviridae are a diverse group of agents producing leukaemia and solid tumours in mammals and birds. Their unique feature is possession of a reverse transcriptase; with this enzyme DNA is produced which is then involved in malignant transformation of the host cell.

Other viruses, which are not yet classified, include viruses of hepatitis A, which is probably an RNA-containing enterovirus, and hepatitis B, which contains double-stranded DNA. The Dane particle, which represents the complete virus of hepatitis B, is 43 nm in diameter and is enveloped (Purcell *et al.* 1973). The virus of Ebola has a unique snake-like structure shared by Marburg fever. The virion contains RNA and may represent a new family.

With the identification of new and exotic diseases in various parts of the world, it is probable that the list of agents involved in human disease will continue to expand and will not be restricted to unusual diseases. For example, current work with non-cultivable viruses involved in enteric illnesses is continuing to result in identification of new agents. It is also probable that additional chronic diseases will be found to have an infectious aetiology, either resulting from an unusual manifestation of a common infection, such as illustrated by

Table 6.8. *Members of family Paramyxoviridae*

Genus	Members
Paramyxovirus	Parainfluenza types 1–4, mumps, Newcastle disease virus (NDV)
Morbillivirus	Measles virus, canine distemper, rinderpest
Pneumovirus	Respiratory syncytial (RS) virus

subacute sclerosing panencephalitis and measles, or from a new virus specific to the process.

Vaccines will continue to be a principal means of prevention of most infectious diseases. New technologies, such as the ability to clone genes coding for specific portions of a virus will allow production of purified antigens of high titre, which will then expand the diseases for which such means of prophylaxis are possible. Live attenuated vaccines are also to be introduced and will have greatest potential against surface infections, in which local immunity is critical. Rapid viral diagnosis, often using monoclonal antibodies, will enable early identification of circulating agents. This in turn should stimulate the search for additional antiviral drugs, or other means of aborting outbreaks already in progress. Thus a number of developments at the molecular level are likely to be employed practically for the control of infectious-disease transmission.

BACTERIA

While viruses are obligate intracellular parasites and as such may cause diseases, most bacteria are autonomously replicating biological entities. In general, if nutritional substrates are provided, bacteria can produce all the components necessary for self-replication. *Rickettsia* and *Chlamydia* are the exceptions to this rule being obligate intracellular parasites.

Nutritional substrates are provided in ecological locations or spaces called habitats. In nature literally all habitats are colonized with bacteria. The substrates and physical components of the habitat dictate the metabolic processes employed by a bacterium and thus define an ecological niche.

In man, bacteria can be found in many habitats most of these being mucosal surfaces. In almost all cases, bacteria and man live together as partners in a mutualistic or symbiotic relationship. Occasionally an ecological imbalance occurs in a habitat and then the so-called commensal or indigenous organisms induce disease. However, most bacteria that induce diseases in man are considered to be true pathogens and can be divided into two classes: (i) organisms that are not indigenous to man and almost always cause disease when in man, such as *Salmonella*; and (ii) organisms indigenous to man but present in a habitat where they are not normally found. Tables 6.9–6.11 list the pathogenic bacteria of public health importance and some of their salient features. These lists, however, are not comprehensive and group bacteria into Gram-positive, Gram-negative, and others.

The resulting diseases are usually based upon the metabolic activities of the organisms and thus upon the niche and habitat. Diseases often occur for example as a result of toxic substances that are by-products of materials synthesized to help obtain the necessary substrates for growth. That the bacterial population survives after the host has either succumbed or rid itself of the organism demonstrates that the organism is simply adapting to the host habitat. Evolutionary freaks also exist where the end result is the loss of life to the pathogen (and often times to the host), such as *Yersinia pestis*. This small group is exemplary of obligate bacterial parasites. Preservation of such populations occurs by direct passage from host to host.

Bacterial virulence is a multifactorial process and certain requirements must be satisfied for expression and induction of disease (Smith 1977). In the following discussion these requirements will be described and when possible, examples will be provided.

Entry

Virulence is dependent upon the method of and portal of entry used by the bacterium. In order to establish itself in a given habitat, it must be able to gain access to that site. Organisms that remain at a mucosal surface are at a particu-

Table 6.9. *Gram-positive pathogenic bacteria*

Organism	Morphology	Diseases*
Corynebacterium diphtheriae	Rod	Diphtheria
Streptococcus pneumoniae	Cocci	Pneumonia, sinusitis, otitis media
Streptococcus pyogenes	Cocci	Pharyngitis, scarlet fever, otitis media, meningitis, peritonitis, pneumonia, acute glomerulonephritis, rheumatic fever
Streptococcus viridans	Cocci	Endocarditis
Streptococcus mutans	Cocci	Dental caries
Staphylococcus aureus	Cocci	Cutaneous abscess, endocarditis, pneumonia, enterocolitis, food poisoning, skin exfoliation
Bacillus anthracis	Spore-forming rod	Anthrax (cutaneous or pulmonary)
Bacillus cereus	Spore-forming rod	Food poisoning
Clostridium botulinum	Anaerobic spore-forming rod	Botulism
Clostridium tetani	Anaerobic spore-forming rod	Tetanus
Clostridium perfringens	Anaerobic spore-forming rod	Gas gangrene, bacteraemia, food poisoning
Clostridium difficile	Anaerobic spore-forming rod	Antibiotic-associated pseudomembranous enterocolitis
Listeria monocytogenes	Microaerophilic rod	Listeriosis

*Does not include all clinical manifestations.

Table 6.10. *Gram-negative pathogenic bacteria*

Organism	Morphology	Diseases*
Neisseria meningitidis	Cocci	Septicaemia, meningitis
Neisseria gonorrhoeae	Cocci	Gonorrhoea
Escherichia coli	Rod	Ascending urinary tract infections, diarrhoea, septicaemia, meningitis, nosocomial infections
Klebsiella pneumoniae	Rod	Pneumonia, diarrhoea, nosocomial infections
Proteus species	Rod	Urinary tract infections
Salmonella enteritidis	Rod	Gastroenteritis
Salmonella typhi	Rod	Typhoid fever
Salmonella paratyphi	Rod	Paratyphoid fever
Salmonella cholerae-suis	Rod	Septicaemia
Shigella species	Rod	Dysentery
Vibrio cholerae	Curved rod	Cholera
Vibrio parahemolyticus	Curved rod	Food poisoning
Campylobacter fetus ssp *jejuni*	Microaerophilic curved rod	Gastroenteritis
Bacteroides fragilis	Anaerobic rod	Abscess, peritonitis, endocarditis
Pseudomonas aeruginosa	Rod	Infections of the urinary tract and burn sites, septicaemia
Yersinia pestis	Rod	Bubonic and pneumonic plague
Yersinia enterocolitica	Rod	Diarrhoea
Francisella tularensis	Rod	Tularaemia
Brucella species	Rod	Brucellosis
Hemophilus influenzae	Small rod	Meningitis, septicaemia
Bordetella pertussis	Small rod	Pertussis
Treponema pallidum	Anaerobic spirochete	Syphilis
Treponema pertenue	Anaerobic spirochete	Yaws
Borrelia recurrentis	Microaerophilic spirochete	Relapsing fever
Legionella pneumophila	Coccobacillus	Legionnaire's disease
Streptobacillus moniliformis	Anaerobic rod	Rat-bite fever
Bartonella bacilliformis	Coccobacillus	Bartonellosis

*Does not include all clinical manifestations.

Table 6.11. *Other pathogenic bacteria*

Organism	Morphology and other traits	Diseases*
Mycobacterium tuberculosis	Small rod	Tuberculosis
Mycobacterium leprae	Small rod	Leprosy
Rickettsia prowazekii	Small coccobacillus	Louse-borne typhus, Brill–Zinsser disease
Rickettsia rickettsii	Small coccobacillus	Rocky Mountain spotted fever
Rickettsia conorii	Small coccobacillus	Boutonneuse fever
Rickettsia akari	Small coccobacillus	Rickettsialpox
Rickettsia tsutsugamushi	Small coccobacillus	Scrub typhus
Coxiella burnetti	Small coccobacillus	Q fever
Chlamydia trachomatis	Very small varies during development cycle	Trachoma, conjunctivitis, urethritis, pelvic inflammation (female), lymphogranuloma venereum
Mycoplasma pneumoniae	Very small spherical to filamentous	Pneumonia

*Does not include all clinical manifestations.

lar disadvantage in this respect since there is usually a single route of entry to that site. Thus, an organism that induces disease in the lung usually must be introduced through some component of the respiratory tract. Conversely, enteric pathogens would not induce a disease if naturally introduced into the respiratory tract. Organisms that are capable of invading mucosal surfaces have the potential to move to literally any organ habitat; however, the success of the invasive organism in gaining access to an internal habitat is usually dependent upon the initial route of entry into the host.

Colonization

Establishment of an organism at a site (usually a mucosal surface) and maintenance of a stable or increasing population size are components of colonization. Most pathogens, whether they are invasive or not, initially colonize mucosal surfaces. In general, the mechanism that promotes a stable interaction at a site is an association of the organism with the mucosal surface (Savage 1972, 1977). Association does not imply direct contact between the bacterium and the host. The extreme example of association is direct bacterial attachment to the mucosa which is analogous to receptor (host)-ligand (bacterium) interaction. The attachment process has been definitely established for very few bacteria. Adherence *in vivo* to mucosal surfaces has been conclusively demonstrated as an essential process in the colonization of pig, sheep, or calf small intestines by some enteropathogenic strains of *Escherichia coli* (EPEC) (Moon *et al.* 1979). Biopsy samples from small intestines demonstrate that some EPEC may adhere to the mucosa and human small intestines. Results from *in vitro* experiments demonstrate the potential adhesiveness of other bacterial species to a variety of tissue and surfaces, however, such results cannot be extrapolated to *in vivo* conditions. Electron micrographs and physical data can be used to establish the concept that association with (not adherence to) mucosal surfaces is a factor involved in colonization.

Although surface association is an important process, it alone will not result in the colonization of a habitat by bacteria. Colonization like virulence is a multifactorial process. Several factors must be fulfilled if the overall process is to occur. Bacteria in a given habitat must have the capacity to survive and proliferate in that habitat. Components of these traits include:

1. The capacity to replicate using the substrates present in the habitat without being adversely affected by other substances.

2. The capacity to replicate at a rate greater than or equal to the rate of washout. The best example of this is in the gastrointestinal tract where fluid is continually flowing from anterior to posterior and may act to dilute the bacterial population.

3. The capacity to evade other host responses that promote bacterial clearance, such as the immune response. This may be facilitated by a variety of cellular components of the bacterium, the most commonly acknowledged structure being the capsule (Davies *et al.* 1980).

These amorphous, poorly antigenic capsules (usually carbohydrate) may act to cover the more highly antigenic sites on the cell surface and thus make them for all practical purposes appear to be non-existent. The trait most commonly associated with bacterial capsules is antiphagocytosis, however, this is likely to be due to the poorly antigenic nature of the capsule.

Capsules clearly are important attributes of virulence. Mutants of *Streptococcus pneumoniae* that do not produce a capsule become avirulent. Capsular revertants obtained by transformation with DNA from capsular strains regain virulence (Avery *et al.* 1944). The M protein of Streptococci may be important in preventing phagocytosis (Fox 1974).

Other bacteria may evade the host immune response by sharing antigenic architecture with the host. Although the role of such properties in virulence has not been established, it has been shown that some strains of *Bacteroides* share antigens with the murine gut mucosa (Foo and Lee 1974). This organism is, therefore, recognized as part of the host and is not subject to immune clearance, at least in the gut. While some organisms try to invade the host immune response, other organisms deliberately present themselves to the host in order to elicite a cellular immune response. Some bacteria are phagocytosed by macrophages, but are insensitive to lysosomal enzymes and therefore persist in the phagocyte ultimately killing it. *Francisella tularensis* enters monocytes and remains there for long periods. This enables it to evade other host responses and ultimately persist (Davis *et al.* 1980). The production of mycosides by Mycobacteria probably makes them resistant to complement-mediated lysis (Davis *et al.* 1980).

Invasion

Some bacteria do not remain on the mucosal surface but invade the mucosa to reach deeper tissue or organ sites. Invasion usually is dependent upon host and bacterial factors. Some pathogens of the family Enterobacteriaceae induce disease by remaining on the mucosal surface (e.g. EPEC) (Moon *et al.* 1979), while others do so by invading through the mucosa (e.g. *Salmonella*) (Davis *et al.* 1980). *Salmonella* species appear to invade by first adhering to the mucosa and then eliciting a message that results in an endocytic response by the host (Jones *et al.* 1981). Inhibitors of microtubule formation such as cytochalasin B prevent invasion by *Salmonella*. Other bacteria such as *Staphylococcus* produce membrane solubilizing toxins (see below) that may aid in invasion. An extreme and rather artificial means of invasion is associated with tissue trauma where exposure to deeper tissues is made directly available. Organisms that use this means of access to tissues may be categorized as opportunistic pathogens. Clostridia that induce gas gangrene require a traumatized portal of entry.

Invasive organisms are subjected to additional stresses by the host and must possess other attributes that permit proliferation. Probably the major non-immune mechanism for controlling bacteria that invade is by regulation of the amount of free iron available for bacterial use. Very potent iron chelators are produced by the host that help maintain low concentrations of free ferrous salts. The serum and tissue proteins, transferrin and lactoferrin, are powerful iron chelators (affinity constants of approximately 10^{30}–Weinburg 1978). With normal body concentrations of iron ($18\mu M$ in the body) the effective concentration of free ferrous ions for bacterial use is 10^8-fold lower than necessary to permit growth. Pathogenic bacteria have evolved their own arsenal of iron-chelating agents, called siderophores, that effectively compete with host chelators for iron. In fact, under the appropriate conditions, the bacterial siderophores can actually take iron away from lactoferrin or transferrin. In the absence of high-affinity siderophores, bacteria simply cannot exist in the mammalian host.

The regulation of iron concentration is one method by which the host effectively combats bacterial infections. During bacterial infections, the host responds by specifically lowering serum iron. Furthermore, some bacteria cannot effectively compete for iron at temperatures above the normal host temperature (Kluger and Rothenburg 1979). Thus, the fever response induced by bacterial endotoxin (see below) prevents the bacteria from obtaining iron and thus the organism dies.

Extracellular products

The production of extracellular substances that in one way or another adversely affect the host may be classified into a general category called toxins, although many of these substances are not generally accepted as exotoxins. Volatile fatty acids secreted by Clostridia in wounds would not be considered as exotoxins, yet they are secreted, toxic, and contribute to the overall virulence of the organism. These secreted products are actually end products of fermentation and putrefaction.

The diversity of true exotoxins is immense. Some exotoxins are enzymes, some are inhibitor- and some detergent-like substances. All exotoxins are secreted. See Table 6.12 for a list of exotoxins. Diphtheria toxin has been intensively studied and will be discussed further as an example of an exotoxin (Collier 1975).

Strains of *Corynebacterium diphtheriae* that are lysogenized by the bacteriophage β have the capacity to produce diphtheria toxin. Toxin is only produced when the concentration of iron in the host is low, a situation expected *in vivo* (see above). The toxin is synthesized as a proteinaceous protoxin requiring activation by a bacterial protease. The toxin attaches to receptors on the target cell surface and then a portion enters the cell. The putative target for diphtheria toxin is within the respiratory tract. The toxic moiety is an enzyme that catalyses the ADP-ribosylation of an important component of eucaryotic protein synthesis; elongation factor 2 (EF2). ADP-ribosylated EF2 is not functional; therefore, cellular protein synthesis is inhibited and the affected cell dies presumably resulting in increased substrate concentration for the *C. diphtheriae* cells.

Interestingly, several other toxins have similar modes of action in that they catalyse the ADP-ribosylation of essential host proteins. The toxin of *Pseudomonas aeruginosa*, PA toxin, affects EF2 (Iglewski and Kabat 1975), while *Vibrio cholerae* enterotoxin (Gill 1979) and *E. coli* heat-labile enterotoxin (Gill and Richardson 1980) affect guanosine triphos-

Table 6.12. *Selected bacterial exotoxins*

Species	Exotoxin	Action
Corynebacterium diphtheriae	Diphtheria	ADP-ribosylation of EF 2
Streptococcus pyogenes	Streptolysisn S	Haemolysin
	Streptolysin O	Haemolysin
	Erythrogenic toxin	Skin rash
	DPNase	Cardiotoxin
	Streptodornase	DNase
Staphylococcus aureus	α, β, γ, and δ toxins	Haemolysins
	Enterotoxin	Gut fluid secretion
	Leukocidin	Leukocidic
Clostridium botulinum	Botulinum toxin	Neurotoxic
Clostridium tetani	Tetanus toxin	Neurotoxic
Clostridium perfringens	$\alpha, \beta, \gamma, \delta, \varepsilon, \eta, \theta, \lambda$	Haemolysins
Clostridium perfringens	κ	Collagenase
	λ	Protease
	Enterotoxin	Gut fluid secretion
Escherichia coli	Heat-stable and heat-labile enterotoxins	Gut fluid secretion
Salmonella enteritidis	Enterotoxin	Gut fluid secretion
Shigella	Shiga toxin	Neurotoxic
Vibrio cholerae	Choleragen	Gut fluid secretion (ADP-ribosylation of a GTP-binding protein)
Pseudomonas aeruginosa	PA toxin	ADP-ribosylation of EF 2
Yersinia pestis	Plague toxin	Necrotizing
Bordetella pertussis	Pertussis toxin	Necrotizing

hate (GTP) binding proteins. Although the reactions cata-
lysed by these toxins are similar, there are vast differences in
the clinical manifestations associated with the toxins and
bacteria. The enterotoxins induce diarrhoea, diphtheria toxin
induces the respiratory disease diphtheria, and the PA toxin
results in tissue desquamation usually associated with burns.

Many toxins have been classified as haemolysins because
they lyse red blood cells. These toxins, whether detergent-like
or enzymes, probably are important because they promote
the solubilization of target cells (usually not red blood cells *in
vivo*) providing the bacterium with additional substrates for
growth. Cardiotoxic, leukocidic, and necrotic activities are all
associated with the various haemolysins.

Neurotoxins are produced by a variety of organisms and
appear to act as inhibitors of nerve message transmission
(Boroff and Das Gupta 1971; van Heyningen and Mellanby
1971). Organisms producing neurotoxins include *Clostridium
botulinum*, *Cl. tetani*, and *Shigella dysenteriae*. Although a
role of toxins in microbial virulence is implicated due to the
effects they have when introduced into the host and in many
cases substantiated, these products are likely produced as a
method for bacteria to be able to survive in the specific host
habitat and thus contribute to the niche.

Endotoxin

The envelope structure of all Gram-negative bacteria includes
an outer membrane (outside of the cell wall) composed in part
of lipopolysaccharide (LPS). The LPS is constructed of a
lipid component, a core carbohydrate, and a carbohydrate
antigen called O-antigen. The O-antigen may enhance the
virulence of the bacteria by making the cell smooth. The
presence of O-antigen makes the cell envelope less hydrophobic thus decreasing cell aggregation and phagocytosis.

The lipid portion of LPS is called lipid A. This has toxic
activity to eucaryotic cells and has also been called endotoxin (Bradley 1979). Endotoxin is different from secreted
exotoxins by a variety of criteria:

1. It is an integral part of the cell envelope and is secreted
into the surrounding environment by pinching off of small
membrane vesicles.
2. The toxin is not very potent when compared to exotoxins. An LD_{50} for endotoxin may be in micrograms while
an LD_{50} for exotoxins may be nano- to picograms.
3. The biological activity of endotoxin is quite diverse and
appears to affect literally all mammalian organs. Among the
activities associated with endotoxin are: pyrogenicity, leuko-
penia, shock, inflammation, and release of histamine.

A Gram-negative organism that produces an adequate
siderophore and can colonize a specific mucosal habitat can
be a pathogen. Capacity to survive and the production of
endotoxin are probably sufficient to induce disease.

Plasmids and resistance to antibiotics

The role of antibiotic resistance in bacterial infections has
been of increasing importance. Although the possession of
genes enabling a bacterium to be resistant to one or more

antibiotics does not make an organism pathogenic, such traits
do contribute directly to the virulence of the organism.

The acquisition of genes conferring antibiotic resistance is
associated, in most instances, with the acquisition of a small
piece of DNA called a plasmid (Helsinki 1973; Levy *et al.*
1981). Plasmids range in size from under 1×10^6 daltons to
larger than 1×10^8 daltons and may code for resistance to
one or more different antibiotics. One of the most important
aspects of plasmids encoding antibiotic resistance (R-factors)
is that these genetic elements are transmissible from cell to cell
within the same species and in many cases to other genera.
Most particularly, many R-factors from Gram-negative
enteric organisms are freely transmissible to any other organism in this group. It is clear that the transmissible nature of
plasmids make them well suited to cause an epidemic spread
of antibiotic resistance to a population of bacterial cells in a
given habitat. Since the acquisition of R-factors contributes to
virulence, poorly virulent organisms are more likely to cause a
disease than previously. This is of particular importance when
one considers the effect this has on the host's attempts to
clear pathogens. As one organism is removed, another one
may acquire the R-factor and may take over. Since these
organisms are resistant to certain antibiotics, treatment must
be with an antibiotic the organism is sensitive to or the host
must actively be able to clear the pathogen.

The widespread and often indiscriminate use of antibiotics
puts extreme selective pressure on bacteria to become resistant
to antibiotics. In nature, there is a diversity of R-factors specifying resistance to different antibiotics. These R-factors
probably evolved in bacterial species that coexisted in habitats
with antibiotic producing fungi. Prior to the use of antibiotics
in medicine, there was no selective advantage for a pathogen
to become resistant to antibiotics and thus the R-factors
remained in bacteria from the environmental habitats. Today,
it is becoming increasingly rare to find bacterial pathogens,
especially the widely disseminated species, that do not possess
resistance to at least one antibiotic. Most bacteria that cause
nosocomial infections are resistant to several antibiotics.
Individuals with gonorrhoea usually are treated with ampicillin. However, strains of *Neisseria gonorrhoea* now exist
that have R-factors specifying the production of β-lactamase
which leads to an inactivation of ampicillin. In such cases the
use of different antibiotics is necessary. However, it is fully
expected that *N. gonorrhoea* strains will ultimately become
resistant to other antibiotics. The scenario that one is left with
is that the use of any antibiotic will result in the ultimate
emergence of resistant strains and thus antibiotics may
become of little use in the not too distant future.

In addition to resistance to antibiotics, other plasmid-
encoded virulence attributes are known including synthesis of
adhesins, toxins, and siderophores (Levy *et al.* 1981).

Diagnosis of bacterial disease

The diagnosis of bacterial diseases has, for the most part,
been dependent upon the cultivation and identification, in the
laboratory, of the pathogen. Cultural requirements among
different organisms differ greatly and thus the reader should
determine the precise protocols necessary for cultivation of

specific organisms. Often, cultivated bacteria are tested for the presence of virulence attributes to determine whether the organism is potentially pathogenic or whether the organism is an avirulent, possibly indigenous organism. *Corynebacterium diphtheriae* must be lysogenized by the bacteriophage β to produce diphtheria toxin and induce the disease diphtheria (Collier 1975). The detection of diphtheria toxin is therefore an important step in determining whether the isolated organism was indeed a pathogen. Some organisms by virtue of their metabolism cannot be cultivated *in vitro*, such as *Treponema pallidum*, while others are so dangerous and readily transmissible that cultivation *in vitro* poses a serious health hazard. Identification of these organisms is usually based on a serologic test (see Table 6.3).

FUNGI

Fungi are divided into moulds and yeasts. Table 6.13 sum-marizes the important species responsible for human disease. Traditionally, *Actinomyces* and *Nocardia* have been grouped with the mycotic agents although they are now generally accepted as Gram-positive bacteria.

Infection in all cases is acquired by exposure to the agent by direct contact with soil containing fungi or by inhalation. It is thus understandable that mycoses are primarily cutaneous, mucocutaneous, and pulmonary with respect to sites of infection. In addition, the immunocompromised host is at major risk for severe, systemic mycotic infections as a result of genetic immune deficiencies, severe malignancies, various acquired immune defects, and chemotherapy. In most cases, fungi are not transmitted from patient to patient, the major exception being those that cause dermatophytosis. Although the mycoses are far less frequent than viral, bacterial, protozoal, and helminthic infections, they remain a significant cause of morbidity and mortality in all regions of the world. Some of the agents are restricted in distribution to

Table 6.13. *Major mycoses of public health importance*

Agent	Disease	Primary sites involved	Diagnosis
*Actinomyces israelii**	Actinomycosis	Cervicofacial, thoracic, abdominal tissues	Gram stain of 'sulphur' granule in biopsy of lesion
*Nocardia asteroides**	Nocardiosis	Lungs, brain, meninges	Gram stain of biopsy of lesion
*Nocardia brasiliensis** *Streptomyces somaliensis** *S. madurae**	Actinomycetoma	Foot, hand	Gram stain of granule in biopsy of lesion
Madurella mycetomi *Acremonium* *Phialophora*	Eumycetoma	Foot, hand	Fungus stain of biopsy of lesion
Others *Aspergillus fumigatus* (moulds)	Aspergillosis	Lungs, other organs	Characteristic hyphae and conidiophores on fungus stain of tissue section
Rhizopus *Mucor* *Absidia* (moulds)	Mucormycosis	Various organs	Characteristic hyphae in tissue sections. Culture required for specific identification
Blastomyces dermatitidis	North American blastomycosis	Various organs	Characteristic yeast forms in tissue sections and exudates. Culture confirms identification
Paracoccidioides brasiliensis	South American blastomycosis	Lungs	Characteristic yeast forms in tissue sections. Culture confirms identification
Candida albicans Other *Candida* sp	Moniliasis, thrush, candidiasis	Cutaneous, mucocutaneous, gastrointestinal infection, other organs	Characteristic yeast forms, hyphae, and pseudohyphae in tissue sections. Culture required for specific identification
Coccidioides immitis	Valley fever, coccidioidomycosis	Lungs primarily, but other organs may be involved	Characteristic sporangium in tissue sections. Culture of tissue aspirates
Histoplasma capsulatum	Histoplasmosis	Lungs	Characteristic yeast forms intracellular in mononuclear phagocytes in tissue sections
Histoplasma duboisii	African histoplasmosis	Skin, bones	Characteristic intracellular yeast forms. Culture aids in specific identification
Sporothrix schenckii	Sporotrichosis	Skin, subcutaneous tissues, lymph nodes	Characteristic yeast forms and asteroid bodies in tissue sections, but frequently not found. Culture of tissue or purulent material is usually positive
Crytococcus neoformans	Crytococcosis, torulosis, European blastomycosis	Central nervous system, lungs	Smear and culture of cerebrospinal fluid
Phialophora sp *Cladosporium* sp	Chromomycosis	Skin, subcutaneous tissue	Culture of tissue or purulent material required for species identification
Trichophyton sp *Microsporum* sp *Epidermophyton* sp	Dermatophytosis, tinea	Skin, nails, scalp hair	Microscopic examination of skin scrapings or hair reveals organisms. Culture provides specific identification

*Bacterial species. These agents and their diseases have traditionally been included with the mycoses.

certain foci in the world but the majority are found world-wide.

Precise diagnosis remains difficult since many smaller laboratories and many less developed countries do not have the facilities nor trained staff to isolate and identify fungi. Thus much of the diagnosis depends upon the clinical picture and identification of characteristic forms of the fungi in properly stained histological sections of biopsy tissues and smears of exudates from lesions. The interested reader should consult specific texts of medical mycology and infectious diseases (Rippon 1974; Al-Doory 1975; Binford and Connor 1976; Emmons *et al.* 1977; Mandell *et al.* 1979) to obtain details on each agent and the disease it causes.

PROTOZOA

Protozoans are single-celled eucaryotic organisms found widely distributed throughout the world in both parasitic and free-living forms. The parasitic forms are agents of diseases, many of which, e.g. malaria, have afflicted humans since ancient times. Their distributions are shown in Table 6.14.

The most important protozoans that are significant causes of morbidity in developed countries will be discussed. Several other agents because of their obvious importance worldwide are additionally described. Tables 6.14 and 6.15 summarize the salient features of most parasites. Complete descriptions of these parasites and the diseases may be found in textbooks of parasitology (Hunter *et al.* 1976; Markell and Voge 1981).

Parasites have evolved elegant strategies to avoid destruction by the host immune response enabling them to persist in humans for years. Thus the prevalence of infection for most species is high although rates of morbidity are variable. Some of the most exciting current research indicates that while strain differences with respect to virulence or pathogenicity do exist, the immunological perturbations occurring during infection (INSERM 1978) and host genetic factors (Skamene *et al.* 1980) are very important determinants of morbidity.

Transmission of protozoan parasites is effected not only from faecal contaminated food and water but also by arthropod vectors. This latter form of indirect transmission is obligatory for *Plasmodium, Babesia, Trypanosoma,* and *Leishmania* providing an extra-human system of parasite amplification and dissemination contributing to the complexity of the dynamics of transmission and difficulty in control.

Parasitic protozoa are either obligate intracellular or extracellular parasites. Their pathogenic effects are best appreciated by their usual habitat in the host, vascular, extravascular, or intestinal. Table 6.15 lists the organisms of public health importance by their habitat and indicates the most appropriate diagnostic test(s). The balance of this discussion will focus on the most important parasitic agents and the major determinants of disease and resistance.

On the global scale, malaria remains the most important parasite. Over 2000 million persons live in malarious areas with high rates of mortality in children (Gramiccia and Hempel 1972). *Plasmodium falciparum* is by far the most important of the four species infecting humans as it causes the most morbidity and almost all of the mortality.

The infective forms (sporozoites) inoculated from *Anopheles* mosquitoes invade liver cells to multiply. Then they burst out and invade erythrocytes progressing through a multiplicative stage (schizogony) forming progeny (merozoites) that burst out of the cell to invade others. Rapid multiplication and the ability to invade all ages of erythrocytes are contributory to the malignant characterization of falciparum malaria. The high density of the gametocytes (sexual forms) that occurs in blood is a prominent factor in the density and distribution of infective mosquitoes.

'Natural resistance' has been recognized for a long time in protozoal (especially malarial) infections although until recently its mechanism(s) eluded clarification. Erythrocytes containing the sickle haemoglobin (Friedman 1978), haemoglobin C (Friedman *et al.* 1979), fetal haemoglobin (Friedman

Table 6.14. *Geographical distribution and prevalence of major parasitic protozoa*

Parasite	Distribution	No. infected (thousands)*
Plasmodium falciparum *P. vivax* *P. malariae* *P. ovale*	Africa, Asia, Latin America	800 000
Trypanosoma brucei gambiense *T. b. rhodesiense*	Tropical Africa	1000
Trypanosoma cruzi	Latin America	14 000
Leishmania donovani *L. tropica* *L. mexicana* *L. brasiliensis*	Asia, Africa, Latin America	12 000
Toxoplasma gondii	Worldwide	500 000
Pneumocystis carinii	Worldwide	(?)
Trichomonas vaginalis	Worldwide	(20–25% of all adult females)
Giardia lamblia	Worldwide	200 000
Entamoeba histolytica	Worldwide	400 000

*Taken from references cited in the text and from Walsh, J.A. and Warren, K.S. (1979). Selective primary health care *N. Engl. J. Med.* **301**, 967.

Table 6.15. *Parasitic protozoa of public health importance*

Parasite	Vector/transmission	Diagnosis
Plasmodium falciparum *P. vivax* *P. malariae* *P. ovale*	*Anopheles*	Peripheral blood smear for parasites
Babesia microti	*Ixodes dammini*	Peripheral blood smear for parasites. Serology
Trypanosoma brucei gambiense *T. b. rhodesiense*	*Glossina* (tse-tse)	Peripheral blood smear, lymph node aspiration, cerebrospinal fluid for parasites. Serology of serum and cerebrospinal fluid (IgM, complement fixation test)
Trypanosoma cruzi	*Triatoma, Rhodnius* (reduviid bugs)	Peripheral blood smear for parasites. Xenodiagnosis ('clean' bugs feed on patient) Serology (complement fixation test)
Leishmania donovani *L. tropica* *L. mexicana* *L. brasiliensis*	*Phlebotomus, Lutzomyia, Sergentomya* (sand-flies)	Biopsy of spleen or bone marrow for *L. donovani* only. Smear of lesion exudate
Toxoplasma gondii	Ingestion of meat containing cysts, or oocysts from cat faeces	Biopsy of lymph node. Serology (methylene blue dye test, immunofluorescence, enzyme-linked immunosorbent assay)
Pneumocystis carinii	Airborne	Smear of tracheobronchial aspirates for parasites. Lung biopsy. Serology (complement fixation test)
Trichomonas vaginalis	Sexual contact	Culture or smears of vaginal fluid, urethral discharge.
Giardia lamblia	Ingestion of cyst-contaminated water	Smear of duodenal aspirate, stool smear for trophozoites and cysts
Entamoeba histolytica	Ingestion of cyst-contaminated water (and perhaps food)	Stool smear for trophozoites and cysts. Serology (immunodiffusion, counter immunoelectrophoresis, indirect haemagglutination)
Cryptosporidium sp.	Ingestion of oocytes (?)	Colonic biopsy, stool smear for oocytes

1979), haemoglobin E (Nagel *et al.* 1981), or deficiency in glucose 6-phosphate dehydrogenase (Friedman 1979) are inimical environments for *P. falciparum* development. The near absence of *P. vivax* from West Africans and descendants from West Africans elsewhere in the world is now thought to be a result of the lack of erythrocytic Duffy factor which serves as a receptor allowing Duffy-positive cells to be invaded (Miller *et al.* 1976). Ovalocytic erythrocytes appear to be another genetic abnormality that prevents invasion of *P. falciparum* and possibly of *P. vivax* and *P. malariae* (Kidson *et al.* 1981).

Specific development of immunity to reinfection is indicated in all epidemiological studies of endemic malaria. The experimental evidence points to the major role of serum IgG antibodies although specific cellular immunity complements the overall picture. Nevertheless, the ability of plasmodial species to subvert the immune process to allow parasite survival provides a dynamic balance between positive and negative forces that is responsible for the outcome of the infection.

Of all the protozoan parasites in humans, infection by *Toxoplasma gondii* is perhaps the most prevalent. Toxoplasmosis is distributed worldwide with a significant proportion of the adult population having experienced exposure as determined by serological tests in immunoepidemiological surveys (Frenkel 1973). *Toxoplasma gondii* is intracellular in mononuclear phagocytes and in immune hosts will form slow-growing cysts in muscle and the central nervous system.

Of greatest significance is that this parasite is intestinal in domestic cats but in all other species of mammal, particularly sheep, *Toxoplasma* exists as cysts in muscle. Depending upon

the ecological conditions human exposure is primarily via environmental contamination by infective cyst-laden cat faeces or by inadequately cooked meat products (Frenkel and Ruiz 1981). Clinically significant morbidity constitutes a very small proportion of the total infected although rates of infection can approach 100 per cent in a few years in certain closed communities (Kean 1972). Although resistance to reinfection develops, the initial infection may persist for years if not throughout a lifetime. The parasites are in cysts in very low density suggesting one possible source of organisms from which disease may result in the immunocompromised host.

Pneumocystosis due to *Pneumocystis carinii* is worldwide. The protozoan appears to inhabit pulmonary alveoli in a latent form. It is found in all mammals as trophozoites and characteristic cysts. The primary mode of transmission is airborne based on experimental studies. This organism is now of great importance since it is a cause of extensive pulmonary morbidity in the immunocompromised host.

Trichomonas vaginalis is a sexually transmitted agent that chronically infects the urogenital tract of men and women. It is estimated to infect 20–25 per cent of the adult female population and 30–35 per cent of women with abnormal vaginal discharge (Jirovec and Petru 1968).

Amoebiasis due to *Entamoeba histolytica* is distributed worldwide but is most prevalent in tropical climates. The amoeba invades colonic mucosa causing extensive dysentery and ulcers and in many the amoebae disseminate to extraintestinal sites, especially to the liver, causing abscesses. Transmission via the oral route is effected by faeces containing infective cysts which contaminate water and food supplies. Historically, it was thought that asymptomatic infection

Table 6.16. *Distribution and prevalence of parasitic helminths*

Species	Distribution	No. infected (thousands)*
Diphyllobothrium latum	North America, South America, Europe, Central Africa, foci in Asia	(?)
Taenia saginata	Worldwide	(?)
T. solium	North America, South America, Europe	
Schistosoma mansoni	Caribbean, South America, Africa	
S. haematobium	Middle East, Africa, Asia	250 000
S. japonicum	Asia	
Paragonimus westermani	Asia	2000
Paragonimus sp	Africa, Latin America	(?)
Clonorchis (Opisthorchis) sinensis	Asia	20 000 (est.)
Fasciolopsis buski	Asia	15 000
Heterophyes heterophyes	Africa, Middle East, Asia	(?)
Ascaris lumbricoides	Worldwide	800 000
Necator americanus	Worldwide	700 000
Ancylostoma duodenale		
Strongyloides stercoralis	Worldwide	40 000
Enterobius vermicularis	Worldwide	500 000
Trichuris trichiura	Worldwide	500 000
Trichinella spiralis	Worldwide (especially North America, Europe)	600
Onchocerca volvulus	Latin America, Tropical Africa	40 000
Wuchereria bancrofti	South America, Africa, Asia, Pacific Islands	250 000
Brugia malayi	Asia	
Loa loa	Tropical Africa	13 000
Dracunculus medinensis	Africa, Middle East, Indian subcontinent	50 000

*Taken from references cited in the text and from Walsh, J.A. and Warren, K.S. (1979). Selective primary health care. *N. Engl. J. Med.* **301**, 967.

predominated but a major proportion of these were due to a morphologically identical but non-pathogenic amoeba *E. hartmanni* which is differentiated on the basis of size (less than 10 μm). Recent advances are the identification of pathogenic and non-pathogenic strains on the basis of isoenzyme pattern differences (Sargeaunt and Williams 1978), and the identification of a cytotoxin-enterotoxin (Lusbaugh *et al.* 1979).

Giardia lamblia inhabits the mucosa of the duodenum adhering to villous surfaces by means of a pair of suctorial discs. Transmission is by the oral route from cysts that have been discharged with faeces contaminating water supplies. The distribution of giardiasis has been changing in recent years especially in the US. Previously infection was thought to be primarily limited to children but now adults are commonly afflicted. Cyst-contaminated water supplies in small communities result from inadequate water processing procedures and from discharge of cysts into water supplies from infected beavers (Juranek 1979). In the US, *G. lamblia* is the primary cause of most waterborne gastrointestinal outbreaks.

HELMINTHS

Helminthic parasites in humans are broadly divided into two groups: flatworms, which include both tapeworms (cestodes) and flukes (trematodes), and roundworms (nematodes). They are widely distributed in the world with most species generally being more prevalent in tropical climates. Table 6.16 lists the important helminths and their general geographical distributions. The most characteristic feature of these parasites is that they may reside in humans for years, in many instances for decades, actively producing eggs or larvae. Almost all species cannot complete their entire life history in the human host and thus the worm burden is directly dependent upon the number of infective eggs or larvae in the inoculum from each exposure.

Modes of transmission are varied and for many species complex, utilizing one and two obligatory intermediate vertebrate or invertebrate hosts. This information is summarized in Table 6.17. The importance of particular parasites in certain regions of the world is reflected in how the infections are transmitted to humans and the types of vectors or intermediate hosts required.

In the human host, almost all helminths induce abnormally high levels of immunoglobulin E (IgE) and eosinophils in the peripheral blood. Both have been regarded as indicative of the induction of parasite-related allergic states, although now the eosinophil increase is thought to be important in the development of immunity to reinfection (Butterworth 1980). Those helminths that migrate through the viscera either via vascular systems or directly through parenchymatous organs

Table 6.17. *Major parasitic helminths of public health importance*

Species	Life span (adult) (years)	Habitat	Mode of transmission	Diagnosis
Diphyllobothrium latum	up to 20	Small intestine	Ingestion of larvae (pleroceroids) in flesh of freshwater fish (first intermediate host is microcrustacean)	Eggs in faeces
Taenia saginata	up to 25	Small intestine	Ingestion of larvae (cysticerci) in beef	Proglottids, eggs in faeces
T. solium		Small intestine	Ingestion of cysticerci in pork	
Schistosoma mansoni	4–20	Mesenteric venules	Penetration of skin by larvae (cercariae) in water (intermediate host is snail)	Eggs in faeces, rectal biopsy
S. haematobium	4–20	Vesical plexus		Eggs in urine and faeces, rectal biopsy
S. japonicum	4–20	Mesenteric venules		Eggs in faeces, rectal biopsy
Paragonimus westermani	6	Lungs	Ingestion of larvae (metacercariae) in flesh of freshwater crabs (first intermediate host is snail)	Eggs in sputum, faeces
Clonorchis sinensis	15–20	Bile ducts	Ingestion of metacercariae in flesh of cyprinoid fish (first intermediate host is snail)	Eggs in faeces
Fasciolopsis buski	? several years	Small intestine	Ingestion of metacercariae on water plants, e.g. caltrop, hyacinth, chestnut (intermediate host is snail)	Eggs in faeces
Ascaris lumbricoides	1–2	Small intestine	Ingestion of eggs	Eggs in faeces
Necator americanus	1–2	Small intestine	Penetration of skin by larvae in soil	Eggs in faeces
Ancylostoma duodenale	1–2	Small intestine	Penetration of skin by larvae in soil Oral ingestion of larvae	Eggs in faeces
Strongyloides stercoralis	30	Small intestine	Penetration of skin by larvae in soil	Larvae in faeces
Enterobius vermicularis	11–35 days	Caecum	Ingestion of eggs	Eggs on perianal skin
Trichuris trichiura	3	Caecum, large intestine	Ingestion of eggs	Eggs in faeces
Trichinella spiralis	30 days	Small intestine (larvae in muscle)	Ingestion of larvae in pork, bearmeat, etc.	Muscle biopsy. Serology (bentonite flocculation)
Onchocerca volvulus	7–20	Subcutaneous	Infective larvae from blackflies *(Simulium)*	Microfilariae in skin biopsy, on eye examination
Wuchereria bancrofti	5	Lymphatics	Infective larvae from mosquitoes *(Culex, Aedes, Anopheles, Mansonia)*	Microfilariae in peripheral blood smear
Brugia malayi	5	Lymphatics	Infective larvae from *Mansonia, Anopheles, Aedes*	Microfilariae in peripheral blood smear
Loa loa	4–17	Subcutaneous	Infective larvae from deerflies *(Chrysops)*	Microfilariae in peripheral blood smear
Dracunculus medinensis	1	Subcutaneous	Ingestion of larvae in microcrustaceans *(Cyclops)*	Adult female worm protruding from cutaneous ulcer

appear to induce the highest levels of eosinophils. Parasites limited to an intra-intestinal existence while in the human elicit minimal host responses. In various ways, parasitic helminths have evolved multiple mechanisms by which they can evade the host defence mechanisms. Interestingly, many helminths in the process of establishing themselves in the human induce protective immunity against further infectious exposures, yet the existing adult worms survive normally. This phenomenon is termed concomitant immunity and the specific strategies used by each parasite species may differ.

Cestode infections

The three important tapeworm species that inhabit the human intestinal tract are *Diphyllobothrium latum* (broad fish tapeworm), *Taenia saginata* (beef tapeworm), and *T. solium*

(pork tapeworm). Of the multitude of intestinal complaints attributed to these organisms, direct competition for vitamin B_{12} by *D. latum* leading to pernicious anaemia is the major pathogenic activity. The other major problem associated with *T. solium* is larval infection, cysticercosis. The hermaphroditic adult tapeworms reside in the small intestine and absorb all of their nutrients from the intestinal contents through their entire body surface, since all species lack alimentary tracts, and live for years attaining lengths of 5–12 m.

Trematode infections

Of all the parasitic organisms, schistosomes are next to the malarial parasites in worldwide importance. Three species are responsible for almost all of the morbidity in schistosomiasis *Schistosoma mansoni, S. japonicum,* and *S. haematobium*

Others infecting humans are *S. mekongi* in South-east Asia and *S. intercalatum* in central Africa. The male and female blood flukes live in constant copulation in the mesenteric venous system (*S. mansoni, S. japonicum, S. mekongi*, and *S. intercalatum*) or the vesical (bladder) venous plexus (*S. haematobium*). Since specific freshwater snails are obligatory intermediate hosts and the skin-penetrating infective larvae (cercariae) are subsequently released, human exposure is dependent upon water contact for acquiring the infection. Infection of the snails is effected by the discharge of egg-containing faeces and urine.

The adult worms cause minimal pathology but the eggs released by the females are trapped in the liver, intestinal wall, and genitourinary tract where they incite a specific cellular immune inflammatory response which is the mechanism of the observed lesions. Severe hepatic fibrosis, colonic bleeding, colonic inflammatory polyposis, anaemia, and chronic obstructive urinary tract disease are commonly encountered depending upon the species and the intensity and duration of infection. *Schistosoma haematobium* is further associated with urinary tract bacterial infections and squamous cell carcinoma of the bladder especially in Egypt (Cheever 1978).

The adult worms become impervious to host defences by the unique strategy of coating their outer surface with host materials. Nevertheless, the human host is able to resist invasion by infective larvae from subsequent exposures. This concomitant immunity enables the host to avoid accumulating large worm burdens and yet allows the resident flukes to survive for years. The infection also modulates the extent of the tissue pathology against the eggs which presumably allows for greater survival of the host.

Nematode infections

In prevalence, infection due to *Ascaris lumbricoides* is one of the most frequent worldwide. Male and female roundworms inhabit the small intestine arriving there after a sojourn by the infective larvae (hatching from ingested eggs) migrating out of the intestine, through the circulation of the lungs, into the air spaces, up the trachea and down the oesophagus back into the intestine. They incite disease as they migrate through the lungs causing eosinophilic pneumonitis. Adults in the intestine can cause intestinal obstruction and can aberrantly migrate into the biliary and pancreatic ducts. Evidence is accumulating implicating ascariasis as a primary determinant of nutritional deficiency leading to poor growth in children (Stephenson 1980).

Hookworm infection is caused by *Necator americanus* and *Ancylostoma duodenale* which live in the small intestine. Adult males and females attach to the mucosa and imbibe blood and tissue fluid for their nutrients. Each worm ingests from 0.03 to 0.15 ml blood per day leading to chronic blood loss and anaemia, the severity of which is directly attributable to the worm burden which may number in the hundreds.

Humans acquire the infection by exposure to skin-penetrating larvae in the soil deposited earlier by faeces containing eggs which rapidly embryonate and hatch. The invading larvae migrate as in *Ascaris* infection to finally reach the small intestine. Oral infection by *A. duodenale* is possible.

And *A. duodenale* has also been shown to undergo a hypo-biotic state during development in the intestine remaining immature for months. Resumption of maturation and egg laying appears to be correlated with optimal environmental conditions for larval survival in the soil (Banwell and Schad 1978).

Infection by *Strongyloides stercoralis* occurs by skin-penetrating larvae in soil originally deposited by faeces containing larvae. This parasite can live entirely as a free-living nematode in soil as well as being parasitic in humans. The invading larvae migrate to the intestinal tract as in *Ascaris* and hookworm infections. The primary clinical problems are gastrointestinal with occasionally pulmonary complications.

The importance of this agent is evidenced by frequent infection in the immunocompromised host leading to extensive morbidity and mortality (Scowden *et al.* 1978). Worms can live asymptomatically for over 30 years with occasional re-activation of disease especially due to larvae migrating in the skin.

Pinworm infection is due to *Enterobius vermicularis* which lives in the caecum and large intestine with the female migrating out of the anus to deposit eggs at night on the perianal skin. These incite pruritis, the major physical problem. The parasite is found worldwide and infection is easily acquired by ingestion of airborne eggs leading to very high prevalence rates especially in children in institutions, hospitals, and families. Infection is self-limited but the high exposure rate leads to frequent re-infection.

Trichuris trichiura ('whipworm') inhabits the mucosa of the caecum and infections can consist of hundreds of worms. Although these parasites can cause some blood loss, their primary importance is in children with massive infections leading to diarrhoea, dysentery, rectal prolapse, and weight loss.

Trichinosis has been long recognized in Europe and North America and is being increasingly reported from tropical countries. The causative agent is *Trichinella spiralis*. Infection is acquired by ingestion of poorly cooked meat especially pork but also in exotic foods such as bear meat and walrus (Juranek and Schultz 1978). Meat contains encysted larvae which emerge and take residence in the small intestine. Females are 3–4 mm in length and deposit live larvae in the mucosa within three days after infection. Larvae enter the circulation and disseminate to the skeletal musculature. The clinical picture is protean but is primarily due to larval invasion and to the intensity of infection. Since infection is acquired only by ingestion of meat, the human infection cannot be transmitted to others. Thus trichinosis is properly a zoonosis.

Onchocerca volvulus the sole agent of onchocerciasis is transmitted to humans by blackflies (*Simulium* sp) inoculating larvae which mature in the subcutaneous tissues where they live frequently in fibrotic nodules. The females lay embryos (microfilariae) which migrate throughout the skin from which they must be ingested by feeding blackflies for larval development to proceed. The mere presence of microfilariae is not harmful but the host antibody response is the determinant of disease. Immune reaction against microfilariae leads to severe chronic inflammatory reactions in skin, producing dermatitis,

Table 6.18. *Larval helminths of public health importance*

Disease	Aetiology	Mode of infection	Diagnosis
Hydatid	*Echinococcus granulosus* *E. multilocularis*	Ingestion of eggs	Serology (indirect haemagglutination, immunofluorescent assay, immunoelectrophoresis), radioisotope imaging methods and radiographs
Cysticercosis	*Taenia solium*	Ingestion of eggs	Serology (indirect haemagglutination), radioisotope imaging methods and radiographs
Swimmer's Itch	Members of the blood fluke family Schistosomatidae	Penetration of skin by larvae (cercariae) in water	Occurrence in known endemic foci combined with clinical picture
Anisakiasis (herringworm disease)	*Anisakia simplex*	Ingestion of larvae in flesh of marine fish	Larvae in surgical specimen (stomach)
Visceral larva migrans	*Toxocara canis*	Ingestion of eggs	Serology (enzyme-linked immunosorbent assay)
Cutaneous larva migrans	*Ancylostoma braziliense* *Uncinaria stenocephala* *Strongyloides*	Penetration of skin by larvae in soil	Clinical picture, history of exposure
Eosinophilic meningitis	*Angiostrongylus cantonensis*	Ingestion of larvae in flesh of terrestrial snails	Larvae in cerebrospinal fluid
Dirofilariasis	*Dirofilaria immitis*	Infective larvae from mosquitoes	Young worm in surgical specimen (lung)

and most importantly in all segments of the eyes, resulting in visual impairment leading to blindness. Since the adult worms live for 20 years, constantly discharging embryos, and the worm burden can be extensive, the severity of disease is correlated with both intensity and duration of infection (WHO 1976).

All animal species harbour their own array of parasites far outnumbering those commonly found in humans. Frequently, human exposure to their infective larvae occurs resulting in disease. In general, the larvae invade the human body, migrate and continue to grow as larvae inciting severe inflammation. The most important species are usually those that parasitize pets or animals with whom close human contact occurs. The most important larval helminthic disorders, the causal organisms, mode of infection, and diagnosis are listed in Table 6.18.

REFERENCES

Al-Doory, Y. (1975). *The epidemiology of human mycotic diseases.* Thomas, Springfield, Ill.

Avery, O. T., MacLeod, C., and McCarty, M. (1944). Studies on the chemical nature of the substance inducing transformation of pneumococcal types. *J. Exp. Med.* **79**, 127.

Bachrach, H. L. (1978). Comparative strategies of animal virus replication. *Adv. Virus Res.* **22**, 163.

Banwell, J.G. and Schad, G.A. (1978). Hookworm. *Clin. Gastroenterol.* **7**, 129.

Bell, J. A., Ward, T. G., Kapikian, A. Z., Shelokov, A., Reichelderfer, T. E., and Huebner, R. J. (1957). Artificially induced Asian influenza in vaccinated and unvaccinated volunteers. *JAMA* **165**, 366.

Binford, C. H. and Connor, D. H. (1976). *Pathology of tropical and extraordinary diseases,* Vol. 2. Armed Forces Institute of Pathology, Washington, DC.

Boroff, D. A. and Das Gupta, B. R. (1971). Botulinum toxin. In *Microbiol toxins* (eds. S. Kadis, T.C. Montie, and S. J. Ajl). Academic Press, New York.

Bradley, S. J. (1979). Cellular and molecular mechanisms of actic of bacterial endotoxins. *Ann. Rev. Microbiol.* **33**, 67.

Butterworth, A. E. (1980). Eosinophils and immunity to parasite *Trans. R. Soc. Trop. Med. Hyg.* **74** (suppl.), 38.

Cheever, A. W. (1978). Schistosomiasis and neoplasia. *J. Na Cancer Inst.* **61**, 13.

Choppin, P. W. (1964). Multiplication of a mysovirus (SV5) wi minimal cytopathic effects and without interference. *Virolog* **23**, 224.

Collier, R. J. (1975). Diphtheria toxin: mode of action and structur *Bacteriol. Rev.* **39**, 54.

Davis, B. D., Dulbecco, R., Eisen, H. N., and Ginsberg, H. (1980). *Microbiology.* Harper and Row, Hagerstown.

Dulbecco, R. and Ginsberg, H. S. (1980). *Virology.* Harper an Row, Hagerstown.

Emmons, C. W., Binford, C. H., Utx, J. P., and Kwon-chung, K. (1977). *Medical mycology.* Lea and Febiger, Philadelphia.

Epstein, M., Boav, Y., and Achong, B. (1965). *Studies with Burkitt lymphoma.* Wistar Inst. Symposium Monograph, Philadelphia.

Foo, M. C. and Lee, A. (1974). Antigenic crossreaction betwee mouse intestine and a member of the autochthonous microflor: *Infect. Immun.* **9**, 1066.

Fox, E.N. (1974). M Protein of group A streptococci. *Bacteriol. Re* **38**, 57.

Frenkel, J. K. (1973). Toxoplasma in and around us. *Bioscience 2* 343.

Frenkel, J. K. and Ruiz, A. (1981). Endemicity of toxoplasmosis i Costa Rica: transmission between cats, soil, intermediate host and humans. *Am. J. Epidemiol.* **113**, 254.

Friedman, M. J. (1978). Erythrocytic mechanisms of sickle ce resistance to malaria. *Proc. Natl. Acad. Sci. USA* **75**, 1994.

Friedman, M. J. (1979). Oxidant damage mediates variant red ce resistance to malaria. *Nature* **280**, 245.

Friedman, M. J., Roth, E. F., Nagel, R. L., and Trager, W. (1979 The role of hemoglobin C, S, and N_{balt} in the inhibition of malari parasite development *in vitro. Am. J. Trop. Med. Hyg.* **28**, 777.

Fujita, N., Tamura, M., and Hotta, S. (1975). Dengue virus plaqu formation on microplate cultures and its application to viru neutralization. *Proc. Soc. Exp. Biol. Med.* **148**, 472.

Gill, D. M. (1979). Cholera toxin catalyzed ADP-ribosylation o erythrocyte proteins: general properties. *J. Supramol. Struct.* **10**, 151.

ill, D. M. and Richardson, S. M. (1980). Adenosine diphosphate-ribosylation of adenylate cyclase catalyzed by heat-labile entero-toxin of *Escherichia coli*: comparison with cholera toxin. *J. Infect. Dis.* **141**, 64.

ramiccia, G. and Hempel, J. (1972). Mortality and morbidity from malaria in countries where malaria eradication is not making satisfactory progress. *J. Trop. Med. Hyg.* **75**, 187.

reenberg, H. B., Valdesuso, J., Yolken, R. H. *et al.* (1979). Role of Norwalk virus in outbreaks of nonbacterial gastroenteritis. *J. Infect. Dis.* **139**, 564.

ayflick, L. (1965). The limited *in vitro* lifetime of human diploid cell strains. *Exp. Cell Res.* **37**, 614.

elinski, D. R. (1973). Plasmid determined resistance to antibiotics molecular properties of R factors. *Ann. Rev. Microbiol.* **27**, 437.

errman, J. E., Hendry, R. M., and Collins, M. F. (1979). Factors involved in enzyme-linked immunoassay of viruses and evaluation of the method for identification of enteroviruses. *J. Clin. Microbiol.* **10**, 210.

oorn, B. and Tyrrell, D. A. J. (1969). Organ cultures in virology. *Prog. Med. Virol.* **11**, 408.

ughes, H. J., Thomas, D. C., and Hamparian, V. V. (1973). Acid lability of rhinovirus type 14: Effect of pH, time and tempera-ture. *Proc. Soc. Exp. Biol. Med.* **144**, 555.

unter, G. W., III, Swartzwelder, J. C., and Clyde, D. F. (eds.) (1976). *Tropical medicine.* Saunders, Philadelphia.

glewski, B. M. and Kabat, D. (1975). NAD-dependent inhibition of protein synthesis by *Pseudomonas aeruginosa* toxin. *Proc. Natl. Acad. Sci. USA* **72**, 2284.

nstitut National de la Sante et de la Recherche Medicale, Collo-quium (1978). *Immunity in parasitic diseases.* INSERM **72**, 1.

acobsson, P. A., Johannson, M. E., and Wadell, G. (1979). Identification of an enteric adenovirus by immunoelectroosmo-phoresis (IEOP) technique. *J. Med. Virol.* **3**, 307.

irovec, D. and Petru, M. (1968). *Trichomonas vaginalis* and trichomoniasis. *Adv. Parasitol.* **6**, 117.

ones, G. W., Richardson, L. A., and Uhlman, D. (1981). The invasion of HeLa cells by *Salmonella typhimurium*: reversible and irreversible bacterial attachment and the role of bacterial motility. *J. Gen. Microbiol.* **127**, 351.

uranek, D. (1979). Waterborne giardiasis (summary of recent epidemiologic investigations and assessment of methodology). In *Waterborne transmission of giardiasis* (ed. W. Jakubowski and J. C. Hoff), p. 150. US Environmental Protection Agency, Cincinnati.

uranek, D. D. and Schultz, M. G. (1978). Trichinellosis in humans in the United States: epidemiologic trends in trichinellosis. In *Proceedings of the Fourth International Conference on Tri-chinellosis, 26–28 August Puznan, Poland* (ed. D. W. Kim and Z. S. Pawlowski). University Press of New England, Hanover.

oprowski, C. and Koprowski, H. (eds.) (1975). *Toward under-standing viruses and immunity: viral immunology and immuno-pathology.* Academic Press, New York.

ean, B. H. (1972). Clinical toxoplasmosis – 50 years. *Trans. R. Soc. Trop. Med. Hyg.* **66**, 549.

idson, C., Lamont, G., Saul, A., and Nurse, G. T. (1981). Ovalo-cytic erythrocytes from Melanesians are resistant to invasion by malaria parasites in culture. *Proc. Natl. Acad. Sci. USA* **78**, 5824.

luger, M. J. and Rothenburg, B. A. (1979). Fever and reduced iron: their interaction as a host defense response to bacterial infection. *Science* **203**, 374.

och-Weser, J., Hirsch, M. S., and Swartz, M. N. (1980). Medical intelligence: drug therapy. *N. Engl. J. Med.* **302**, 903.

Lennette, W. W. and Schmidt, N. J. (eds.) (1979). *Diagnostic procedures for viral, rickettsial and chlamydial infections.* Am. Public Health Assoc., Washington, DC.

Levy, S. B., Clowes, R. C., and Koenig, E. L. (eds.) (1981). *Mole-cular biology, pathogenicity and ecology of bacterial plasmids.* Plenum, New York.

Lusbaugh, W. G., Kairalla, A. B., Cantey, J. R., Hofbauer, A. F., and Pittman, F. E. (1979). Isolation of cytotoxin-enterotoxin from *Entamoeba histolytica. J. Infect. Dis.* **139**, 9.

Mandell, G. L., Douglas, R. G., Jr, and Bennett, J. E. (1979). *Principles and practice of infectious diseases.* Vol. 2, Part III, Section F. Wiley, New York.

Markell, E. K. and Voge, M. (1981). *Medical parasitology.* Saunders, Philadelphia.

Maynard, J. E. (1978). Passive immunization against hepatitis B: a review of recent studies and comment on current aspects of control. *Am. J. Epidemiol.* **107**, 77.

Melnick, J. L. (1980). Taxonomy of viruses. *Prof. Med. Virology* **26**, 214.

Miller, L. H., Mason, S. J., Clyde, D. F., and McGinnis, M. H. (1976). The resistance factor to *Plasmodium vivax* in blacks: the Duffy-blood-group genotype, FyFy. *N. Engl. J. Med.* **295**, 302.

Mirkovic, R. R., Kono, R., Yin-Murphy, M. *et al.* (1973). Entero-virus 70: the etiologic agent of pandemic acute hemorrhagic conjunctivitis. *Bull. WHO* **49**, 341.

Monto, A. S. and Cavallaro, J. J. (1972). The Tecumseh study of respiratory illness. IV. Prevalence of rhinovirus serotypes, 1966–1969. *Am. J. Epidemiol.* **96**, 352.

Monto, A. S. and Lim, S. K. (1974). The Tecumseh study of respira-tory illness. VI. Frequency and relationship between outbreaks of coronavirus infection. *J. Infect. Dis.* **129**, 271.

Moon, H. W., Isaacson, R. E., and Pohlenz, J. (1979). Mechanisms of association of enteropathogenic *Escherichia coli* with intestinal epithelium. *Am. J. Clin. Nutr.* **32**, 119.

Murphy, B. R., Phelan, M. A., Nelson, D. L., Yarchoam, R., Tierney, E. L., Alling, D. W., and Chanock, R. M. (1981). Hemagglutinin-specific enzyme-linked immunosorbent assay for antibody to influenza A and B viruses. *J. Clin. Microbiol.* **13**, 554.

Nagel, R. L., Raventos-Suarez, C., Fabry, M. E., Tanowitz, H., Sicard, D., and Labie, D. (1981). Impairment of the growth of *Plasmodium falciparum* in HbEE erythrocytes. *J. Clin. Invest.* **64**, 303.

Nahmias, A. and Roisman, B. (1973). Infections with herpes-simplex virus 1 & 2. *N. Engl. J. Med.* **286**, 667.

Odagiri, T., DeBorde, D. C., and Maassab, H. F. (1982). Cold-adapted recombinants of influenza A virus in MDCK cells: 1. Development and characterization of A/Ann Arbor/6/60 × A/Alaska/6/77. *Virology* **119**, 82.

Osterholm, M. T., Kantor, R. J., Bradley, D. W., *et al.* (1980). Immunoglobulin M-specific testing in an outbreak of foodborne viral hepatitis, type A. *Am. J. Epidemiol.* **12**, 8.

Purcell, R. H., Gerin, J. L., Almeida, J. B., and Holland, P. V. (1973). Radioimmunoassay for the detection of the core of the Dane particle and antibody to it. *Intervirology* **2**, 231.

Rafferty, K. A. Jr. (1975). Epithelial cells: growth in culture of normal and neoplastic forms. *Adv. Cancer Res.* **112**, 249.

Raghow, R. and Kingsbury, D. W. (1976). Endogenous viral enzymes involved in messenger RNA production. *Ann. Rev. Microbiol.* **32**, 21.

Rippon, J. W. (1974). *Medical mycology.* Saunders, Philadelphia.

Rossen, R. D., Kasel, J. A., and Couch, R. B. (1971). The secretory immune system: its relation to respiratory viral infection. *Prog. Med. Virol.* **13**, 194.

Sargeaunt, P. G. and Williams, J. E. (1978). Electrophoretic iso-enzyme patterns of *Entamoeba histolytica* and *Entamoeba coli*. *Trans. R. Soc. Trop. Med. Hyg.* **72**, 164.

Savage, D. C. (1972). Survival on mucosal epithelia, epithelial penetration and growth in tissues of pathogenic bacteria. In *Microbial pathogenicity in man and animals.* (ed. H. Smith and J. H. Pearce) p. 25. Published for the Society for General Microbiology by the University Press, Cambridge.

Savage, D.C. (1977). Microbial ecology of the gastrointestinal tract. *Ann. Rev. Microbiol.* **32**, 107.

Scowden, E. B., Schaffner, W., and Stone, W. J. (1978). Overwhelming strongyloidiasis, an unappreciated opportunistic infection. *Medicine* **57**, 527.

Shelokov, A., Vogel, J., and Chi, L. (1958). Hemadsorption (absorption-hemagglutination) test for viral agents in tissue culture with special reference to influenza. *Proc. Soc. Exp. Biol. Med.* **97**, 802.

Skamene, E., Kongshavn, P. A. L., and Landy, M. (eds.) (1980). *Genetic control of natural resistance to infection and malignancy.* Academic Press, New York.

Smith, H. (1977). Microbial surfaces in relation to pathogenicity. *Bacteriol. Rev.* **41**, 475.

Stephenson, L. S. (1980). The contribution of *Ascaris lumbricoide* to malnutrition in children. *Parasitology* **81**, 221.

van Heyningen, W. E. and Mellanby, J. (1971). Tetanus toxin. I *Microbial toxins* (ed. S. Kadis, T. C. Montie, and S. J. Ajl) p. 69 Academic Press, New York.

Vogt, M. and Dulbecco, R. (1960). Virus-cell interaction with tumor-producing virus. *Proc. Natl. Acad. Sci. USA* **46**, 365.

Weinberg, E. D. (1978). Iron and infection. *Microbiol. Rev.* **42**, 4.

World Health Organization (1976). *Epidemiology of onchocerciasis report of a WHO Expert Committee.* WHO Technical Repor Series, No. 597, Geneva.

Yates, V. J., Dawson, G. J., and Pronovost, A. D. (1981). Serologi evidence of avian adeno-associated virus infection in an unselec ted human population and among poultry workers. *Am. J Epidemiol.* **113**, 542.

Yolken, R.H., Kim, H.W., Clem, T., Wyatt, R.G., Chanock, R.M Kalica, A. R., and Kapikian, A. Z. (1977). Enzyme-linke immunosorbent assay (ELISA) for detection of human reovirus like agents of infantile gastroenteritis. *Lancet* **ii**, 263.

7 The social environment

M. G. Marmot and J. N. Morris

INTRODUCTION

This chapter deals with man as a social being. Health and disease are very unequally distributed in relation to social life, which implies that social factors have a powerful influence on health status. Here we shall first use differences in life-styles, health, and disease across the different social classes in England and Wales to illustrate this. Social class, however, is only a beginning. 'Class' encompasses differences in economic reality, culture, and social relations (all of which affect life-style), in environmental exposures, and in the use of health services. This chapter will consider in some detail the first three of these: economic position, culture, and social relations. In addition, a major concern of public health should be the impact of social change; rising chronic unemployment is presented as an example, which illustrates the methodological difficulties of studying this important area.

In what sense can any of these influences and factors be considered as 'causal' of health and disease states? Do they have the same status as physical or biological causes? The chapter closes with some discussion of this issue.

KEY CONCEPTS

Personal and environmental factors and their interaction

First, we will look at a few terms. 'Environment' may be defined as all influences on life that are not genetic; but concerned as we are with health, and mainly with aetiology, it is more useful to consider personal factors, environmental factors, and their interactions.

Personal factors

Personal factors, here equivalent to host susceptibilities, in health are initially defined by genetics, and subsequently by other biological factors, such as normal growth or the decline in immune competence that occurs with age. But 'personal' factors include also the influence of socialization and life-history, including medical history, that can transform ways of living. Thus, personal factors include anatomical, physiological, hormonal and metabolic profiles, and predispositions, as well as personality structure, behaviour, homeostatic and coping mechanisms, and so on. Nature, society, and culture all contribute to the personal characteristics of an individual.

Environment

The multiple environments of concern to public health may be described simply as either natural or man-made; and more usefully as physical, chemical, biological, and social.

Much that is regarded as 'personal' in fact integrates what is innate, genetically determined, with the past and/or contemporary environment to which the individual has been and is exposed, and his or her experience to produce the 'constitution' or phenotype: for example, stature; IQ; value of $\dot{V}O_2$ max (oxygen transport capacity); levels of blood pressure; or of serum lipids; ethnicity. Each of these manifestly has a genetic, biological base, but its expression is influenced by environmental and behavioural influences or factors. Standard of living has an influence on stature; appropriate stimuli on IQ; aerobic exercise and training on $\dot{V}O_2$ max; salt consumption on blood pressure; fat intake on serum lipids; 'culture' on ethnicity.

These *interactions* of personal factors with the environment continue throughout the life-cycle, from birth to death as illustrated by the examples below:

Family development
Patterns of child-bearing and of family-size in a society; birth rates; family life and the emotional development and social relations of children; educational achievement; innate and learned behaviour; social roles; the 'internalization' among its people of society's values and norms.

Adolescence
Rapid growth and abundance of hormones, oxygen, and energy; individual variation of bodily growth occurring in the context of nutritional norms of the society; male/female difference, that is gender, emerging from the biological substrate of 'sex' after conditioning in society; self-image, that is the identity adolescents seek, developing as they break away from the family and interact with peer groups in the transition to adult society; the larger society's provisions, or failures often even to offer a job, and its expectations of them – all these combine to produce the typical adolescents of a particular society and culture.

Personal–social environmental interaction in disease
Examples are legion and the following are a pertinent selection:

Phenylketonuria

The early detection by mass screening of the gene defect that causes this condition, followed by dietary manipulation (excluding the amino acid that cannot be digested) permits the child to develop normally or near normally.

Improved medical and social care

This has led to increased survival of children with juvenile diabetes, cystic fibrosis, achondroplasia, Down's syndrome, and so to relaxation of the forces of natural selection.

Social status

That is, unequal advantage and disadvantage, are reflected in mortality throughout the life-cycle.

Errors of refraction

These are a simple illustration of low technology overcoming a biological defect.

Social (that is cultural, political, economic) availability

The availability of alcohol or firearms, or of housing, creates the setting of individual alcoholism, violence, or homelessness and of their prevalence in the population.

Cigarette smoking and asbestos

The deadly mixture of personal cigarette smoking and environmental–occupational exposure to asbestos puts an individual at high risk of asbestosis.

Psychosocial environment

At a complex level, work in California suggests that conditions of the 'psychosocial' environment, such as competitive challenges in an acquisitive society and deadline pressure, interact with a particular *personality* type to produce the 'Type A' behaviour pattern, which is accompanied by physiological changes, such as excess sympathetic responses and higher serum cholesterol levels. Repeated sufficiently often, it is postulated, these can cause organic cardiovascular impairment. In other words, a combination of adverse social environment, with host predispositions developing on a biological substrate, are translated through the central nervous system into neurological, neuroendocrine, and biochemical maladjustment (Susser and Watson 1971; Jaco 1972; Morris 1976; Kasl 1977; United Nations 1979; Eisenberg and Kleinman 1981; Rothschild 1981; Parron *et al.* 1982; Starfield 1983).

What is the social environment?

The social environment may be described under the headings economy, culture, and political system. We have to examine the pressures and influences these systems bring to bear upon us, how we respond and what potentials they present for effecting change (Susser and Watson 1971; Morris 1976; Rothschild 1981).

Economy

This concerns material conditions and the provision of the basic necessities of life in terms of food and shelter and health services – *commodae vitae* – and of the 'hierarchy' of material needs and wants beyond. At another level, the economy includes systems of production; the occupational and class structure with its differential power, resources, and opportunity; income and wealth over the life-cycle; social security and other safety nets (Westergard and Resler 1975) and the psychosocial factors that are associated with these.

Culture

This includes the mode of life of the society, its customs, 'mores', language, and prevalent symbols; morals, values, and beliefs; people's assumptions and expectations; the spirit of the age, that is tradition, the learned as distinct from the biological inheritance. Plural subcultures have to be identified, of social class, ethnic group, region, profession, etc.

'Psychosocial' factors that influence health operate through all of these facets of culture, for example in child rearing and family relations, the climate of consumerism, the urge to autonomy and to self-fulfilment, the decline of the work ethic, or of the social acceptability of cigarettes (Kluckhohn 1949; Paul 1955; Rothschild 1981).

Political, legal, and administrative framework and institutions

These are critical in controlling the environment – urban and occupational, for example – and in effecting or resisting change. The political system influences personal behaviour, in determining the degree of smoking and alcohol exposure, for example, or the price and availability of various foods (Simon 1980).

For our purpose of describing connections with health and disease, we shall be considering the social distribution of health in terms, primarily of social class – as this involves economy, culture, and the political system; then, in more detail, culture and social relations, and aspects of social change. We will make only brief reference to health services – they are fully considered elsewhere (see Chapters 13 and 14) – and introduce the concept of 'life-styles' that transcend all these ways of looking at social reality and health.

Health services

Two issues are central: first, society's policy choices and its capacity to provide services; and secondly, their utilization by the population according to needs. 'Access' which represents the synthesis of the two is complicated, and little understood. It involves education, the ability of individuals to find their way about the system and to articulate their needs (and not feel intimidated by staff and bureaucracy); and illness-behaviour, thresholds, and attitudes. All these are class-bound. How far do available services in fact meet potential consumers' varied and particular needs? For example, those of the ethnic minorities? Do they positively discriminate in favour of those individuals or populations in greatest need? That is, are they concerned with equity and not only with equality? Arising out of these is the crucial issue whether, and if so in what measure, health services can and should aim to make good the damage of social disadvantage. Other social aspects of health services that cannot be considered here are 'institutionalism'; community care; health services as agents of social control; and iatrogenic ills as a major element in the modern mode of life.

Life-styles

Ways of living, habits, and behaviour patterns are so critical for health and for normal and abnormal function of the whole person, that they require drawing out. They may be regarded as on-going interactions of *host*, the individual, with *environment*; the former with his or her inherited and acquired dispositions; and, plainly, the economic, cultural, and political pressures of the latter (Morris 1976; Rothschild 1981). Reference groups and opinion leaders, the media, fashion, powerful commercial and ideological anti-health interests – and the extent to which public policy is enabling and supportive – all these diverse social forces can influence life-style. That is, life-styles are *sociobehavioural* or, more correctly, *sociocultural-behavioural*: though the natural environment, too, is influential.

Adult life-styles relevant to health, with much interaction among them, may be identified today in: diet and nutrition; exercise in leisure-time; weight control; gardening, do it yourself, and other hobbies; smoking, alcohol, and drug use; self-care; stress management techniques; birth control; social networks and support systems; family/household structures and relationships.

These life-styles include most of the range of personal behaviours, both protective and self-destructive, and of personal responsibilities ('look after yourself!') that are now regarded in western societies as vital for health. Built upon knowledge and a new confidence that good health and longevity can be achieved, they form the basis of modern policies for health promotion and maintenance (though as old as Hippocrates and Galen and the regimen of Salerno), and for preventing the dominant chronic, non-communicable diseases of adult life (OPCS, annually; Lalonde 1974; Doll and Peto 1976; Breslow 1978; Surgeon General 1979; Morris *et al.* 1980).

The direct content of *mental health* and *interpersonal relations* in current thinking about healthy life-styles is limited – for lack of consensus. Birth-control excepted, there is still widespread confusion in accommodating *psychosexual conduct* to the new freedoms. The life of the *arts* and *imagination* have to be disregarded, as have *spiritual* ways of living – for lack of data, despite today's extraordinary flowering of the former.

All these aspects of social structure and social action have multiple connections with the health of the population. In any particular situation – whether home or neighbourhood, factory or university, village or city – social factors are many and mixed, as are their effects on aetiology and outcome.

SOCIAL DISTRIBUTION OF HEALTH

We will start by discussing 'social class', because of its long tradition, the abundance and comprehensiveness of the data relating class to health, and its demonstrable power to illumine health issues. The economy, culture, and political system, are expressed in class structure, and social class is associated with differences in life-styles and mortality and

Table 7.1. *Child mortality: England and Wales*

Social class*	1978–79 Perinatal mortality ‡	Post-neonatal ‡	1970–72 1–14 Years † Boys	Girls
I (4.8)§	11.2	3.1	74	89
II (20)	12.0	2.9	79	84
III N (16)	13.3	2.9	95	93
III M (33)	14.7	4.1	98	93
IV (19)	16.9	4.8	112	120
V (7.6)	19.4	7.6	162	156

*Of father.
I Leading professions, and managerial, business.
II Lesser professions, and managerial, business.
III Non-manual skilled workers.
III Manual skilled workers.
IV Part-skilled workers.
V Unskilled workers.
† Rates per 1000 relevant legitimate births.
‡ Standardized mortality ratios; all in England Wales = 100.
§ Per cent of 'heads of households' in the different social classes, Census of 1971.
Sources: 1970–72 data from OPCS (1978).
　　　　1978–79 data from OPCS (weekly *Monitors*) and OPCS (personal communication).

morbidity throughout the life-cycle. Before discussing what is meant by social class and its impact, infant mortality rates in England and Wales will serve to illustrate its importance.

Infant mortality rates (Table 7.1), and in particular post-neonatal rates which classically are among the most sensitive of health indicators to social factors, show the familiar deterioration between Class I and Class V. Respiratory and alimentary infections have been the main contributors to the excess mortality in Class V. Domestic living space and sanitary conditions are distributed similarly across the classes to infant mortality rates.

Absolute levels of mortality are much lower than at the time when the National Health Service and welfare state were instituted: the period was one of great scientific advance and standards of living more than doubled. However, the social gradient has remained largely unchanged.

Figures for the crucial factor of birth weight correspond to current patterns of death rates (Table 7.2). This is the most obvious mechanism or precursor whereby 'social class' affects the death rate (OPCS, weekly). Table 7.3 displays

Table 7.2. *Birthweight and social class: England and Wales 1980*

Social class	Per cent of legitimate live births ≤2500 g	≤1500 g	2000–2499 g
I	5.3	0.8	3.7
II	5.3	0.6	3.6
III N	5.8	0.7	4.0
III M	6.6	0.7	4.7
IV	7.3	0.8	5.2
V	8.1	0.6	6.2

Source: OPCS weekly *Monitors*; OPCS (personal communication).

Table 7.3. *Biological and social factors in stillbirth: England and Wales. Rates per 1000 total (live and still) births, 1949–50*

Social class	Mothers age (years)		
	Of all ages and parities	20–24 bearing second child	≥40 bearing sixth or later child
I	16	–	–
II	19	11	52
III	21	12	56
IV	23	12	56
V	26	13	56

Single, legitimate births.
– Nos. too few.
Source: Morris (1976).

how in extreme situations, in this case, mother's parity and age related to stillbirths, personal biological factors predominate over social class (Morris 1976).

Social class and socio-economic status

Most of the information about the social distribution of health and life chances in England and Wales is ordered in terms of the Registrar General's social classes (SC) or 'socio-economic groups' (SEG). These are statistical aggregates or constructs, that are a shorthand for the standard of living. Both are based on occupation. Social class is defined mainly by the level of skills required in a given occupation, the responsibility (as well as working conditions) these involve, and their status and prestige in society. In the socio-economic groups classification, a deliberate attempt is also made to bring together similar life-styles. Both gradings thus are based on a mixture of objective criteria and value judgements, hallowed through long usage by government statisticians. (Occupational class and group would be more appropriate terms for this particular way of looking at society.) Earnings, and capital, are stratified into income groups in much the same way as social class. However, the difference between high- and low-income groups was even greater earlier in this century than today, and comparisons over the lifetime therefore would be more illuminating for health related issues. The same applies to housing conditions and the quality of neighbourhood. Levels of education (and educational opportunity) today are salient; the record of the two lowest classes stand out (Table 7.4) as they would doubtless also on elementary literacy and numeracy. Breakdown by age does not significantly affect this table.

Both social class and socio-economic group classifications involved intimate psychological relations, as will be seen, as well as larger scale psychosocial relationships in support systems, and in the feeling of powerlessness and low self-image of the poor (Orr 1937; Vernon 1939; Susser and Watson 1971; *Social Trends* 1975; Wastergard and Resler 1975; Brown and Harris 1975; United Nations 1975; OPCS 1978, weekly; Black 1980; Morris 1980; Rothschild 1981; Parron *et al.* 1982).

Table 7.4. *Education: highest qualification† attained, b socio-economic group for economically active men, not i full-time education, ages 16–69 years – Britain 1975–7 (weighted means) (per cent)*

Socio-economic group*	Degree and other higher	A level	O level/CSE	None
Professional	76	9	8	3
Employers and managers	22	10	30	33
Other non-manual groups	from 39 to 9	12	29	32
Skilled manual workers, etc.	(2)	6	33	55
Semi-skilled manual workers, etc.	(1)	2	18	75
Unskilled manual	1	1	10	85

*15 SEG are aggregated into six to correspond with the social classes.
( ) – small numbers.
†Foreign qualifications are disregarded.
Source: OPCS, London.

Social forces and life-styles

These socio-economic disparities interact with culture i determining the attitudes and personal behaviour, the value and horizons, that give rise to life-styles affecting health throughout life. At the very beginning there are social dispari ties in attitudes to family planning, promptness of antenata booking, and rates of breast-feeding, and family size i inversely correlated to social class (Morris 1979). In the following sections the relation of social factors to various life-styles that particularly influence health status will be discussed in detail.

Smoking

Table 7.5 shows the record for smoking among the mal population in the UK since the pioneer report of the Roya College of Physicians in 1962 (RCP 1962, 1971, 1977, 1983) concern with life-style in Britain may be dated from this. A Table 7.5 illustrates, a social class gradient has rapidl developed for this newly recognized health hazard.

Smoking is a 'disadvantage' that is liable to be 'trans mitted' to the children of smokers (Brown and Madg 1982) and, in general, the twentieth century habit of cigarette smoking provides a model for exploring environmental and personal factors in behaviour and health. Manifestly there ar character traits that make smoking more likely and, later, lead to pharmacological dependency, and personal needs tha are met by smoking. In addition, the childhood experience i the family, and adolescent peer-group pressures are influen tial, particularly in the critical smoking-initiation phase. Bu as Table 7.5 shows there are large-scale social forces, beyond the individual that are encouraging or discouraging of smoking. These are evident in the prevailing cultural pattern of smoking as an acceptable relaxant and as a means of personal communication, by exchange of gifts for example; in price (the persisting relative cheapness of cigarettes); in

Table 7.5. *Cigarette smokers (percentage) by social class – Britain 1958, 61 and 1975–76*

Social class	1958, 61	1975–76
	54	29
	59	42
	60	47
	57	49
	62	55
All	58	46

In 1980, the General Household Survey found that the rate in professional SEG was 21; among the unskilled manual 57; and among all aged 6+, 42 per cent.

Source: General Household Survey; Morris (1980).

Table 7.6. *Cigarette smoking, by education (percentage) among men and women aged 16 years and over – Britain, 1975–76*

Highest qualification attained	Current smokers Male	Female
Degree	26	26
Other higher	34	34
A level	38	29
O level/CSE	41	32
Lesser CSE	51	41
None	56	47
All	47	39

Source: General Household Survey.

the relentless pressure of advertising and sports sponsorship (The social models and opinion-leaders of many?); in the power of the tobacco lobby and of the Treasury over politicians who would like to take action, even if at a low level of priority. The pattern of smoking according to attained educational level mirrors the findings for social class (Table 7.6). One might explain part of the other.

We tend however to forget that in the UK, for example, there are eight million ex-smokers (and 17 million smokers). The implications of these figures for preventive policy or strategy have not been analysed sufficiently (Tobacco Research Council 1978; Royal College of Physicians 1962, 1971, 1977, 1983; Brown and Madge 1982).

Diet

Diet has now assumed a prominent place in public concern, as an important influence on health. There are substantial differences in type and quantity of foods purchased, according to income group (Table 7.7) although the amount of money spent overall on food for the home is remarkably similar across these groups. These correlate fairly closely with social class and socio-economic group, but it is necessary to 'disaggregate' the mother bringing up young children on her own (if indeed she is an earner at all and not relegated to group E) from the middle-aged unskilled manual worker, both of whom are liable to be locked in the poverty of group D. Subsections of the populations, for example minority ethnic groups, with their very different dietary cultures will also be

lost in such broad aggregates. Crossing all these, another range of social factors and life-styles affect diet and nutrition, as exemplified in the importance of the body image and fashion for adolescents, or of social networks and support systems, and physical activity patterns, among the elderly.

Income group differences in diet have been consistent through the 40-year history of the National Food Survey of Britain, so the long-term cumulative effects have to be reckoned with. In general, poorer people consume more refined carbohydrates (and suffer more dental caries and obesity); Group A, the most affluent 10 per cent, eat much more fresh and other fruits and more fresh vegetables. This is interesting because of the observation made in several countries that cancer of the stomach, so class-bound and full of mystery, is associated with low intakes of these foods and of vitamin C (one of whose actions is to interfere with the breakdown of nitrates into nitrosamines). The other feature of fruit consumption is the inverse trend with size of family, producing a nearly threefold range between group A households without children and group D with 4 or more. Intake of beta-carotene again is greater for the high-income groups. This is of interest since it may be a protective factor against malignant disease and may thus contribute to the observed social class distribution of these conditions. Food and nutrient data by education level are not available (Home Office, annual; Doll and Peto 1981; *Am. J. Clin. Nutr.* 1982; Schottenfeld and Fraumeni 1982).

Exercise

Table 7.8 gives some figures for the social distribution of exercise in leisure-time – another activity postulated to be protective against some forms of ill health. The widespread deficiency of this element of bodily (and possibly mental) health is increasingly unlikely to be made up at work; and among some groups who exercise too little, like the elderly, this does not apply at all. Representative measures of aerobic power, or any other aspect of physical fitness, are not available for any civilian group in the UK; and this is the typical situation for too many of the functional capacities involved in the epidemiology of health (Social Trends, annual; General Household Survey annual).

Social class – specific or general?

Social class, socio-economic group, and income group, are very broad categories and imprecise guides to social and behavioural differences. We do not know how much the associations with health are obscured and attenuated by the inevitable misclassification. The cross-connections and the overlap between the many aspects of class present enormous problems in interpretation and in developing hypotheses of health and the social environment. On the one hand, we must 'unpackage' social class; we need far more data on the relationships with defined aspects of health of particular components of class like education and income, in uni- and multivariate analysis.

At the same time, the diverse elements of class invariably cluster and interact, and perhaps it is as a general, non-specific cause of health and disease, the standard of living and how human needs are met, that social class has its primary

Table 7.7. *Food purchases for domestic consumption – Britain, 1979–80, weighted means (Food in ounces per person p week unless otherwise stated)*

Income group*	White bread	Brown and wholemeal bread	Cheese	Fruit	Sugar and preserves	Vitamin C (mg/day)	Beta-Carotene† µg/day	Weekly expenditure‡
A (high)	15.6	6.2	4.8	37.2	10.8	69	2303	7.30
B	21.5	5.0	4.0	27.7	11.6	56	2237	6.66
C	25.2	4.6	3.6	22.8	13.2	52	2183	6.64
D (low)	27.7	4.3	3.2	19.9	14.5	50	2145	6.47

*Households with one or more earners.
†1975–80.
‡per person, pounds and pence.
Source: Morris (1979, 1980); Household Food Consumption and Expenditure (annual, and personal communication).

Table 7.8. *Participation in active outdoor sports (percentage) in Britain, 1977 – men and women ages 45–64 years*

Socio-economic group	Male	Female
Professional	42	30
Intermediate	34	27
Skilled manual, etc.	23	17
Semi-skilled manual	17	14
Unskilled manual	15	11
All*	28	20

*7153 respondents.
Source: GHS (1977).

significance. Hence its value as shorthand for the whole and not merely its parts (for the wood as well as the trees). The issue is critical for social policy whether to adopt general or specific measures (Morris 1976, 1980).

Community studies

Comparative studies of health indicators and social factors within the populations of administrative areas is another approach to the investigation of social factors in health and disease. Here we will discuss one such example of a community study in which infant mortality rate is the health indicator. Plainly, in an investigation into the usually wide variation in infant mortality rates observed in community studies, it is necessary first to consider the distribution of birth weights among areas, as this is likely to be a major factor in producing local differences (Chalmers *et al.* 1978). If such standardization is not carried out other social factors in infant mortality are liable to be swamped (new ones not detected at all); and it would be difficult to detect achievements of local health services in overcoming the consequences of social inequalities (Morris 1980).

An analysis of this kind was conducted in England and Wales (Knox *et al.* 1980). Birth weight accounted for over 60 per cent of the variance of perinatal mortality in the 90 Health Areas of England and Wales during 1974–77; birth weight in turn was strongly associated with indices of local economic advantage/disadvantage. Weight-adjusted proportional mortality ratios (PMRs), were further associated with social indices (urbanization, poverty, housing

conditions) that did not appear to operate through bir weight.

Interestingly, local obstetric and paediatric facilities we not a significant factor in the small residual variance (Knox al. 1980). This, however, is a limited way of examining t contribution of health care. Its quality could only crudely measured by the inputs of manpower and facilities that we analysed; and whereas equity of provision in relation *population* needs could be studied, there is no way assessing whether *individuals* in greatest need received speci service.

A study of 27 of the 28 areas of Cleveland, Ohio (Brook 1980) found that low birth weight accounted for 39 per cent the variance of *neonatal,* and 59 per cent of *post-neonate* mortality. Low birth weight was very strongly associated wit local rates of illegitimacy and the proportion of Blacks in th community, though not directly with the figures for lo income.

Missing from all these analyses are such factors as materna physical and mental health, and protective factors like th quality of parenting and family attitudes. A case-contro study would be required to investigate these factors. If avail able, however, such information might further illumine th social distribution (giving also pointers for policy), and th interaction of personal with environmental factors: fo example, who among the socially vulnerable do in fac become casualties (Orr 1937; OPCS 1975, 1978; Morris 1976 1980; United Nations 1979; Black 1980; DHSS 1980).

Social class and mortality of working men

Occupational mortality

To return to social class, much of the data for England and Wales come from the analysis of occupations recorded at death for the years around the decennial census; the estimate of denominators coming from the census. Again substantia deterioration from Class I to V is evident for the overall death rate of men during working years (Table 7.9). There are suggestions also of a divide between Classes I and II (the 'middle classes') and all other groups. The gradient is steeper at younger ages, peaking in the late twenties with a death rate in Class V three times that of Class I. This indicates the importance of 'cohort' effects in such analyses, for example

Table 7.9. *Mortality in men and women in England and Wales, ages 15–64, 1970–72*

| Social class | All causes* | | | Coronary heart disease* |
	Men	Married women†	Single women	Men
I	77	82	(110)	88
II	81	87	79	91
III N	99	92	92	114
III M	106	115	108	107
IV	114	119	114	108
V	137	135	138	111

*Standardized mortality ratios.
†Classified by husband's occupation.
Source: OPCS (1978).

of early life during the Second World War. It has now been demonstrated that only about one-fifth of the 'variance' in general death rate between the social classes is accounted for by the particular occupations of which they are comprised, and that most of it is explained by more general social and environmental conditions (Fox and Adelstein 1978).

Writing in 1983 about the experience of 1970–72 (the most recent years for which complete data are available) is frustrating since death rates in general have been falling throughout the 1970s. The effect on class gradients mostly can only be conjecture; for infant mortality in 1978–80, the difference between upper and lower classes was substantially smaller than in 1970–72. Unemployment, too, starting in the late 1970s, could – it may be postulated *will* – affect some of the death rates. It is too early to discuss.

Mortality from bronchitis and pneumonia, all malignant disease, lung cancer (cf. Table 7.5) and many other cancers, peptic ulcer (both gastric and duodenal), cerebrovascular disease and a wide variety of other conditions, show the classical I to V gradient with minor variations.

The figures for coronary heart disease (CHD), in its modern social metamorphosis, again look somewhat like the middle professional and business classes versus the rest (Marmot *et al.* 1978) (Table 7.9). The mortality rates for coronary heart diseases seem to be the embodiment of multiple errors in the modern social environment and culture patterns – and mass failure to adjust to them. Will developing countries learn in time? And achieve 'primordial prevention' (Morris 1982).

As to the possible causes of the social class gradient for coronary heart disease and the coronary 'risk profile', smoking and physical activity patterns by social class (Tables 7.5 and 7.8) are sharper than the gradient of mortality. However, total consumption of fats at the several income levels (despite the figures for cheese consumption) is rather uniform – high on current understanding – and this may modify upwards the risk profile, and hence mortality in the higher social classes. Close to half the fat consumed across classes is saturated, and there is a low ratio of about 0.24 polyunsaturated:saturated (P:S) fatty acids. The modal national palate, that is the social and cultural norm, is unhealthy; and such diet is the most likely environmental factor in the high and

high-risk national serum cholesterol level. The result, it may be postulated, is mass coronary atherosclerosis; the degree of this varying with personal, possibly genetic, responsiveness to the lipid loads.

Data on social class differences in coronary heart disease have been assembled from a study of civil servants in London. Men in the lowest grade of employment have nearly four times the mortality of men in the highest grade. The lower grade men are shorter, more obese, smoke more, report less leisure-time physical activity, as well as having higher blood pressure. These differences provide part but not all of the reason for the higher mortality. We need better measures of, among other things, dietary intake and psychosocial factors (Rose and Marmot 1981).

Cancer of the colon, another disease of 'advanced industrial societies', with only a few other sites (including the mysteriously increasing carcinoma of the pancreas), shows similar rates across the social classes. Overall consumption of cereal fibre is probably greater at lower incomes because of the bulk of white bread that is eaten (though this contains only about half the fibre of brown bread and a third of wholemeal); but intake of dietary fibre from fruit and vegetable overall is positively associated with income, though potatoes are eaten more by the poorer.

The intake of fats has just been mentioned and this is increasingly being considered also as a possible aetiological factor in female cancer of the breast.

A gradient, increasing from Class I to V of mortality from cancer of the stomach, a disease in long decline, has also been found in the UK as well as in the USA, Japan, Norway, Iceland, and Hawaii, using sundry indicators of 'socio-economic status' from residential district, census tract, and occupation.

Myeloid leukaemia, lymphosarcoma, and Hodgkin's disease are among the few sizeable malignancies with highest death rates in Class I. This applies also to melanoma which seems to be rising in incidence. There is evidence that successive generations of Whites have received gradually more exposure to ultraviolet light. Cancer of the testis is also more common in Social class I than V; there has been a rise in incidence only among younger men (OPCS 1978; Doll and Peto 1981; Schottenfeld and Fraumeni 1982).

Longitudinal study

The previous discussion is based on 'cross-sectional' data of deaths at one time with the estimates of the population at that time. There are several potential biases and drawbacks to this approach (OPCS 1978) which can be overcome in a longitudinal study.

A 1 per cent random sample of the UK population was identified in the 1971 census and is likely to be a major source of data linking mortality and social factors. This random sample is now being followed, allowing record-linkage of subsequent mortality not merely to initial occupation, but to other relevant information on individuals available in the census. At the same time, the technical snags in using the occupations of death certificates for numerator, and those of the census as denominator, are overcome. Moreover, the

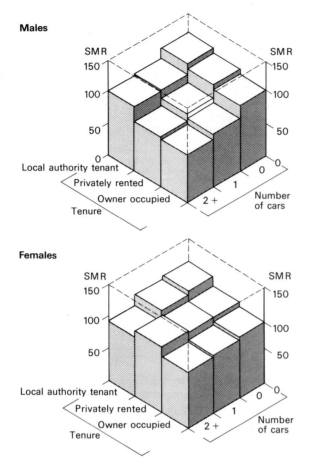

Fig. 7.1. Standardized mortality ratios in 1971–75 of persons in private households by tenure and access to cars. Ages 15–64 years.

employment 'career' from census to death certificate may also be informative.

Analysis to date of this sample confirms the main observations of Table 7.9, for 1971–75. Two additional variables, *housing tenure and car ownership* have also been introduced representing wealth and property, which may be analysed within the same class and so at similar broad levels of income (Fig. 7.1). This raises questions on attitudes and priorities, of short- vs long-term goals; a little over half the whole population own or are buying their own homes, and 60 per cent own a car. The combination of housing and access to cars has a remarkably strong – and thought provoking – connection with mode of life and health. There are corresponding data in the National Food Survey on food budgeting by household 'tenure' which should be worth analysing in detail.

Space forbids any attempt at comprehensive treatment, for example by *region* and by such factors as *density of population* – urban/rural, etc. With regard to *sex* the findings in single women are generally similar to those for men (see for example Table 7.9), though at lower levels. But sex differences in this social context is altogether too big a subject to consider. It would have to start with classification of *married women* according to their own and not merely their husband's em-

ployment (OPCS 1975), as will be possible in the longitudinal study.

Inequality and poverty

Plainly, there are several general issues in these adult death rates. The most important may be exemplified in the unequal experience of the great phalanx of skilled manual workers, Social Class III manual, who represent 40 per cent of the population: their record is close to 40 per cent worse than that of Class I. This is a group where explanations such as simple notions of absolute poverty, or of relative difficulty for economic reasons in access compared to population norms are inadequate (Townsend 1979). We have to seek explanations in, for example, education, life-styles, and environmental exposures over the lifetime and to consider the known stronger defences of Class I, with higher education, favourable living conditions, a better diet, taking more exercise, supported more strongly by social networks, making greater use of preventive health services – as well as less exposure to known hazards. Moreover, the more enterprising, and the healthier of lower social classes are more likely to be upwardly mobile, into Classes II and I, with the modern expansion of professional, technical, managerial, and service occupations (Illsley 1980).

On the other hand, absolute poverty as deprivation of primary needs for health, even if now above subsistence level – there is no hunger and no bare feet – has to be postulated at the lower end, in Class IV and in particular V, where lack of money is the most obvious of the multiple disadvantages commonly present (Black 1980; Morris 1980, 1982).

The lowest class

In several of the tables, Table 7.1 and 7.9 for example, Social Class V shows up particularly badly. This group experiences all the typical features of social deprivation: unskilled and dirty work, poor pay, heavy unemployment, minimal education, and inferior housing and local environment (overlapping thus with problems of urban decay and inner city areas, etc., Table 7.10). Correspondence in life-styles has already been illustrated.

Two main components may be identified in Social Class V. First are those at the low end of the normal gradation of job skills and status. Secondly, there are the assortment of chronic sick who have drifted down, and the diverse deviants, isolates, the down-and-outs – social class overlapping thus with social disorganization and its casualties; the underclass of family disruption, mental disorder, crime, violence, racial conflict, drug addiction, alcoholism. Cutting across both are small numbers representing the 'cycle of deprivation' again by no means limited to Class V, of families who are not coping and who originate in homes that likewise often failed to cope (Askham 1969; Auletta 1982; Brown and Madge 1982).

Plainly, the contribution of social Class V to misery, morbidity, and mortality, to social dependence and incompetence, and the consequential load on health and welfare services is out of all proportion to their numbers in the population. Routine official health statistics, as so often, indicate issues for research, for policy – and for the very notion of a good society (Morris 1976, 1982).

Table 7.10. *Social deprivation, social pathology, 1960s*

Population	Social Class IV and V (%)	Housing Households no hot water tap (%)	Shared WC (%)	Over-crowding (%)	Health Infant mortality (‰)	TB cases (‰)	Mental hospital discharges (‰)	Children At school at 16 (%)	Received into care (‰)	Juvenile delinquency (‰)	Old people Pensioners living alone (%)
England and Wales	26	12	6	3	18	7	4	36	5	20	20
Inner London Borough Tower Hamlets*	37	35	21	8	17	12	6	20	25	37	27
One ward in this borough*	43	55	32	10	22	27	9	16	27	46	42

*Population, 1966, 200 000; of the ward, 11 730. Age-compositions are unremarkable.
Source: Morris (1976).

Well-being, working capacity, illness, and disability

Two broad concepts of 'health' have been found helpful. The 'medical' model or paradigm, labelling health as absence of pathology, disease, and disability, is concerned mainly with the body as machine, which of course it is. The 'social' model (so called, even if invented and mainly propagated by physicians) is concerned with the whole person, mind and body, one of a family, and a member of society and culture. The social model recognizes the multiple interactions of these, and emphasizes well-being, fulfilment, independence, functioning in society, and social roles; that is it is comprehensive and 'positive'.

Data on combining these two aspects of health are beginning to be available from the GHS (Table 7.11). Such subjective, self-assessed, and self-reported acute data show the familiar social class gradient after 15 years of age; in children, largely mother-reported, it is remarkably equal across the strata. There is some excess of chronic illness among children of the lower classes, and the usual class distinctions at 15–64 years. What is reported will vary so manifestly with age as well as social circumstances and subculture, that understanding of such findings must wait on follow-up research, including case study and cohort analysis.

CULTURE AND HEALTH

The previous section charted the social distribution of disease and showed examples of the likely influence of social and

Table 7.11. *Daily living, well-being among males in Britain*

Socio-economic group	Acute* 0–14	45–64	Chronic† 0–15	45–64
Professional	12	13	50	198
Managerial	14	13	51	176
Other non-manual	13	21	67	279
Skilled manual, etc.	12	23	65	278
Part-skilled manual, etc.	12	21	65	310
Unskilled manual, etc.	10	29	61	377

*Days of restricted activity p.a. 1974–76.
† Rates per 1000 reporting limiting long-standing illness, 1979–80.
Source: OPCS *General Household Survey*, various years.

economic position on life-style that may contribute to this pattern. In this section we widen the scope by looking, in the most general terms, at patterns of disease in relation to type of social organization. In addition, within one society, there are variations in health and disease that cannot be described solely by social class, occupation, or economic indicators. Cultural differences go some way in aiding the search for explanations of health and disease differences among, for example, ethnic minorities. Finally, as a link with the section to follow on social relations, an example is pursued that illustrates the association between culture and social relations.

Concept of culture

Ideas and practices that affect health 'penetrate deeply into the domains of politics, philosophy, etiquette, religion, cosmology, and kinship . . . we would do well to adopt a way of looking at the community that gives some coherence and depth to the array of observable details. The concept of culture fills part of that need' (Paul 1955). Culture may be thought of as the way of life of members of a social group or 'that part of the environment that is the creation of man' (Kluckhohn 1949). Many aspects of culture are explicit: the various behaviours that we have listed under 'life-style', as well as patterns of dress, of housing, and patterns of family and social interaction; and other aspects of culture are implicit and form the values, the ethos, the world view which members of a group share. For anthropologists, culture is, by definition, acquired: learnt not genetic. Cultural differences, therefore, are not synonymous with racial differences. The latter include both cultural and genetic differences.

The distinction between cultural and social is somewhat artificial. Culture cannot exist without society, and in humans, if not in animals, the converse is true. The distinction between social and cultural is useful because they convey somewhat different information and raise different questions. As detailed below, the socio-economic position of a group is an insufficient guide to the practices of that group relevant to health. Economic position *per se* explains only part of the social variation in diet, in alcohol consumption, in use of health services, in acceptance of the work ethic. The fact that Americans preceded the British by several years in taking up jogging on a massive scale, and increasing their consumption of polyunsaturated fats, cannot easily be explained without resort to a concept such as culture. Of course, cultural practices may arise as a result of economic forces, but they then take on a dynamic *influence* of their own; for example, the high alcohol consumption in France, Spain, and Italy may well be a partial result of their large production of grapes and wine and the ready availability of cheap (and good!) wine; but wine drinking is now clearly a part of the culture – and a likely cause of the high mortality from cirrhosis of the liver in those countries.

Culture, life-styles, and health

Culture may affect health in a variety of ways:

1. Practices that lead to exposure to or protection from human hazards – for example: diets over-rich in sugar, calories and fat, and low in fibre or vitamins; culturally accepted high intake of alcohol; sun-bathing leading to increased risk of skin cancer; liability to aggression and violence of particular groups.

2. Reaction to health education and/or medical services – cultural barriers to change, for example: desire to maintain traditional diet with all its symbolism; not wishing to refrain from excess food, alcohol, or smoking in subcultures where these are the norm; women from certain cultures may not be examined by male doctors; cultural barriers to contraception.

3. Psychosocial – patterns of child-rearing; family and social relations; Type A behaviour; stress arising from clash of values (for example the generation gap, or immigrants in a new culture). These may all affect mental and physical health.

Examples follow, but first we shall touch on the notion that diseases may only arise under certain cultural conditions.

Culture and social organization

The knowledge that smallpox virus causes smallpox by itself explained little of the distribution of smallpox in human populations where the virus was prevalent: the existence of an effective smallpox vaccine was insufficient to lead to the eradication of smallpox as a human disease. This major public health triumph of the 1970s was made possible by among other things, an understanding of the way cultural and social behaviour influence person-to-person contact and hence virus transmission; and an understanding of the strategies most appropriate to redress the failures of previous mass vaccination campaigns.

Fenner (1971) provides a summary of how historic changes in culture and social organization have affected patterns of infectious disease (Table 7.12). Although this labelled 'historical', examples of these various cultural types exist today. In hunter–gatherers, the group size is too small to sustain person-to-person transmission of a virus that has no animal reservoir. Hence infections such as measles cannot affect such a population unless introduced from outside it. In a society based on agriculture, the size of the population is no longer limited by the availability of food. Larger populations allow transmission and sustaining of enteric and respiratory viruses.

An illuminating example of the interplay of culture and biology in determining the prevalence of disease is provided by Wiesenfeld (1976). There is good evidence that possession of the sickle-cell trait (for haemoglobin S) confers partial protection against falciparum malaria (see also Chapter 3). As a result the distribution of sickle-cell trait in the population is largely influenced by the distribution of malaria. Wiesenfeld shows quite plausibly that a particular style of slash-and-burn agriculture – the Malaysian agricultural complex – by providing breeding grounds for *Anopheles gambiae* mosquitoes was likely to be associated with the spread of malaria. Hence, the introduction of this particular cultural form to Africa, about 1900 years ago, was associated not only with the spread of disease, but by selecting for sickle-cell trait, probably changed the gene frequency of the population of Africa in the tropical rain forest belt. In consequence the sickle-cell gene has survived and sickle-cell disease affects people of African origin in the US, the Caribbean and the UK, as well as in Africa.

Another likely consequence of denser human settlements is

Table 7.12. *Pattern of infectious disease in relation to cultural state and community size*

Years before present	Cultural state	Size of human communities	Infectious disease patterns
1 000 000	Hunter-gatherer	Scattered nomadic bands of < 100 persons	Only human viruses with latency of recurrence e.g. herpes simplex, chickenpox, arthropod-borne, 'animal' viruses, TB, wound infections
10 000	Development of agriculture	Villages of < 300; few cities of 100 000	Irrigation → arthropod-borne viruses and malaria Human viruses: enteric and respiratory, smallpox, measles Enteric bacteria
250	Introduction of steam power – rapid urbanization	Some cities of 500 000; many of 100 000; many villages of 1000	Crowding, poverty → increased respiratory infections + Malnutrition → TB Water contamination → cholera, dysentery
140 to present	Sanitary reforms modern cities	Some cities of > 5 000 000; many of 500 000; fewer villages of 1000	Decrease in infectious disease mortality Decrease in sexually transmitted diseases Respiratory viruses Emergence of diseases of affluence

Adapted from Fenner (1971).

...e contamination of communal water supplies with and hence ...fection caused by enteric bacteria. The accelerated movement ...to cities at the start of the industrial revolution was associated ...ith great poverty and unsanitary conditions. With sanitary ...form and improvement in housing and nutrition, infectious ...iseases declined in the cities of industrialized countries and ...ade way for mass non-communicable diseases of modern ...dustrialized societies. Diseases of affluence may arise, to ...me extent, as diseases of adaptation. Humans are biologic... ...lly adapted to more primitive conditions with recurrent ...carcity. Many modern industrialized disease problems are ...iseases of plenty.

...Western' diseases

...rowell and Burkitt (1981) reviewed studies from Africa, ...North America (Indian), Australia (Aborigines), New Zealand ...Maoris), Pacific Islands, Israel, Japan, Taiwan, and Hawaii, ...nd produced a tentative list of diseases that are uncommon ...n non-western countries and that increase in incidence ...luring the economic and social development of westernization. ...These include: hypertension, obesity, diabetes, gall-stones, ...enal stones, coronary heart disease, appendicitis, haem-...rrhoids, varicose veins, colorectal cancer, hiatus hernia, and ...liverticular disease. The fact that migrants increase their rate ...of many of these diseases when they move from a non-western ...o a western environment is evidence against a genetic ex-...planation of these differences. More likely, these diseases are ...elated to the way of life of a country – the culture. Trowell ...nd Burkitt suggest that western diets low in fibre products, ...nd high in sucrose and saturated fats, together with increased ...igarette consumption and reduced exercise, may bear major ...esponsibility for the increase in these diseases. There may be ...a genetic/environmental interaction. As hinted above, human ...enotypes may not be completely adapted for western living.

As with the example of alcohol above (p. 106), such dietary, ...moking, and exercise patterns are complex in their origin. ...These life-styles are bound up with the economy, culture, and ...political system of a society, and consequently pose complex ...problems for making changes in the interests of public health. ...Dietary patterns, and hence the diseases affected by them, are ...haped by economic forces dictating production, pricing ...including government subsidies), agricultural policy, and the ...distribution of food. However, once a food pattern becomes ...part of the culture, it in turn affects production and avail-...ability. For example, in many non-western countries, a mark ...of achievement of affluence is the ability to buy white bread, ...made from highly processed flour. Similarly in the UK, when ...post-war controls ceased, the consumption of brown bread ...fell and the consumption of white bread increased – a symbol ...also of the end of post-war shortages. Until and unless ...economic policies are pursued that change the type of bread ...produced, attempts to promote the eating of wholemeal ...bread should take into account the symbolic value placed on ...the type of bread consumed, as well as the force of established ...custom. A new symbolism now attaches to bread: wholemeal ...bread is seen as a health food with connotations of appealing ...mainly to special subgroups of the population.

Subcultures – ethnic differences in health and disease

The concept of culture is useful not only in comparing patterns of health and disease in different countries, or the changing pattern as westernization proceeds, but also in examining sub-cultures within one society. The UK, for example, is now a multi-ethnic society and its different subcultures, with different life-styles, may be expected to have different patterns of health and disease, throughout the life-cycle. Some examples follow (Marmot *et al.* 1984).

Birth

There are marked differences among ethnic groups, starting at the beginning of life, in *birth rates*. Table 7.13 shows total period fertility rates in England and Wales, 1971, for women classified according to their country of birth. At current rates of fertility, women born in the UK would expect to bear an average of 2.3 children during their reproductive period, women in England and Wales born in the Caribbean 3.4, and women born in India, Pakistan or Bangladesh 5.4.

Age of mother at birth affects the outcome of pregnancy, and this too varies among ethnic groups as shown in Table 7.14 (Immigrant Statistics Unit 1978). Of the women from the Caribbean who gave birth in 1976 a relatively high proportion were in high-risk categories: 18 per cent were aged less than 20 years, compared to the national (England and Wales) average or 10 per cent; and 4 per cent of Caribbean mothers were 40 years or over, compared to the national average of 1 per cent. By contrast, a smaller than average proportion of the Indian and Pakistani mothers were very young. (The percentage distribution of age of mothers is not merely a function of the age-distribution of women in the population as is shown by age-specific fertility rates.)

Childhood

Rickets, due to vitamin D deficiency, has become rare in the British population. There is, however, a higher prevalence among Asians in Britain (Sheiham and Quick 1982). The explanation for this appears to be a complex mix of the cultural and biological. Much of the vitamin D in the British diet comes from fortified margarine and from eggs. Because

Table 7.13. *Total period fertility rates*, 1971, England and Wales*

Birthplace of mother	Total period fertility rate
United Kingdom	2.3
All birthplaces outside UK	3.1
India, Pakistan, Bangladesh	5.4
Africa	2.9
Caribbean	3.4
Malta, Gibraltar, Cyprus	2.9

*Sum of age-specific fertility rates in 1971. It is a measure of the average number of live births that would result if women survived to the end of their reproductive period and throughout the period were subject to the age-specific fertility rates in 1971. It therefore standardizes the differences in age structure.

Source: OPCS (1978).

Table 7.14. *Per cent distribution of live births in England and Wales, 1976, according to age of mother and country of origin mother*

Birth place of mother	Age of mother at birth of child (years)						
	All ages	Under 20	20–24	25–29	30–34	35–39	40 and over
All birthplaces (including England and Wales)	100	10	31	38	16	4	1
India, Pakistan, and Bangladesh	100	7	37	29	15	8	4
Africa	100	5	33	38	18	5	–
Caribbean	100	18	32	23	15	9	3
Malta, Gibraltar, Cyprus	100	10	37	33	14	6	–

Source: OPCS (1978).

traditional Indian cooking relies more on ghee (purified butter) than margarine and because some Asian vegetarians avoid eggs, the Asian diet – particularly vegetarian – contains less vitamin D than the British diet. There is some scepticism that this difference in vitamin D intake is sufficient to account for the difference in prevalence of rickets. An alternate, genetic, hypothesis is that dark-skinned people need greater exposure to ultraviolet radiation than white to produce the same amount of vitamin D. Against this as an explanation for Asian rickets is the observation that the prevalence of rickets and/or low vitamin D blood levels is only marginally higher in Caribbean than White schoolchildren in Britain and much lower than in Asian schoolchildren.

An interesting three-way hypothesis has been proposed: Asian and Caribbean children produce less vitamin D for a given amount of ultraviolet exposure; Asian children in Britain are not exposed to the sun more, and possibly less, than white children; Caribbean children compensate for this lack by a high dietary intake of vitamin D, but Asian children have a relative deficiency of this vitamin in their diet. If this is true, we have a good example of the personal–environmental interaction described at the beginning of the chapter: a cultural pattern (diet and protection from the sun), interacting with an aspect of the physical environment (less sunshine in Britain than in India), and with a specific genetic biological trait (relative resistance to ultraviolet radiation).

Maternal mortality

Maternal deaths are, to a large extent, avoidable. In England and Wales, deaths associated with pregnancy, labour, and the puerperium declined from 54 per 100 000 births in 1952 to 10 per 100 000 in 1978. This low level of mortality is not 'rock-bottom'. In Denmark, in 1971 for example, the maternal mortality was 5.3 per 100 000 and in Sweden 7.9 (in England and Wales in 1971, it was 13.5). Regular confidential enquiries into maternal deaths have been conducted. The 1976–78 report concluded that, of the 227 deaths directly due to pregnancy, 58 per cent could have been avoided by some change in behaviour of the woman or of the medical care personnel involved (DHSS 1982).

Against this background of avoidable deaths should be set Table 7.15(a) which compares maternal mortality in England and Wales among immigrant women with the England and Wales *average* (Marmot *et al.* 1984). Women from Asia

Table 7.15. *Standardized maternal mortality ratios (SMMR in England and Wales according to (a) birthplace of moth 1976–78 and (b) social class 1970–72*

(a) Birthplace of mother	SMMR	(b) Social class	SMMR
All birthplaces (including England and Wales)	100	All classes	100
		I	79
India, Pakistan, and Bangladesh	188	II	63
		III N	86
Africa	396	III M	99
		IV	147
Caribbean	255		
Malta, Gibraltar, and Cyprus	99	V	144

*The maternal mortality/100 000 live births has been standardized take account of age differences, by the indirect method using England an Wales as the standard.
Source: (a) Marmot *et al.* (1984).
        (b) OPCS (1978).

have nearly twice the risk of dying a maternal death of British women, women from the Caribbean two-and-a-half time the risk, and women from Africa four times the risk. The high mortality of immigrant women is likely to be the resul of a combination of social and cultural influences. Table 7.15(b) shows that for 1970–72 (the latest available) standardized maternal mortality ratios (SMMRs) vary by socia class, but not nearly to the extent that they vary by country of birth. The high SMMRs of Caribbean, Asian (Indian), and African women cannot simply be explained by social and/or economic causes, in so far as these are captured by conventional social classification (I–V).

If the majority of these extra deaths were avoidable, why were they not avoided? Immigrant women appear to a disproportionate extent among deaths from induced abortion – almost all of which are avoidable (DHSS 1982). Similarly, there is a disproportionate number of immigrant women among deaths from ectopic pregnancy. About half of deaths due to ectopic pregnancy are considered to be due to delay in diagnosis and operation.

These examples indicate that women from these sub-
ltures – Asia and the Caribbean – are not benefitting from
alth services in England and Wales to the same extent as
itish women. These cultural barriers to care may arise both
m the women's behaviour and attitude to medical care,
d from the treatment they receive from medical staff who
not fully understand how to cross the cultural gap as well
the general 'social distance' factor, and administrative
ndness to their different needs.

lture and social relations

e previous examples have dealt with *some* aspects of
lture: patterns of child-bearing, diet, and use of health
rvices. A quite different aspect is the pattern of social
lations in different cultures, and the effects that these may
ve in generating or modifying stressful influences and,
bsequently, on stress-induced disease. Various aspects of
cial relations and health will be taken up in the next section,
it first an example is presented that links social relations to
seases of 'westernization'.

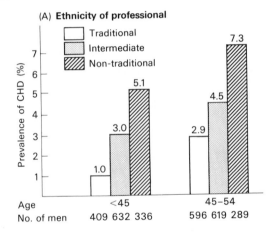

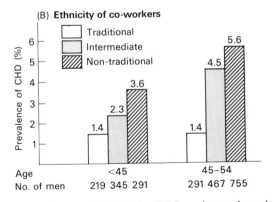

ig. 7.2. Prevalence of CHD (by ECG and questionnaire) in
apanese-Americans in California according to culture of upbring-
ng and two measures of social assimilation based on answers to the
uestions: (A) Do you go to a Japanese doctor, dentist, lawyer?
B) Are most of the people you work with Japanese? Traditional =
Japanese' score on both measures; non-traditional = 'western' score
n both measures; intermediate = the rest.

Japan has the lowest mortality rate from coronary heart
disease (CHD) of any industrialized country and the US one of
the highest. Japanese who have migrated to the US have intermediate rates. In fact among men of Japanese ancestry, there
is a gradient in CHD occurrence: low in Japan, intermediate
in Hawaii, and highest in California (Robertson *et al.* 1977).
It is likely that the low dietary intake of fat in Japan and the
higher intake by Japanese-Americans provides part of the
explanation of the change in heart-disease rates.

A different kind of explanation has been proposed that
may contribute further to the apparent protection from
coronary heart disease in Japan (Matsumoto 1970). An important feature of Japanese culture is the tightly-knit social
group – both in the family and at work. This pattern of social
relations by providing emotional and social support may act
as a buffer against stress. Another feature of American culture
seems to be singularly lacking in Japanese culture – the Type
A, or coronary-prone behaviour pattern. This is characterized
by hard-driving, personally ambitious, aggressive, competitive
behaviour and has been shown to be related to the occurrence
of CHD. In Japan, competitiveness is between groups (the
factory, the business) rather than individuals, and individual
striving tends to be on behalf of the group.

The hypothesis that traditional Japanese culture is associated
with a lower prevalence of CHD received support from a
study of Japanese-Americans living in California (Marmot
and Syme 1976). Japanese who were brought up exposed to a
high degree of traditional Japanese culture had a low CHD
prevalence, more westernized Japanese a higher prevalence
(Fig. 7.2). These differences between traditional and non-
traditional men were independent of differences in smoking,
obesity, plasma cholesterol, or blood pressure.

These notions of a supportive culture owe much to
Durkheim's classic formulation in 1897 (reprinted 1952) of
the link between suicide and lack of social integration.

SOCIAL RELATIONS AND HEALTH

How people live together in society, their social ties, and
social group membership are of manifest significance for
health. Of main concern are the family (now in flux); neighbourhood, school, and work situation (this, too, increasingly
in flux); and local and dispersed, formal and informal, social
networks and support systems.

Roles represent the individual behaviour that is expected by
society and its culture. Multiple roles have to be described:
for example, the adult role-playing of the adolescent that
prompts his or her smoking behaviour, which has already
been instanced, vs the role-models of his or her sporting
heroes who (hopefully!) don't smoke. Social roles of the
individual are inherent in today's key concept of disability.

Provocation and predisposition

Relations between people may affect health by transmission
of infections or, in the case of families, by transmission of
genes or of learned health-related behaviour. Social and
family relations also have a symbolic meaning. Obviously,
they can lead to the whole gamut of emotions and feelings.

This 'symbolic' side of social relations may affect health in at least two different ways: as a 'provoking' agent – pushing a predisposed individual from health to ill health, mentally or physically; or by contributing to host resistance – affecting predisposition. Dubos (1965) has argued, that in an age and society where the major infectious diseases have been conquered, exposure to environmental agents are not, *per se*, the determinants of human disease. Of major importance is the level of host resistance or defences. This may take the form of immunity to a specific infection, for example induced by prior exposure or immunization; or it may be a more general resistance to disease, for example provided by good nutrition.

Cassel (1976) has postulated that the social environment, specifically the relation between people, may affect the level of host resistance and hence be one of the determinants of whether an 'exposed' individual develops clinical disease. In this section we shall present examples of the social environment both as provoking agent, and as it affects host resistance, at various stages of the life-cycle.

We attempt to do this with minimum resort to the use of the word 'stress'. As originally used by Selye it referred to a general, non-specific state of arousal of the organism that could be elicited by a variety of stimuli – 'stressors'. The conceptual and methodological problems in defining stressors and stress have kept many investigators in disagreement for years, and have led others to abandon this as a field of scientific enquiry. The examples below bypass this issue, by relating a social/psychological feature, such as, maternal deprivation, to a health outcome, for example in mental health, without seeking a direct physiological/biochemical measure of stress, although much of psychosomatic research has been devoted to such measures. The question of how to determine 'stress' is taken up again in the discussion of life events.

Maternal deprivation

A variety of studies have shown that disrupted family life can affect personality development and mental health of offspring. A drastic form of this is complete deprivation of mothering. Bowlby (1951), in an influential report, brought together much of the work on this topic from western countries. He concluded that maternal deprivation could produce in the child an affectionless and psychopathic character and could increase the risk of subsequent juvenile delinquency. More specifically, this type of character could be brought about by three somewhat different experiences: (i) lack of an opportunity for forming an attachment to a mother-figure during the first three years of life; (ii) deprivation for a limited period – at least three months and probably six months during the first three years; and (iii) changes from one mother-figure to another during this period.

Fierce controversy surrounded Bowlby's thesis. The response to these criticisms (Bowlby 1965) left intact the central thesis of the importance of maternal deprivation, but a number of issues were clarified: maternal deprivation was seen as either insufficient, discontinuous, or disturbed mothering; although continuity is important, other carers may play a role in healthy development; damage to the child does not inexorably follow deprivation and the degree of

damage varies; not all the effects of maternal deprivation need be permanent.

Bowlby proceeded from a psychoanalytic perspective emphasizing the importance of the relationship with parent on personality development and subsequent behaviour. It perhaps too simple to ascribe all the effects of maternal deprivation to interference with this relationship. Maternal deprivation is liable to be associated with a number of other factors that also may affect the child: disrupted family life, psychological instability of parents, poverty, social instability, long-term stay in an institution. With a number of interrelated variables such as these it is difficult to isolate one factor that is the 'cause' of personality disturbance.

A less psychoanalytic and more social perspective is to ask about the causes of maternal deprivation and disrupted family life – their distribution in society, their relation to such experiences as unemployment, and to the level of social and welfare services.

Disturbance in children

An important part of Bowlby's message was that one should not expect to find a 1:1 relationship between maternal deprivation and disturbance in children. Parenthetically, we are familiar with this problem in chronic disease. Too little research has been done on what keeps people healthy in the face of hazards. Bowlby recognized that the association between maternal deprivation and mental disorder was a crude one and required further delineation.

Rutter and his colleagues, in a series of studies using the methods of psychiatric epidemiology, have added subtlety and detail to the study of the relation between family factors and mental illness in children (Rutter and Quinton 1981). They examined characteristics of the family rather than simply maternal deprivation. In early work they found an increased risk of psychiatric illness in offspring of parents with psychiatric illness, both in clinic-based studies and in surveys in the general population.

The effect on the child of parental mental illness may not have been direct but have resulted from the disruption of family life and relationships caused by mental illness. Some support for this was found in a subsequent study: among families with mental illness in the parents, children were more likely to show psychiatric disorder if there was serious marital discord than if not. Nevertheless, the close intermingling of psychiatric symptoms, personality difficulties and problems in interpersonal relationships make it very difficult to isolate the effects of any one of these or to show that a change in family characteristics results in a change in the child's mental disorder (Rutter and Quinton 1981).

Returning to the question of maternal deprivation, Rutter and his colleagues made detailed assessment of family life and relationships. Separation from mother was shown to be associated with family discord and disharmony. It was more likely that these were the cause of disorders in children rather than separation *per se*.

A striking finding from this work is the number of children from disrupted backgrounds who, by the measures used, were not disturbed. As indicated above, such a finding is

ble 7.16. *Comparison of children with and without psychiatric disorder on the Isle of Wight and in an Inner London Borough
er cent who have the characteristics listed)*

vironmental factor	Isle of Wight children		Inner London Borough children	
	Normal	Psychiatric disorder	Normal	Psychiatric disorder
vere marital discord	2.7	17.9	5	26.5
ychiatric disorder mother	6.0	50.0	29.6	39.0
ther – offence against the law	12.5	29.0	24.1	47.3
ur or more children in household	12.9	35.1	33.3	37.1
ther has unskilled/semi-skilled job	14.1	30.6	19.4	45.2
achers in school > 3 yrs	25.8		43.3	
oportion of children changing school/yr	6.8		10.8	
oportion of children absent each day	6.6		8.6	

Source: Rutter *et al.* (1974).

pical of research into health and disease. The factors relating
such host resistance are not understood and should be an
portant area of enquiry.

The relation between these family characteristics and the
cial environment is shown by the studies of emotional and
nduct disorders in 10-year-old schoolchildren by Rutter *et
*(1974, 1975). The prevalence of disorder was higher in an
ner London Borough than it was on the Isle of Wight. In
eking an explanation for this, in both areas, childhood
isorder was found to be related to four sets of factors: family
iscord, parental deviance, social disorder, and unfavourable
aracteristics of the school attended.

All of these were more common in London (Table 7.16).
/hy the urban environment, particularly the inner city,
ould be associated with these indicators of social disruption
open to analysis. There is no shortage of potential explan-
tions: high-rise housing, poverty, prevalent crime and
iolence, instability and geographical mobility, downward
cial drift of the sick. Whatever the reason, there appears to
e a link between inner-city living and parental deviance,
arital discord, and social disorder; and between these
ctors and childhood disorder. In Chicago in the 1930s,
aris and Dunham (1939) had similarly linked the occurrence
f mental illness to inner city problems.

tressful life events, social, and personal factors in adult
mental illness

he link between social and personal factors and adult mental
llness is shown by the studies of depression in women in inner
London by Brown and Harris (1978). They argue that the
ccurrence of depressive illness, clinical depression, can be
nderstood as a result of a 'vulnerable' or predisposed indi-
idual being exposed to a 'provoking' agent and that both
hese, the level of resistance or defences, and the precipitant,
ave social origins.

The provoking agents are severe life events involving long-
erm threat to the individual, and major personal difficulties,
hat is of a chronic not acute type, such as with housing,
amily, or work. The methodological question that surrounds
ny work in this field is of the form: who decides what is
tressful (or threatening or major)? Brown (1981) characterizes

two types of measure of life events: respondent-based and
investigator-based. Questionnaires are put into the first
category, because the respondent makes the decision as to
whether to include an occurrence as an event, or as stressful.
Brown and colleagues opt for investigator-based measures in
which it is the investigator, following a predetermined schema,
who decides if an event involves threat to the particular
subject or if a difficulty is major. This approach allows the
investigator greater insight into people's lives and the possible
causal links with mental illness, but has attracted some criticism
as being more open to interviewer and coding bias than a
standard questionnaire (Brown and Harris 1979). Presumably
for some events, death of a spouse, loss of job, etc., respondent-based and investigator-based methods would agree.

Armed with these measures, Brown and colleagues find a
clear relation between the onset of depressive illness and
preceding life events or major difficulties. The social link is
shown markedly by the higher rate of depression of working-
class than of middle-class women, (whether measured by the
Registrar-General's Classes I to V, or other social class
indices), and women with children at home are at higher risk
than women without. Provoking agents, that is life events
and difficulties, occur with greater frequency in working-class
than middle-class women, but this difference did not account
for the higher rate of depression (Table 7.17).

The data in Table 7.17 led to two related questions: (i) Why
does a provoking agent only lead to depression in one in five
of women exposed? What protects the other four out of five?
(ii) What other factors lead working-class women to be more
vulnerable to depression? Their answers to these questions are
tentative, but Brown *et al.* found four interrelated factors
that are associated with increased vulnerability: not having an
intimate relationship with husband or other confidant, no job
outside the home, loss of mother at an early age, and having
three or more children under 14 years old at home. These
vulnerability factors, except no outside job, were more
common in working-class women and went a long way to
'explaining' the higher incidence of depression in response to
a severe life event or major difficulty.

Replication of findings is an important part of research. In
particular, the social environment may have very different
meaning cross-culturally. In related studies in the Hebrides

Table 7.17. *Per cent of women developing depression by whether they have children at home, social class, and whether they had a severe event or major difficulty prior to onset of depression*

	Severe event/ major difficulty	No severe event/ no major difficulty	Total
Women with child at home			
working class	31	1	16
middle class	8	1	3
Women without children at home			
working class	10	2	5
middle class	19	1	7
All women			
working class	25	2	12
middle class	13	1	5
total	20	2	9

Source: Brown and Harris (1978).

Islands, off the coast of Scotland, Brown and Prudo (1981) found that similar provocations were related to depression as was the case in London, but there was no social class difference in occurrence of depression. Indeed, in the Hebrides, as compared to London, social class was likely to mean different things socially and psychologically. Instead, they found that the more integrated women were into the traditional rural life of the islands the greater their resistance to developing depression in the face of a severe life event or major difficulty.

The Hebrides study provided partial support for the vulnerability factors identified in London: the lack of confiding relationship with husband or boyfriend, three or more children under 14 years old at home, in the presence of provoking agents, were associated with depression.

This research has also provided insight into the greater rate of childhood accidents in working class families. Brown and Davidson (1978) found that both social class and depression in the mother were associated with an increased risk of childhood accidents (Fig. 7.3). The greater rate of serious difficulties – poor health, shortage of money, marital tensions – in working-class households, further increased the rate of childhood accidents.

Social and family factors and organic disease

There is little disagreement that, in principle, the psyche can affect the soma, resulting in psychosomatic disorders. There is much disagreement as to which disorders are psychosomatic, and the extent to which organic diseases with clear physical/biological causes also have a psychosomatic component in causation. Traditionally, there has been scanty information relating psychosomatic disorders to the social environment.

Among the current generation of researchers interested in social/psychological factors and disease, cardiovascular diseases have attracted attention away from peptic ulcer and rheumatic diseases. This work will serve to illustrate attempts to move from a psychological to a social focus. In a recent review, Jenkins (1982) classifies the huge literature on social/psychological factors and coronary heart disease into four categories: sustained disturbing emotions; Type A behaviour; work overload; and socio-economic disadvantage. The first

of these, including anxiety, depression and neuroticism m⟨
be related to the social environment, as detailed in t⟨
previous section, but much of the research has failed explici⟨
to make the link.

The second category, Type A behaviour, because of i⟨
strong relation to coronary heart disease, has excited muc⟨
interest. Only recently have concerted attempts begun ⟨
determine how much the Type A behaviour pattern is relate⟨
to basic personality structure formed early in life and hen⟨
fairly resistant to change, and how much to the contempora⟨
social environment, culture, and work environment.

The third category, work overload, is clearly an interactic⟨
between objectively verifiable pressures arising in the socia⟨

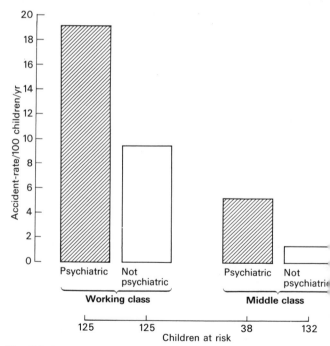

Fig. 7.3. Number of serious accidents per 100 children at risk pe⟨ year by psychiatric state and social class of mother. Based o⟨ findings in 420 children under 16 years. (Source: Brown and David⟨ son 1978).

rk environment and personal factors relating both to ·ception of work-load and ability to deal with pressure. It ·l therefore not necessarily be the social groups with ·parently the highest work pressure who succumb, if their ·ources to deal with the pressure are greater. The higher ·ronary heart disease mortality rates in working-class (IV ·d V) compared to executive-class men (I and II) (Marmot *et* · 1978) is therefore not a refutation of a work-stress hypo- ·sis. To some extent people select themselves into jobs, and ·ecutives, for example, may find apparently high-pressure ·os not to be stressful, and indeed to be healthful. Recent ·dies have classified work not only according to the degree ·· pressure involved, but along an extra dimension: decision ·itude, that is the degree of flexibility and independence a ·rker has in governing the way the work is done. Prelim- ·ary evidence shows a higher rate of coronary heart disease ·nong men in jobs involving high demands and low decision ·itude (Karasek *et al.* 1982).

The fourth category, socio-economic disadvantage, has ·en discussed *in extenso* previously, in relation to relevant ·e-styles, education, etc. It is a possibility, but it has yet to be ·early shown, that one of the contributors to the higher ·ronary death rates in working-class men and women, ·asses IV and V, is a greater perception of stressful demands ·om the environment with fewer resources to cope with those ·mands (Marmot 1982).

The question of resources to deal with stressful demands is · relevant to physical disease as it is to mental illness, dis- ·ssed above: why when faced with stressors, physical and ·notional, do a majority of people not break down and ·come ill (Antonovsky 1979)? Support for Cassel's thesis ·at the social environment can contribute to host resistance ·mes from work on social supports. In Alameda County, ·alifornia, for example, a sample of men and women were ·assified according to various measures of social support and · nine-year mortality follow-up was conducted. Higher ·ortality was observed among the non-married (as shown by · any others), among people with little contact with friends or ·latives, among non-members of a church or other group ·sociation. Combining these into a social network index ·ig. 7.4) showed a clear association in men and women: ·ose with fewer social 'connections' had a higher all-cause ·ortality rate (Berkman and Syme 1979). In this population, ·ople of lower income and education had, on average, fewer ·cial 'connections' than the better off, but the two factors, ·cial network and socio-economic status, were independently ·sociated with mortality.

The data on lower heart disease rates in Japanese-Americans ·ho retain traditional Japanese culture may relate, in part to ·e protective effects of social supports in Japanese culture ·Marmot and Syme 1976). Other work suggests that social ·upport may moderate life-stress and affect outcome of ·regnancy, rheumatic disease, recovery from illness, and the ·ttempt at stopping excessive drinking (Cobb 1976).

In this section on organic disease, we have paid less atten- ·on to stressful life events, because the data are not as strong ·nd consistent as with mental illness. There is, nevertheless, ·ome evidence that life events such as bereavement, migration,

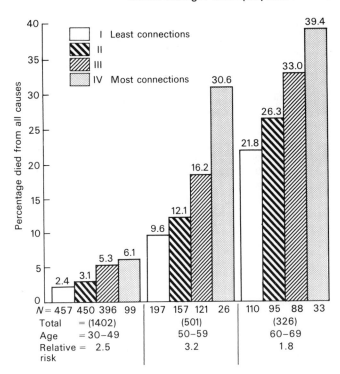

Fig. 7.4. Age-specific mortality rates/100 from all causes (men) according to an index of 'social networks'. (Source: Berkman and Syme 1979.)

increased work-load, or job loss can increase cardiovascular risk (Theorell 1982), and perhaps general mortality.

SOCIAL CHANGE: UNEMPLOYMENT

Unemployment a specific factor?

As conditions of the social environment change, we might expect health and disease patterns to change. The most dramatic change facing capitalist and 'mixed' economies is chronic high unemployment. There are at least two reasons for speculating *a priori* that unemployment may have an impact on morbidity and mortality. First, it can be an indi- cator of conditions and standards of living (Morris and Titmuss 1944). As the level of unemployment rises, more and more people have their material conditions markedly worsened. Second, unemployment is a stressful life event. In a work-oriented society, work has social and psychological meaning, that goes beyond its economic import. To become unemployed is to be deprived of a social role and function. The self-image of the unemployed person is changed as is the pattern of social relationships.

The existence of plausible theoretical reasons why unemployment might affect health status is no guarantee that such a relationship can be demonstrated. One difficulty comes in isolating the effects of unemployment from the effects of other social or economic conditions. In a sense, this is an artificial question. If unemployment leads to increased mortality rates for the first of the above reasons – that it increases poverty – then it becomes difficult to separate the effects of unemployment from the effects of poverty: poverty is the effect of unemployment which anyhow is particularly likely to affect the poor. The unemployment question is then seen as part of the general question: does increased poverty lead to increased morbidity and mortality? In the second case, unemployment as stressful life change, it will again be difficult to isolate the health effects of this particular stress from the other stresses associated with poverty – as described above in the work of Brown and colleagues on depression.

One might argue that unemployment is unlikely to have the same effect on all societies at different times. This is theoretically true, but the same argument might be raised about social class. Remarkably, social class, despite the crudity of the measures employed, has been a strong predictor of mortality since it was first measured as such in England and Wales in 1911 and the same is true of other industrialized countries.

Two potentially important distinctions should be made, however. First that between temporary and long-term unemployment (>1 yr). These are likely to affect different people by age, skills, social class, and health record and may have different associations with ill health. And secondly, whether only the health of the unemployed is being considered, or whether the health of employed and unemployed people is considered in relation to unemployment rates.

Methods of study

Broadly, two approaches have been taken to studying the impact of unemployment on morbidity and mortality: (i) correlational studies of whole populations or subgroups thereof, and (ii) studies of unemployed people. Each has advantages and limitations as detailed below.

Correlation

Among the earliest of these was the study by Morris and Titmuss (1944) of rheumatic heart disease mortality in young people in the county boroughs of England and Wales, related to the depression of the 1930s. They showed a correlation between increase in overall unemployment rates and change in rheumatic heart disease mortality – the towns worst hit by unemployment had the worst mortality record. The correlations were strongest with a 'lag' period of up to three years, and were apparent even after standardizations for an index of poverty and overcrowding.

Best known among recent studies is the series by Brenner (1977, 1979). He has argued that increases in unemployment affect not only the unemployed, but also those still in employment, that is, a rise in unemployment is a general indicator of economic instability, which leads to loss of income, social status, and close personal attachments, and to stress in employees of firms experiencing economic difficulties (Brenner 1979). In his American studies, Brenner (1977) claimed that peaks in mortality from a variety of causes follow peaks in unemployment with a lag period of between 0 and 5 years. One of his major critics, Eyer (1977), agrees that peaks in mortality rate do correspond with the business cycle, but he comes to the opposite conclusion to Brenner. He argues that *troughs* in unemployment correspond to peaks in

mortality, with no lag period. Eyer did not use the sa complex multivariate statistical models as Brenner, w rejected this interpretation.

Brenner (1979), has applied a similar statistical anal to mortality trends in England and Wales. He analysed m tality for the period 1936–76, that is before current recessi and mass unemployment. His statistical model to 'expla trends in mortality – both the long-term secular decline a short-term fluctuations – includes four components: (i) e nomic growth trend; (ii) rate of unemployment; (iii) ra economic growth (that is, deviations from the long-te exponential trend in· real per-caput income); and, fina (iv) government expenditure on 'welfare' as a percentage total government expenditure. Unemployment is built i the statistical model with a variable lag period.

The results, on the surface remarkable, are very difficult interpret. The R^2 value (a perfect correlation has an R^2 of no correlation: $R^2 = 0$) of his multiple regression equation 0.97. Interpreted literally, this means that these fo economic indices 'account for' 97 per cent of the variance death rates, over the period in England and Wales. Similar in a regional analysis of counties in England and Wales, 197 Brenner finds that economic indices including unemployme 'explain' 95 per cent of the variance in total death rates.

It is not the present purpose to enter a general discussion regression analyses, but to put these results in perspective, should note that completely different variables also find hi orders of correlation. For example, in England and Wales t mortality rate is higher in winter than in summer and t winter excess is greater in severe winters (defined by weath not economics), with high rates of influenza, than in mi winters.

For arteriosclerotic heart disease mortality in England a Wales, over the period 1950–62, the correlation between t winter excess in mortality and coldness of the winter is 0.95 95 per cent of the variance, the year to year fluctuations winter *excess*, can be 'explained' by temperature (Rose 196 It is similarly possible to show that trends in heart disea mortality are correlated to a high order with consumption various foods and cigarettes (Armstrong *et al.* 1975).

Brenner's high order geographical correlation betwe economic factors, economic growth, unemployment, etc and mortality in England and Wales can also be reproduce with other variables. For example, an analysis of mortali 1969–73 from cardiovascular disease in 253 towns England, Wales, and Scotland found the following correla tion coefficients with mortality (SMR): water hardness −0.6 mean daily maximum temperature −0.70; total annual rai fall 0.58; latitude 0.74; longitude 0.68; air pollution (mea annual smoke) 0.54; blood group (per cent A – frequenc −0.59 (Pocock *et al.* 1980).

If economic indices including unemployment account fo all the variation in mortality over time and over place, ho can it be true that this same variation is also 'explained' b variations in temperature, longitude, water hardness, a pollution, and consumption of flour and fresh vegetables There may be several answers. Many of these variables ar highly inter-correlated and a multiple regression equation i not the appropriate tool to tell us which of these variables i

sally related to mortality. It is too affected by circum-
nces and quality of measurement to sort out biological
ootheses. Second, by allowing for variable lag periods
ween unemployment and mortality, as Brenner does, and
selecting some variables (for example, percentage of
rkers in chemical industries, and farm employment) but
t others, it is possible, *post hoc*, to fit a curve to the data
h a high order of precision.

An important test of the statistical model is its ability to
dict mortality beyond the period for which it was developed.
avelle and colleagues (1981) have criticized Brenner's
alysis on a number of grounds. For example, the strong
rrelation between unemployment and mortality seen in the
riod 1936–76, is no longer evident if the period is extended
include 1922–76. Further lack of 'robustness' is demon-
ated by the failure of the model to predict mortality
bsequent to the period over which it was developed, better
an a simple extrapolation.

The lesson from this exchange is not that unemployment
s no relation with general mortality, but that such a relation
difficult to tease out of a number of inter-correlated
riables. Certainly few would find difficulty in accepting
at the long-term downward trend in mortality in England
d Wales, the US and other countries, is related to general
provements in standard of living. Whether short-term
actuations in mortality are related to fluctuations in
onomic fortunes has not been demonstrated unequivocally
this type of analysis (Kasl 1979). There are other diffi-
lties apart from methodological ones. For example,
employment, since the depression of the 1930s, has not
en a reflection of *general* economic decline. Those in
nployment (close on 90 per cent in England and Wales) have
ntinued to enjoy an increased standard of living, at least
til now – although this may change.

tudies of unemployed people

hese studies present different problems. It has commonly
en found that unemployed people have a higher morbidity
rate than those in employment (Stern 1981). For example, in
the General Household Survey (1976) in Britain, the proportion of males reporting a long-standing illness was nearly
40 per cent higher for the unemployed. This finding is consistent with three alternative explanations: (i) the unemployed
differ from the employed with respect to other characteristics
that account for their ill health; (ii) ill health causes
unemployment; (iii) unemployment causes ill health. There is
some evidence in support of all three of these.

Several studies in England and Wales have shown that
unemployment affects selectively people in low social class
and low incomes (Stern 1981). For example, a 1978
survey showed that half the entrants to unemployment had
prior incomes in the bottom 20 per cent of the earning distribution. This makes it difficult to separate the effects of
unemployment from the effects of prior poverty and thus to
see if unemployment increases further the disadvantage of
this high-risk group. A major British study of the 1930s found
difficulty in separating the effects of unemployment from the
effects of working-class life on a low income, but emphasized
the likely ill-effects of the latter (Pilgrim Trust 1938).

Clearly, ill health can also lead to unemployment. The
'healthy worker' effect is well recognized in epidemiology.
People in employment have lower mortality rates than those
out of employment. For example, Table 7.18 from the OPCS
longitudinal study (Fox and Goldblatt 1982) shows that
among men aged 15–64 years, those actively in work have an
SMR of 86, that is 86 per cent of the average mortality. With
the exception of students, all other groups of men have a
higher mortality than the average – at least in part because the
non-working group includes people off work, sick (SMR =
392). Findings for women were similar. If the definition of
'unemployment' is restricted to people not off sick and
seeking work, the SMR is still raised for men (130) but not for
women (80). Even this latter group of men could include
some people who lost their jobs through ill health.

These national data for England and Wales illustrate the
problem. Unemployed men and women have a higher

Table 7.18. *Mortality 1971–75 of men and women in the OPCS Longitudinal Study according to age and economic position at the time of the 1971 census*

Economic position	Men (15–64 years)			Women (15–59 years)		
	Observed	Expected*	SMR	Observed	Expected*	SMR
Active						
Employed	3021	35087	86	682	884.4	81
Off work, sick	211	65.3	323	48	11.1	432
Seeking work	165	126.9	130	20	25.0	80
Inactive						
Retired	91	59.4	153	37	26.2	141
Permanently sick	370	94.5	392	101	20.1	502
Student	26	1.5	83	16	17.5	91
Other inactive	43	410	105	646	605.9	107
Total	3927	3927.3	100	1550	1550.2	100

*Expected deaths are calculated separately for each sex using death rates for 1971–75 (in five-year age groups)
for all males/females in the Longitudinal Study 1971 Census sample.
Source: Fox and Goldblatt (1982).

mortality than the employed, but sickness is one reason for being out of work. From a study that examines employment status at one time, it is difficult to distinguish ill health as a cause or effect of unemployment. Longitudinal data on health status before and after jobs are lost are few. One American study of this type reported an increase in blood pressure after unemployment (Kasl and Cobb 1970).

These studies have all been based on relatively 'hard' end-points. Clearly, unemployment can have a major impact on family life, on general well-being, and on the children of the unemployed, whether or not this is reflected in usual measures of morbidity and mortality.

The failure to demonstrate unequivocally that unemployment has an independent effect on health and disease does not exonerate unemployment. No evidence does not equate with no effect. At the very least, one can conclude that the failure to show clearly such an effect of unemployment is due, in part, to the strong harmful effects of poverty. As Stern (1981) comments: 'The incidence of unemployment is non-random and reflects wider economic inequalities. High unemployment reveals the consequences of low incomes more starkly'.

SOCIAL FACTORS AS CAUSES

The notion of 'necessary' cause is not generally very helpful in studying human health and disease. Infectious diseases have necessary causes because, by definition, we do not label a chest disease tuberculosis unless the tubercle bacillus is judged to be its cause. Comparable situations are found in single-gene defects, nutritional deficiencies, and the effects of toxic substances, alcohol, asbestos, etc. But for most prevalent diseases, and certainly for health, disability, or handicap, we are not able to identify necessary causes. More useful is the notion of 'sufficient' cause, made up of a complex of unfavourable conditions. For tuberculosis to develop after exposure to Koch's bacillus, a range of social-environmental and personal factors also have to be present. Nor is smoking a sufficient cause of lung cancer; a number of other conditions also contribute. The recognition that health states and diseases have many causes means that the failure to find a 1:1 relationship between factor and disease is not a crucial argument against the causal nature of an association.

Terminology is loose here, and these other conditions that contribute to make up the *sufficient* cause, are themselves often labelled as causes: for example, malnutrition is called a cause of tuberculosis, vitamin A deficiency (possibly) a cause of cancer. Where do social causes fit into this picture? It is not enough to state that if an individual is infected with the tubercle bacillus, or smokes, his risk of tuberculosis, or lung cancer, is increased. For a start it is relevant to ask why the individual became exposed to infection, why he smoked, or why the many other conditions leading to disease were met. The social/psychological determinants of infection, smoking, nutrition, and stress, all may play a part.

How do we find our way out of this morass? The operation of any of the conditions making up the sufficient cause may be viewed for simplicity as a chain (Fig. 7.5). For the biochemist, the study of causes may be the study of chemical

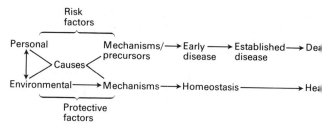

Fig. 7.5. Simplified model of chain of causation.

reactions in the body – 'mechanisms' in the figure. For public health the focus is further back in the causal chain, on environment and behaviours; a cause is any part of the sufficient complex which, when altered, leads to a change in the frequency of the disease.

In general, the procedures for establishing that a condition is causal are the role of epidemiology and, although vitally important, need not concern us here: a salient example is whether social class is truly causal or merely an artefact of social mobility, etc. (DHSS 1980). The main justification for regarding social conditions as causes is the overwhelming evidence that these influence disease rates, and that change in social conditions is associated with change in the frequency of such rates.

Focus on social conditions as causes need not exclude simultaneous focus 'further down' the causal chain. If lowering the tar content of cigarettes lowered the frequency of lung cancer, it would be useful to consider tar as contributing to cause. If reducing the high prevalence of smoking in men and women of Classes IV and V, compared to Classes I and II, reduced their mortality from lung cancer towards that of I and II, social class could usefully be considered as contributing to the sufficient cause of the disease.

Two related characteristics of social conditions as causes should be noted: their degree of *proximity*, and their *specificity*. Compared to physico-chemical conditions such as smoking, low vitamin A, and air pollutants, social conditions tend to be further back on the causal chain, less proximate, and their relation to particular diseases may therefore be less consistent. For example, it is true that in 1970–72 in England and Wales, Classes IV and V had higher mortality from coronary heart disease than Classes I and II. But in England and Wales this represents a change from the picture in the 1950s, presumably because the relation of social class to suspected causal conditions, such as smoking and physical activity, have changed. Specificity of social conditions is also likely to be low: being poor, and the cluster of conditions involved in social class and the standard of living, is likely to be related to a greater range of pathological processes than, say, smoking or inhaling pollutants. However, despite this relative lack of specificity, if it is possible to do something about these social–environmental, and personal contributions to 'cause', they are of crucial importance to public health.

REFERENCES

American Journal of Clinical Nutrition (1982). Symposium on nutrition and ageing. *Am. J. Clin. Nutr.* **36(5)**, 977.

ntonovsky, A. (1979). *Health stress and coping: new perspectives on mental and physical well-being.* Josey-Bass, San Francisco.

rmstrong, B.K., Mann, J.I., Adelstein, A.M., and Eskin, F. (1975). Commodity consumption and ischaemic heart disease mortality with special reference to dietary practices. *J. Chronic Dis.* **28**, 455.

skham, J. (1969). Delineation of the lowest class. *J. Biosoc. Sci.* **1**, 327.

uletta, K. (1982). *The underclass.* Random House, New York.

erkman, L.F. and Syme, S.L. (1979). Social networks, host resistance and mortality: a nine-year follow-up study of Alameda County residents. *Am. J. Epidemiol.* **109**, 186.

owlby, J. (1951). *Maternal care and mental health.* WHO Monograph Series No. 2, Geneva.

owlby, J. (1965). *Child care and the growth of love,* 2nd edn. Penguin, Harmondsworth.

renner, M.H. (1977). Health costs and benefits of economic policy. *Int. J. Health Serv.* **7**, 581.

renner, M.H. (1979). Mortality and the national economy: a review, and the experience of England and Wales 1936–76. *Lancet* **ii**, 568.

reslow, L. (1978). Risk factor intervention for health maintenance. *Science* **200**, 908.

rooks, L.H. (1980). Social economic and biologic correlates of infant mortality in city neighborhoods. *J. Health Soc. Behav.* **21**, 2.

rown, G.W. (1981). Life events, psychiatric disorder and physical illness. *J. Psychosom. Res.* **25**, 461.

rown, G.W. and Davidson, S. (1978). Social class, psychiatric disorder of mother, and accidents to children. *Lancet* **i**, 378.

rown, G.W. and Harris, T. (1978). *Social origins of depression.* Tavistock, London.

rown, G.W. and Harris, T. (1979). The sin of subjectivism: a reply to Shapiro. *Behav. Res. Therapy* **17**, 605.

rown, M. and Madge, N. (1982). *Despite the welfare state.* Heinemann Educational, London.

rown, G.W. and Prudo, R. (1981). Psychiatric disorder in a rural and an urban population. I. Aetiology of depression. *Psychol. Med.* **11**, 581.

assel, J. (1976). The contribution of the social environment to host resistance. *Am. J. Epidemiol.* **104**, 107.

halmers, I., Newcombe, R., West, R. *et al.* (1978). Adjusted perinatal mortality rates in administrative areas of England and Wales. *Health Trends* **10**, 24.

obb, S. (1976). Social support as a moderator of life stress. *Psychosom. Med.* **38**, 300.

HSS (1980). *Research into services for children and adolescents.* HMSO, London.

HSS (1982). *Report on confidential enquiries into maternal deaths in England and Wales 1976–1978. Report on health and social subjects 26.* HMSO, London.

HSS (1980). *Inequalities in health. Report of a research working group* (chairman D. Black). DHSS, London.

oll, R. and Peto, R. (1976). Mortality in relation to smoking. *Br. Med. J.* **ii**, 1525.

oll, R. and Peto, R. (1981). *The causes of cancer.* Oxford University Press.

ubos, R. (1965). *Man adapting.* Yale University Press, New Haven.

urkheim, E. (1952). *Suicide.* Routledge and Kegan Paul, London.

isenberg, L. and Kleinman, A. (eds.) (1981). *The relevance of social science for medicine.* Reidel, Dordrecht.

yer, J. (1977). Does unemployment cause the death rate peak in each business cycle? A multifactor model of death rate changes. *Int. J. Health Serv.* **7**, 625.

Faris, R.E.L. and Dunham, H.W. (1939). *Mental disorders in urban areas.* Chicago University Press.

Fenner, F. (1971). Infectious disease and social change. *Med. J. Austr.* **1**, 1043.

Fox, A.J. and Adelstein, A.M. (1978). Occupational mortality: work or way of life? *J. Epidemiol. Community Health* **32**, 73.

Fox, A.J. and Goldblatt, P.O. (1982). *Longitudinal study: 1971–75.* HMSO, London.

Gravelle, H.S.E., Hutchinson, G., and Stern, J. (1981). Mortality and unemployment: a critique of Brenner's time-series analysis. *Lancet* **ii**, 675.

Illsley, R. (1980). *Professional or public health? Sociology in health and medicine.* Nuffield Provincial Hospitals Trust, London.

Immigrant Statistics Unit (1978). Marriage and birth patterns among the New Commonwealth and Pakistani population. *Population Trends* **11**, 5.

Jaco, E.G. (ed.) (1972). *Patients, physicians and illness.* Free Press, New York.

Jenkins, C.D. (1982). Psychosocial risk factors for coronary heart disease. *Acta Med. Scand. (Suppl.)* **660**, 123.

Karasek, R.A., Theorell, T.G.T., Schwartz, J., Pieper, C., and Alfredsson, L. (1982). Job, psychological factors and coronary heart disease. Swedish prospective findings and US prevalence findings using a new occupational inference model. In *Psychological problems before and after myocardial infarction* (ed. H. Denolin) *Adv. Cardiol 29,* p. 62. Karget, Basel.

Kasl, S.V. (1977). Contributions of social epidemiology to studies in psychosomatic medicine. *Adv. Psychosom. Med.* **9**, 160.

Kasl, S.V. (1979). Mortality and the business cycle: some questions about research strategies when utilising macro-social and ecological data. *Am. J. Public Health* **69**, 784.

Kasl, S.V. and Cobb, S. (1970). Blood pressure changes in men undergoing job loss: a preliminary report. *Psychosom. Med.* **32**, 19.

Kluckhohn, C. (1949). *Mirror for man.* McGraw Hill, New York.

Knox, E.G., Marshall, T., Kane, S., Green, A., and Mallett, R. (1980). Social and health care determinants of area variations in perinatal mortality. *Community Med.* **2**, 282.

Lalonde, M. (1974). *A new perspective on the health of Canadians.* Government of Canada, Ottawa.

Marmot, M.G. (1982). Socio-economic and cultural factors in ischaemic heart disease. In *Psychological problems before and after myocardial infarction. Adv. Cardiol. 29.* (ed. H. Denolin) p. 68. Karger, Basel.

Marmot, M.G., Adelstein, A., and Bulusu, L. (1984). *Mortality of immigrants to England and Wales. OPCS. Studies on Medical and Population subjects.* HMSO, London.

Marmot, M.G. and Syme, S.L. (1976). Acculturation and coronary heart disease in Japanese-Americans. *Am. J. Epidemiol.* **104**, 225.

Marmot, M.G., Adelstein, A.M., Robinson, N., and Rose, G.A. (1978). Changing social-class distribution of heart disease. *Br. Med. J.* **ii**, 1109.

Matsumoto, Y.S. (1970). Social stress and coronary heart disease in Japan: a hypothesis. *Milbank Mem. Fund Q.* **48**, 9.

Ministry of Agriculture, Fisheries and Food (annually). *Household food consumption and expenditure.* HMSO, London.

Morris, J.N. (1976). *Uses of epidemiology.* Churchill-Livingstone, Edinburgh.

Morris, J.N. (1979). Social inequalities undiminished. *Lancet* **i**, 87.

Morris, J.N. (1980). Social inequalities undiminished. *Health Visitor* **53**, 361.

Morris, J.N. (1982). Epidemiology and prevention. *Milbank Mem. Fund Q.* **60**, 1.

Morris, J.N. and Titmuss, R.M. (1944). Health and social change.

1: the recent history of rheumatic heart disease. *Medical Officer* **72**, 69.

Morris, J.N., Everitt, M.G., Pollard, R., Chave, S.P.W., and Semmence, A.M. (1980). Vigorous exercise in leisure-time: protection against coronary heart disease. *Lancet* ii, 1207.

OPCS (1975). *Social trends No. 6.* HMSO, London.

OPCS (1978). *Occupational Mortality 1970–2. Decennial Supplement.* HMSO, London.

OPCS (annually). *General Household Survey.* HMSO, London.

OPCS (weekly). *OPCS monitors.* HMSO, London.

Orr, J.B. (1937). *Food, health and income.* Macmillan, London.

Parron, D.L., Solomon, F., and Jenkins, C.D. (1982). *Behavior, health risks, and social disadvantage.* National Academy Press for Institute of Medicine, Washington, DC.

Paul, B.D. (1955). Review of concepts and contents. In *Health, culture and community* (ed. B.D. Paul), p. 459. Russel Sage Foundation, New York.

Pilgrim Trust (1938). *Men without work.* Macmillan, London.

Pocock, S.J., Shaper, A.G., Cook, D.G. *et al.* (1980). British regional heart study: geographic variations in cardiovascular mortality, and the role of water quality. *Br. Med. J.* **280**, 1243.

Robertson, T., Kato, H., Rhoads, G.G. *et al.* (1977). Epidemiologic studies of coronary heart disease and stroke in Japanese men living in Japan, Hawaii and California: incidence of myocardial infarction and death from coronary heart disease. *Am. J. Cardiol.* **39**, 239.

Rose, G. (1966). Cold weather and ischaemic heart disease. *Br. J. Prev. Soc. Med.* **20**, 97.

Rose, G. and Marmot, M.G. (1981). Social class and coronary heart disease. *Br. Heart J.* **45**, 13.

Royal College of Physicians (1962, 1971, 1977, 1983). *Reports on smoking and health.* Pitman Medical, London.

Rothschild, H. (ed.) (1981). *Biocultural aspects of disease.* Academic Press, New York.

Rutter, M. and Quinton, D. (1981). Longitudinal studies of institutional children and children of mentally ill parents (United Kingdom). In *Prospective longitudinal research.* (eds. S.A. Medrick, A.E. Baert, and B.P. Bachman) p. 297. Oxford University Press.

Rutter, M., Cox, A., Tupling, C., Berger, M., and Yule, W. (1975). Attainment and adjustment in two geographical areas. I – the prevalence of psychiatric disorders. *Br. J. Psychiatry* **126**, 493.

Rutter, M., Yule, B., Quinton, D., Rowland, O., Yule, W., a[nd] Berger, M. (1974). Attainment and adjustment in two ge[o]graphical areas. III – some factors accounting for area differenc[e]. *Br. J. Psychiatry* **125**, 520.

Schottenfeld, D. and Fraumeni, J.F. (eds.) (1982). *Cancer e[pi]demiology and prevention.* Saunders, Philadelphia.

Sheiham, H. and Quick, A. (1982). *The rickets report.* Harring[ton] Community Health Council, London.

Simon, J. (1980). *English sanitary institutions.* Cassell, London.

Starfield, B. (1983). Social factors in child health. In *Ambulato[ry] pediatrics III* (eds. M. Green and R. Haggerty). Saunders, Phi[la]delphia.

Stern, J. (1981). *Unemployment and its impact on morbidity a[nd] mortality.* Centre for Labour Economics, London School [of] Economics. Discussion paper 93.

Surgeon General (1979). *Healthy people. The Surgeon-Genera[l] report on health promotion and disease prevention.* DHE[W] Washington, DC.

Susser, M.W. and Watson, W. (1971). *Sociology in medicine,* 2nd edn. Oxford University Press.

Theorell, T.G.T. (1982). Review of research on life events a[nd] cardiovascular illness. In *Psychological problems before a[nd] after myocardial infarction.* Adv. Cardiol 29. (ed. H. Denoli[n]) p. 140. Karger, Basel.

Townsend, P. (1979). *Poverty in the United Kingdom.* Allen Lan[e], London.

Townsend, P. and Davidson, M. (1982). *Inequalities in health. T[he] Black Report.* Penguin, Harmondsworth.

Trowell, H.C. and Burkitt, D.P. (1981). *Western diseases.* Edwa[rd] Arnold, London.

United Nations (1979). *Proceedings of the meeting on soci[o] economic determinants and consequences of mortality, Mexi[co] City.* United Nations, New York.

Vernon, H.M. (1939). *Health in relation to occupation.* Oxfo[rd] University Press, London.

Westergard, J. and Resler, H. (1975). *Class in a capitalist societ[y].* Penguin, London.

Wiesenfeld, S.L. (1967). Sickle-cell trait in human biological a[nd] cultural evolution. *Science* **157**, 1134.

8 Natural and man-made disasters

M.F. Lechat

NATURAL DISASTERS

Natural disasters can be defined as ecological disruptions which exceed the community's capacity of adjustment so that outside assistance is needed. There are many types including earthquakes, floods, tidal waves, landslides, and volcanic eruptions. Natural disasters are generally of sudden onset and constitute unforeseen, serious, and immediate threats to health. At times, they exert an heavy toll in terms of mortality (Table 8.1).

In recent years public health officials have become increasingly concerned with natural disasters and their human consequences. There are two main reasons for this. First, major disasters necessitating international aid are reported several times a year; as a result of better reporting by the mass-media they appear to occur more frequently. They also become more devastating as the population density in disaster-prone areas increases. Secondly, there is a feeling that nowadays disasters, even natural ones, should be amenable to some kind of management to prevent their occurrence, mitigate their impact, or at least to improve rescue and relief.

The types of health problems associated with natural disasters can best be viewed in terms of a time scale (Fig. 8.1). For the sake of simplicity, five successive epochs in the disaster process can be identified and the health measures needed at each phase are discussed below.

Pre-disaster phase

This phase, often referred to as the *interdisaster phase*, is the time for prevention and preparedness. For most natural hazards, the respective risks according to geographical areas can be mapped, i.e. the identification of zones of tectonic instability.

The study of the ratio of deaths to numbers of houses badly damaged in various regions of Iran and Turkey has indicated that high case-fatality rates from earthquakes in these countries are associated with the introduction of cheap new building methods. The use of large concrete slabs supported by walls made of sun-dried bricks (adobe) insufficiently reinforced with concrete blocks is associated with a

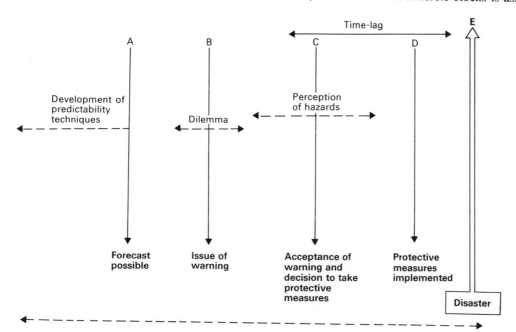

Fig. 8.1. Relationship between prediction and prevention of disasters (Source: Lechat 1974).

Table 8.1. *Natural disasters in Europe and the world in the twentieth century. (From Velimirovic, personal communication)*

Year	Disaster	Place	Deaths
1908	Earthquake	Messina	+100 000
1912	Earthquake	Turkey	3000
1915	Earthquake	Arezzano (Italy)	30 000
1930	Earthquake	Naples (Italy)	2000
1939	Earthquake	Turkey	33 000
1959	Earthquake	Algeria	1500
1960	Earthquake	Agadir (Morocco)	12 000
1963	Earthquake	Skopje (Yugoslavia)	+1000
1966	Earthquake	Turkey	2500
1970	Earthquake	Gediz (Turkey)	1000
1971	Earthquake	Turkey	1000
1975	Earthquake	Lice (Turkey)	3–5000
1976	Earthquake	Friuli (Italy)	1000
1976	Earthquake	Turkey	3790
1977	Earthquake	Bucharest (Romania)	1570
1979	Earthquake	Montenegro (Yugoslavia)	91
1980	Earthquake	El Asnam (Algeria)	10 000
1980	Earthquake	Irpinia (Italy)	+3000

Year	Disaster	Place	Deaths
1906	Earthquake	San Francisco	60
1907	Earthquake	Kingston (Jamaica)	140
1908	Flood	Yangtze-Kiang (China)	100 00
1920	Earthquake	Kansu (China)	180 00
1923	Earthquake and fire	Tokyo (Japan)	+20 00 41 0
1927	Earthquake and fire	Narka (China)	200 00
1931	Flood	Hoangho (China)	1 000 00
1932	Earthquake	Canton (China)	70 00
1935	Cyclone	India and Pakistan	60 00
1939	Earthquake	Chile	40 00
1939	Earthquake	Erxigan (Iran)	23 00
1939	Typhoon	Trentin (China)	200 00
1949	Earthquake	San Juan (Argentina)	10 00
1949	Earthquake	Equador	60
1949	Flood	Guatemala	40 00
1950	Earthquake	Assam (India)	26 00
1951	Earthquake	El Salvador	60
1953	Earthquake	Phillipines	4
1956	Earthquake	Afghanistan	20
1957	Earthquake	Iran	25 0
1959	Flood	China	2 000 0
1960	Earthquake	Arequipa (Peru)	1
1962	Earthquake	Iran	12 4
1963	Earthquake	Libya	30
1964	Earthquake	Indionage (Harka)	1
1964	Earthquake	Taiwan	1
1968	Earthquake	Iran	11 5
1970	Earthquake	Yungay-Chimbote (Peru)	70 00
1970	Cyclone	East Pakistan	206 00
1971	Earthquake	Los Angeles	?
1972	Earthquake	Managua (Nicaragua)	60
1974	Earthquake	Pakistan	53
1975	Earthquake	China	655 00
1976	Earthquake	Guatemala	22 7
1978	Earthquake	Tabas (Iran)	15–20 00
1978	Earthquake	Kerman (Iran)	25 0
1981	Earthquake	Kerman area	100
1981	Earthquake	Kerman	4–800
1981	Earthquake	Golbaft (Iran)	200

high death rate. Anti-seismic engineering has also made remarkable advances during recent decades and deaths from earthquakes can now be prevented to some extent by appropriate techniques, especially in public buildings. These are expensive, however, and add at least 15 per cent to the cost of the building.

It is increasingly recognized that the appropriate management of natural disaster requires advance planning. To ensure that health services are prepared for disasters, requires a careful analysis of past disasters in order to determine hazards amenable to prevention and mitigation. Most countries have drawn up plans for action in the event of various natural disasters. These plans may vary greatly in detail and quality. At times, although health problems represent a major component of disasters, the health authorities are not adequately represented. In all disaster-prone countries, there should be multidisciplinary planning for disasters in which the health aspects should be fully integrated. Such planning presupposes advance information on health facilities and supplies, localization and mobilization of manpower, distribution and accessibility of the populations, mapping of environmental hazards, as well as transport and communication. Detailed provision should also be made for co-ordination with other levels of governments and the Red Cross, control of aid from diverse origins (non-governmental organizations and channelling of foreign aid. Special attention should be given to hospitals and other health institutions, which generally serve as focal points for the convergence of the population, even when they have been destroyed or damaged (as frequently happens after earthquakes). Hospitals from adjacent or more accessible areas therefore should be linked into a network, with appropriate and autonomous means of communication and transport.

Pre-impact phase

This corresponds to the period during which indications of an imminent disaster are accumulating. Many but not all disasters are preceded by preliminary signs. This is the time for warnings based on appropriate prediction techniques. The mber of deaths will depend for a large part on the early cognition of an impending disaster which would allow the population enough time to take measures. The timing of the warning is all important. A decision has to be made whether to be on the safe side and run the risk of giving a false alarm, or to wait for definite signs of a disaster and perhaps give the alarm too late. The problem is similar to the dilemma of sensitivity versus specificity in the methods used for case-detection surveys in preventive medicine. For example, the 00 000 or so deaths from the cyclone in the Gulf of Bengal 1970 (Sommer and Mosley 1972) were partly due to a decision to delay the warning because an alarm had been given a few days previously for a threat which failed to materialize.

Epidemiological studies following a disaster can also help to identify high-risk population groups for whom special protection should be planned. In the 1976 earthquake in Guatemala, for example, mortality was higher in the 5–9 than in the 0–4 years age groups (Fig. 8.2). This seems to suggest that children aged 5–9 are left to take avoiding action by themselves (De Ville De Goyet *et al.* 1976; Glass *et al.* 1980). Clearly, this is an area where proper education of parents before the event can save lives.

Impact phase

This is the period during which the disaster strikes. Destruction and deaths occur in this phase. It may last from a few seconds (as in the 1976 Guatemala earthquake which lasted 30 seconds with a human toll of over 22 000 deaths) to weeks (the 1973 floods in Pakistan in which five millions were made homeless).

Relatively little is known about the health effects in the few minutes or hours after impact. This is owing to the lack of reliable observations, for there are obvious emotional objections to the gathering of data during an emergency, when relief is the top priority. A number of observations indicate (Sommer 1972) that external aid, however prompt it might be, comes too late to have a significant impact on the prevention of early deaths and that insufficient use is made of local resources for rescue and immediate relief in the affected community (De Ville De Goyet *et al.* 1976).

That the disaster-stricken community can make an effective contribution to immediate rescue and relief is demonstrated by a number of observations made by sociologists. In some earthquakes, it has been observed that within half an hour up to 75 per cent of the survivors are engaged in some kind of rescue activity. The pattern is characterized by low individual efficiency but probably high overall effectiveness. A number of other issues have also been identified, which can affect patterns of survival. Amongst them are a general absence of panic, convergence behaviour, role conflict, professional identification, emergence of new leadership, withdrawal behaviour, personalization of disasters, changing frames of reference, and dependency. All this should be taken into account for planning rescue and relief.

To be effective immediate rescue and relief for natural disasters should be a part of primary health care. This calls for decentralized pre-disaster planning at the community level and education of the community in preparedness for disasters.

Relief phase

This phase begins when assistance from outside starts to reach the disaster area. This stage is often characterized by the intervention of ill-informed and unprepared personnel. Provision and aid may be based on stereotypes and myths, such as the need for sophisticated field hospitals, teams of highly specialized physicians, large quantities of medical supplies, and vaccines for non-existent diseases. As a consequence, useless and unsorted drug samples, airlifted by the ton, pour in. Swarms of well-intentioned volunteers invade the disaster area bringing with them no appropriate skills whatsoever, simply clogging the area and needing to be accomodated, fed, and provided with transport. The major preoccupation is with promptness of reaction; with urgent help however non-specific.

Immediate aid can indeed be rather non-specific, calling for rescue materials, shelters, and survival items (such as food and blankets). But subsequently, relief should be more carefully directed. In reality, the sacrifice in promptness required to collect the information necessary to provide apt and well-directed aid is more than justified by the improved results. An immediate assessment of needs and damage is vital, including the number, type, and localization of casualties, the risk of transmissible diseases, environmental hazards (gas, fire, powerlines, storage of toxic materials), as well as an inventory of preserved structures, facilities, supplies, and manpower. It should be stressed that such an evaluation is essential for effective relief, and the need for relevant information should not be sacrificed to ill-considered hastiness, especially in view of the fact that however prompt the aid given from outside it will have minimal or no effect on early deaths and casualties.

Methods for conducting such assessments under the adverse conditions of disasters have not yet been fully developed and discussion continues. Aerial surveys have proved valuable in identifying areas most affected. It is obvious, however, that ground surveys are essential to

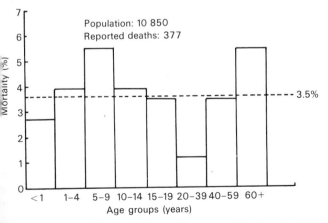

Fig. 8.2. Age-specific mortality in Sumpango, Guatemala, 1976. (Source: De Ville De Goyet *et al.* 1976.)

Table 8.2. *Indices proposed for assessing the health effects of natural disasters and the related needs. (Source: Lechat 1979)*

Indices	Use
Deaths	
Number of impact-related deaths/population of disaster area	– Rough assessment of the importance of the disaster – Evaluation of pre-disaster prevention or mitigation measures – Evaluation of adequacy of warning
Number of impact-related deaths/population of given age	– Identification of vulnerable groups for further contingency planning
Number of impact-related deaths/population within given habitat or given location	– Vulnerability analysis of building structures or location for improvement of preventive measures
Number of deaths/number of houses destroyed	– Assessment of adequacy of building structures
Number of impact-related deaths per unit of time after the disaster/population of disaster area	– Determination of rescue measures required and evaluation of rescue measures – Evaluation of self-reliance of community – Evaluation of pre-disaster community rescue training
Casualties	
Number of deaths/number of casualties	– Determination of rough indices for estimating the numbers of casualties (and emergency supplies required) in different types of disaster
Number of casualties/population of disaster area	– Evaluation of pre-disaster and mitigation measures – Evaluation of adequacy of warning – Estimation of emergency care and relief needs
Distribution of types of casualty	– Estimation of emergency care and relief needs – Identification of risk factors for planning pre-disaster prevention or mitigation
Morbidity	
Number of consultations/surviving population	– Estimation of the type and volume of medical relief and resources needed for immediate action – Evaluation and feedback regarding the relevance of relief given – Identification of remote population groups affected by the disaster – Gross assessment of health needs for further contingency planning
Time distribution of consultations	– Scheduling of medical relief – Identification of remote population groups affected by the disaster – Assessment of the profile of utilization of emergency and relief care by local populations
Distribution of types of complaint	– Identification of critical services to be maintained in emergencies
Incidence of communicable diseases	– Epidemiological assessment for establishing surveillance and control measures – Identification of disaster-related risks of communicable diseases for further contingency planning
Hospital bed occupancy and duration of stay in hospital	– Monitoring of health facilities and evaluation of the adequacy of care
Geographical origin of hospitalized patient	– Assessment of needs for relief supplies including field hospitals and location of extra facilities

evaluate the health needs of a disaster-stricken community. This requires the development of appropriate survey methods and unsophisticated and easily applied health indicators. A number of standard indicators have been proposed, whose relevance, reliability and sensitivity need further testing in actual disaster conditions (Lechat 1979) (Table 8.2). The development of such indicators is not easy and there is a great need for research in this new epidemiological field. The challenge is not unlike the one raised by the development of an appropriate information system for primary health care.

Full evaluation also requires well-trained personnel. The organization of standby epidemiological assessment teams is one area in which international co-operation, possibly set-up as TCDC (technical co-operation between developing countries) could yield immense benefits.

The constitution of health teams sent to disaster areas is very important. It should be firmly repeated that relief teams should be self-sufficient and never constitute an additional burden on the affected community. Highly specialized physicians are generally not appropriate; GPs, hygienists, sanitation experts, and epidemiologists are more useful. In many instances, nurses and sanitation experts will better meet the immediate needs than doctors.

Rehabilitation phase

The final phase in a disaster should lead to the restoration of pre-disaster conditions. Much could be said about the junction between short-term relief and rehabilitation. Suffice it to say that rehabilitation starts from the very first moment of a disaster. Too often, measures decided in a hurry tend to obstruct the re-establishment of normal conditions of life. Provision by foreign agencies of sophisticated medical care for a temporary period has negative effects. On the with rawal of such care the population is left with a new level of expectation which simply cannot be fulfilled.

It has been said that disasters can also have positive effects in the long run. They can be considered as an opportunity to get rid of obstacles to development and to develop new attitudes. This is perhaps an over-optimistic view. But there is no doubt that more research should be conducted on ways of integrating the short-term objectives of immediate relief with the long-term objectives of restoring or improving health in the affected populations.

Disease associated with natural disasters

There is considerable misunderstanding of the association of communicable diseases and natural disasters. The danger of decomposing human bodies has been grossly misrepresented as a source of epidemics. It should be stressed that unless a person has died from a communicable disease such as cholera or plague, a corpse presents no risk of spreading epidemics.

Contrary to common belief, *disasters are not necessarily followed by major epidemics* (Vijil 1973; Western 1975; De Ville De Goyet 1977; Zeballos 1981). Yet, mass immunization against typhoid fever is widely practised at the scene of disasters, although the usefulness of this practice has never been evaluated. The result is to divert useful and badly needed personnel from more important activities and to foster a sense of false security. In countries where cholera is prevalent, contrary to the general assumption that the disease will spread in the aftermath of such calamities like tidal waves, the immediate effect is for human excreta to be diluted in a larger area than the confined surroundings of the domestic compound. If cholera has been associated with disasters, it has been due to overcrowding and promiscuous defecation in refugee camps. A few outbreaks of leptospirosis have been reported following large floods (Simoes *et al.* 1969). Although stray dogs are reported to be numerous in earthquake-stricken areas, no case of rabies has ever been documented. Anthrax has been reported occasionally following handling or consumption of animal carcasses in disaster zones.

Disasters can, however, increase the transmission of communicable disease through three mechanisms: (i) overcrowding and poor sanitation in temporary resettlements; (ii) the disruption of routine control programmes; and (iii) the multiplication of breeding-places for vector-transmitted diseases (the severe malaria epidemics following hurricane Flora in Haiti in 1963 being a dramatic example – Mason and Cavalie 1965). Malnutrition, especially in camps for refugees and displaced persons, is widely recognized as an associated factor increasing susceptibility to and death from communicable diseases. Special attention must be given to measles among children whose natural resistance is impaired. The lack of basic sanitary facilities after a disaster leads to faecal contamination and outbreaks of diarrhoeic diseases, among which dysentery has been repeatedly reported. Hence the strict control of sanitation and rapid restoration of a safe water supply should be major priorities following disasters.

Control of communicable diseases following disasters should be based on *epidemiological surveillance*, which calls for the setting up of a system of early notification and prompt investigation of suspected cases (Romero *et al.* 1978). Such a surveillance system cannot be improvised. It requires facilities and manpower, such as appropriate channels of communication, access to public health laboratories, and personnel trained in epidemiology. It is of course impossible to assess the significance of any reported increase in the number of cases if no pre-disaster baselines are available on the incidence of diseases. It should, therefore be geared into an existing system of reporting for communicable diseases.

Public pressure for medical procedures in the aftermath of a disaster can be used to advantage in carrying out or launching routine immunization programmes for common diseases, such as diphtheria–pertussis–tetanus and poliomyelitis.

The consequences of the disruption of routine health services in disasters are often overlooked. It has been the experience of many medical teams that demands for current non-disaster-related ailments, such as ischaemic heart disease, obstetrics and renal failure, can often represent a significant part of the need even in the short-term after the disaster. In some countries, especially following earthquakes, mental health has constituted an important problem, requiring the inclusion of psychiatrists in relief teams.

Conclusions

The health management of disasters has thus definitely moved beyond rescue and short-term relief, to encompass the whole disaster process, from pre-disaster planning and preparedness to long-term rehabilitation. Natural disasters have major and dramatic consequences in the field of health, being major causes of deaths, casualties, and permanent disability, but they are far from being exclusively a health problem. The interaction between their various aspects, including the major health implications is extremely complex.

To be effective, the planning of health care in natural disasters must be closely associated with planning in other fields. There is still much to be done to ensure proper communication between health and other disciplines in order to achieve better disaster management.

MAN-MADE AND TECHNOLOGICAL DISASTERS

In man-made disasters, human action results in the disruption of living conditions with a considerable number of deaths and casualties. War and social disorders cause special problems which will be considered separately. They are distinguished from other man-made disasters in that damage is the intended goal of the action.

Although natural and man-made disasters raise many of the same problems, particularly regarding acute short-term assistance, they also have a number of distinctive characteristics. Man-made disasters are sometimes predictable and preventable. Industrial accidents or accidents in the transport of dangerous materials are examples. They may have specific, for instance toxic, effects. And they are eventually amenable to calculation of risks, which introduces psychological and political dimensions in what becomes almost a game context.

Man-made disasters can develop suddenly or slowly. They may have a technological or ecological origin. They may have effects over the short or the long term. Their diversity ranges from sudden technological catastrophes such as the crash of a wide-body jet plane (e.g. the crash at Ermenonville, France, in 1974 with 346 deaths) or the explosion in a chemical factory (Flixborough, UK, 1974) to the delayed effects of techno-logical failures (industrial effluents resulting in the passage of methyl-mercury through the food chain, Minamata, Japan, and the disposal of toxic wastes at Love Canal, Michigan) and slowly developing ecological catastrophes such as possible thawing of glaciers with deadly avalanches as a result of warming of the climate following the increase of carbon dioxide in the atmosphere.

In some instances, it is hard to make a sharp distinction between natural and man-made disasters. The collapse of a dam may result from an earthquake. Conversely, earthquakes may be triggered by large water reservoirs (e.g. at Lice, Turkey, 1975). Droughts causing starvation and death in hundreds of thousands of nomads are an extreme case of this inter-relationship. They are associated with population increase, overgrazing, lack of veterinary care, deforestation, and changes in social and political conditions.

The following are examples of well-publicized man-made disasters in the last 40 years:

1. The fire at Coconut Grove, in Boston in 1942, in which 450 died (about 1000 people crowded into a night club, a match thrown away on to a paper palm-tree, panic, and revolving door and other exits not visible in the smoke).

2. Vamont Dam, Italy in 1963 in which 1189 died (land-slide in the artificial reservoir above the dam causing a gigantic wave, overflooding of the dam, flashflood in the valley downstream).

3. Lima football match in 1964, with 300 deaths and 500 injured (panicking spectators crushed to death against the doors).

4. Aberfan landslide, Wales in 1966 with 145 deaths among them 116 schoolchildren (collapse of a slag heap, engulfing houses and a school).

5. São Paulo fire in 1974 with approximately 500 deaths (fire in a high-rise building with parking on the first six floors, non-fireproof material, television declaration that the fire could not be controlled provoking a massive convergence of cars in the adjacent street blocking arrival of fire brigades, insufficiency of fire-fighting equipment, panic).

Owing to the wide variety of potential disasters associated with human activities, it is very difficult to delineate the subject. In addition, the development of technologies whose consequences often cannot be foreseen opens the way for new types of disasters which still remain unidentified. Disaster prevention and mitigation are difficult precisely because the cataclysm cannot be described in advance.

Some examples of disasters which have been recognized after the event are outbreaks of insecticide poisoning, toxic accidents such as the dioxine release in the atmosphere at Seveso, Italy, effects of low-level radiation, or cigarette smoking. Other disasters could and will arise in the future

from present changes in ecology, new technologies, styles of life and occupations. Only an epidemiological approach will allow these insidious disasters to be recognized in time. For the moment, it is appropriate to omit them from this discus-sion, and to concentrate on events of sudden onset such as fires, dam collapses, mass-transport accidents, building collapse and the like, for emergency health measures. Management of this category of man-made disasters should concentrate on two types of measures: advance measures and mitigation.

Advance measures

When hazards are identified, appropriate advance measures might include: (i) appropriate engineering or other techno-logical measures (building techniques, dam design, contain-ment of toxic material, etc.); (ii) early warning if appropriate and (iii) protection against human errors.

Prevention

The implementation of preventive measures of a technical nature raises the crucial issue of risk assessment and subse-quent decision-making. Although this problem is not basically a health matter, several points should be clarified:

1. Zero risk does not exist. There is only calculated risk. The development of technology and indeed all human activi-ties, are inherently linked with risk. Life is dangerous. The pursuit of zero risk is a fallacy, particularly apparent in the dreams of some eco-activists. While buildings are not supposed to collapse for centuries or more, dams are built to undergo major accidents such as an overflow once a given number of years, for example 10 000 years. That means that among 100 dams one will possibly be overflooded in one hundred years.

2. Setting a level of risk implies measurements of the consequences occurring if and when the threshold is exceeded. These consequences may include a number of health effects such as deaths, casualties, diseases, handicaps, disruption of services, destruction of health facilities, together with other factors affecting industry, agriculture, loss of natural resources and the economy, or leading to social disruption, etc. This raises the problem of measuring health in economic terms, i.e. to calculate the financial value of life, death, and suffering. Health economists have faced this issue for a long time and it will be a long time before it is resolved. What is the economic value of a person? Is it different according to age, social status, educational background, or the type of job he or she is performing? It could even be argued that some individuals have a negative economic value, for example children in a country with an accelerating demography, the unemployed or the elderly.

Rather than measuring the economic value of life in absolute terms, it is probably more efficient, and less shocking for the medical profession, to study it in compara-tive terms. In the Netherlands, opposition to the construction of a chemical plant in the vicinity of a town has been success-fully countered by demonstrating that, with the safety measures which had been taken, the risk of death was equal that faced by the vast amount of the population protected by dams while living below sea-level.

3. Like the assessment of value, the appreciation of risk is subjective rather than an absolute judgement. This introduces the concept of acceptable risk. However, a new difficulty arises here, i.e. a risk acceptable to whom – the population exposed, the governments, the experts?

Acceptability to a population is an intriguing matter. Studies have shown that there is a great difference in acceptability between voluntary and involuntary risks. Individuals are quite ready to take risks as long as these are voluntarily taken: climbing mountains, smoking cigarettes, riding motorcycles. It has been estimated that a one per thousand risk of death in a year represents quite an acceptable risk for an individual when it is voluntarily taken. Risks imposed by the community are quite another matter. The figure which people are ready to accept is much lower (one per million per year). If the risk has something 'nuclear' involved (nuclear plants, etc.), the acceptable figure is as much as three orders of magnitude below (one in one billion chances of death per year).

The problem for governments is different since other factors have to be taken into account. These are of no or little interest to the individual and include matters such as industrial development, economics of the country, and defence.

4. Individuals at risk may differ from governments in the time scale within which they are prepared to contemplate risks.

5. A cost–benefit analysis of risks is further complicated by the fact that the advantages and disadvantages are often distributed unequally between population groups. Toxic wastes from expanding rich industrial areas of a country will be evacuated to poor rural undeveloped areas, if not to the countries of the Third World. The construction of a large dam will expose hundreds of thousands of people to risk of dam collapse (not to say displacement of villages, schistosomiasis, and social disruption) in order to provide electrical energy to industry employing thousands of workers hundreds of miles away.

6. There is considerable confusion in the public's mind between risk and detriment. While advanced technology is associated with a constant decrease in the probability of accident, the consequences of such an accident, should it occur, are increasing by orders of magnitude. When a small earth-dam collapses in a rural area it might affect only a dozen people. If the 209 m high Auburn Dam in California gives way, it will flood the city of Sacramento. (Put in another way, it is much safer to fly in a 'jumbo' jet than a small single-engined aircraft, but in the event of a crash, the number of victims is 100 times greater.) Risk-assessment and decision-making regarding acceptable risks must be placed within this context.

Early-warning

For a number of potentially disaster-generating man-made hazards, early warning systems can be designed. Examples are nuclear plants, natural gas refineries, and chemical industry plants. An alarm given in appropriate time can save a number of lives, either by limiting the process, or evacuating the population.

The problem here is when, to take action. The dilemma is quite similar to the one raised by the setting of criteria of disease in preventive medicine, that is whether to be specific or sensitive. It is complicated by the fact that measures are generally quite costly, for example, the evacuation of a population. It is also costly to stop an industrial process and to get it restarted (restarting in itself might present hazards). Setting too specific criteria which will decide that a disaster is imminent embraces the risk of giving the alarm too late. Sensitive criteria result in costly action and generate a loss of credibility. The multiplication of surveillance systems can also decrease the specificity of the system by increasing the risk of failure of redundant devices.

Protection against human failure

Finally, whatever the complexity, relevance, or appropriateness of prevention and prediction, all systems are open to human failure. Although it is perhaps premature to term it a disaster, an example is given by the PBB (poly-bromobiphenyl) poisoning of several millions of people in Michigan, where a fireproof ingredient was packed in wrongly coloured bags supposed to contain food additives for cattle. It is likely that despite the increasing complexity of monitoring and warning devices, the ever-present unplanned human factor will contribute to man-made disasters in the future.

Although they have no direct responsibility for prevention and early warning, the medical profession should be aware of the issues involved. They also have the responsibility to assess the effects of potential hazards on human health. Furthermore, identification of the hazards calls for the development of epidemiological surveillance systems of the population in relation to environmental factors.

Mitigation

Man-made disasters have up to now with a few notable exceptions been on a small scale. The casualties have usually numbered in the hundreds. They have been localized. Health facilities were not damaged and services around the affected area were fully operative.

There are four main ways in which medical efforts can be directed: (i) mobilization and deployment of rescue medical teams; (ii) preparedness of medical facilities (hospital planning); (iii) handling of the casualties; and (iv) identification of the dead.

Medical teams

There are differences of opinion regarding the contribution which can be made by rescue medical teams at the site of a disaster. When the number of casualties is relatively small and the victims can be easily moved and transported, the injured should be sent to hospital as rapidly as possible. In other circumstances, the number of casualties might be so high that it exceeds the capacity of one hospital. This is especially so when some casualties need to receive care (for burns for example) which is available only in specialized centres. In other disasters, such as railway catastrophes, the victims are trapped and need help on the spot.

The need to send a medical team to the site of a disaster should be decided on the basis of the first reports received, i.e. number of casualties, conditions of disaster, and presumed types of injuries. Mobile hospital-based medical teams for disasters have two duties: resuscitation, and when appropriate, surgery. After a disaster most of those who have not been hurt leave the scene as quickly as possible. On arrival, the medical team is faced only with those victims who have been trapped, seriously injured, or who are unconscious. The task of the resuscitation team will be to give first aid and to maintain vital functions while the victims are extricated. Resuscitation is the first priority. It aims to keep the victims alive until appropriate care can be given. Surgery on site is required only when the victims are inextricably trapped. Surgical teams should therefore be sent only as a back-up for the resuscitation teams. One of the major responsibilities of the team sent to the scene of a disaster is triage. This is the determination of priorities for treatment and the allocation of victims to those hospitals where adequate facilities are available.

Great attention must be given to the equipment of mobile medical rescue teams. Special clothing is essential, to offer protection to the members of the team as well as to help identify them in the *mêlée*. Equipment should include: (i) resuscitation equipment; (ii) transfusion sets; and (iii) oxygen apparatus. This equipment should be adequately packed, ready to use, and clearly labelled.

Detailed plans should have been laid down specifying the composition, equipment, and distribution of tasks for medical teams. They should be consulted and incorporated into the planning for disaster of every hospital. The deployment of rescue medical teams should be an integral part of disaster rescue planning in the community, and carried out in close co-operation with other interested services such as the fire department, police, and civil defence.

Hospital planning

Hospital disaster planning should be included in the general disaster planning of the community. Each hospital should know exactly what place it will be assigned in case of a massive emergency, since the role of different hospitals can vary according to their size, location, and type of available services. Disaster planning by hospitals is best carried out by a committee representing all concerned parties as well as representatives of the public authorities. The function of this committee (Savage 1979) should be:

1. Development of the hospital plan.
2. Co-ordination of the hospital disaster plan with community plans.
3. Development of departmental plans in support of the hospital disaster plan.
4. Assignment of duties.
5. Establishment of standard emergency care.
6. Conduct and supervision of training programmes.
7. Supervision of drills to test the hospital disaster plan.
8. Review and revision of the disaster plan at regular intervals.

A disaster manual must be prepared, spelling out the indivi-dual responsibilities of each member of the staff and definin the hospital's place in the total plan, in such a way that all th individuals not only know their duties but also have an unde standing of how the total plan is supposed to work. The task should be defined in different ways according to the type o personnel concerned. While individuals in key position should be given flexible instructions, allowing enough initia tive in their sphere of influence to adapt to unexpecte situations, other individuals should be given detailed instruc tion to avoid uncoordinated action. This is best achieved k using 'action cards' incorporating written informatio advice and orders for members of the hospital staff, a recommended by Savage (1979). These cards describe th essential responsibilities of members of the staff and can k easily related to the master plan. Precise instructions shoul be provided for alert mobilization and reporting of personne

Hospital admission procedures in case of emergency diffe from regular admissions. Special attention should be given t access to the emergency department, which should b prepared to receive a massive influx of casualties. Arrang ments should be made in advance for admitting mass casua ties by enlarging the emergency department and equipping for the rapid registration of victims. Hospitals should have special area where patients can wait before being directed t the various departments. Supervision of traffic outsid (ambulances) and within the hospital is of great importanc Provision should be made to handle a large convergence o people (relatives, press, and officials seeking news, bot personally or by telephone). In this respect, disaster exercise in hospitals are often unrealistic because they do not take in account this large flow of people.

Appropriate identification and recording of the victim throughout the hospital, including procedures and treatmen administered, is of the utmost importance.

It is generally necessary to make room for the victims b sending home those in-patients whose stay in hospital is no absolutely necessary. A list of such patients should be kept u to date and appropriate provision made to discharge them.

In order to implement the hospital plan, the comman structure should be clearly defined. Finally, it should b stressed that no plan can be expected to work in an actua disaster if it has not been strenuously tested in advance.

Handling of casualties

Handling of a large number of casualties in a minimum tim under adverse conditions and with scarce resources require the sorting of victims in such a way that the greatest help ca be given to the maximum number. This procedure, whic comes from military medicine, is called triage. In triage th highest priority is granted whenever some simple intensiv care may modify dramatically the immediate or long-ter prognosis. Moribund patients who require much attention fo a questionable benefit have the lowest priority. Triage is th only approach to provide a maximum of benefit to most o the injured in the aftermath of a disaster.

Casualties can be sorted into a number of categorie according to their chances of survival and expected effective ness of treatment to be applied. In military medicine, fou

iage categories are commonly used (Savage 1979). These
re:

nmediate treatment: casualties for whom the available
medical care can be expected to save life or function if performed as soon as possible.

Delayed treatment: casualties who, after emergency medical
care, incur little increased risk by limited delay in further
treatment.

Minimal treatment: casualties who do not require in-patient
treatment and can be discharged following first aid.

Expectant treatment: casualties so critically injured that only
complicated and prolonged treatment offers any hope for
improving life expectancy.

For the sake of simplicity, Spirgi (1979) distinguishes three
categories:

1. *Victims who require urgent hospital care.* They should
be prepared for evacuation by a skilled emergency resuscita-
ion team and evacuated as soon as possible. In the reception
area these patients are immediately reassessed so that those
equiring urgent operation are resuscitated (or resuscitation is
continued or intensified) and transferred to the operating area
as soon as possible. The classical injury belonging to this
category is the intracranial haemorrhage.

2. *Victims whose injuries are minor and do not require
urgent life-saving treatment.* These patients can either wait
for evacuation or make their own way to a clearing station or
to a hospital. Many of them can be treated on an out-patient
basis.

3. *Moribund patients who are beyond the scope of medical
care likely to be available in a disaster area.* It is useless to
evacuate and/or treat a victim with multiple and severe
injuries and in shock who could only be saved by the most
sophisticated intensive care when only simple facilities are
available. It is not rational to cope with these hopelessly
injured to the detriment of those in the first category who
could be saved. These patients must, however, be reviewed
every hour on the scene of disaster or after arrival in the
hospital since some injured whose condition seemed
desperate may, on a second assessment, be saved when
evacuated with the first category or, after second review in the
hospital, operated right away.

Triage is a most difficult task, which needs a combination
of authority, confidence, and considerable expertise. It
should always be carried out by the most experienced
clinicians available. The concept of triage is anathema to the
working ethics of most physicians, who will expend the
maximum of efforts in order to save the worst affected
patients. It is therefore important that triage be the responsibility of one or several persons respected by their colleagues.

In addition to triage, standard procedures should be
adopted. This is especially important in view of the fact that
patients are channelled through various services, from
outposts to hospital, and the multiplicity of medical personnel,
precludes to some extent individualized care. Continuity of
care under a changing team is possible only when procedures
are standardized.

Triage and standard procedures require appropriate

identification of the patient, including all relevant information. An essential principle of the management of casualties is
'tag first, then treat'.

Identification of the dead

Taking care of the dead is an essential part of disaster
management. A large number of dead can also impede the
efficiency of the rescue activities at the site of the disaster.
Care of the dead includes: (i) removal of the dead from the
disaster scene; (ii) reception in the mortuary; (iii) identification; (iv) autopsy when feasible; and (v) reception of bereaved
relatives. Identification requires great expertise and is best
performed by specialists. Visual identification may be
augmented or replaced by dental records, finger prints, and
skeletal X-rays.

Proper respect for the dead is of great importance. Every
effort should be made to provide appropriate burial ceremonies. This is particularly important in certain cultures
where the lack of adequate ceremonies can be strongly
resented by the relatives and considerably add to their grief.

NUCLEAR WAR

Medical care in war resembles that needed in disasters but the
scale is usually much larger. To cope with this huge load, the
victims have to be dealt with *en masse* not as individuals. In
the face of needs far exceeding resources, the aim is to save as
many lives as possible. Maximum efficiency in the mobilization of those resources which are available, and optimal
effectiveness in technical procedures is therefore essential.
The basic principles are: (i) assessment of needs; (ii) triage;
(iii) evacuation from disaster area to reference health facilities;
and (iv) appropriate emergency care.

Military medicine for conventional war has been extensively developed, and will not be reviewed here. Much less is
known about the immediate care which would be appropriate
after a thermonuclear attack. Since there is a risk that future
wars will be fought with nuclear weapons, medical care after
a thermonuclear attack on the civil population will be briefly
discussed in terms of the principles outlined above.

Assessment of medical care requirements after a nuclear attack

Estimates of the number of casualties, types of injuries, and
location of the victims will form the basis of any assessment
of medical care needs. The number and types of immediate or
short-term casualties resulting from a thermonuclear attack
depend upon a number of factors. These include the type of
weapon, explosive yield, altitude of the burst, number of
warheads, density and distribution of the population, nature
of the terrain, type of buildings, number and density of
ignition points, and meteorological conditions. Precise estimates cannot be made. All that can be said is that even after a
limited attack the number of victims will run into hundreds of
thousands or millions (Ervin *et al.* 1962; Lewis 1979). The
injuries will include the direct effects of the blast (mainly to
the lungs, thorax, and abdomen) and heat (burns), lacera-
tions of soft tissues and fractures (by collapse of building,

Table 8.3. *Predicted distribution of kinds of injuries in a nuclear war (Source: Geiger 1964)*

Single injuries 30–40%	Radiation injuries (including fall-out)	15–20%
	Burns	15–20%
	Mechanical injuries	up to 5%
Combined injuries 65–70%	Burn + wound + radiation injury	20%
	Burn + radiation injury	40%
	Mechanical injury + radiation injury	5%
	Mechanical injury + burn	5%

displacement of bodies, impact of flying objects), acute radiation sickness (from early radioactive fall-out), and psychological effects.

A large proportion of the victims will suffer from several types of injury. It has been estimated that more than half the victims will sustain combined injuries (Table 8.3). The proportion of survivors with combined injuries will not necessarily decrease with distance from the blast. Indeed, it may increase, since most of the people close to the hypocentre will be killed immediately. The chances of survival in victims with multiple types of injuries will be considerably decreased.

Not all the types of injury mentioned above will necessarily be observed. The relative ranges of lethal effects of the three energy forms released by a thermonuclear bomb, i.e. overpressure, thermal radiation, and ionizing radiation, depend on the energy yield (Fig. 8.3). For relatively small bombs of 1 kt, the range of radiation exceeds the range of the pressure blast and of the thermic wave. With increasing yield, blast, and particularly thermal effects, increase in comparison to radiation. As a result, with large bombs of 100 kt and over, the number of people suffering from initial nuclear radiation (neutrons and high-energy gamma-rays) will be comparatively small, because most of them will die from the mechanical or thermal effects. Similarly, the outbreak of fires (firestorms and conflagrations) will engulf most of the people who have survived the blast, resulting in a high incidence of burn injuries. Radiation sickness will depend mostly on the type of

weapon, altitude of the burst, and prevailing meteorological conditions, which determine the intensity, spread, and time distribution of early fall-out. Enhanced fall-out can also be engineered by selecting a suitable combination of weapon, meteorological conditions, and burst altitude.

Taking these limitations into account, the distribution of injuries will vary with the distance from the hypocentre. The concept of LD_{50} (median lethal dose) reflects the relation between distance and probability of death. It corresponds to the dose (be it radiation, overpressure, or heat) where the number of survivors equals the number of those killed. Another concept is the lethal area, which is defined as the circular area within which the number of survivors is equal to the number of people killed outside. For a one megaton bomb, the lethal area for the initial radiation will be 2.8 km. For a similar bomb, exploded at an altitude of 300 m, the lethal area for blast will be 5 km, and 11.5 km for severe third-degree burns. The areas of lethal damage due respectively to blast, heat, and radiation, with different explosive yield are given in Table 8.4.

Table 8.4. *Areas of lethal damage from various effects (in km².) (From Rotblatt 1981)*

Type of damage	Explosive yield				
	1 Kt	10 Kt	100 Kt	1 Mt	10 Mt
Blast	1.5	4.9	17.7	71	313
Heat	1.3	11.2	74.2	391	1583
Radiation	2.9	5.7	11.5	22	54

The probability of injuries from displacement of the human body against a hard surface following the blast has been calculated for a 100 kt bomb (Table 8.5). Buildings are much more sensitive to overpressure from the blast than human bodies. While human bodies can withstand pressure over 200 kPa (about 2 atm), it has been shown during the Nevada test that brick structures will cave in at much lower overpressures. It is estimated that 35 kPa is the relevant value for calculating the lethal effects of the blast wave. For a 1 m bomb, this pressure is reached at 5 km from ground zero. According to the types of dwelling, collapse of 50 per cent of the buildings will take place at respectively 3 km, 4 km, and 6 km for concrete skeleton structures, houses with concrete ceilings, and dwellings with wooden ceilings. This however is below the range of second degree burns (15 km). For a bomb with a yield under 20 kt, the range of effects to buildings will exceed the range of second-degree burns (Table 8.6).

The injuries caused by buildings collapsing, bodies being hurled against immobile surfaces, and flying debris, will be similar to those caused by earthquakes (fractures, crush syndrome, etc.). However, in Hiroshima and Nagasaki severe incapacitating fractures were uncommon because only those who could walk escaped the later fires.

Injuries from glass fragments will presumably occur at a larger distance. While 50 per cent of the concrete buildings are expected to collapse at a distance of 1.2 km for a 100 kt bomb, the probability of 50 per cent serious wounds by glass

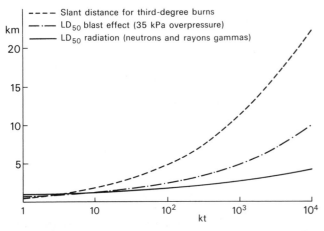

Fig. 8.3. Effects of thermonuclear bomb according to distance from burst at ground-zero and explosive yield. (From Rotblatt 1981.)

Table 8.5. *Injuries from displacement of the human body with impact on a hard surface (after 3 m of travel). (From US Department of the Army 1969)*

Type of injury	Peak over-pressure (atm)	Velocity (m/s)	Distance from ground-zero (km)		
			1 kt	10 kt	100kt
Mostly safe (whole body)	0.21–0.35	3.0	0.75	1.8	4.5
Skull fractures (threshold)	0.28–0.42	4.0	0.65	1.6	4.0
Fractures of the extremities	0.28–0.42	4.3	0.60	1.5	3.6
Skull fractures in 50 per cent	0.35–0.49	5.5	0.55	1.4	3.5
First fatalities	0.42–0.56	6.0	0.52	1.3	3.1
Skull fractures in 100 per cent	0.42–0.63	7.0	0.49	1.2	3.0
Lethality in 50 per cent	0.49–0.70	8.0	0.45	1.1	2.8
Lethality in 100 per cent	0.56–0.77	9.1	0.40	1.0	2.5

Table 8.6. *Maximum ranges (km from ground-zero) of immediate effects from atomic weapons of different yield (air burst). (From Buhl 1968)*

Yield	Range (km) at which 50% of houses are destroyed by blast			Range (km) at which 50% of windows and roofs damaged	Range (km) for thermal radiation burns, second degree	Range (km) for 2–3 Gy nuclear radiation
	Concrete skeleton structure	Dwellings with concrete ceilings	Dwellings with wooden ceilings			
1 kt	0.2	0.3	0.6	1.0	0.8	1.0
20 kt	0.6	1.0	1.5	3.0	3.0	1.5
100 kt	1.2	2.0	3.0	6.0	6.0	2.0
1 Mt	3.0	4.0	6.0	12.0	15.0	3.0
Pressure (atm)	1–1.5	0.5–1	0.3–0.5	0.1–0.2		

fragments has been put at 4 km, and the probability of 100 per cent serious wounds at 2.5 km (Messerschmidt 1979).

Since most of the people directly affected by the blast and/or thermal wave will be killed, ruptured eardrums, a minor effect, could possibly constitute a common complaint in the survivors at larger distances from ground zero.

The timing and intensity of early local fall-out will depend on the type of weapon used and the meteorological conditions (wind and rain). According to the distance, it will occur in a matter of hours after the explosion, the intensity decreasing with time. It may extend over thousands or tens of thousands of square kilometres. It will generally be distributed in an ellipsoidal shape, according to the direction and the velocity of the wind. Very little fall-out occurred in Hiroshima and Nagasaki (Committee 1979), but techniques of weapon assemblage and detonation are now available to minimize or maximize fall-out.

Gamma rays from fast-decaying radionuclides in the early fall-out will induce radiation sickness, whose symptoms may occur within minutes or days, according to the dose received. Since early fall-out will occur at large distances from the hypocentre, possibly at several hundreds of kilometres, it is likely to affect a very large number of people, at least in metropolitan and densely populated areas. The obvious symptoms of radiation sickness such as anorexia, nausea, vomiting, and in the more severe cases diarrhoea and other gastrointestinal disorders, will severely tax medical services. Psychological effects which may simulate the signs of radiation sickness, and panic, will increase the demand for care. Owing to the large awareness of the danger of radiation

in the population, this effect will by far exceed the limits of fall-out. Moreover, since the area of fall-out might be highly irregular due to the meteorological conditions, it will be difficult to delineate the area where people were actually exposed.

Organization of triage

Based on the experiences of Hiroshima and Nagasaki, and from the theoretical considerations developed above, it appears that the only prediction that can be made about the state of affairs which will face health personnel is that it will be utter chaos. No appropriate and efficient deployment of rescue teams or alert of hospitals can be planned. The optimal emergency location for first-aid stations cannot be identified beforehand. Casualties will have to be dealt with on a first-found first-served basis. Most of the victims will not come into contact with rescue teams. Self-help and mutual help immediately after injury will have to be given by the injured themselves or by unskilled survivors. Many people will be made permanently or temporarily blind by burning of the retina or from the lightflash of the fireball, especially if the explosion occurred at night, and this effect will extend far beyond the range of the blast and thermal waves. Many casualties will be left with no medical attention of any kind.

To have an effect on survival, triage must be as sensitive and specific as possible, aiming at minimizing the number of false-positive and false-negative decisions regarding chances of survival under medical treatment. For conventional war, rules of thumb have been developed to assess the chances of survival in association with treatment. From lack of experience, no such rules exist for nuclear war. On theoretical assumption, it appears that effective triage of nuclear casualties would meet a great deal of difficulties. The signs and symptoms of lesions resulting from the blast wave are unspecific. Shock is the most consistent sign in case of pulmonary and abdominal lesions, the two most common effects resulting from over-pressure. In the absence of appropriate diagnostic procedures, no assessment of the severity of lesions and judgment on the consequent potential efficacy of medical procedures on survival can generally be made.

Triage of burn victims is another matter. It also calls for much expertise. In optimal conditions cases with third-degree burns affecting less than 50 per cent of the whole body can be saved with appropriate care. Under the catastrophic conditions of a nuclear attack, it is estimated that the threshold for survival could be decreased to 20 per cent of the body surface, especially if there is additional stress in the form of combined injuries from blast and/or radiation.

Regarding indirect blast injuries, the major effects will be fractures, lesions to internal organs, soft-tissue wounds, and crushing.

Triage will be particularly important in the areas of fall-out. The following criteria for victims of fall-out have been proposed according to the accumulated doses received:

above 6 Gy: survival improbable;
between 2 and 6 Gy: survival possible;
below 2 Gy: survival probable.

These criteria are based on dosimetric parameters. They correlate with the expected development of radiation sickness. Above 20 Gy, victims develop a central nervous syndrome and death may occur within hours or a few days; between 6 and 20 Gy, a gastrointestinal syndrome leads to death after a matter of days or a few weeks. Between 2 and 6 Gy, in the absence of treatment, the haemopoietic syndrome is lethal after one month or more (Gerstner 1958; Schild 1967; Messerschmidt 1979). Having said this, only the identification of the haemopoietic syndrome (following exposure to 2–6 Gy)

has practical significance since it alone can be influenced by therapeutic measures.

Unfortunately, the prodromal signs of radiation sickness are remarkably similar irrespective of the dose received (Table 8.7). The overlap of response and the similarity of symptoms in people who have been lethally irradiated and those who have received smaller doses will create major difficulties in triage. People who have received high doses, over 20 Gy, in the initial moments of the fall-out, will be incapacitated in a matter of minutes. But, for people who have received lower doses, the diagnosis will be difficult. Anorexia, vomiting, and nausea are the most consistent signs (Table 8.8). The onset of these symptoms may give a guide to prognosis. Vomiting occurring sooner, being more pronounced, and accompanied by early diarrhoea and circulatory failure, may to some extent identify the individuals exposed to higher doses who have a poor prognosis. Nevertheless, although victims with the gastrointestinal syndrome will usually die in the first week, they will contribute to the immediate medical emergency problems.

The only way to make triage possible for victims of fall-out would be to have continuous dosimetric measures for everyone exposed, from the moment fall-out started. This would amount to equipping in advance every person in the population with an individual dosimeter. This clearly an unrealistic prospect. Thus, there are no early criteria to indicate whether or not the prodromal signs of radiation sickness announce the haemopoietic form with possibilities of survival. Continuous observation of the patients, supported by laboratory examinations (counts of platelets and lymphocytes) may help, but such procedures do not fall within the context of triage. No adequate laboratory facilities will be accessible, trained technicians will be scarce if available at all, and there will be no opportunity to follow-up survivors systematically for weeks.

The whole population exposed to fall-out should therefore be treated in the same way as potential survivors, except for those with clear early signs of massive contamination, presenting neurological symptoms. All others should be

Table 8.7. *Clinical and haematological symptoms after neutron-gamma whole-body irradiation and conclusions. (Source Messerschmidt 1979)*

Symptoms	Survival assured to probable (50–200 rad)	Survival possible to questionable (200–600 rad)	Survival improbable (more than 600 rad)
Initial symptoms	Vomiting and nausea absent or slight within 2–6 hours	In 70–100% severe vomiting within 1–2 hours, weakness	In 100% severe, retching vomiting within one hour, diarrhoea, severe exhaustion
Duration of initial symptoms	Absent or of short duration	12–24 hours	Up to two days
Early erythema	None	Slight reddening	Distinct reddening
Duration of latency period	More than three weeks	10–20 days	Up to one week
Lymphocytes	Slight to moderate decrease in 1–2 days to $1200/mm^3$	Moderate to large decrease within first day to $300–1200/mm^3$	Large decrease within hours down to $300/mm^3$
Granulocytes	Decrease to 40–50% of normal in 45 days	Initial granulocytosis, decrease in 7–20 days to about 20% of normal	Initial granulocytosis, decrease in 4–10 days, nadir 10% of normal
Platelets	Decrease to 50% of normal within 30 days	Decrease to 10–30% within 25 days	Decrease to almost 0% within 14 days
Reticulocytes	Unchanged	Slight decrease after several days	Definitive decrease after a few hours

Table 8.8. *Radiation doses (in Grays) which produce early radiation sickness symptoms. (Source: Rotblatt 1981)*

Affected symptom	Percentage of exposed population		
	10	50	90
Anorexia	0.4	1.0	2.4
Nausea	0.5	1.7	3.2
Vomiting	0.6	2.1	3.8
Diarrhoea	0.9	2.4	3.9

considered as potential survivors provided adequate treatment is administered. The large number of people exposed will raise horrifying problems.

No quick triage, compatible with timely care, therefore, can be envisaged after a nuclear attack (Sidel *et al.* 1962; Lechat 1981).

Evacuation

Owing to the chaotic situation resulting from a nuclear attack, no efficient 'treatment chain' can be organized for the referral of those casualties sorted for subsequent care. In potential fall-out areas, that is in a radius of hundreds of kilometres, people would try to run away, as soon as the explosion had occurred. Once the fall-out has started, crossing hot spots in contaminated areas may involve a substantial increase of radiation exposure, especially in the first few hours when the radionuclides of fall-out have not yet decayed to a substantial extent (Fig. 8.4).

Evacuation will be impeded by the convergence to hospitals of victims with slight or minor injuries (ruptured eardrums, contusions, burns to the skin from beta-rays, and psychological effects) or merely believing that they have been injured. These people will clamour for attention before the most

severe casualties arrive. This convergence will possibly be increased by epidemics of mimicked radiation sickness, such as psychogenic diarrhoea and vomiting in non-exposed people. Owing to the lack of specificity of prodromal symptoms in radiation sickness, it will be most difficult to distinguish between genuine and spurious reactions in the absence of physical measurements of the radiation actually received.

Second-level care

Treatment of nuclear casualties raise specific problems. Effective treatment will be hampered and delayed for lack of prior efficient triage. For direct blast injuries, with patients in shock, prolonged clinical, laboratory, and X-ray diagnostic procedures will be required.

To a large extent, indirect blast injuries are similar to common accident injuries, albeit on a massive scale. Shock treatment will be required for many victims, with infusion of large amounts of plasma and other replacement fluids, a time-consuming and personnel-intensive procedure.

Patients with burns have a chance of surviving only if the most elaborate care is provided. The treatment for burns requires: (i) maintenance of vital functions; (ii) control of shock; (iii) alleviation of pain; (iv) prevention of infection; and (v) specific wound treatment, for example skin grafts. Treatment of burns must be carried out under sterile conditions, which will be hard to maintain in the context of a nuclear attack.

Victims presumed to be suffering from radiation sickness will constitute the bulk of patients admitted to hospital. Owing to the clinical impossibility of conducting an efficient triage for radiation sickness in the aftermath of the attack, triage will have to be carried out again at the hospital level. This second-level triage will be rendered particularly difficult because hospital facilities will be clogged with people not suffering from fall-out exposure but presenting with similar psychogenic symptoms. There is no specific therapy for radiation sickness.

The stark conclusion is that treatment of nuclear casualties will stupendously overtax the available health services. Under normal conditions, facilities for treatment of radiation sickness and even for treatment of burns are quite limited in any country. The levy imposed on health facilities by a nuclear attack is therefore several orders of magnitude larger than the resources existing under normal conditions.

REFERENCES

Natural disasters

De Ville de Goyet, C., Del Cid, E., Romero, A. *et al.* (1976). Earthquake in Guatemala: epidemiologic evaluation of the relief effort. *Bull. Pan. Am. Health Organ.* **10**. 95.

De Ville de Goyet, C., Lechat, M. F., and Boucquey, C. (1977). Attitude face au risque d'épidémie lors de désastres soudains. *Rev. Epidemiol. Santé Publique* **25**, 185.

Glass, R. I., Craven, R. B., Bregman, D. J. *et al.* (1980). Injuries from the Wichita Falls tornado: implications for prevention. *Science* **207**, 734.

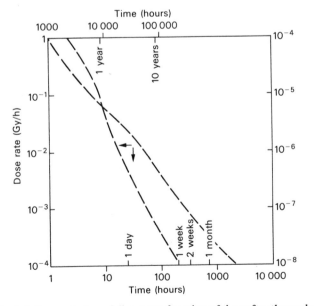

Fig. 8.4. Dose rate from fall-out as a function of time after the explosion. (From Rotblatt 1981).

Lechat, M. F. (1974). An epidemiologist's view of earthquakes. In *Engineering seismology and earthquake engineering* (ed. J. Solnes) p. 285. NATO advanced study institutes series, Series E: Applied Sciences (3).

Lechat, M. F. (1979). Disasters and public health. *Bull. WHO* **57**, 11.

Mason, J. and Cavalie, P. (1965). Malaria epidemic in Haiti following a hurricane. *Am. J. Trop. Med. Hygiene* **14**, 533.

Romero, A., Cobar, R., Western, K. A., and Mayorga Lopez, S. (1978). Some epidemiologic features of disasters in Guatemala. *Disasters* **2**, 39.

Simoes, J., Fraga de Azevedo, J., and Maria Palmeiro, J. (1969). Some aspects of the Weil's disease epidemiology based on a recent epidemic after a flood in Lisbon (1967). *An. Esc. Nac. Saude Publ. Med. Trop.* **3**, 19.

Sommer, A. and Mosley, W. H. (1972). East Bengal cyclone of November, 1970 – epidemiological approach to disaster assessment. *Lancet* **i**, 1029.

Vijil, C. (1973). The earthquake in Managua. *Lancet* **i**, 146.

Western, K. A. (1975). Epidemiology of communicable diseases in disaster situations. (Summary.) Proceedings of an International Colloquium Antwerp, 5–7 December.

Zaballos, J. L. (1981). *Desastres naturales sus efectos en la salud con enfasis en las enfermedades prevenibles.* Oficina de Preparativos para socorros de Emergencia OPS/OMS. (Unpublished.)

Manmade and technological disasters

Savage, P. E. A. (1979). *Disasters—hospital planning: a manual for doctors, nurses and administrators.* Pergamon Press, New York.

Spirgi, E. D. (1979). *Disaster management: comprehensive guidelines for disaster relief.* Hans Huber Verlag, Bern.

Nuclear war

Buhl, A. (1968). *Atomwaffen, Baden Honnef.* Osang-Verlag.

Committee for the Compilation of Materials on Damage caused by the Atomic Bombs in Hiroshima and Nagasaki (1979). *Hiroshima and Nagasaki: the physical, medical and social effects of the atomic bombings.* Iwanami Shoten, Tokyo.

Department of the Army (1969). *Nuclear handbook for medical service personnel.* Technical Manual, TM8-125. US Department of the Army, Washington, DC.

Ervin, R. F., Glazier, J. B., Aronow, S. *et al.* (1962). Human and ecologic effects in Massachusetts of an assumed thermonuclear attack in the United States. *N. Engl. J. Med.* **266**, 1127.

Geiger, K. (1964). *Grundlagen der Militärmedizin.* Deutscher Militär Verlag, Berlin.

Gerstner, H. B. (1958). Acute radiation syndrome in man. *US Armed Forces Med. J.* **9**, 313.

Lechat, M. F. (1981). Epidemiological approach to nuclear war. *Proc. Med. Assoc. Prev. War* **3**, 178.

Lewis, K. N. (1979). The prompt and delayed effects of nuclear war. *Scient. Am.* **241**, 27.

Messerschmidt, O. (1979). *Medical procedures in a nuclear disaster.* Karl Thiemig Verlag, Munchen.

Rotblatt, J. (1981). *Nuclear radiations in warfare.* Taylor and Francis, London.

Schild, T. E. (1967). *Nuclear explosion casualties.* Alimquist and Wiksell, Stockholm.

Sidel, V. W., Geiger, H. J., and Lown, B. (1962). The physician's role in the post-attack period. *N. Engl. J. Med.* **266**, 1137.

Determinants of health and disease

Disease control and health promotion

Governmental and legislative control of environmental hazards – the UK approach

Central Directorate on Environmental Pollution,
Department of the Environment

INTRODUCTION

In the UK, measures to protect or improve the environment in the interests of public health have been taken for many years. The Public Health Act of 1848, for instance, led to improvements in water and sewerage services, and the Alkali Act of 1863 was introduced to control the emission of noxious gases from alkali works. The present system of environmental control has developed gradually and pragmatically over the years as new environmental hazards have arisen or old ones have come into sharper focus and action has been taken to counter them.

Within the Government, the Secretary of State for the Environment has a general responsibility for environmental protection. He co-ordinates central government activity in this field, ensuring that control in one part of the environment is not exercised at the expense of another and that an overall view is taken of priorities.

Many of the overall statutory responsibilities for specific aspects of environmental protection also lie with the Environment Departments.* They are the Departments mainly concerned with air and freshwater pollution, noise (except for aircraft, traffic, and occupational noise); the disposal of solid, liquid, and radioactive wastes; and whatever may be washed ashore by the sea. The control of marine pollution by oil and chemicals, and pollution from civil aviation activities (including noise and emissions) lies with the Department of Transport, which is also responsible for control of vehicle emissions and traffic noise. The Agriculture Departments† have responsibility for controlling pollution caused by agriculture and for the safe use of agricultural pesticides; they also protect fisheries, both freshwater and marine, which involves control over dumping at sea and the oversight of marine pollution at large. The Health and Safety Commission (HSC) has certain responsibilities for pollution control as part of its general remit to secure health and safety in and around the work-place.

Central government prepares the statutory framework for environmental protection and issues advice to public pollution control authorities – usually by means of circulars but also through codes of practice. It can further influence events through the financial control which it exercises over such authorities. In certain circumstances (for example, in relation to particularly difficult industrial emissions to air, lead smelting, or the processing of radiochemicals), it controls industrial pollution directly through central inspectorates.

But for the most part, pollution control is delegated to a local level – principally to water authorities (river purification authorities in Scotland) and to local authorities. Within a local authority, the chief environmental health officer usually takes executive action, but the medical officer of environmental health provides medical advice and liaises with the local health authority as necessary.

Within industry, under Section 3 of the Health and Safety at Work etc. Act 1974, every employer has a duty to conduct his undertaking in such a way as to ensure, so far as is reasonably practicable, that his activities do not pose a risk to his employees or, through the contamination of the wider environment, to the general public. (Occupational hazards are not, however, covered in this chapter, which is more general in scope.)

OBJECTIVES AND PRINCIPLES

Public health in its widest sense is more than the absence of disease or infirmity – it incorporates all aspects of human welfare. The UK Government's environmental protection policy not only protects human health in a narrow sense but also seeks to safeguard plant and animal life and in general to maintain and, if possible, improve the quality of human life. But tackling potential hazards to human health is the cornerstone on which all else is built.

Some environmental hazards are natural – rivers flood, earthquakes take place, and the coastline erodes. Land-use planning policy in the UK takes account of the need to avoid

*Throughout this chapter the phrase 'Environment Departments' means the Department of the Environment, the Welsh Office, the Scottish Office, and the Department of the Environment, Northern Ireland.
†'Agriculture Departments' means the Ministry of Agriculture, Fisheries and Food, the Department of Agriculture and Fisheries for Scotland, and the Department of Agriculture, Northern Ireland. The phrases 'Environment Ministers' or 'Agriculture Ministers' have corresponding meanings.

the use of parts of the environment which are naturally hazardous; restrictions may be introduced or permission to develop refused altogether.

Environmental hazards which have been introduced by man can also be skirted round: land contaminated by a former use need not, for example, be re-used. But often the most economic solution is to tackle and resolve problems of environmental pollution* rather than to avoid them, for in many cases environmental pollution cannot safely be left alone. The remainder of this chapter concentrates on how environmental pollution is tackled in the UK, with particular reference to public health.

Environmental pollutants hit various kinds of 'targets' – people, animals, plants, or property – through the medium of water, air, land, or biological food chains. The impact of a particular pollutant or combination of pollutants on a particular target varies with the concentration and toxicity of the pollutant, the duration of exposure, and the susceptibility of the target. When seeking appropriate remedies or controls, other factors also have to be taken into account – the availability of substitutes for the polluting substances or processes, the public's perception of the risk entailed and the consequent political concern, and the costs involved in remedy or control. A careful balance has to be struck, based on a 'prudent public health' foundation.

This will lead to different controls in different circumstances. For example, radioactivity has well-documented effects on health and is subject to comprehensive statutory controls. The policy in the UK is to keep man-made radioactive discharges as low as is reasonably achievable and to no more than a fraction of the natural background level. At the other end of the spectrum, the noise made by street vendors advertising their wares is rarely dangerous and can be dealt with by a simple code of practice.

Besides 'ALARA' (as low as reasonably achievable), two other acronyms and the approaches which they denote are essential components of the UK system of pollution control:

BPM (best practicable means) – the application to a particular problem of the best practicable means of resolving or mitigating it. This was built into legislation and applied as early as 1874 to the control of emissions to the atmosphere from particularly troublesome industries. It enables account to be taken of, among other things, local conditions and circumstances, the current state of technical knowledge and the financial implications; and is particularly apt where the pollution medium is unbounded (like air) and the pollutants are serious but not especially dangerous.

'The EQO/EQS (environmental quality objectives/standards) approach' – which concerns the present or potential use of water, e.g. for drinking, for fisheries, or for recreation, and the quality of discharges permitted to sustain that use. Thus, depending on the EQO chosen, local environmental quality standards can be set and discharge consents carefully tailored

to meet those standards. This is generally achieved, in accordance with water pollution legislation, by attaching conditions to a consent governing the quality of effluent. This approach has been developed for fresh water since the 1920s and will gradually be applied to estuarial and other waters as legislative controls are extended under Part II of the Control of Pollution Act 1974.

The aim in the UK is to apply to each pollution problem the solution which seems most appropriate to it. This flexible approach contrasts with that traditionally adopted by most of the UK's partners in the European Community, who, perhaps as a consequence of their more codified legal systems, have tended to adopt fixed, national maximum emission standards. European Community directives lay down environmental standards in quantitative terms; but as a result of the UK consistently urging the case for an EQO approach, the main framework directive on dangerous substances in the aquatic environment provides for 'parallelism' (*either* uniform emission standards *or* an EQO approach). This has also been followed in an offspring directive on mercury. However, even with parallelism, the gradual adoption of Community directives means that standards are increasingly being prescribed rather than, as has historically been the case in the UK, being left to the discretion of pollution control authorities. In the course of time continental and UK views can be expected gradually to converge, leading to greater uniformity of approach by pollution control authorities in Britain (and, indeed, in the Community).

The UK approach is different in style from that in the US. In the UK there is close and informal co-operation between government, pollution control authorities, and industry – even though this may mean that progress is sometimes slow. In the US (see Chapter 10), relations are more formal: legally binding standards can only be set after statutory public hearings, and pollution limits for individual plants are set during formal negotiations between the US Government's Environmental Protection Agency (EPA) and the company concerned.

The UK plays a full part in international discussions leading to conventions and actions under the European Community, United Nations (UN), and other auspices – not least because of the growing importance of trans-frontier pollution questions. These include marine oil pollution, sea dumping, movement of wastes, 'acid rain' (the deposition in rainfall of sulphuric and nitric acids derived from the products of fossil fuel combustion, often at a considerable distance away), and the possibility of the increasing release of CO_2, leading to climatic change, and of chlorofluorocarbons, leading to depletion of the ozone layer.

Most of the UK's grosser air and water pollution problems have now been resolved. Measures to reduce further the risk of contamination of land and water from waste-disposal activities continue to be strengthened through tighter control and improved standards of operation. Increased emphasis is being placed on tackling past dereliction of land, particularly so as to regenerate healthy economic and social conditions in urban areas. But the emphasis is shifting from remedial measures to measures designed to anticipate and avoid

*Defined as 'the introduction by man into the environment of . . . [factors] . . . liable to cause hazards to human health, harm to ecological systems, damage to structures or amenity, or interference with legitimate uses of the environment' (Holdgate, M.W. (ed.) (1979). *A perspective of environmental pollution*. Cambridge University Press).

oblems; and most of the country's remaining environ-
ental problems will involve assessing the significance of
ng-term low-level exposure to substances which may or may
ot be toxic if experienced in small doses. The next section
escribes how one persistent environmental hazard – lead –
as been tackled so far; and also illustrates how the UK is
etting about preventing new chemicals and pesticides from
ecoming hazards.

CONTROL IN PRACTICE

Many pollutants reach their target through one or at most
wo environmental media, or sectors. This chapter describes
he UK system of general control in each of the sectors, air,
ater, and land, with a concluding section on noise. But a
umber of pollutants affect all the environmental sectors and
eed to be considered separately before being left to their own
evices (because they pose insufficient of a problem),
ontrolled through the setting of sectoral standards, or
anned altogether. The following paragraphs illustrate a
ross-sectoral approach by the UK, with reference to specific
xamples: lead (a typical heavy metal), new toxic chemicals,
esticides, and radioactivity.

Control of cross-sectoral pollutants

Lead

Lead is widely dispersed throughout the UK environment to
arying degrees and has long been known to be toxic at rela-
vely high levels of human exposure to it. The current WHO
evel of concern' (i.e. level at which positive action to reduce
uman exposure is recommended) is 40 μg of lead per 100 ml
f blood, but there is increasing, if inconclusive, evidence to
uggest that even below that level lead may impair normal
ctivity and in particular affect the development of children.
Research is continuing, both in the UK and elsewhere, in an
ttempt to clarify matters. Meanwhile, UK Government
olicy is to reduce exposure to lead from all sources,
ollowing the BPM (best practicable means) approach
escribed above, and concentrating on measures to protect
ritical groups (e.g. children) and to deal with known likely
hot spots' (e.g. down-wind of lead smelters).

For most people, food is the main pathway for lead,
ommonly accounting for 80–90 per cent of the human body-
urden. Most of the lead in food derives from other sources,
rimarily:

1. Plant intake from soil (where it occurs naturally and
has been added to by fall-out from centuries of coal-burning,
ometimes by contaminated sewage sludge deposited as fertil-
zer, and, in some places, from car exhausts).
2. Fall-out from air onto crops.
3. Absorption from plumbosolvent water flowing through
ead pipes and used for drinking or cooking.
4. From lead used to solder certain food cans, which dis-
olves into the food.

The maximum permissible amount of lead in food for sale
s laid down in national regulations which are enforced by
ocal authority trading standards officers in England and

Wales, by Consumer Protection Departments of regional
and islands councils in Scotland, and by environmental
health staffs of district councils in Northern Ireland.
Following a review by the Ministry of Agriculture, Fisheries
and Food's advisory Food Additives and Contaminants
Committee the general limit has been reduced to 1 mg/kg,
with higher specific limits for certain foods, particularly
shellfish and canned foods. The limit for foods specially
prepared for young children is now 0.2 mg/kg. Setting of
statutory maximum permitted concentrations compels
producers to aim for average levels below the nominal limits;
and, in effect, manufacturers use completely lead-free
packaging for babyfoods.

For most people, lead inhaled in air provides the balance of
the normal body-burden of lead. The UK has adopted a lead-
in-air quality standard (also proposed in a draft European
Community directive) of 2 μg/m^3 on an annual average for
places where people are continuously exposed to lead for long
periods.

Since 90 per cent of the lead in UK air comes from petrol,
reductions of airborne concentrations depend largely on
action on petrol-lead. Regulations made under the Control of
Pollution Act 1974, and enforced by trading standards
officers in England and Wales, Consumer Protection Departments of regional and islands councils in Scotland, and
environmental health staffs of district councils in Northern
Ireland, lay down the maximum permitted lead content of
petrol. This was set at 0.4 g/l from 1981 (as required by EC
Directive 78/611). The recently introduced Motor Fuel (Lead
Content of Petrol) Regulations 1981 require the lead content
to be further reduced to 0.15 g/l by the end of 1985.

Industrial sources can give rise to significant amounts of
lead in the air (and in dust: lead-workers risk taking leaded
dust into their homes). In relation to environmental pollution,
most lead-using works are controlled by district councils
using 'statutory nuisance' powers under the Public Health Act
1936 (there are equivalent powers in Scotland). A number of
works, however, have processes scheduled under the Alkali
etc. Works Regulations Act 1906 for control by the Industrial
Air Pollution Inspectorate (in Scotland HM Industrial Pollution Inspectorate). Exposure to lead at work is controlled by
HM Factory Inspectorate under the Health and Safety at
Work etc. Act 1974, using in particular the Control of Lead
at Work Regulations 1980 and related Approved Code of
Practice.

A number of consumer goods have their lead content
controlled by Regulations made under the Consumer Protection Act 1961 and enforced by trading standards officers in
England and Wales, Consumer Protection Departments of
regional and islands councils in Scotland, and environmental
health staffs of district councils in Northern Ireland. These
include cooking utensils and tableware, toys (lead in the dried
paint film must not exceed 2500 p.p.m.), pencils, etc. (soluble
lead must not exceed 250 p.p.m.), and cosmetics (where lead
is banned except lead acetate in hair darkening preparations).
There will soon be requirements under an EC Directive for
the distinctive labelling of paints containing more than 0.5 per
cent lead; meanwhile members of the Paintmakers Association have decided voluntarily to meet these requirements.

In some areas, particularly in Scotland, drinking water supplied to dwellings can dissolve considerable amounts of lead from plumbing. A survey in 1975–76 showed approximately 4 per cent of households in Great Britain (but 21 per cent in Scotland) with daytime water–lead concentrations above 100 $\mu g/l$ – the level set in a recent EC Directive. This standard is not specifically set out in UK legislation, but the water undertakings are working to achieve it wherever possible, through treatment of the water supply. Grants are available to help with the cost of bypassing or replacing lead plumbing between the water main and the drinking water tap, where water treatment cannot solve the problem.

New chemicals

Over 50 000 chemicals are manufactured and marketed worldwide. All but a few may find their way, eventually, to any or every sector of the environment. For many of them, very little is known about their behaviour in the environment and their effects. It would be difficult to examine retrospectively all existing chemicals. But under a European Community Directive of 18 September 1979 (for the Classification, Packaging and Labelling of Dangerous Substances), with certain exceptions, new chemicals must be tested before they are put on the market and information must be provided to national authorities concerning the likely effect on man and the environment. Testing includes both toxicological and ecotoxicological studies and, in the UK, the results must be reported to the Department of the Environment and the Health and Safety Executive, who act jointly as the competent authority. When the data have been assessed, summaries are to be sent to the European Commission for the information of other European Community states. The main objectives of the scheme are to assess the potential of a chemical to cause harm both to man and the environment and to alert industry and pollution control authorities to that potential at the earliest possible stage. The test guidelines used in this work have been developed and agreed under the auspices of the Organization for Economic Co-operation and Development (OECD) to ensure that data generated in one country are acceptable in others. The Control of Pollution Act 1974 contains fall-back provisions to prevent the use of unacceptable chemicals.

Pesticides

Control of pesticides in the UK is exercised principally through the Pesticides Safety Precautions Scheme, which was set up in 1957. This is a non-statutory scheme, formally agreed between Government and industry under which the Agriculture and Health Departments,* the Department of the Environment, and the Health and Safety Executive consider the safety of pesticides before they go into general use. It is supervised by the Advisory Committee on Pesticides, an independent body appointed by the Secretary of State for Education and Science.

The Pesticides Safety Precautions Scheme covers almost all

*The Department of Health and Social Security; the Welsh Office; the Scottish Office; and the Department of Health and Social Services, Northern Ireland.

pesticides, including those used in agriculture, forestry, horticulture, home gardening, in and around the home, and wood preservatives. The scheme determines the particular uses for which pesticides should be sold and lays down conditions of use. It also includes machinery to ensure that the use of any pesticide may be reviewed by the Advisory Committee in the event of any new scientific evidence coming to light about risks which could not have been envisaged when the pesticide was originally cleared. Pesticides used in other industrial or manufacturing processes (i.e. other than food storage, wood preservation, or public health) are gradually being brought into the scheme after consultation with interested parties. The Farm and Garden Chemical Act 1967 empowers the Agriculture Ministers jointly to make regulations governing the labelling of pesticides intended for sale for plant protection purposes in agriculture or garden. The Farm and Garden Chemicals Regulations 1971, require farm and garden pesticides to be labelled clearly and conspicuously with the names of any scheduled active ingredients which they contain. The small amounts of pesticides used in medical and veterinary products are subject to statutory control under the Medicines Act 1968.

The Health and Safety at Work etc. Act 1974 and related legislation, which makes provision for the health and safety of persons employed and others who may be affected by the work activity, apply in places where pesticides are manufactured, formulated, and used, including agriculture.

A European Community Directive on pesticide residues in fruit and vegetables has been adopted together with a directive harmonizing national provision in the member states on the classification, packaging, and labelling of dangerous pesticide preparations.

Radioactivity

Responsibility for protection against environmental hazards especially from civil radioactive waste lies with the Environment Ministers. An independent Radioactive Waste Management Advisory Committee (RWMAC) advises the Environment Ministers for that purpose. The Secretary of State for Defence has responsibility for wastes from defence installations. To ensure that man-made radioactive releases are kept as low as is reasonably achievable (on the ALARA principle, see above p. 136), before all but the smallest amounts of radioactive waste (which includes gaseous, liquid, and solid wastes), are discharged into the environment or disposed of, the formal authorization of the Environment Ministers is required under the Radioactive Substances Act 1960. In the case of the UK Atomic Energy Authority (AEA) establishments and licensed nuclear sites, this is issued by the Environment and Agriculture Ministers acting jointly. Furthermore, the holding of radioactive substances other than on sites in the latter category, is controlled by the Environment Ministers. The Secretaries of State for the Environment and Wales are assisted in administering the Radioactive Substances Act 1960 by the Radiochemical Inspectorate (RCI) which has inspection, enforcement, and advisory functions. The Industrial Air Pollution Inspectorate advises both the RCI and the operator directly on methods of reducing radioactive discharges to the atmosphere. Scotland and Northern Ireland have their own ollution Inspectorates with overall regulatory and advisory functions in this field. The Environment Ministers are responsible for ensuring that adequate research and development is carried out into methods of disposal of radioactive wastes.

The UK regulations controlling the transport of radioactive materials, including all types of radioactive waste, conform with the model regulations developed by the UN International Atomic Energy Agency (IAEA) and are administered by the Department of Transport. The UK operations to dispose of radioactive wastes at sea are subject to the Convention on the Prevention of Marine Pollution by Dumping of Waste and Other Matter 1972 (the 'London Convention'), and take place under a consultation and surveillance mechanism operated by the OECD. A licence is needed from the relevant Agriculture Minister under the Dumping at Sea Act 1974, in addition to the authorizations under the Radioactive Substances Act 1960. The IAEA has drawn up a specification of wastes unsuitable for sea disposal and has determined limits on the quantities of radioactive materials which may be disposed of at any one site and within any one ocean.

Responsibility for nuclear health and safety lies with the Health and Safety Commission (HSC) and it's Executive (HSE) who, for this purpose, report to the Secretary of State for Energy. The Nuclear Installations Inspectorate (NII), forms part of the HSE and is responsible for determining safety standards and for the licensing and inspection of nuclear installations apart from those operated by the AEA and the Ministry of Defence. The HSE's other Inspectorates are responsible for ensuring safety in the use of radioactive materials in workplaces other than licensed nuclear installations. A directive on basic safety standards for health protection against ionizing radiation has been adopted under Article 31 of the Euratom Treaty by the Council of the European Community, but has not yet been fully implemented by all member states.

Control of air pollutants

Certain processes that give rise to particularly noxious or offensive substances are regulated in England and Wales under the Alkali etc. Works Regulations Act 1906 and the Health and Safety at Work etc. Act 1974 by the Industrial Air Pollution Inspectorate (IAPI). In Scotland, similar functions are exercised through an agency agreement between the HSC and the Secretary of State for Scotland by HM Industrial Pollution Inspectorate (IPI) on behalf of the Health and Safety Commission. The Inspectorates ensure that works use the best practicable means (BPM: see above p. 136) for preventing the discharge of emissions and for rendering such emissions, where discharged, harmless and inoffensive. Emissions from other commercial and industrial processes and from domestic sources come under the control of local authorities (see below). The Department of Transport is responsible for legislation to control air pollution by motor vehicles and emissions from aircraft engines.

Local authorities use the Public Health and Clean Air Acts to control noxious or offensive emissions. They have a duty under the Public Health Act 1936 to inspect their district for nuisances and take action to require their abatement.

Nuisances include 'any dust or effluvia caused by any trade, business, manufacture or process and being prejudicial to the health of or a nuisance to the inhabitants of the district'. Similar provisions (under the Public Health (Scotland) Act 1897) apply to control of nuisance in Scotland. Certain trades, mainly concerned with the processing of animal residues, are expressly declared in the Public Health Acts to be 'offensive trades' and may be carried on only with the consent of the local authority. The Clean Air Acts 1956 and 1968 replaced and extended the provisions relating to smoke nuisance in the Public Health Acts.

Dark smoke from any trade or industrial premises or from the chimney of any building is in general prohibited, and new furnaces must as far as practicable be capable of smokeless operation. The height of the chimney serving a new furnace has to be approved by the local authority, and an approved grit and dust arrestment plant has to be installed. Regulations made in 1971 prescribe specific limits to the quantities of grit and dust which may be emitted from certain furnaces. Other furnaces must satisfy the requirements of the local authority. The Control of Pollution Act 1974 gives powers to local authorities to acquire information about emissions from industrial processes. In addition, this Act controls by regulations the sulphur content of oil fuels for furnaces or engines, and the lead content of petrol.

Where an area is specified in a smoke control order made under the Clean Air Acts 1956 and 1968, all smoke is generally forbidden within the area – whether from commercial or industrial premises or from homes. Householders who as a result of a smoke control order have to change their means of cooking or heating are eligible for grants from the local authority of at least 70 per cent of the cost of installing new appliances. Four-sevenths of the grant is refunded to the local authority by the Government.

Emissions from motor vehicles are controlled principally by the Motor Vehicles (Construction and Use) Regulations 1978 made under the Road Traffic Act 1972 [in Northern Ireland the Road Traffic (Northern Ireland) Order 1981]. These Regulations require motor vehicles to be so constructed that no avoidable smoke or visible vapour from them causes injury to other road users or damage to property. The Regulations also incorporate controls over the emission of carbon monoxide, unburnt hydrocarbons, and nitrogen oxides from petrol engines. These controls are being progressively amended to tighten the emission standards further. The Department of Transport tests heavy goods vehicles annually for emission of smoke and in addition carries out checks at the roadside and at operators' premises.

A European Community directive imposes an obligation on member states to ensure that specific levels of smoke and sulphur dioxide are not exceeded. The limits for these pollutants are based on evidence of health effects available from the WHO.

Control of water pollutants

Freshwater

Under the Water Act 1973, the Environment Ministers have a duty to promote a national policy for water and to secure:

1. Effective treatment and disposal of sewage and other effluents.

2. The restoration and maintenance of the wholesomeness of rivers.

3. The enhancement and preservation of amenity in connection with inland water.

Nine regional water authorities in England and the Welsh Water Authority are responsible for the management of all water services in England and Wales. In Scotland, water supply, sewerage, and sewage disposal are the responsibility of the local authorities. Prevention of water pollution is the function of the Scottish river purification authorities which were established under the 1973 Act. In Northern Ireland, water and sewerage services and prevention of water pollution are the responsibility of the Department of the Environment for Northern Ireland under the Water and Sewage Services (Northern Ireland) Order 1973 and the Water Act (Northern Ireland) 1972.

Under the Water Act 1973, statutory water undertakers are required to supply wholesome water. Local authorities are responsible for ascertaining that consumers in their area receive sufficient supplies of such water. They also have powers in relation to private supplies. Wholesomeness has been defined in part by reference to the WHO European Standards for Drinking Water 1970, and also to the more recent quality standards contained in the EC Directive on Quality of Water for Human Consumption 1980. The European Community has adopted a series of directives establishing appropriate quality objectives in relation to the intended use of water for bathing, for supporting freshwater fish and for supporting shellfish as well as for drinking purposes.

From a public health point of view, particular attention has been paid to: the nitrate and lead content of water at the tap; nitrate in water resources, particularly groundwater, coming from intensively cultivated agricultural land; and lead stemming from plumbosolvent water. But many water supplies also contain organic contaminants in very small amounts derived from industrial activities which, it is suspected, may have health implications if consumed over long periods. Little is known so far about this; but discharges can be controlled to limit the escape of organic substances to the aqueous environment. Comprehensive water treatment reduces organic matter in water supplies to very low levels, although chlorination of some of this organic matter produces trihalomethanes (such as chloroform) which have been alleged to carry a small health risk.

Modern methods of sewage treatment aim to convert raw sewage into an effluent which may safely be discharged to a watercourse. Sewage may contain industrial effluents (including farm wastes) as well as domestic sewage. Chemicals can enter the water system by run-off from some waste landfills and contaminated pasture, by leakages from storage tanks, and by accidents during the transport of hazardous chemicals. The Rivers (Prevention of Pollution) Acts 1951 and 1961 (and the Scottish equivalent), largely superseded by the Control of Pollution Act 1974, make it an offence to cause or knowingly permit poisonous, noxious, or polluting

matter to enter a stream and prohibits new or altered outlet for discharges of industrial (including farm) or sewa, effluents into streams and new discharges without the conse of the appropriate water authority (in Scotland, river puri cation authority). The 1951 Act originally applied only non-tidal waters, but the Clean Rivers (Estuaries and Tid Waters) Act 1960 also brought under control new or altere discharges to most estuaries; there was a similar extension controls in Scotland. Under Part I of the Control of Pollutic Act 1974, licensing controls for new landfills require pri consultation with the appropriate water authority to ensu proper water protection.

Part II of the Control of Pollution Act 1974 covers virtual all forms of water pollution and will strengthen existir legislation as it is progressively implemented. Broadly ensures that all discharges of trade or sewage effluent made t rivers, the sea, specified underground waters, or land a subject to the control of the water authorities (and corre ponding Scottish authorities). Moreover, regulations can b made to ensure that specified precautions are taken to prever polluting substances from reaching water.

Marine

Responsibility for controlling or dealing with aspects c marine pollution affecting the UK is divided between sever; Ministers. The Agriculture Ministers have a general respons bility for safeguarding fishing interests, with a specifi responsibility for controlling marine pollution by dumping a sea under the Dumping at Sea Act 1974. Part II of th Control of Pollution Act 1974 will extend water authorities powers of control over land-based discharges to all tidal estuarial, and coastal waters up to three miles from the coas (and beyond in the case of pipeline discharges). The Secretar of State for Transport is responsible for legislation governin, the control of oil and chemical pollution, primarily from ships and for remedial action at sea (the principal Act being th Prevention of Oil Pollution Act 1971). The Secretary of Stat for Energy is responsible for the control of off-shore oil an gas development operations, including the control o pollution from such operations under the Continental Shel Act 1964 and its associated regulations. And the Environmen Ministers have responsibilities in relation to oil and chemical on beaches. The Department of Transport Marine Pollutio Control Unit takes direct action when oil or chemicals at se; threaten serious coastal pollution; and local and port authori ties have a (non-statutory) responsibility for clearing anythin which comes ashore. In the case of an unknown or ar unidentified product, any authority concerned can contac the Chemical Emergencies Centre at the Atomic Energ Research Establishment, Harwell. Pollution of the sea i: covered by a number of International Conventions. The Oslc Convention controls dumping in the north-east Atlanti Ocean – which includes all the waters around the UK – while the Paris Convention relates to marine pollution from land based sources. Oil pollution of the sea has been the subject of several International Conventions of the UN Inter-Govern mental Maritime Consultative Organization (IMCO), of which the UK is a member.

Control of land pollutants

Land can be contaminated either accidentally or deliberately. The use of land for a particular purpose (for example as the site of a gas-works or lead smelter) can result in contamination as an incidental by-product. Careful consideration has to be given to the purpose for which such land is to be recommissioned, and appropriate measures taken to make it safe for that purpose. In the UK normal land use planning procedures apply (see above, p. 136) under the Town and Country Planning Act 1971 (and its Scottish and Northern Irish counterparts), conditions may be imposed before permission to re-develop is granted, including conditions which require remedial works on a particular site. Appropriate government departments are represented on an Interdepartmental Committee on the Redevelopment of Contaminated Land (CRCL). The Department of the Environment provides the secretariat for this committee and gives advice on the treatment of contaminated land.

'Deliberate contamination' – for example through controlled landfilling of waste – is, of course, intended to safeguard the environment as a whole; and the sites in question can be, and often are, subsequently used for another purpose. Controlled waste disposal can, indeed, be a means of restoration of sites like old mineral workings which have no other use. But environmental hazards can arise both during and after the depositing of wastes if this is not carefully planned and controlled. The strict site licensing provisions of the Control of Pollution Act 1974 are designed to prevent such problems.

In England collection of household and commercial waste the responsibility of the district authorities and the county authorities are responsible for waste disposal. The district councils in Wales and Northern Ireland, and the district councils and islands councils in Scotland are responsible both for the collection and disposal of such wastes. Industrial wastes are generally dealt with by the private sector. Farm wastes are mostly disposed of in accordance with good agricultural practices which the Agriculture Departments promote through their advisory services. Mining and quarrying wastes are controlled to a large extent by planning consent for exploitation.

Part I of the Control of Pollution Act 1974 deals with waste on land and provides the statutory framework for a systematic and co-ordinated approach to waste collection and disposal. Because of restraint on local authority expenditure the relevant provisions are being implemented progressively. The Act provides for a duty to be placed on waste disposal authorities to ensure that satisfactory arrangements are made for the disposal of wastes in their areas and to prepare waste disposal plans. Regulations made under Section 17 to provide for special controls from 'cradle to grave' for the more difficult or dangerous wastes came into operation in March 1981 in England, Scotland, and Wales; and in January 1982 in Northern Ireland. Provision is made for a register containing a record of the despatch, conveyance, and disposal of special waste by each of the parties handling it and for a permanent record to be kept of the location of deposits of special wastes. Under the same Act, however, local authorities are encouraged to reclaim and/or recycle waste as far as possible.

Four EC Directives dealing with land waste have been adopted. They are generally intended to protect human health and safeguard the environment by reducing pollution and to encourage recycling within the Community.

Control of noise levels

In England, the Secretaries of State for Transport and the Environment are responsible respectively for legislation concerned with traffic and vehicle noise (including that from civil aircraft), and neighbourhood noise (the Secretaries of State for Wales and Scotland are responsible for traffic and neighbourhood noise within Wales and Scotland), and are advised by two main research establishments: the Transport and Road Research Laboratory and the Building Research Establishment. The Secretary of State for Defence is responsible for controls on military aircraft. The Secretary of State for Employment is responsible for legislation on noise within work places.

Under Part III of the Control of Pollution Act 1974 local authorities have a general duty to control environmental noise and specific powers to require abatement of noise where this amounts to a statutory nuisance. In practice the majority of noise problems are dealt with informally. The Act also makes specific provisions for noise control on construction and demolition sites, and enables local authorities to establish noise abatement zones, within which it is an offence for registered noise levels from classified premises to be exceeded without permission.

The Motor Vehicles (Construction and Use) Regulations 1978 (as amended), made under the Road Traffic Act 1972, require vehicles to be fitted with efficient and well-maintained silencers, prohibit the causing of excessive noise by motor vehicles and trailers, and control the use of motor horns.

The Regulations place limits on the amount of noise which vehicles can make. The Noise Insulation Regulations 1975, made under the Land Compensation Act 1973 (in Scotland, the Noise Insulation (Scotland) Regulations 1975 and the Land Compensation (Scotland) Act 1973), give the power, and in certain circumstances impose a duty, to provide or pay grants for noise insulation in residential properties at the highway authority's expense where noise from new or altered roads exceed a specified level.

The Air Navigation (Noise Certification) Order 1979, made under the Civil Aviation Act 1949, details noise certification requirements for aircraft taking off and landing in the UK and is administered by the Civil Aviation Authority.

The Civil Aviation Act 1971 gives the Secretary of State for Transport power to designate airports and assume direct responsibility for the control of noise from aircraft taking off and landing at them. Heathrow, Gatwick, and Stansted are designated airports and noise abatement measures introduced include maximum day and night noise limits, minimum noise routes, restrictions on night movements, and grants towards the insulation of homes. Control of noise at non-designated airports lies with the owners or operators, who have introduced similar controls at the busier airports. Noise Insulation Grants have been provided at some airports run by the British Airports Authority and local authorities.

European Community Directives set noise level standards for motor vehicles and aircraft applicable to all Member States.

SUMMARY AND CONCLUSION

There is now a fairly comprehensive system of environmental hazard control in the UK, the framework of which has developed over a century and more in response to particular problems.

There is no uniform methodology, and the ALARA, BPM, and EQO/EQS approaches described earlier in this chapter have been variously applied to specific problems as has seemed most appropriate.

The determination of a particular environmental standard normally involves close consultation between Government (in one or more of its manifestations) and industry, which helps to ensure that adequate account is taken of economic factors.

Central government lays down the statutory framework for pollution control. But, in general, limits on emissions or discharges of pollutants are set and enforced at local level – principally by local authorities and regional water authorities, although some controls are exercised by national bodies such as the Industrial Air Pollution Inspectorate, or special agencies such as the Health and Safety Executive. The most recent legislation is the Control of Pollution Act 1974, which is being implemented progressively. The Act gives a wide range of new powers to local and water authorities affecting many aspects of pollution control, amending existing legislation where this has become outdated, and tackling problems for which comprehensive legislation had not previously existed.

There have been distinct improvements in the UK environment, especially in recent years and particularly in relation to air and water. The air is now some 60 per cent cleaner than it was 20 years ago, and hours of winter sunshine are the same in Central London and Manchester as in Kew Gardens. River quality has steadily improved and lengths of grossly polluted rivers have decreased by over 50 per cent. Water fit for drinking can be abstracted from more than 80 per cent of UK rivers, and fish have returned to the lower reaches of the River Thames.

The UK has participated over many years in attempts to promote environmental improvement on an international basis. It actively contributes to the work in this field of the EC, the OECD, the European Commission for Europe (ECE), and the International Civil Aviation Organization (ICAO), and to the collation of scientific data and recommendations on health limits which are made by bodies such as WHO and IAEA. This will continue, and UK standards can as a result be expected increasingly to reflect the recommendations of such bodies.

In general, the grosser problems of the past are now well under control in the UK, even if they have not yet been solved in their entirety. Attention is increasingly now being focused on environmental hazards whose effects are much le dramatic and less well understood. The most careful scienti and technical analysis will need to be coupled with the keen of economic assessment if resources are not to be wasted. F in this area, as in any other, over-reaction is to be avoided ju as much as under-reaction.

THE PRINCIPAL LEGISLATION CONCERNED

General

Public Health Acts 1936 and 1961
Town and Country Planning Act 1971; Town and Count Planning (Scotland) Act 1972; The Planning (Northe Ireland) Order 1972
Control of Pollution Act 1974
Dumping at Sea Act 1974
Health and Safety at Work etc. Act 1974

Heavy metals – lead

Public Health Acts (Northern Ireland) 1878 to 1967
Public Health (Scotland) Act 1897
Alkali etc. Works Regulations Act 1906
Consumer Protection Act 1961
Factory Act (Northern Ireland) 1965
Cooking Utensils (Safety) Regulations 1972
Water Act (Northern Ireland) 1972
Pencils and Graphic Instruments (Safety) Regulations 1974
Toys (Safety) Regulations 1974
Glazed Ceramic Ware (Safety) Regulations 1975
Vitreous Enamel Ware (Safety) Regulations 1976
Consumer Safety Act 1978
Cosmetic Products Regulations 1978
Health and Safety at Work (Northern Ireland) Order 1978
Materials and Articles in Contact with Food Regulations 197
Pollution Control and Local Government (Northern Irelanc Order 1978
Lead in Food Regulations 1979
Control of Lead at Work Regulations 1980 and Approve Code of Practice
Motor Fuel (Lead Content of Petrol) Regulations 1981

Pesticides

Protection of Animals Acts 1911–1927
Protection of Animals (Scotland) Act 1912
Pharmacy and Poisons Act 1933
Hydrogen Cyanide (Fumigation) Acts 1937 and 1974
Rivers (Prevention of Pollution) Acts 1951 and 1961
Protection of Birds Act 1954
Food and Drugs Act 1955 as amended
Food and Drugs (Scotland) Act 1956
Factories Act 1961
Animals (Cruel Poisons) Act 1962
Farm and Garden Chemicals Act 1967
Farm and Garden Chemicals Regulations 1971
Poisons Act 1972

r Navigation Order 1976 and Rules of the Air and Air
affic Controls Regulations 1976
ealth and Safety (Agriculture) (Poisonous Substances)
egulations 1975
ported Food Regulations 1978
edicines Act 1978
ildlife and Countryside Act 1981

adioactivity

adioactive Substances Acts 1948 and 1960
tomic Energy Authority Acts 1954 and 1971
uclear Installations (Licensing and Insurance) Act 1959
ctories Act 1961
uclear Installations Acts 1965 and 1969
nising Radiation Regulations 1968 and 1969
adiological Protection Act 1970

ir

ablic Health Acts (Northern Ireland) 1878 to 1967
lkali etc. Works Regulations Act 1906
ablic Health (Recurring Nuisances) Act 1969 and
ablic Health (Scotland) Act 1897
lean Air Acts 1956 and 1968
adioactive Substances Act 1960
oad Traffic Acts 1972 and 1974
ollution Control and Local Government (Northern Ireland)
rder 1978
ocal Government Planning and Land Act 1980
lean Air (Northern Ireland) Order 1981
oad Traffic (Northern Ireland) Order 1981

Vater

etroleum (Production) Act 1934
ublic Health (Drainage of Trade Premises) Act 1937
/ater Acts 1945 and 1948 and Water (Scotland) Act 1980
oast Protection Act 1949
almon and Fresh-water Fisheries (Protection) (Scotland)
ct 1951
ivers (Prevention of Pollution) Acts 1951 and 1961
ivers (Prevention of Pollution) (Scotland) Acts 1951 and 1965
lean Rivers (Estuaries and Tidal Waters) Act 1960
/ater Resources Act 1963
ontinental Shelf Act 1964
ea Fisheries Regulations Act 1966 (England and Wales only)
ewerage (Scotland) act 1968
Aerchant Shipping (Oil Pollution) Act 1971
Aineral Working (Off-shore Installations) Act 1971
revention of Oil Pollution Act 1971
Vater Act (Northern Ireland) 1972
ocal Government (Scotland) Act 1973
Vater Act 1973
Aerchant Shipping (Oil Pollution) Act 1974 (Part II)
etroleum and Submarine Pipelines Act 1975
almon and Fresh-water Fisheries Act 1975

Land

Public Health Acts (Northern Ireland) 1878 to 1967
Burgh Police (Scotland) Acts 1892–1903
Local Government (Development and Finance) (Scotland)
Act 1964
Water Act (Northern Ireland) 1972
Water Act 1973
Pollution Control and Local Government (Northern Ireland)
Order 1978

Noise

Civil Aviation Acts 1949, 1963, 1978, and 1980
Road Traffic Acts 1972 and 1974
Land Compensation Act 1973 (amended 1975)
Land Compensation (Scotland) Act 1973
Airports Authority (Consolidation) Act 1975
Motor Vehicles (Construction and Use) Regulations 1978
Pollution Control and Local Government (Northern Ireland)
Order 1978
Air Navigation (Noise Certification) Order 1979
Road Traffic (Northern Ireland) Order 1981

REFERENCES

General

Ministry of Housing and Local Government (1970). *Protection of the environment. The fight against pollution.* Cmnd 4373. HMSO, London.
Royal Commission on Environmental Pollution (1971). *First report.* Cmnd 4585. HMSO, London.
Royal Commission on Environmental Pollution (1972). *Second report: three issues in industrial pollution.* Cmnd 4894. HMSO, London.
Declaration of the Council of the European Communities on programme of action on the environment (1973). *Official Journal of the European Communities* 16 (C112).
Control of Pollution Act (1974). Chapter 40. HMSO, London.
Royal Commission on Environmental Pollution (1974). *Fourth report. Pollution control: progress and problems.* Cmnd 5780. HMSO, London.
Department of the Environment, Central Unit on Environmental Pollution (1974). *The monitoring of the environment in the United Kingdom.* (Pollution Paper No. 1.) HMSO, London.
Department of the Environment Central Unit on Environmental Pollution (1975). *Controlling pollution: a review of Government action related to recommendations by the Royal Commission on Environmental Pollution.* (Pollution Paper No. 4.) HMSO, London.
Department of the Environment (1977) *Environmental standards: a description of United Kingdom practice. A report of an interdepartmental working party.* (Pollution Paper No. 11.) HMSO, London.
The Council of the European Communities (1977). Resolution on the continuation of a European Community policy and action programme on the environment. *Official Journal of the European Communities* 20 (C139).
Commission of the European Communities (1979). *State of the environment. Second report.* CEC, Brussels.
Department of the Environment. Central Directorate on Environ-

mental Pollution (1979). *The United Kingdom environment 1979: progress of pollution control.* (Pollution Paper No. 16.) HMSO, London.

Organization for Economic Co-operation and Development (1979). *Organization for Economic Co-operation and development and the environment.* OECD, Paris.

Organization for Economic Co-operation and Development (1979). *The state of the environment in OECD Member Countries.* OECD, Paris.

Department of the Environment (1980). *Digest of environmental Pollution and Water Statistics* (No. 3). HMSO, London.

Organization for Economic Co-operation and Development (1980). *Environment policies for the 1980s.* OECD, Paris.

Department of the Environment (1982). *Digest of environmental pollution and water statistics* (No. 4). HMSO, London.

Lead and other heavy metals

Department of the Environment: Central Unit on Environmental Pollution (1974). *Lead in the environment and its significance to man. A report of an interdepartmental working party on heavy metals.* (Pollution Paper No. 2.) HMSO, London.

Department of the Environment: Central Unit on Environmental Pollution (1976). *Environmental mercury and man. A report of an interdepartmental working group on heavy metals.* (Pollution Paper No. 10.) HMSO, London.

Department of the Environment (1977). *Lead in drinking water. A survey in Great Britain 1975–76. A report of an interdepartmental working group.* (Pollution Paper No. 12.) HMSO, London.

Department of the Environment: Central Unit on Environmental Pollution (1978). *Lead Pollution in Birmingham. A report of the Joint Working Party on pollution around Gravelly Hill.* (Pollution Paper No. 14.) HMSO, London.

Department of the Environment: Central Directorate on Environmental Pollution (1980). *Cadmium in the environment and its significance to man. An interdepartmental report.* (Pollution Paper No. 17.) HMSO, London.

Department of Health and Social Security (1980). *Lead and Health, the report of a DHSS Working Party on Lead in the Environment.* HMSO, London.

Pesticides

Department of Education and Science: Advisory Committee on Pesticides and other Toxic Chemicals (1969). *Further review of certain persistent organochlorine pesticides used in Great Britain: report by the Advisory Committee.* HMSO, London.

Organization for Economic Co-operation and Development: Study Group on Unintended Occurrence of Pesticides (1971). *The problem of persistent chemicals: Implications of pesticides and other chemicals in the environment.* OECD, Paris.

Department of the Environment: Central Unit on Environmental Pollution (1974). *The non-agricultural uses of pesticides in Great Britain: a report.* (Pollution Paper No. 3.) HMSO, London.

Ministry of Agriculture, Fisheries and Food (1975). *Agricultural chemical approval scheme. Annual list of approved products and their uses for farmers and growers.* MAFF, London.

Royal Commission on Environmental Pollution (1979). *Seventh report: agriculture and pollution.* Cmnd 7644. HMSO, London.

Radioactivity

Ministry of Housing and Local Government (1959). *Control of radioactive wastes.* Cmnd. 884. HMSO, London.

Radioactivites Substances Act (1960). Chapter 34. HMSO, London.

Medical Research Council (1960). *The hazards to man of nucl[e] and allied radiations. Second report.* Cmnd 1225. HMS[O] London.

International Commission on Radiological Protection: Committ[ee] 4 on the Application of Recommendations: Task Group [on] Environmental Monitoring (1966). *Principles of environmen[tal] monitoring related to the handling of radioactive materials: [a] report adopted by the commission on 13 September 1965.* (ICR[P] Publication 7.) Pergamon Press, Paris.

Department of the Environment (1975). *Code of practice for t[he] carriage of radio-active materials by road.* HMSO, London.

Royal Commission on Environmental Pollution (1976). *Sixth repo[rt] Nuclear power and the environment.* Cmnd 6618. HMS[O] London.

Department of the Environment (1977). *Nuclear power and t[he] environment, the Government's response to the sixth report [of] the Royal Commission on Environmental Pollution.* Cmnd 682[?] HMSO, London.

International Commission on Radiological Protection (197[7]) *Recommendations of the International Commission on Radi[o]logical Protection. Annals of the ICRP; 1. No. 3.* (ICRP Pub[li]cation 26.) Pergamon Press, Paris.

National Radiological Protection Board (1977). *Recommendatio[ns] of the International Commission on Radiological Protecti[on] (1977). ICRP Publication 26: a summary.* National Radiologic[al] Protection Board NRPB-R63. HMSO, London.

Nuclear Energy Agency and Organization for Economic Co-operati[on] and Development (1977). *Objectives, concept and strategies f[or] the management of radioactive waste arising from nuclear pow[er] programmes. Report by a NEA Group of Experts.* NEA/OEC[D] Paris.

Department of the Environment (1978). *Annual Survey of radi[o]active discharges in Great Britain 1977.* DOE, London.

National Radiological Protection Board (1978). *Radiation exposu[re] of the UK population.* National Radiological Protection Boa[rd] Report NRPB R77. HMSO, London.

Department of the Environment (1979). *Annual survey of radi[o]active discharges in Great Britain 1978.* HMSO, London.

Department of the Environment (1979). *A review of Cmnd 88[4] 'The Control of Radioactive Waste'. A report by an Expe[rt] Group to the Radioactive Waste Management Committee.* DO[E] London.

Department of the Environment and Department of Transpo[rt] (1979). *Review of research on radioactive waste management an[d] radioactivity in the environment.* DOE/DTP Research Repo[rt] 32. HMSO, London.

International Commission on Radiological Protection (197[9]) *Radionuclide release in the environment: assessment of Do[se] Man. Annals of the ICRP Vol. 2, No. 2* (ICRP Publication 29[.]) Pergamon Press, Paris.

International Commission on Radiological Protection (1979). *Limi[ts] for intakes of dionuclides by workers. Annals of the ICRP Vol. [2] Nos. 3/4.* (ICRP Publication 30.) Pergamon Press, Paris.

Department of the Environment (1980). *Annual survey of radio[active] active discharges in Great Britain 1979.* DOE, London.

International Commission on Radiological Protection (1980). *Bio[logical] logical effects of inhaled radionuclides. Annals of the ICRP Vo[l.] 4, Nos. 1/2.* (ICRP Publication 31.) Pergamon Press, Paris.

Ministry of Agriculture, Fisheries and Food (1980). *Radioactivity i[n] surface and coastal waters of the British Isles 1978. Aquati[c] Environment Monitoring Report.* MAFF Directorate of Fisherie[s] Research, London.

National Radiological Protection Board (1980). *The application o[f] cost benefit analysis to the radiological protection of the public [–] a consultative document.* HMSO, London.

dioactive Waste Management Advisory Committee (1980). *First annual report.* HMSO, London.

dioactive Waste Management Advisory Committee (1981). *Second annual report.* HMSO, London.

partment of the Environment (1981). *Annual survey of radioactive discharges in Great Britain 1980.* DOE, London.

nistry of Housing and Local Government: Working Party on Grit and Dust Emissions (1969). *Report of the Working Party on Grit and Dust Emissions.* HMSO, London.

partment of the Environment (1971–75). *Annual reports on alkali etc. works nos 107–111. 1970–1974.* Presented by the Chief Inspectors. HMSO, London. (Issued jointly with the Scottish Development Department and the Welsh Office.)

arren Spring Laboratory (1972–76). *National survey on air pollution (1961–71).* HMSO, London.

  Vol. 1. General introduction; United Kingdom—a summary— East Region (exclusive London): Greater London Area (1972).
  Vol. 2. South-West Region; Wales Region; North-West Region (1973).
  Vol. 3. East Anglia; East Midlands and West Midlands (1973).
  Vol. 4. Yorkshire and Humberside Region; Northern Region (1976).
  Vol. 5. Scotland and Northern Ireland. Accuracy of Data, Index. (1976).

ean air Council (1973). *Information about industrial emissions to the atmosphere: report by a working party of the Council.* HMSO, London.

ntral Office of Information (1973). *Towards cleaner air: a review of Britain's achievements.* HMSO, London. (Prepared by the Central Office of Information for the Department of the Environment and the British Overseas Board.)

epartment of the Environment: Working Party on Grit and Dust Emissions (1974). *Report of the second Working Party.* HMSO, London.

epartment of the Environment (1974). *Clean air today.* HMSO, London.

epartment of the Environment: Working Party on the Suppression of Odours from Offensive and Selected Other Trades (1974 and 1975). *Odours: report Part 1. Assessment of the problem in Great Britain: Part 2. Best present practice in odour prevention and abatement.* Warren Spring Laboratory, Stevenage.

ealth and Safety Executive (1975). *Health and safety. Industrial air pollution 1975.* HMSO, London.

oyal Commission on Environmental Pollution (1976). *Fifth report. Air pollution control: an integrated approach.* Cmnd 6371. HMSO, London.

ealth and Safety Executive (1978). *Health and safety. Industrial air pollution 1976.* HMSO, London.

arren Spring Laboratory (1980). *Odour control—a concise guide.* Warren Spring Laboratory, Stevenage.

ealth and Safety Executive (1981). *Health and safety. Industrial air pollution 1979.* HMSO, London.

ealth and Safety Executive (1982). *Health and safety. Industrial air pollution 1980.* HMSO, London.

Water

Ministry of Housing and Local Government: Central Advisory Water Committee: Trade Effluents Sub-Committee (1960). *Final report.* HMSO, London.

Ministry of Housing and Local Government (1968). *Standards of effluents to rivers with particular reference to industrial effluents.* HMSO, London.

Ministry of Housing and Local Government: Working Party on Sewage Disposal (1970). *Taken for granted. Report of the Working Party on Sewage Disposal.* HMSO, London. (Joint publication with the Welsh Office.)

Department of the Environment, Central Advisory Water Committee (1971). *The future management of water in England and Wales.* HMSO, London.

Department of the Environment (1971–74). *Report of a River Pollution Survey of England and Wales.* HMSO, London.
  Vol. 1. Report (1971).
  Vol. 2. Discharges and forecasts of improvement (1972).
  Vol. 3. Discharges of sewage and industrial effluents to estuaries and coastal waters excluded from Volume 2 of the 1970 survey and a summary of all effluent recorded in the survey and to other coastal waters.

Water Pollution Research Laboratory (1971). *Annual report of the Water Pollution Research Laboratory Steering Committee with the report of the Director of Water Pollution Research 1970.* HMSO, London.

Water Pollution Research Laboratory (1971 and 1974). *Notes on water pollution 1971 (No. 52) and March 1974 (No. 64).* Water Pollution research Laboratory, Stevenage.

Department of the Environment (1972). *River pollution survey of England and Wales. Updated 1972. River quality.* HMSO, London. (Issued jointly with the Welsh Office.)

Royal Commission on Environmental Pollution (1972). *Third report: pollution in some British estuaries and coastal waters.* Cmnd 5054. HMSO, London.

Scottish Development Department (1972). *Towards cleaner water, rivers pollution survey of Scotland.* HMSO, Edinburgh.

Department of the Environment: Standing Technical Committee on Synthetic Detergents (1973). *14th Progress report.* HMSO, London.

Department of the Environment (1973). *Report of a survey of the discharges of foul sewage to the coastal waters of England and Wales.* HMSO, London. (Issued jointly with the Welsh Office.)

Department of the Environment (1973). *Background to water reorganisation in England and Wales.* HMSO, London.

Royal Commission on Environmental Pollution (1973). *Pollution in four industrial estuaries, studies in relation to changes in population and industrial development: four case studies undertaken for the Royal Commission on Environmental Pollution: by Elizabeth Porter.* HMSO, London.

Ministry of Agriculture, Fisheries and Foods (1973). *Farm waste disposal short-term leaflet No. 67.* MAFF, London.

Waste Research Centre (1974). *Annual report, nineteenth for the 15 months ended 31 March 1974.* Water Research Centre, Marlow, Bucks.

Department of the Environment (1975). *River pollution survey of England and Wales. Updated 1973. River quality and discharges of sewage and industrial effluents.* HMSO, London. (Issued jointly with the Welsh Office.)

Scottish Development Department (1976). *Towards cleaner water 1975. Report of a second rivers pollution survey of Scotland.* HMSO, Edinburgh.

Department of the Environment (1978). *River pollution survey of England and Wales. Updated 1975. River quality and discharges of sewage and industrial effluents.* HMSO, London. (Issued jointly with the Welsh Office.)

National Water Council (1981). *River quality: the 1980 survey and future outlook.* National Water Council, London.

Royal Commission on Environmental Pollution (1981). *Eighth report. Oil pollution of the sea.* Cmnd 8358. HMSO, London.

Land

Ministry of Housing and Local Government: Technical Committee on the Experimental Disposal of House Refuse in Wet and Dry Pits (1961). *Pollution of water by tipped refuse. HMSO, London.*

Ministry of Housing and Local Government: Working Party on Refuse Collection (1967). *Refuse storage and collection: Report of the Working Party on Refuse Collection.* HMSO, London.

Ministry of Housing and Local Government: Technical Committee on the Disposal of Solid Toxic Wastes (1970). *Report of the Technical Committee.* HMSO, London. (Issued jointly with the Scottish Development Department.)

Department of the Environment: Working Party on Refuse Disposal (1971). *Refuse Disposal: report of the Working Party.* HMSO, London.

Department of the Environment: Standing Committee Research into Refuse Collection (1973). *Storage and disposal. First report.* HMSO, London.

Department of the Environment: Working Group on the Disposal of Awkward Household wastes (1974). *Report.* HMSO, London.

Department of the Environment (1974). *War on waste. Policy for reclamation.* Cmnd 5727. HMSO, London. (Issued jointly with the Department of Industry. A Green Paper.)

Department of the Environment: Library (1975). *Occasional Paper No. 61. Waste management research.* Department of the Environment, London.

Department of the Environment (1976). *Waste Management Advisory Council, 1st report.* HMSO, London. (Issued jointly with the Department of Industry.)

Department of the Environment. Policy Review Committee (1978). *Co-operative programme of research on the behaviour of hazardous wastes in landfall sites.* HMSO, London.

Department of the Environment (1980). *Report of the Committee on Waste Paper Supply, PI.* Issued jointly with the Department of Industry, London.

Department of the Environment. *Waste Management Papers.* HMSO, London. (23 published to date, dealing with a wide range of topics, including reclamation, treatment and disposal of many wastes, preparation of plans and surveys, statistics and definitions of special wastes. Available from HMSO, London.)

Noise

Office of the Ministry for Science: Committee on the Problem of Noise (1963). *Final report.* Cmnd 2056. HMSO, London.

Noise Advisory Council (1971). *Aircraft noise: flight routeing near airports, report by a working group of the Council.* HMSO, London.

Noise Advisory Council (1971). *Neighbourhood noise: report by the working group on the Noise Abatement Act.* HMSO, London.

Office of Population Censuses and Surveys: Social Survey Division (1971). *Second survey of aircraft noise annoyance around London (Heathrow) Airport.* HMSO, London. (Prepared by MIL Research Ltd. for the Social Survey Division on behalf of the Department of Trade and Industry.)

Health and Safety Executive (1972). *Code of practice for reducing the exposure of employed persons to noise.* HMSO, London.

Noise Advisory Council (1972). *Aircraft noise: should the noise and number index be reported? Report by the Research Sub Committee of the Council.* HMSO, London.

Noise Advisory Council (1972). *Traffic noise, the vehicle regulations and their enforcement: report by a working group of the Council.* HMSO, London.

Department of the Environment (1973). *Structure and local plans*

—your opportunity. HMSO, London. (Prepared jointly with the Welsh Office and the Central Office of Information.)

Department of Trade and Industry (1973). *Action against aircraft noise: Progress report 1973.* Department of Trade and Industry, London. (Prepared jointly with the Central Office of Information.)

Department of the Environment (1974). *A guide to noise units (Prepared by the Noise Advisory Council.)* Department of the Environment, London.

Noise Advisory Council (1974). *Aircraft engine noise research report by the Research Sub-Committee at the Council.* HMSO, London.

Noise Advisory Council (1974). *Aircraft noise: review of aircraft departure routeing policy: report by a working group of the Council.* HMSO, London.

Noise Advisory Council (1974). *Noise in public places: report by a working group of the Council.* HMSO, London.

Noise Advisory Council (1974). *Noise in the next ten years: report by the Panel on Noise in the Seventies.* HMSO, London.

British Standards Institution (1975). *Code of practice for noise control on construction and demolition sites.* BSI. (Obtainable from: Newton House, 101 Pentonville Road, London N1 9ND.)

Department of the Environment (1975). *Calculation of road traffic noise.* HMSO, London. (Joint publication with the Welsh Office.)

Noise Advisory Council (1975). *Noise units: report by a Working Party for the Research Sub-Committee of the Council.* HMSO, London.

Noise Advisory Council (1976). *Bothered by noise? How the law can help you.* Noise Advisory Council, London.

Noise Advisory Council (1977). *Concorde noise levels: report by a working group of the Council.* HMSO, London.

Department of the Environment (1977). *Hearing hazards and recreation: prepared by the Noise Advisory Council.* Department of the Environment, London.

Department of the Environment (1977). *Land compensation—your rights explained. 2. Your home and nuisance from public development.* Department of the Environment, London. (Prepared jointly with the Welsh Office and the Central Office of Information.)

Department of the Environment (1977). *Land compensation—your rights explained 5. Insulation against traffic noise.* Department of the Environment, London. (Prepared jointly with the Welsh Office and the Central Office of Information.)

Noise Advisory Council (1977). *Helicopter noise in the London area. Report by a working group of the Council.* HMSO, London.

Noise Advisory Council (1978). *A Guide to Measurement and Prediction of the equivalent continuous sound level leq. Report by a working party for the Technical Sub-committee of the Council.* HMSO, London.

Noise Advisory Council (1978). *Noise implications of the transfer of freight from road to rail.* HMSO, London.

Department of Trade (1979). *Action against aircraft noise: progress report 1979.* Department of Trade, London.

Noise Advisory Council (1980). *The third London airport. Report by a working group of the Council.* HMSO, London.

Noise Advisory Council (1980). *Hovercraft noise. Report by a working group of the Council.* HMSO, London.

Noise Advisory Council (1981). *A study of government noise insulation policies. Report by a working group of the Council.* HMSO, London.

Noise Advisory Council. (in press). *The Darlington quiet town experiment. Report by a working group of the Council.* HMSO, London.

0 United States governmental control of environmental health hazards

J.Z. Bernstein and M. Freedman

INTRODUCTION

Until recently the history of public health has been punctuated by dramatic outbreaks of specific diseases that are caused by micro-organisms, such as typhoid and cholera. Many of these infectious diseases no longer pose serious threats to western society. Modern water filtration and disinfection systems have arrested the spread of water-borne diseases like cholera and diphtheria. Similarly, sanitation and modern medicine have drastically reduced the threat once posed by typhus, pneumonia, influenza, and tuberculosis.

As these hazards have diminished, however, a new and serious threat to the public health has arisen from toxic chemicals. Exposure to toxic chemicals has increased significantly since the Second World War, with the general growth of industry and the rapid growth of synthetic organic chemical production in particular. In 1941 the US produced less than one billion pounds of synthetic organic chemicals; nearly 40 years later, she produced 172 billion pounds of the top 50 organic chemicals alone (US Toxic Substances Strategy Committee 1980).

Toxic chemicals are linked to a variety of health problems, including chronic lung disease, heart disease, sterility, depression, birth defects, and kidney, liver, brain, nerve, and other damage. As Russell E. Train, a former Administrator of the US Environmental Protection Agency (EPA), stated:

Most Americans had no idea, until relatively recently, that they were living so dangerously. They had no idea that when they went to work in the morning, or when they ate their breakfast – that when they did the things they had to do to earn a living and keep themselves alive and well – that when they did things as ordinary, as innocent and as essential to life as eat, drink, breathe or touch, they would, in fact, be laying their lives on the line. They had no idea that, without their knowledge or consent, they were often engaging in a grim game of chemical roulette whose result they would not know until many years later (US Congress, Senate 1976)

The disease with the most publicized association with chemicals is cancer. The National Cancer Institute has estimated that 60–90 per cent of the cancers occurring in the US were caused by environmental factors (US Congress, Senate 1976), which many have argued would include toxic chemicals, as well as diet, cigarette smoking, and natural radiation

(Zener 1981). According to the National Cancer Institute the highest incidence of cancer generally occurs in industrial centres, where chemical concentrations are greatest. The National Institute of Occupational Safety and Health, the National Cancer Institute, and the National Institute of Environmental Health Sciences recently estimated that in the next few decades workplace exposures will account for 20 per cent or more of all cancers (US Toxic Substances Strategy Committee 1980).

The hazards associated with toxic chemicals that threaten modern industrial society differ in a number of respects from earlier public health problems caused by micro-organisms. This chapter will first discuss some of the identifying characteristics of these modern-day hazards, focusing on their industrial origin, the uncertainties associated with their assessment, and the potential geographical scope of their impact. It will then analyse the implications of these characteristics for the control of such hazards in terms of the participants in the regulatory and legislative process, the difficulties of arriving at and justifying regulatory decisions in this area, and the federal role in addressing such problems. Finally, the chapter reviews current legislative and regulatory controls in the US governing particular environmental hazards at the federal level.

THE CHARACTERISTICS OF MODERN ENVIRONMENTAL HEALTH HAZARDS

The industrial origin of such hazards

As suggested above, the current threat posed by toxic substances is rooted in modern industry. Unlike the micro-organisms that historically threatened the public health in developed countries, the sources of contemporary hazards provide social benefits as well. Synthetic organic chemicals, confined to a minor role before the Second World War, have been used to make many products considered beneficial and even essential to modern society, such as weed killers, furnishings, structural materials, and fabrics. Sales in the chemical industry exceed $100 billion a year and approximately 1000 new chemicals are expected to enter the marketplace each year (US Congress, Senate 1976).

Uncertainties associated with environmental health risks

Although the causal relationship between acute diseases, such as typhoid and cholera, and biological contaminants has been quite clear, the risks posed by chemical contaminants are far more difficult to assess. There are profound uncertainties in assessing whether a substance poses a risk and, in addition, the extent of that risk.

Several factors contribute to the difficulty of identifying risk. First is our ignorance concerning how harm occurs – the physiological mechanisms of action in response to environmental exposures. Such ignorance was a significant factor underlying the enactment, in 1958, of the Delaney or anti-cancer clause governing food additives in the Federal Food, Drug, and Cosmetic Act, 1938. This clause prohibits the marketing of any substance that causes cancer when ingested by animals, regardless of available human data related to the substance. The Delaney Clause reflects the assumption – not necessarily outdated – that scientific understanding of physiological mechanisms is not sufficient to distinguish animal from human carcinogens.

A second factor contributing to uncertainty is the long latency period between exposure and symptoms. For cancer this is usually measured in decades, while the mutagenic effect of a chemical may take several generations to appear. Thus, latency is usually sufficiently long that risk is borne unknowingly and is difficult to trace when injury eventually occurs.

Third, the fact that many environmental diseases have multiple causes also makes isolating or disentangling contributing factors more difficult. Thus, for example, an increase in diet-related cancers would not exclude the possibility that environmental contaminants significantly contribute to such cancers as well. As a result of all of these factors, epidemiological data do not easily permit linking of particular hazards with discrete substances.

Animal studies, which are relied on to a great extent for toxicological information, also cannot provide definitive evidence of risk. The predictive value of such studies would be seriously limited even if one could assume complete comparability between human and animal physiological mechanisms of action. This is because, among other reasons, test animals are maintained under ideal conditions and, unlike human beings, are not subjected to numerous pollutants, debilitating diseases, and stress. In addition, animal studies are able to reveal only those physical effects readily observable by pathologists, and those mental impairments that are revealed by physical effects.

The most serious obstacle to predicting health effects on human beings based on animal tests derives from the high costs of testing, which limit the numbers of animals or sample sizes that can be tested. Because carcinogens, for example, typically affect only a small percentage of an exposed population, unless the sample size is quite large, a carcinogen has a good chance of escaping detection altogether.

Ignorance about whether a risk exists also leads to ignorance of the extent of that risk. Animal studies may suggest the existence of a risk confronting human beings, but the size of the risk suggested by animal studies may differ from human risks over many orders of magnitude. For example, women are 100 times more sensitive to the drug thalidomide than rats and 700 times more sensitive th hamsters (Verrett and Carper 1975). Thus ignorance ab physiological response mechanisms, long latency perio multiple causation, sampling problems, and differen between human and animal susceptibility all contribute the toxicological uncertainties associated with chemical s stances.

The geographical scope of the potential harm

The risks accompanying toxic chemicals are potentially wide geographical scope. Where commercial products such pesticides are widely marketed, the risks posed to users others potentially benefited, such as consumers of food, a widespread as well. Also, some substances pose potentia catastrophically broad effects because of the indirect cons quences of ecological changes they set in motion. F example, scientific evidence indicates that the release chlorofluorocarbons from aerosol propellants into t atmosphere threatens the protective layer of stratosphe ozone surrounding the earth. This may increase UV radiati reaching the earth's surface, which in turn may result significantly higher rates of disfiguring and fatal skin canc (Environmental Law Institute 1982).

THE IMPLICATIONS FOR REGULATORY CONTROL

The characteristics of modern toxic substances outlined abo have a number of implications for their control. The include the presence of industrial participants in the regulato process and the forces they exert, various problems associat with selecting and justifying different kinds of regulato controls, and the federal role in controlling these substances.

As discussed below, federal control mechanisms in the L have been premised on the assumption that profit incentiv lead industry to engage in conduct that ignores importa social goals with respect to environmental quality, health ar safety and that state and local authorities cannot be relied to control that conduct because of competition among stat and regions for economic development, resource limitation and the existence of national markets. In almost all instance both Congress and the courts have developed national contr mechanisms and formal adversary procedures to govern reg latory decision making. This political solution, grounded congressional distrust of administrative power, facilitated tl participation of affected parties in the regulatory process.

Participation of industry in the regulatory process

Because no segment of society manufactured, supported, derived benefits from the typhus or cholera bacilli, both tl costs and benefits of preventing infectious disease were born by the same party, the general community. Thus historically public health regulation was governed largely by a share interest. This is not true of toxic chemical regulation wher costs and benefits accrue to different parties. Whereas th greater community experiences the hazards associated wit toxic chemicals (or the benefits of regulation), industry bear immediate regulatory burden. Without a shared community of interests, the regulatory process has become adversarial, with industry and other parties, such as local communities that would bear disproportionate costs of regulation through unemployment, espousing their own united interests. All vie to persuade the decision maker.

That the business community bears the immediate cost of regulation while not generally deriving regulatory benefits accounts in large part for the positions assumed by industry in the regulatory process. For example, industry generally advocates incorporating costs in calculating appropriate regulatory standards, rather than basing standards purely on health considerations. Thus, in the recent Clean Air Act debates, the business community advocated introducing cost-benefit analysis into the process of setting air quality standards, and has advocated greater consideration of cost in the technological standards applicable to new industrial sources of pollution in areas containing clean air.

The past few years also have brought a growing concern that the burdens of total compliance have adversely affected the ability of American industry to market new products or improve processes to produce at less cost. For these reasons, the Congress, and increasingly the agencies concerned, are attempting to develop flexible regulatory approaches without abandoning social goals.* This direction, however, is in its infancy and tensions over costs, benefits, and market innovation continue.

Developing rational policies based on estimates of the costs of control has also been inhibited by industry, which has tended to rely on generous estimates of regulatory costs or the social advantages derived from the unregulated product. Such estimates are frequently based on the apparent and immediate social advantages of the product, but may exaggerate the actual costs of regulation by measuring short rather than long-term benefits. Short-term benefits ignore the positive effects that control or regulation of a substance may have on promoting the availability of substitutes. For example, the rise in production costs caused by prohibition of a substance may stimulate research into new techniques of production, and encourage development of new and safer alternatives. In the long run, the costs associated with regulation of a substance are likely to be far less than those suggested by its immediate market impact.

The difficulties of selecting and justifying environmental health hazard regulations

As indicated above, both the benefits and risks of substances are far from straightforward and are clouded in uncertainty. The costs of regulation, however, frequently appear more easily measured: they may be presented as immediate, pecuniary, and apparent. The risks, on the other hand, may be remote in time, dispersed among the population, not necessarily directly evident to bearers, difficult to disentangle

from other forces, and difficult to quantify. Thus, while the costs of regulation often appear obvious and clear, the reduction in risks they purchase are far less visible. Unlike the dramatic reduction in infectious disease stemming from chlorination and filtration of public water systems, the public cannot point to what effects, if any, have occurred as a result of the discontinued manufacture of polychlorinated biphenyls, a dielectric and heat transfer fluid; Red dye #2, a colour additive used in food; or Tris, a chemical flame-retardant applied to children's pyjamas.

The difficulties of discerning the benefits of environmental regulations, even when the hazards are serious and irreversible, coupled with the apparent costs they entail make the regulatory agency particularly vulnerable to pressures from opposition. Moreover, the juxtaposition of immediate costs and remote and non-quantifiable benefits jeopardizes the credibility of the regulatory agency.

Even if reliable data on the relevant benefits and risks are available, selecting an appropriate standard is made more difficult by ignorance of the preferences of the public as to what risks are worth enduring in exchange for what benefits. The absence of a measure of the public's value system and the public's susceptibility to promotional distortions add to the vulnerability of regulatory agencies. The only available substitute for the preferences of the public is the leadership delegated by the electorate to the executive branch, which is charged through various mechanisms with establishing priorities and implementing political decisions.

Reliance on federal control of environmental health hazards

Much of the environmental health regulation in the US occurs at the federal rather than state or municipal level. There are various factors stemming from the effects of toxic chemicals that contribute to federal, rather than local, regulation.

Federal regulation is more appropriate where environmental health effects are widespread and not restricted to any locality. For example, as stated above, scientific evidence indicates that the release of chlorofluorocarbons from aerosol propellants into the atmosphere could result in increased skin cancer rates. This potential threat affects all human beings and is not restricted to any particular nation, and certainly not to any locality. Local control is therefore ineffective.

Also, because environmental health risks are frequently geographically widespread, whereas the costs of regulation are experienced locally in the form of reduced sales, employment, and tax revenues, the federal government is in many cases the appropriate control unit. It, rather than local or state government, is in the best position to balance the total costs and benefits of regulation for the general community. Even if health effects in the first instance are confined to the locality confronting the costs of regulation, the benefits of regulation none the less frequently extend beyond this locality. With a mobile population, those suffering from diseases with a long latency period are likely to face medical costs in jurisdictions other than the one which contained the health hazard.

Moreover, the concentration of costs in the local community together with the more widespread distribution of

*This has included, for example, the 'bubble' policy designed to limit overall plant air pollution emissions rather than individual stack emissions, thus granting plants the flexibility to select the most cost-effective emission reduction programme.

benefits encourages competition among localities in the national market to implement more permissive environmental controls. Thus, in the absence of federal regulation, reliance on state and local regulations may induce a level of regulation less rigorous than that which the community as a whole would favour.

In fact, the inadequate protection against toxic chemicals provided by many localities across the country has been responsible for the enactment of much national environmental health legislation imposing federal controls or standards. The Safe Drinking Water Act was enacted by Congress to authorize the federal government to set national standards for safe drinking water in part because evidence demonstrated that many local public water systems failed to meet existing guidelines for drinking water. The Comprehensive Environmental Response, Compensation and Liability Act, which authorizes federal authorities to respond to releases of hazardous wastes from inactive hazardous waste sites that endanger the public health, was explicitly enacted to compensate for inadequate state and local response to such threats. The legislative history of the Federal Water Pollution Control Act reflects a similar intent to establish federal minimum regulatory standards where historically local authorities had not.

FEDERAL LAWS REGULATING ENVIRONMENTAL HEALTH HAZARDS

The environmental health hazards posed by chemical substances are subject to regulation under a wide variety of federal laws in the US. In fact, Congress has enacted more than two dozen statutes regulating the various uses of chemicals that can threaten the public health, for example, exposure to air and water pollution, pesticides, food additives and contaminants, consumer products, work-place hazards, and hazardous wastes. These laws are administered primarily by several federal regulatory agencies, including the Environmental Protection Agency, the Food and Drug Administration, the Consumer Product Safety Commission, the Food Safety and Quality Service of the Department of Agriculture, the Occupational Safety and Health Administration, and the Department of Transportation. The predominant regulatory approach underlying federal legislation is reduced exposure to toxic substances, through such methods as required engineering controls, maximum allowable emissions, prohibitions on production or use, and requirements for safe disposal. A brief review follows of some of the primary and presently controlling legislation enacted to regulate environmental health exposure.

The Clean Air Act

The Clean Air Act Amendments of 1970 were explicitly enacted to extend protection of the public health. In its report on the amendments, the Senate Public Works Committee, which reported the legislation, stated:

The Committee's concern with direct adverse affects upon public health has increased since the publication of air quality documents

for five major pollutants . . . These documents indicate that the pollution problem is more severe, more pervasive, and growing a more rapid rate than was generally believed (US Congress, Sen: 1970).

The foundation for the regulatory programme of the Cle; Air Act is found in nationally uniform air quality standard known as National Ambient Air Quality Standards,* for tl control of major air pollutants. These standards establish prec: numerical levels of acceptable concentrations of pollutan To date, they have included carbon monoxide, hydrocarbor lead, nitrogen dioxide, ozone, total suspended particulate and sulphur dioxide.

Each state is required to develop a comprehensive Sta Implementation Plan (SIP) for attaining, maintaining, a enforcing these standards. This is a continuous process, tl SIP being changed each time a state seeks to alter the requir ments applicable to a particular industrial pollution sourc The Environmental Protection Agency (EPA), the respo sible federal agency, may substitute a federal plan for tl state's plan if that is deemed inadequate.

Particularly hazardous air pollutants are subject to mo stringent controls than other pollutants that are governe by ambient air quality standards. However, as of 1982, on four pollutants – asbestos, beryllium, mercury, and vin chloride – have been subject to such controls.

The Act also governs emissions from mobile sources suc as automobiles, buses, and trucks. It includes provisio: designed to reduce vehicle emissions, promote reduce automobile use, and encourage maintenance of vehicles ar their emission control equipment.

The Occupational Safety and Health Act

The Occupational Safety and Health Act enacted in 1970 w: the first comprehensive federal attempt 'to assure so far : possible every working man and woman in the Nation sa1 and healthful working conditions. . .'† Under the Act tl Secretary of Labor is authorized to set various kinds of safe1 and health standards, to inspect work-places, cite violation: and propose penalties and abatement periods.

The Act authorizes the Occupational Safety and Healt Administration (OSHA) to set permanent standards to regu late occupational health and safety hazards which 'mu: adequately assure, to the extent feasible, . . . that no employ will suffer material impairment of health or function: capacity . . .'; and short-term emergency standards when th Secretary determines that employees are exposed to grav danger and that such emergency standards are necessary t protect employees from such danger. To date, OSHA ha promulgated few permanent standards – for example, thos relating to asbestos, vinyl chloride, coke oven emissions, and group of 14 carcinogens – and has proposed standards for small number of other substances including arsenic, beryllium and trichloroethylene.

---

*Clean Air Act §108(a) (1), 42 USC §7408(a) (1) (1981 Suppl.).
†OSHA Act §2(b), 29 USC §USC §651(b) (1981 Suppl.).

The Federal Water Pollution Act

The Federal Water Pollution Control Amendments of 1972 were enacted to control all pollutant discharges into navigable waters of the US. The basic regulatory structure of the Act is designed to control 'point source' discharges through permits; provide federal assistance to localities for the construction of publicly owned treatment works or sewerage plants; and facilitate state and regional planning to control non-point source pollution discharges such as agricultural run-off.

Under the point source programme, EPA issues on an industry-by-industry basis numerical limits on effluent discharges. These are applied to individual industrial sources through permits under the federal permit system, called the National Pollutant Discharge Elimination System (NPDES). Every company discharging pollutants into surface waters must obtain an NPDES permit from the EPA or from the state that has been authorized to issue such permits by EPA. In a related programme the Act provides EPA with the authority to clean up hazardous waste spills into navigable waters and assess costs to those responsible. It may also require companies to adopt plans to prevent and control such spills.

The effluent limitations applicable to particularly toxic pollutants are potentially more rigorous. The 1977 Amendments to the Act required EPA to establish standards for 65 compounds characterized as toxic pollutants. Although the deadline for meeting these standards is July 1984, progress in setting them has been quite slow.

The Construction Grants Program, the second component of the Act, has provided over $30 billion to help finance the building of public sewage treatment plants. The EPA also finances state and local planning programmes which are intended to identify controls for non-point source pollution and to obtain and maintain water quality standards.

The Safe Drinking Water Act

The Safe Drinking Water Act, 1974, was enacted in response to reports of chemical contamination of drinking water in major cities. The legislation required the Administrator of EPA to prescribe national interim primary drinking water standards for contaminants that may adversely affect the public health. Such regulations were to be revised based on the study to be undertaken by the National Academy of Sciences to determine the maximum contaminant levels for drinking water that would be considered safe. Where it was not possible to specify contaminant levels, EPA was authorized to specify technology to control particular chemicals.

Because the National Academy of Sciences report failed to specify safe contaminant levels, EPA continued the interim regulations in force. Since 1977, EPA has established only one new primary standard, for trihalomethanes, which are carcinogenic substances formed by a reaction between chlorine and organic matter in water.

The law also required notices to consumers whenever violations of the regulatory scheme occur – when contaminant levels exceed permissible levels or mandatory monitoring is not carried out. This notice requirement was intended to make water problems more visible and thus protect consumers from health hazards, as well as build political support for safe drinking water.

The Toxic Substances Control Act

The Toxic Substances Control Act was enacted in 1976 to close a number of regulatory gaps in environmental health protection that remained despite enactment of various Acts including the Clean Air Act, the Federal Water Pollution Control Act, and the Occupational Safety and Health Act. None of these statutes had provided a mechanism for discovering or controlling the adverse effects of chemicals on health or the environment before manufacture.

Specifically, the Toxic Substances Control Act requires the manufacturers of new chemical substances to notify EPA of such substances in advance of manufacture and to provide test data, if required by EPA. Manufacturers of existing chemical substances for 'significant new uses' must also notify EPA with accompanying information. The Act also authorizes EPA to require companies to test any chemical substance they manufacture or process. Such information may then be used to decide on appropriate regulation of the substance.

The Act also requires manufacturers and processors to keep records and make various kinds of reports. Companies are obligated to report adverse information concerning the risks accompanying any chemicals they manufacture, process, or distribute. Finally, the Act authorizes EPA to regulate the manufacture, processing, distribution, labelling, commercial use, or disposal of any chemical that presents an unreasonable risk. To date, EPA has only imposed control provisions on a few chemicals under this Act, e.g. fully-halogenated chlorofluoroalkanes and polychlorinated biphenyls.

The Resource Conservation and Recovery Act

In 1976 Congress passed the Resource Conservation and Recovery Act (RCRA) to regulate waste, including hazardous waste. Passage of the law represented the first direct federal role in hazardous waste management.

Subtitle C of the Act, which concerns hazardous wastes, establishes a system for 'cradle to grave' management of hazardous wastes. The objective is to ensure that hazardous wastes are safely handled from original generation to ultimate disposal. Under the Act, the generator must determine which wastes are hazardous in accordance with EPA regulations, and ensure that such wastes are properly transported and arrive at permitted facilities for their disposal. It also establishes a permit system for treatment, storage, and disposal facilities. The issuance of permits turns on the facilities' ability to comply with performance criteria. In addition, the Act sets up a manifest requirement under which wastes must be labelled from original production to disposal. The statute also provides that administration of the hazardous waste programme may be undertaken by the states. As of mid-1982, the Agency was completing work on performance standards for land disposal facilities and would then be equipped to issue permits for these and all other treatment, storage, and disposal facilities.

This Act does not provide funds or mechanisms for the cleaning of abandoned disposal sites. This was the basis for enactment of the Comprehensive Environmental Response, Compensation and Liability Act of 1980, which is discussed below.

The Comprehensive Environmental Response, Compensation and Liability Act, 1980

This law, known popularly as Superfund, authorizes federal response to releases from inactive hazardous waste sites and more generally to environmental spills of hazardous substances. States are required to compile and up-date an inventory of inactive sites to be submitted to the Administrator of EPA. Then EPA must rank the sites requiring action based on relative danger. In addition, Superfund requires the person in charge of a facility to report any release of a hazardous substance to EPA.

Superfund authorizes the Administrator to relocate, contain, clean up, and take other remedial action in response to the release of a hazardous substance. Alternatively, when a release may pose an imminent and substantial danger, the Administrator may order a responsible private party to take such remedial action.

In addition, the Act establishes a hazardous substance response fund derived primarily from a tax on the petroleum and chemical industries, monies received under liability provisions, reimbursements, and penalties collected under the Act. Such monies may be used for emergency response, containment, clean-up, and other actions necessary to fulfill the goals of the Act.

Although hundreds of millions of dollars have already been collected in the fund, EPA has initiated such actions at a relatively small number of sites. Furthermore, EPA has been slow in promulgating regulations implementing the Act, most notably in publishing the National Contingency Plan which under the Act serves as the blueprint for government clean-up action.

CONCLUSIONS

We see, therefore, that an impressive statutory framework has been erected to provide protection from the effects of hazardous chemicals. But in regulatory effect, because of factors noted above – the disparity of interests involved, the timing and incidence of costs and benefits, general uncertainties about sources and natures of hazards and quantitative effects of programmes, the tentative groping for what costs are worth enduring for what benefits, and the general magnitude of the problem – the outcomes by 1982 were less comprehensive than envisioned in the enabling legislation. As suggested, the number of regulatory actions taken to reduce risks has been far less than intended or necessary.

PRINCIPAL UNITED STATES ENVIRONMENTAL REGULATORY STATUTES

Air

Clean Air Act, Pub. L. No. 86–206, 77 Stat. 392 (1963).

Clean Air Act Amendments of 1966, Pub. L. No. 89–675, Stat. 954 (1966).
Clean Air Act Amendments of 1970, Pub. L. No. 91–604, Stat. 1676 (1970).
Clean Air Act Amendments of 1977, Pub. L. No. 95–95, Stat. 685 (1977).

Water

Federal Water Pollution Control Act, ch. 927, 66 Stat. 7 (1952).
Federal Water Pollution Control Act Amendments of 196 Pub. L. No. 87–88, 75 Stat. 204 (1961).
Federal Water Pollution Control Act Amendments of 197 Pub. L. No. 92–500, 86 Stat. 816 (1972).
Clean Water Act of 1977, Pub. L. No. 95–217, 91 Stat. 15 (1977).
Safe Drinking Water Act, Pub. L. No. 93–523, 88 Stat. 16 (1974).
Safe Drinking Water Amendments of 1977, Pub. L. No. 9 190, 91 Stat. 1393 (1977).

Wastes and toxic substances

Federal Hazardous Substances Act, Pub. L. No. 86–613, Stat. 372 (1960).
Solid Waste Disposal Act, Pub. L. No. 89–272, Title II, Stat. 997 (1965).
Federal Environmental Pesticide Control Act of 1972, Pu L. No. 92–516, 86 Stat. 973 (1972).
Toxic Substances Control Act, Pub. L. No. 94–469, 90 Sta 2003 (1976).
Resource Conservation and Recovery Act of 1976, Pub. I No. 94–580, 90 Stat. 2795 (1976).
Federal Pesticide Act of 1978, Pub. L. No. 95–396, 92 Sta 819 (1978).
Used Oil Recycling Act of 1980, Pub. L. No. 96–463, Stat. 2055 (1980).
Comprehensive Environmental Response, Compensation an Liability Act of 1980, Pub. L. No. 96–510, 94 Stat. 27 (1980).

Miscellaneous

Federal Food, Drug, and Cosmetic Act, ch. 675, 52 Sta 1040 (1938).
Food Additives Amendment of 1958 (Delaney Clause), Pu L. No. 85–929, 72 Stat. 1784 (1958).
National Environmental Policy Act of 1969, Pub. L. Nc 91–190, 83 Stat. 852 (1970).
Environmental Quality Improvement Act of 1970, Pub. L No. 91–224, Title II, §§202–205, 84 Stat. 114 (1970).
Occupational Safety and Health Act of 1970, Pub. L. Nc 91–596, 84 Stat. 1590 (1970).
Noise Pollution and Abatement Act of 1970, Pub. L. Nc 91–604, §14, 84 Stat. 1709 (1970).
Noise Control Act of 1972, Pub. L. No. 92–574, 86 Stat. 123 (1972).

Quiet Communities Act of 1978, Pub. L. No. 95–609, 92 Stat. 3079 (1978).

REFERENCES

Environmental Law Institute (1982). *Air and water pollution control law: 1982.* Environmental Law Institute, Washington, DC.

US Congress, Senate. Committee on Commerce (1976). *Toxic Substances Control Act.* S. Rept. 698, 94th Cong., 2d Sess.

US Congress, Senate. Committee on Public Works (1970). *National Air Quality Standards Act of 1970.* S. Rept. 1196, 91st Cong., 2d Sess.

US Toxic Substances Strategy Committee (1980). *Report to the President. Toxic Chemicals and Public Protection.* US Government Printing Office, Washington, DC.

Verrett, J. and Carper, J. (1975). *Eating may be hazardous to your health.* Doubleday Anchor Press, New York.

Zener, R.V. (1981). *Guide to federal environmental law.* Practising Law Institute, New York.

11 Government and legislative control of environmental hazards – private sector

A. Stein

INTRODUCTION

The attitude of the private industrial sector toward environmental hazards has changed drastically over the past two decades. In the industrial boom which followed the Second World War few companies were aware of environmental risks associated with their activities and thus able to take steps even to inform their employees and customers of the potential health hazards. Since the early 1960s, however, private firms have come to be cognizant of and to recognize responsibility for environmental hazards associated with their activities.

Most large companies have employed professionals since the 1960s who are responsible for identifying potential environmental hazards related to the company's activities and for monitoring and abatement programmes to reduce them. These persons often participate in forming the policy and direction of the company with respect to these important matters.

Some contend that this change in direction has been caused by legislative and regulatory control of environmental hazards by governments. In part they are right, but these governmental actions have been far from efficient and effective in reducing environmental hazards. Unnecessarily stringent environmental regulations based on poor science, expensive unproven control technology, and unrealistic schedules for complying with environmental regulations have consumed a large amount of time and resources of the private sector. In many instances the legislation and regulations have even been regressive, prolonging the effort to reduce environmental hazards. Moreover, the evolutions in product liability laws and in occupational safety and health regulations have been separate and very substantive motivating forces in the private sector's efforts to reduce environmental hazards.

In the following section we describe the industrial situation in the private sector to which government regulation of environmental hazards applies. We then go on to consider private and non-environmental action to reduce health risks in the private sector, and the private sector response to government regulation of environmental hazards.

THE INDUSTRIAL SITUATION

An understanding of the response of private firms to governmental control of environmental hazards requires an appreciation of the industrial circumstances to which the controls apply. Ideally the government regulators should thoroughly investigate and consider the impact of the regulations in the private sector before the regulations are issued. Indeed, in the UK several years of industrial experience have been required as a qualification for employment as a government official in environmental permitting. However, in practice, and in other parts of the world and most notably in the US, environmental regulations appear to have been written with little or no consideration of their practical effect or effectiveness. In some circumstances, as with health-related national ambient air quality standards in the US, such considerations of economic and technological feasibility are even forbidden by law.

The plant

The modern industrial plant is analogous to a city in microcosm and similarly exists in myriad sizes and shapes. Raw materials flow in and products and waste flow out at several levels. No matter how tight the management structure and the level of care exercised, it is simply not possible to identify the constituents of all materials flowing in and out of the plant, or even the environmental implications of the known constituents.

Material potentially environmentally hazardous may reach the plant through purchased materials and process water, or may be generated in the plant by operating activities. In either event, the materials may leave the plant as products, as solid waste, or as discharges into the air or water. Analysing all of these on a continuous basis is simply not possible.

It is not even possible to monitor completely the materials purchased for the plant. There are always some materials that are not secured by the agent responsible generally for purchasing. Moreover, the purchasing agent has little control over the compositions of the materials that he or she purchases for the plant. Many are bought through commercial distributors who have little, if any, knowledge of the ingredients or associated health hazards. Even where the constituents are specified, the supplier may be unaware of impurities or variations in composition that may be crucial to control for environmental hazards.

The professionals that monitor private plants, attempt to determine the materials flowing in and the products and ste flowing out for environmental hazards, to the extent ssible. However, industrial activity is so extensive and mplex that the monitoring cannot be exhaustive. Even with entified materials, the environmental implications are not vays clearly known or understood.

terrelationship of controls

nother important consideration in assessing the impact of vernment regulations in controlling environmental hazards the modern plant is the interrelationship of such regulations th other government controls of environmental and non-vironmental hazards. In many respects, the problem can be ened to pressing on a balloon: when the balloon is pressed at e location it must bulge out at another. Similarly the control one environmental hazard may create a different and ssibly worse environmental, occupational, or consumer alth hazard.

Industrial activity necessarily generates wastes that must ter the environment in some form, either as an air or water scharge or as a waste product. Government controls rarely volve a value judgement as to which is least hazardous. ather, the government controls focus on reduction of one rticular air emission, waste discharge, or solid waste without nsideration of whether that may create an equal or worse vironmental hazard elsewhere. For example, the control of lphur dioxide emissions with scrubbers results in the rmation of a sulphate or sulphuric liquid or a solid sulphate dge that presents a waste disposal problem. There are any examples that could be given where the potential en-ronmental hazards are ignored at the expense of reducing e immediately identified environmental hazard.

Another aspect is the interrelationship of government ntrol of environmental hazards with government control of ccupational health hazards. It makes little sense to try to duce an environmental risk when the result is an equal or orse health hazard to employees in the work-place. An cample of this was the conflict in the US in the early 1970s etween two federal agencies, the Environmental Protection gency and the Occupational Safety and Health Adminis-ation, over whether enclosures ('sheds') should be retrofitted n existing by-product coke-oven batteries to capture fugitive missions from pushing operations. The Environmental rotection Agency insisted on sheds for compliance with air ollution regulations, while the Occupational Safety and Iealth Administration banned the use of sheds as creating an itolerable and unhealthy working environment.

Still another aspect of this interrelationship involves the se of large amounts of energy to eliminate environmental azards. Many of the abatement processes are energy intensive, or example, high-efficiency scrubbers. Frequently the large mount of energy required to reduce the environmental azard may involve creation of even greater emissions in enerating electricity and/or additional hazards in transporting lectricity, gas, or other energy supplies to a control site. This roblem is in addition to the increased economic burden and epletion of finite natural sources that occurs in use of the nergy, and the inevitable conflict with government energy onservation policies.

There is little evidence that government control of environmental hazards takes cognizance of these limitations and interrelationships; yet this is essential if the health and other environmental risks of today's society are to be intelligently managed. The day is past in most of the industrialized countries when the massive air and water pollution evident in the early part of this century (and in some countries into the 1960s and sometimes even into the 1970s) could be dealt with in individual abatement programmes. In short, control of environmental hazards can no longer be addressed with *ad hoc* programmes.

PRIVATE AND NON-ENVIRONMENTAL GOVERNMENT ACTION TO REDUCE HEALTH HAZARDS

In the last two decades, several developments have had an accumulatively greater effect in reducing environmental health hazards than direct government environmental regulation. Of particular impact have been the evolution of product liability laws in protecting the physical health of consumers and users, and the emergence of substantive government controls of occupational safety and health. In part because of these developments, the private sector has voluntarily taken steps to anticipate and avoid potential hazards. Also, to a considerable extent, the occupational safety and health controls incorporated earlier, and continuing, private efforts to develop and maintain good industrial health standards.

Product liability

Many governments have made the seller of products liable for physical harm to users and consumers. In the US, this has taken the form of court-made state law adopting (in some variant) Section 402A of the Restatement of the Law, second (Torts 2d) of the American Law Institute. That Section provides that 'one who sells any product in a defective condition unreasonably dangerous to the user or consumer or to his property is subject to liability for personal harm thereby caused to the ultimate user or consumer, or to his property . . .' (American Law Institute 1965).

By this rule of law, the seller is made strictly liable to the user and consumer even though he or she has exercised all possible care in the preparation and sale of the product. The justification for the rule is said to be that the seller, by marketing the product for use and consumption, has undertaken and assumed a special responsibility toward any member of the consuming public who may be injured by it; and that public policy demands that the burden of accidental injuries caused by products intended for use or consumption is placed upon those who market them and should be treated as a cost of production against which liability insurance can be obtained. Application of such laws to assertedly hazardous substances has led to the emergence of a new body of law that has come to be known as 'toxic torts'.

This application of product liability laws originated with asbestos. Ironically asbestos was once considered to be one of the safest and most useful of all substances, and, beginning in the early part of this century, came into wide use for its insulating and fire-repellant properties. Numerous lives were saved during the Second World War by the use of asbestos to reduce shipboard fires. By 1965, although the evidence was not firm, published articles had appeared suggesting asbestos was associated with the diseases of asbestosis, lung cancer, and mesothelioma in insulation workers (for example, Selikoff *et al.* 1965). This led in 1973 to the celebrated Borel court decision from the State of Texas that held an asbestos manufacturer strictly liable for failing to warn an insulation worker of the danger involved in handling asbestos (Federal Reporter, 2nd Series 1973). Since then there have been over 20 000 lawsuits filed by asbestos workers in the US seeking compensation for harm and sometimes death based on exposure to asbestos. It is estimated that total claims against asbestos companies in the US may reach $50 billion within 20 years.

From the asbestos litigation has come a multitude of health injury claims under the same product liability laws for asserted exposure to a host of substances: birth defects attributed to the mother's use of the generic drug diethylstilbestrol (DES); sterility and liver ailments in agricultural workers exposed to pesticides and herbicides; lead poisoning based on inhalation of fumes by workers in battery plants; leukaemia based on exposure to radiation leaks; and various ailments based on wartime exposure to Agent Orange (dioxin). And this is only the beginning: hundreds of chemicals have recently been identified as probable or suspected carcinogens.

These product-liability laws, which have their counterparts in most of the major industrialized nations of the western world, have had a salutary effect on the private sector in attempting to identify and avoid suspected health hazards. Indeed, under some laws, it is not even possible to defend on the basis that the hazard was unknown or could not have been known at the time the exposure occurred. It is deemed that the manufacturer should have had knowledge of the hazard through the application of developed human skill and foresight, and having that knowledge, should have provided an adequate warning of the harm the hazard could produce. As might be expected, these laws have been a substantial incentive for private firms to spend a great deal of time and energy in identifying and reducing possible health hazards involved in their products and operations.

Occupational safety and health

Industrialized countries throughout the world have adopted strong laws controlling health hazards in the workplace. These laws have mainly come into being since 1960. In the US, the most far-reaching law of this kind was the Occupational Safety and Health Act of 1970 (US Code, Title 29, §651 *et seq.*). The act which took effect in April 1971 covered approximately 55 million workers throughout the country, and now applies to every employer with one or more workers and whose business affects interstate commerce. Prior to this Act, the laws in the US regulating occupational safety and health were mainly ineffective and poorly enforced state laws, and federal laws that applied only to a limited number of employees and to particular industries.

The stated purpose of the Occupational Safety and Health Act is 'to insure so far as possible every working man and woman in the Nation safe and healthful working conditions

and to preserve our human resources' (United States Cod Title 29, §7656). The Act created the Occupational Safety an Health Administration (OSHA) under the US Department Labor to: (i) encourage employers and employees to redu hazards in the workplace and to implement new or impro existing safety and health programmes; (ii) establish 'separa but dependent responsibilities and rights' for employers an employees for the achievement of better safety and heal conditions; (iii) establish reporting and recordkeeping proc dures to monitor job related injuries and illnesses; (i develop mandatory safety and health standards and effe tively enforce them; and (v) encourage the states to assun the fullest responsibility for establishing and administeri their own occupational safety and health programmes, whic must be 'at least as effective as' the federal programmes. Tl Assistant Secretary of Labor in charge of OSHA was give broad powers under the Act to implement these objectives.

These laws have been applied to reduce levels of variou potentially hazardous substances in the work-place. Regul tions have been applied to substances such as asbestos, cottc dust, benzene, lead, vinyl chloride, acrylonitrile, 1, dibromo-3-chlorpropane, coke-oven emissions, ionizir radiation, and carcinogens. These regulations also require, i varying detail, that employers measure and maintain recor of employee exposure to such substances, and that medic examinations be provided to the employees.

These occupational safety and health regulations are n designed to produce a risk-free work-place. Unlike many the government controls of environmental hazards, th occupational safety and health laws have been interpreted t require achievable controls and not the elimination of a potential hazards even to healthy workers. Yet, these contro have had a direct impact in reducing exposure to healt hazards. Whether these controls have actually reduced illne and injury may be too early to fully assess, but the associate probabilities of health hazards have been substantially reduced

Private action

Aside from the substantial incentives described above, the has been in addition a continuing effort by the private secto to take steps voluntarily to reduce health hazards. Part of th is a sensitivity of professionals on the scene. Another part the broader recognition by private firms of their respons bility to anticipate and reduce potential health hazard associated with their activities (in part no doubt in sel interest).

In broad focus, it must be recognized that the evolution i both environmental and non-environmental governmer controls originated with private organizations. At least sinc the 1940s, the American Conference of Governmental an Industrial Hygienists (ACGIH) has issued guidelines o threshold limit values for hazardous substances and accept able work standards. These efforts, which have continued b the ACGIH, have been largely adopted by government inside and outside the US as controls for health hazards particularly in the workplace. The American National Stan dards Institute (Z-37 Committee) has also been active in thes efforts.

Similarly the American Society for Testing and Materials (ASTM) prepares standards for monitoring and analytical testing. These private standards have often been incorporated as the norm for monitoring and analytical procedures specified in government regulations of both environmental and non-environmental hazards.

Another private source of identification and control of environmental hazards has been labour unions. An example of this activity is the research into the health effects associated with hazardous substances supported by the US Rubber Workers.

In all, the private sector has participated a great deal in voluntarily identifying and reducing health hazards. This is obvious in countries like the UK where both environmental and non-environmental governmental controls are a direct product of co-operative efforts between government and industry. In the US, where the positions have been more formal and adversarial, government is still in the process of recognizing that greater progress can be made in reducing health hazards by co-operative efforts with responsible industrial representatives. In large measure this progress is necessarily based on recognition of the substantial contributions the private sector has made in reducing real health hazards.

PRIVATE RESPONSE TO GOVERNMENT ENVIRONMENTAL CONTROLS

The private sector involvement in government control of environmental hazards usually comes by participation during proposal or revision of regulations. Such participation may be formal or informal, oral or written, and typically involves presentation of scientific data and analyses indicating errors in the proposed regulations or in the basis for them. Opportunities are also available in regard to proposed legislation and enforcement proceedings, but these are much more restricted.

Certain fundamental issues recur in review of actual and proposed government control of environmental hazards, namely, the spectre of reducing to nil the risk of the environmental hazard, scientific accuracy and integrity in interpretation of data on which the control is based, and technological and economic feasibility of the control. These problems are discussed below. Also, as observed below, the prospects for legal and political action are limited.

The zero-risk syndrome

One of the greatest difficulties for the private sector is the prevailing belief of the governmental sector that actual and potential environmental hazards can be reduced to or near zero with scientific certainty. The private sector is put in the impossible position of firmly proving a negative, that is, that a substance is without effect at a given level. This is most clearly manifested by the implementation of legislation directing the setting of ambient and emission standards for air and discharge standards for water. As interpreted by the regulations, the standards are said to represent 'safe' levels below which there are no adverse effects on public health and welfare. The health-related national ambient air quality standards in the US even require that the standard levels incorporate an 'adequate margin of safety' to provide 'a reasonable degree of protection . . . against hazards which research has not yet identified' (US Code, Title 42, §7408; US Senate, 1970).

The data from which environmental controls are derived are not susceptible of indicating absolute, risk-free levels with regard to environmental hazards. 'Safe' levels and standards, which are for the most part health-related, are based on the interpretation of epidemiological studies and toxicological studies. There is no mechanism for inferring unequivocally from epidemiological studies on humans or toxicological tests on animals that a pollutant is or is not adverse to health. One can only compare response rates between subjects exposed to different levels of the pollutant, and infer from those observations whether the data support the hypothesis that the pollutant is adverse to health.

An illustration of the risk-free objective is the Delaney Amendment to the US Food, Drug and Cosmetic Act, which regulates environmental carcinogens present in food additives. The so-called 'Delaney Clause' states:

Provided, that no additive shall be deemed to be safe if it is found to induce cancer when ingested by man or animal, or if it is found, after tests which are appropriate for the evaluation of the safety of food additives, to induce cancer in man or animal . . . [US Code, Title 21, §348(b) (3) (A)]

The regulation of carcinogenic substances under the Delaney Clause seems simple and straightforward. A food additive either induces cancer or it does not. The dose level at which carcinogenic effects are observed is not at issue; the power of analysis at which effects occur is not at issue; and metabolic differences between the animal species tested and man are not at issue. Nor are the benefits of the use of the food additive in reducing health hazards weighed against the cancer risks at the levels of use. It also should be recognized that as analytical techniques have improved, the ability to find incredibly small amounts of suspected carcinogens has increased dramatically.

Aside from the Delaney-type legislation, the inferences for purposes of determining 'safe' levels are typically drawn by analysing data using statistical techniques. The null hypothesis assumes that the observed differences in responses between study groups is due entirely to chance. The probability that a difference resulting from chance is perceived as real is a type I error or false-positive. An acceptable type I error level is traditionally 1 or 5 per cent. The minimum response rate differential to reject the null hypothesis is then calculated. If the observed differential exceeds the minimum, the test is statistically significant at the specified error level and the health impact of the pollutant is considered real – within the specified percentage chance of error. Simply stated, the power of the analysis is its ability to differentiate between chance and real associations.

These analyses are also compounded by the need to take into account the presence of other potential causes of the observed response difference that may co-vary with the pollutant in the study. If these co-variables are not accounted for in the analysis, the association calculated between the health-response and the pollutant will reflect the combined impacts of all of the co-variables and in turn will present an inaccurate and misleading indication of the impact of the pollutant. In such an analysis there is a very substantial chance that the health response attributed to the pollutant is totally an aberration caused by the analysis, since the apparent response may have resulted entirely from sources other than the pollutant.

Another difficulty with these analyses is the failure to recognize limitations in the performance of the study. Epidemiological studies in particular are known for deficiencies in data gathering. These may involve simple omission in the study design such as failure to gather data on a co-variable, or a deviation of the data gathering from the study design. In either case, the performance of each study must be carefully scrutinized before the study is used for evaluation of health hazards to be sure that the perceived hazard is not an aberration resulting from the way in which the study was performed.

It is absolutely essential in evaluating environmental hazards, and notably levels for standards, that all of these aspects in the collection and analysis of the data be fully considered. Yet, to this point, it can be stated that in general governmental regulations have not made these evaluations as thoroughly as they should have.

Also, in making decisions on 'safe' levels for purposes of standards, and other environmental hazards, one must identify the population group to be protected. It makes no sense to control outdoor environmental hazards based on anticipated responses from those dependent upon controlled internal environments, such as occur in intensive care and other clinical units. Further, by reason of the nature of the data, such standards are not to be based on the sensitivity of single individuals. Also, what may be an environmental hazard to particular, especially sensitive groups may not be a hazard to the population in general. The focus in assessing environmental hazards, particularly for purposes of ambient standards, should involve identifiable subgroups of the general population that are apparently affected by exposure to the environmental hazard in question (for example, bronchitis patient to respiratory effects from high ambient levels of air pollution).

Further, rational consideration should be given to the type of health response that should be given cognizance in the setting of 'safe' levels for environmental hazards. Obviously, a prospect of death in the general population is of greater concern than the hastening of the death of persons already *in extremis*. Similarly, the prospect of widespread acute illness in the population is of far greater concern than an increased number of common colds among children or simple discomfort among chronic bronchitic and emphysema patients. Yet government control of environmental hazards to date have focused generally on 'safe' levels to protect the public health or welfare, with the indication that some scintilla of response is enough. This approach in the US has led to such esoteric discussions as whether a slight bronchial constriction in clinical studies of acute bronchial asthmatics, with no further manifestation of illness, is a sufficient response to take cognizance in setting 'safe' levels.

Use of these data in determining 'safe' levels by governments has generally resulted in standards and other controls that are unrealistically stringent. The levels are set at or near those that naturally occur and the regulator believes he or she cannot be faulted in minimizing the risk from the environmental hazard. But these 'safe' levels make little, if any, sense as achievable levels in an industrialized country. If 'safe' levels and standards are to be set, the focus must be a competent realistic appraisal of the nature and extent of the environmental hazard in the real world based on an objective accurate assessment of the demonstrable effects from the available scientific information.

Scientific accuracy and integrity

The nature of the analysis described above places a premium on the scientific competence and integrity of both the investigators who perform the studies and the regulators who evaluate and interpret them in formulating regulations for the control of environmental hazards. This has been the source of extreme consternation to the private sector in the US and Europe in responding to government regulation of environmental hazards.

Investigators have in the past been under various pressures to find positive results. In the reports of any number of studies limitations in the performance of the study have been downplayed or ignored, or the analysis has been skewed, in an effort to show positive results. In other studies, conclusions reporting positive results in glowing terms simply are not supported by the data and the analysis. Also, there are studies where the data have been found to be 'doctored' to support given results.

Then, there are the regulators who view their task of setting governmental controls for environmental hazards with a certain fervour. They may be less than scientifically objective in their scrutiny and appraisal of a study reporting positive associations of adverse effects with a pollutant under consideration – particularly at low levels. The regulator may also overinterpret the findings from good studies stretching the data far beyond permissible bounds, and often even over the strong objection of the researchers who performed the studies.

All of this has combined to produce enormous controversy in the placing of governmental controls on environmental hazards. Safeguards have been introduced in an effort to try to reduce the problems. The legislation in the US has provided for scientific advisory committees to oversee these activities in an effort to provide a more objective scientific appraisal (US Code, Title 42, §7409(d)), but even this has been politicized. The members of these advisory panels are often selected by the regulators whose work they are reviewing – regulators who are also allocating research monies to outside scientists. This is not to say that these advisory committees do not have a salutary effect on the process, but it must be recognized at the same time that the impact is only as good as the competence of the scientists and the degree to which they are permitted and are motivated to be involved in the process.

The extent to which these matters have gone is illustrated by the US Environmental Protection Agency's Community Health and Environmental Surveillance System (CHESS) programme. Between 1969 and 1975 the Agency spent over

1 million in the conduct of a series of epidemiological studies of the health effects of air pollution in several cities across the US. The first year's results of these studies were reported in a monograph (EPA 1974), in the course of consideration of the validity of the national ambient air quality standard for sulphur dioxide. Controversy surfaced surrounding this monograph particularly in a series of newspaper articles charging that the head of the project had distorted the data and had otherwise conducted himself unprofessionally. This led to a Congressional investigation in 1976 which concluded that the data-collection methods were so inadequate the data should not even have been analysed, and that further the data were analysed incorrectly (US House of Representatives 1976). When the Environmental Protection Agency took no substantive action in response, the Agency was directed by statute in 1978 (Environmental Research, Development and Demonstration Authorization Act of 1978) to implement the recommendations of the Congressional investigation. Unfortunately, the CHESS programme is only indicative of the misuse of science in formulation and maintenance of bad government decisions in regulating environmental hazards.

In the final analysis, the process of government control of environmental hazards requires the utmost in scientific integrity and accuracy from all involved (government and private sector alike). It must be recognized that all have a common stake in appropriate government control of real environmental hazards. Otherwise, governments and the private sector will expend their limited resources in over-controlling lesser and imaginary hazards.

Technological and economic feasibility

Many environmental controls issued by governments are not capable of being achieved, or are capable of being achieved only at the expense of enormous economic and social disruption. The technology to control discharges to regulation levels is often not available, and where it is available, the cost of the technology is frequently so great that it is economically impractical.

This is not surprising where standards and other environmental control levels are set, as above described, at or near naturally occurring levels. And even where the levels are reasonable, the impact on the private sector may be the same. If, as often occurs, substantial hazards are created by activities operated or controlled by local governments, where enforcement is politically impalpable (for example, dust emissions from streets and roads), the impact of reducing overall the hazards disproportionately falls on the private sector.

Moreover, government regulations are in some cases expressly designed to force regulated sources to develop pollution control devices that may at the time appear to be economically or technically infeasible. This is, for example, the situation with the health-related national ambient air quality standards in the US. The Administrator of the US Environmental Protection Agency is forbidden by the Clean Air Act from considering the technological and economic feasibility of implementing standards in setting them. The legislators expressed the value judgment that 'the health of people is more important than the question of whether the early achieve-

ment of ambient air quality standards protective of health is technically feasible . . .' (US Senate 1970).

The 'technology-forcing' legislation was put in place in the early 1970s at a time when the prevailing view was that technological solutions would inevitably occur given the pressure of circumstances. (The US had just placed a man on the moon and returned him to earth safely, after declaring it a national objective a decade before.) In the decade of the 1970s we have learned differently. The technology does not develop that quickly and is often enormously expensive – particularly when balanced with the environmental hazard against which the control is designed to protect. The result has been a contraction of industries and higher costs for goods and services in countries, such as the US, that take seriously the government environmental regulations. For this reason alone, it is essential that the available resources be used for efficient and effective controls appropriate for protection of real environmental hazards.

Legal and political action

The ability of the private sector to respond to government control of environmental hazards in judicial or legislative proceedings is most limited. Action by the European Communities is by proposal of the Commission of the European Communities and adoption by the Council of the European Communities, under the authority of the Rome Treaty. In the US, court review of a regulation imposed by the Environmental Protection Agency is essentially limited to whether the regulation is arbitrary, capricious, an abuse of discretion or otherwise not in accordance with law (US Code, Title 42, §7607(d)). In both cases, the governmental regulation is implemented by subsequent legislation by member countries or states, where there again is no opportunity for independent review of the substantive validity of the regulations.

The ability of the private sector effectively to present substantive evidence in the legislative process is limited by the emotional and political aspects of environmental hazards. Few legislators and even fewer members of the public have an appreciation for the nature of the data addressing environmental hazards; and even fewer are inclined to speak out in favour of reliance on objective science. For this reason, legislative decisions tend to be broadly framed, deferring the hard decisions to an administrative body such as an environmental protection agency or department. When the legislative considerations become focused, the proceedings tend to become politically packed events with little chance for considered, rational deliberation. In any event, public health and welfare are not served by the resulting politically expedient decisions that all too frequently are based on bad science or distortion of good science.

CONCLUSION

Direct government controls serve an important function in reducing environmental hazards, but the time has passed in most industrialized countries where particular environmental hazards can be regulated *ad hoc* in isolation. If the controls are to be effective and efficient, it is essential that the regulations be based on an accurate, objective interpretation of reliable scientific information, and be interrelated in a meaningful way with other environmental and non-environmental regulations and laws, with voluntary action by the private sector, and with energy conservation policies. Also, they must realistically take into account the industrial situation in which the government regulations are to be applied.

Current government controls of environmental hazards do not generally reflect these considerations. If such controls are to do so in the future, it is essential that ways be found to involve more directly the competent, responsible segments of the private sector in the government decision making, and that governments in preparing the control regulations realistically weigh the nature and extent of the environmental hazard against the impact of the regulation in the private sector and in the community as a whole.

REFERENCES

American Law Institute (1965). *Restatement of the Law, Second (Torts 2d) by the American Law Institute,* Volume 2, §402A.

EPA (1974). *Health consequences of sulfur oxides: a report fro CHESS, 1970–1971.* EPA-650/1-74-004. US Government Prin ing Office, Washington, DC.

Federal Reporter (1973). *Borel v. Fibreboard Paper Products Co poration, United States Court of Appeals, Fifth Circuit.* Feder Reporter, 2d Series 493: 1096. US Government Printing Offic Washington, DC.

Selikoff, Churg and Hammand (1965). The occurrence of asbestos among industrial insulation workers. *Ann. NY Acad. Sci.* **13** 139.

US House of Representatives (1976). *The Environmental Protectic Agency's Research Program with primary emphasis on the Com munity Health and Environmental Surveillance System (CHESS An investigative report.* (Prepared for the Subcommittee on Speci Studies, Investigations and Oversights and the Subcommittee c the Environment and the Atmosphere of the Committee O Science and Technology, US House of Representatives). U Government Printing Office, Washington, DC.

US Senate (1970). *Report* No. 91-1196. US Government Printin Office, Washington, DC.

12 Governmental and legislative policies to control and direct the promotion of health

Hugh H. Tilson

INTRODUCTION

Health promotion may be the greatest policy opportunity available to public health – it may also pose the toughest challenges: conceptual, scientific, political, and programmatic. There is the opportunity not only to prevent or defer onset of chronic disease but also to help people in all stations in life and in all parts of the globe to get more out of their lives. The level of public debate on the subject suggests the great importance of these issues and the evolving public expectation to enhance the quality of life. Yet society continues to fall short of reaping the full benefits of health promotion. This apparent paradox finds its explanation in the characteristics of the policy-making process itself. These are presented in this chapter as challenges which must be met if society is to achieve the full potential of health promotion.

THE CONCEPTUAL CHALLENGE

To achieve governmental policies for the promotion of health, the world of public health needed clarification (especially in the minds of the people who thought they already knew); what is meant by 'health'?; what is different about the 'promotion of health' from the accepted concepts of preventive medicine?; and what exactly is or is not a 'government policy'? To the relative newcomer into public health, it must be hard to believe that these three questions were ever really matters of hot debate – their answers seeming so obvious in the sunlight of the 1980s. Indeed, it must seem even stranger that these three questions had not been asked – at least not so boldly – and certainly not associated with one or the other until very recent years. And most striking of all, it may be surprising that the answers which seem so straightforward, are not so – at least not yet.

The World Health Organization (WHO) has set the world-wide tone for health promotion, following the wisdom of antiquity by defining health as not simply the absence of disease but the presence of physical, social, and emotional well-being. In the years intervening since the articulation of this definition of health, volumes have been written about the need for efforts which advance health and not simply treat or even prevent specific illnesses. Indeed, pages in this textbook are devoted elsewhere to this subject, for example, wellness models versus medical models and environmental or social strategies in contrast to medical or health care efforts. And although the terminology of health and health care is now part of the vocabulary of every person trained in those pursuits, the disciplines involved with health promotion, which we now designate as 'health professionals' were called as recently as a decade ago the medical and 'ancillary professions' – not exactly equal partners in the health challenge.

If the great sanitary reforms of the nineteenth century represent the first public health revolution, the new idea that something specific and positive can be done by individuals, groups, or populations to *promote* health represents the second major conceptual advance – one seemingly small step for man but a great conceptual leap forward for mankind from the Benjamin Franklin aphorisms about 'early to bed and early to rise'. This crystalization of a series of ideas occurred in the super-saturated solution of countless programmes in search of a frame of reference. These disparate ill-integrated but well-meaning and often well-conceived programmes for health embodied many of the notions subsequently evolved ('re-discovered') under the umbrella and tagged with the name of health promotion. Many of the programmes currently counted in official inventories of health promotion programmes had existed before in another form and/or with a different name – often as parts of health education, community health nursing, health screening programmes, school hygiene programmes and the like. To some, this restatement was regarded as nothing short of a 'second public health revolution'; to others it was regarded as a great opportunity to capture people's imaginations and advance existing causes; and to still others it was regarded as the 'emperor's new clothes'.

Finally, for *policy* to emerge, a greater self-consciousness regarding health policy was needed. Stated conversely, just because you have practised policy all your life does not mean that it is a policy until you call it one. The absence of a statement: 'it shall be the policy of these united provinces or states or municipalities . . .' is no more a statement of the lack of activity (or indeed even implicit policy) than is the presence of such a statement any indication that the activity which follows will embody the spirit of the policy (or even that any activity will actually follow). With the evolution of the social sciences, especially political science, over the past 30 years has come the emergence, within the health professions, of health social scientists, and a body of scholarly logic regarding emerging health policy. This has led to a more rigorous, structured approach to the understanding and resultant proposal of such policies.

However, even if it is correct that policies explicitly directed at health promotion represent a new breakthrough, this is in no way to imply that policies governing or materially influencing health and health status are at all new. Dating back to the very beginnings of governmental policies and practices, and indeed to the roots of orthodox religious practices before their codification, policies and laws have been created to protect health and prevent disease, to insulate us from our own weaknesses, and to quarantine away those hazards which can be contained in no other way. Generally speaking, governmental policies or practices, including those influencing health, tend to balance the rights of the individual against the rights of the collectivity. In such instances, the value system of that society tends to determine the extent to which it is willing to abridge individual freedoms for collective good. Thus, in the presence of great central control or shared sentiment regarding the prior claim of the collectivity over the individual (for example, certain Communist countries), a central policy which requires changes in individual behaviour is feasible, for example, the eradication of syphilis in the Peoples Republic of China. One attempt at such policy in the US – the prohibition of alcoholic beverages – was less successful, at least in part rooted in the fundamental American principle of the 'inalienable rights' of the individual.

A current debate raging in the US balances the right of the individual motorcyclist to expose himself or herself to a potentially fatal injury versus the right of a society to require more responsible behaviour (that is, the use of helmets) to insulate itself against excessive financial and moral exposure. This is especially controversial in light of the conflicting scientific evidence concerning the possible risks as well as benefits from helmet use.

Perhaps a more classic case in point is society's decision to intervene in the parent–child relationship to require a parent, whatever his or her health beliefs and practices, to have a child immunized to protect that child against an unseen and otherwise sinister environment and, in the process to protect others who might be exposed to an unimmunized infected child from that liability.

Public funding of family planning and contraceptive programmes may represent a step closer to the issue of public policies which ensure the promotion of health. That is, family planning can be viewed not as a conscious decision on the part of an individual to change her personal risk status for a single condition – unwanted pregnancy – but rather as a commitment by a society to reducing the risk to a future generation of the various conditions excessively prevalent in the unwanted products of reproduction. In the developing world, an emerging nation may establish such policies to protect itself against the otherwise inevitable ravages of an unsustainable population. At this end of the spectrum, such policies could be viewed as health promotion policies. In their pragmatic form as public activities in Europe and North America, the public policy debates about family planning

programmes generally 'duck' these broader and more controversial social issues. They are, instead, quite specific and addressed to an individual prevention agenda, not health promotion or social reform.

An additonal arena for health policy-making, which nowadays is claimed (often in retrospect) to be part of the province of programmes for the promotion of health, is the enhancement of the physical and social environment. Social policies which result in economic, social, educational, and physical well-being, influence overall health status without being directed at a specific disease condition and quite independent of healthful behaviour of any individual. Thus, in classic economic development efforts, the investment of resources into proper environmental sanitation, reductions in speed limit, or proper highway safety features, human factors, engineering in housing, and, most fundamentally, adequate jobs, proper habitat, proper nutrition and a hope of a meaningful future are all circumstances associated favourably with reduction in the risk of excessive prevalence of major diseases and early disability and death. And they may therefore represent, using a different name, the 'real' governmental policies addressing the promotion of health – if so, they are hardly new!

THE SCIENTIFIC CHALLENGE

One of the great barriers to establishing programmes directed more specifically at health promotion has been the world-wide failure of such efforts to capture the imagination and gain the support of physicians. This lack of support (while certainly attributable to one or more of: political agendas, economic motives, lack of education and insight – issues to be discussed further – and competing priorities for the spotlight) may be ascribed at least in significant measure to the emergence of science in medicine. The medical professions in the twentieth century are taught to require reasonable evidence of scientific validity to assertions regarding effectiveness of methods to promote the health of people. There has been an ever-increasing awareness of and emphasis upon professional content of the practice of medicine since the Flexner Report (Flexner 1910) and the demise of the proprietary medical education system in the US in the early part of the twentieth century. Medicine has increasingly emphasized its science and embraced its role in helping the public to recognize and eliminate quackery, charlatans, and unscientific practices. Therefore the need is to *measure* and not simply define health. However, it is not simple to quantify the impact upon health status of various measures alleged to be promotive of the health. Disease end-points are easier to measure than the absence of disease, and the dimension on the other end of the sickness scale – namely health – is essentially uncharted. Thus, while the scientific standard is both an understandable and a commendable phenomenon of the latter half of the twentieth century, it has been a major stumbling block for progress as the science of health promotion has been emerging.

The demand for scientific rigour, while delaying the emergence of health promotion practice, has, paradoxically, also strengthened it. Progressively, society has achieved more pecific definitions of the tools for the advancement of health nd, more rigorous measurement of the effect of those tools. Notable have been health hazard appraisal and health risk ssessment which have resulted in recent programmes for risk eduction and health self-help, the holistic health movement nd biofeedback, to name but a few. These, in turn, are beginning to emerge from the application of well-honed epidemiological analytic tools to the morbidity and mortality statistics of the decades since infectious diseases have been controlled. The new challenges of the second public health evolution have been world-wide, spearheaded by the articuation by Minister of Health, LaLonde of new protection against threats to the health of Canadians (LaLonde 1974), and repeated in the new promise of community medicine in the Third World to address so-called diseases of unhealthy life-style prominently appearing in the precepts of Chairman Mao (Barefoot Doctor's Manual 1977).

At least in part the redefinition of emphasis occurred as a result of disappointments with the new technology of medicine, however scientific and more readily counted, and however dramatic as processes. Heavy investments in treatment of disease had *not* succeeded in bringing about the dramatic outcomes – that is, reductions in morbidity and mortality – which have been hoped for. The focus has gradually (though only slightly) shifted, at least in part, because of the immensity of the cost. In America a nationwide network of programmes to conquer heart disease, cancer, and stroke (the Regional Medical Programs), initially concentrated on the very costly 'centres of excellence' approach with a heavy emphasis upon the distribution of high technology, tertiary medical care for the medical treatment of these major causes of disability and death. The approach has now been redefined in terms of prevention. The focus in the 1970s became individual behaviours that influence the risk of these serious medical outcomes in definable (for example, so-called 'high-risk') populations. By inference, persons who carry the attributes of the population with increased risk are, therefore, themselves at increased risk of the adverse outcome if they practise the 'bad' behaviour. Epidemiological analysis – coupled with cost–benefit logic borrowed from the social sciences – examined the link between behaviours and those outcomes associated with the greatest morbidity and mortality. By inference, health could be improved if one could change behaviour. And if society could help individuals to change, society would also benefit.

The emergence of the 'big five' health life-styles to be targeted by health promotion programmes followed from assessment of factors associated with the greatest morbidity and mortality: stress reduction; smoking cessation; alcohol intake moderation; proper diet; and exercise. Though still modest in comparison with investments in research in curative medicine, relatively major nationwide appropriations in the US and in other western countries have been made for research studies to document the effectiveness of large scale programmes for intervention into specific risk factors, such as the 'Mr Fit' (MRFIT: Multiple Risk Factor Intervention Trial) programmes in the US, the North Karelia Programme in Finland, the Oslo Coronary Heart Disease Project (all described elsewhere in this text, see Volume 3).

THE POLITICAL CHALLENGE

The process of development of public policies and their derivative public appropriations and programming varies dramatically from nation to nation. In the US, there is a long history of competition between the public and the private sector for primacy in health. There is an unquestioned political dichotomy, represented by the difference in the prevailing political parties between a predominant centrism – that is federal responsibility for public health – and decentralized public policy, with primary implementation responsibilities at the state or local levels. And finally there is the ever-present competition for resources between the vested interests in curative medicine and those in preventive medicine (the 'politics' of the profession). In the next several sections, the context is drawn for the emergence of health promotion policy in the US. Readers from other nations are invited to compare and contrast differing political situations as they might influence the emergence of similar policies elsewhere.

The role of government

The USA is a huge diverse decentralized entrepreneurial nation founded by mavericks and pioneers. There is an ever-present tone of sentiment (sometimes louder, as at present) against government intervention in all forms of human commerce including health care. This includes an article of economic and political faith among some that government is inherently large, bureaucratic, inefficient, inept, and lacks the incentives to improve itself or its productivity. Reinforcing this, an occasional programme 'failure', such as ill-fated attempts at nationwide protection against swine-flu, invariably attracts vastly more attention than do the manifold more frequent and more meaningful unsung successes of government programmes. Then, too, there is an inherent pride in the distinction between the 'American way' and the 'un-American way' – which in its polar extreme attempts to paint those approaches used in other nations, especially the developing world and Communist nations, as inherently evil, essentially letting the ends (which are often certainly political and controlled) taint the means. Thus in the 1950s, planning was viewed as communistic, since the Russians created five-year plans. In the 1960s, when the Swedes aggressively institutionalized prevention of sexually transmitted diseases, it was considered socialistic. And in the 1970s as the Chinese emphasis upon judicious use of folk practices and indigenous health workers (the barefoot doctors), became better understood, there were those foes who saw the movement as 'Maoist'. Therefore for a public health policy to evolve in this context in the US, it must aim to be understood as non-interventionist, non-propagandistic, and non-organizational.

The evolving role of government in health

Within the general political framework in America there is a very specific set of principles which give primacy for medical interventions to the private practising physician and his or her associates. Government's role is expressly not to intervene in the private practice of medicine. Thus policy statement after policy statement embodies the proviso: 'except insofar as this policy is not intended to interfere with the existing practice of medicine . . .'. Within this strong political context, a system of local, state and federal public health has evolved, the role of which is to identify gaps in the health care delivery system and when the existing private resources cannot fill them, stimulate or actually undertake activities to meet the needs, but only insofar as direct competition with the strong private sector is not identified as an issue. The conflicts engendered by this phenomenon have been the subject of hortatory literature for decades. Whether advocating one or another possible chief role or emphasis for public health, all the exhortations have a common denominator of provider of last resort or 'residual guarantor' as the role for government in health.

Often this role translates into the clinic for the poor, this population being the most under-served. All too often, however, the result is the bureaucratic substitution of means for ends. People forget the basic role, and instead stereotype the health departments as programmes for poor people. This makes difficult the re-emergence of government in an arena in which often the major beneficiary is the overweight and overwrought middle class.

The local level

Public health in cities, towns, counties, and municipalities in the US usually means the four walls of an institution, the local health department. Funded variously by local property tax, mixtures of state and local funds or in some states entirely through state funding, these represent the embodiment of public health policy at the local level. What health departments actually do or occasion to get done in their local communities, therefore, represents the expression of that health policy at the local level. Yet these institutions in the simplest sense, are creatures of their local political environment – city and county politics, local medical politics, and the politics of community action. There is no clear national charter in the US which enfranchises all people at the local level to a certain minimum set of community preventive health services, despite countless efforts to establish this minimum entitlement set. What counties themselves provide, then, must be determined locally on the basis of professional wisdom and political imperative. What gets financed, of course, is determined by the elected politicians on Boards of County Commissioners, often buffered by a local politically-appointed Board of Health. To get programmes started, therefore, there must be clear and unambiguous leadership at least somehow recognized by a budget proponent, a constituency to support an effort in the field, and political support. The local health department over the past 20 years has become the agency which does what no one else wants to do. The corollary is that often there is no one outside the health department who cares enough about the programme to understand it and fight for it against competing priorities. Further, as revenues at the local level have become progressively more difficult to raise – especially in the era of the American tax revolt which started at the local level – more and more, local health departments have addressed those needs for which there are outside funding. Local com-

munities, then, which had been very independent of state control and policy self-determining, along with those who had always been supported by the states, have become progressively dependent upon state financing for continued programming.

The state level

State financial support for local public health programmes comes in three forms: programmatic or categorical grants; reimbursement for services; and (less prevalent) general support. These, in turn, are determined by the state political apparatus again in the American federal configuration of independent (though united) states without declared national cohesive policy for health. State public health policies are determined by negotiation between professional and political concerns and are usually resolved at the state budget table. With notable exceptions, policy ping pong has been an easy game to play, with counties blaming lack of resources on the state and states blaming lack of programming on the counties. Depending on tradition, innovation, level of resources, and political imperatives, direct programming for public health has also been conducted by state health departments in lieu of, in conjunction with, and sometimes in spite of local public health. A corollary to the political axioms governing what local health agencies may expect in health policy is that the same problems confront the programme innovator at the state level, except that the 'pay-off' of good programming is even more remote and harder to sell.

The federal role

Federal health policy in the US, after two centuries of evolution, experienced a major watershed, and re-infused a major new emphasis upon curative medical care with Title 18 (Medicare) and Title 19 (Medicaid) of the Social Security Acts of 1965. And with Medicaid came large mandatory state-match appropriations and a major emphasis not on health promotion and disease prevention as had been evolving as the national agenda but once again upon curative services for the poor. This was not an unprecedented role for public health in the US. Indeed, the US Public Health services was originally created to provide care for the Merchant Marine.

Indeed, funded through separate bureaucracies and managed outside of the traditional public health apparatus, these new programmes actually prohibited use of these resources for preventive and health promotive services. With cash flow compromised at the local level, and with the ability of states to generate the large sums of money needed for general public health programming hindered by a hefty state match in Medicaid, health departments have turned, in the past decade, more and more toward fee-for-service disease-oriented curative medicine for which the appropriations were available. These programmes, detailed elsewhere in this text, have met – to a varied degree – crying medical needs. However, one of the costs of this progress has been the demise of many an appropriations bill and a serious crimp in the potential health promotion fabric.

Parallel with its neighbour to the north, Canada, as budget

ts have been needed in the US during the early 1980s, a block grant consolidation of what remained of the traditional Public Health projects with transfer of jurisdiction back to e states has been the policy of America's 'New Federalism' Brandt 1981). In contrast to Canada, no taxing authority has een transferred with programme. The result has been pro- essively less money in public health programmes, including ealth promotion, even in an era of escalating rhetoric to the ontrary.

And yet it may be the very experience of the 'uncontrolla- lity' of national expenditures on curative medicine which ill drive the balance of appropriations back toward preventing ese illnesses for which we cannot afford to pay the medical lls. Despite the fifty years since the report of the US Com- ittee on the Costs of Medical Care (CCMC 1933), the rhetoric ill outstrips the reality. Why?

Perhaps the answer lies beyond the financial political hallenge on a far more fundamental political one – America's read of propaganda. The new 'stuff' of which health prom- tion is made is not something which communities do to their nvironment or doctors do with patients. It is rather a funda- ental restructuring of the individual's approach to himself r herself and life-style. And this, in turn, strikes at perhaps e most vital part of freedom – the ability to structure and pply one's own values. The mentality which 'wants govern- ent off our backs' and cherishes separation of church (that , values) and the state (that is, programmes) as a fundamental overning principle of the nation can hardly embrace un- uestioningly governmental programmes in behaviour modi- ication which apply the best which is known in the health ducation and behavioural literature. Yet among other xioms of health education, perhaps none is more fundamental han the lesson that the facts alone will rarely change a erson's behaviour. Rather the message must be persuasive . . . ven compelling. Yet this may appear – or be vulnerable to ttempts to make it seem – to step over the fine line between ducation and manipulation. Proof of this paradox was hown by the demise of a substantively excellent but politically imply unacceptable federally-funded series of anti-smoking advertisement' on commercial television. Designed to offset he enormous impact of cigarette commercials, the advertise- ents were aimed at behaviour changes through affective ppeal. They were withdrawn.

THE PROGRAMMATIC CHALLENGE

Trick Question: 'When does policy really become policy?'
Quick Answer: 'When it leads someone to do something!'

One underlying rule – generalizable across most public health programming – is the policy of pragmatism. The public health official, tied as he or she is to the 'real world' often cannot wait for full consensus and/or scientific documentation. Rather, certain programmatic entrepreneurship is required. This becomes especially true in the face of public demand for service or action and particularly so given the politics of public health in the 1970s and 1980s – in which the expectation for bureaucratic survival in a political climate is to provide services for everybody'. Finally, part of the politics of prag-

matism among many public health professionals is to get on with 'doing' rather than all of the preliminaries of 'talking' even if the latter is the embodiment of policy development. As a result, implementation of health promotion ideas in public health programmes precedes the development of national, state, and local official policies literally by decades, though often under another guise and even for purposes which might have been stated quite differently.

Published speeches of public leaders including Presidents and Mayors on the campaign trail, and Secretaries and Commissioners of Health or Human Resources have left an inspirational trace of wonderful words regarding health promotion over the past decade. Translating those words into programmatic action has had to await implementation strategies which are sensitive to the politics which eschew propaganda. Likewise they required adjustment to the American balance between public health and private medicine. Yet policy now seems to be catching up with pragmatic imple- mentation, and rhetoric with reality. These implementation programmes are described below under three broad headings: health education strategies; risk reduction programmes; and research and demonstration strategy.

HEALTH EDUCATION STRATEGIES

Health information strategy

An important constituency for health promotion programmes is that group of public health professionals whose prog- rammes, under a different name, have long been inadequately supported, namely health educators. In its most rudimentary forms, health education represents the application of edu- cational techniques to the distribution of health messages. Pamphlets, brochures, booklets, books, films, slide shows, audio tapes, synchronized slide shows, video tapes, lecture outlines, curriculum guides, media centres, speakers bureaux, classroom techniques, small group, self-help, peer education approaches – these are the stock in trade of effective efforts to help people to receive, comprehend, and incorporate messages essential to their health. The literature is replete with discouraging, though often amusing, examples of well-meant but ill-conceived efforts at information transmission which fail to recognize the science of health education. Classroom educators ill-prepared in health or health workers ill-prepared in education continue to fail to recognize the gaps in their com- petence and fail to reach their audience with effective health messages. Much of the current leadership for health promotion programming comes from the specialist community of health educators who recognize the sensitivity of the messages and the complexity of motivational techniques, especially for the modification of personal health behaviours.

Physical fitness and health strategies

Another important health constituency, currently vitally invested in the advance of health promotion – at least in part as professional defence – is the recreational and physical activity specialist. Following the realization of the conquest of communicable disease, the focus on social gerontology around the world has resulted in emphasis upon programmes of social and physical activity for elders. Part of the awareness of the potential preventability of degenerative disease was stimulated by the findings of the physical examination screening programmes of the US military during the Korean War, in which high levels of physical unfitness were found in America's youth. Also from the autopsy table the grisly evidence of physical unfitness – the presence of early degenerative cardiovascular disease in the symptomatically healthy young battle casualty – became a grim reminder that something needed to be done. The response in America and elsewhere, was a resurgence of interest in sports and physical activity, less for the winning of the game and more for the winning of the battles – those military and health-related. School sports curricula and physical fitness programmes were re-justified on their relationship to reduction of long-term disease and disability. And coaches' and physical education experts' salaries and roles were justified not solely on the basis of sport but also for health reasons in the governmental budgets of state and local school districts. Perhaps as important as any event to precipitate a new culture of joggers and runners was a coronary occlusion of an American President (Eisenhower) and a physically fit cardiologist (Paul Dudley White) suddenly holding the nation's pulse. And as jogging and running as part of cardiovascular fitness have been advocated (even practised) in more recent years by more important medical opinion leaders, public funding for parks, recreation and running facilities have been justified on the basis of health and public councils and commissions on physical fitness and health from national to local levels have sprung up.

Health awareness strategy

A relatively inexpensive way to 'get the ball rolling' is to assemble meetings, conclaves, conferences, think tanks, and the like at national or state levels to encourage participants in their organizational or daily professional lives and/or to generate good ideas for other peoples' (unfunded) implementation – for example, recommendations of commissions. Over the past decade, the US has witnessed many of these efforts, including an extensive objective setting process involving hundreds of interested experts and opinion leaders in the development of objectives for the Nation, resulting in the publication *Promoting Health, Preventing Disease* (DHHS, 1980). The development of President's and Governor's Councils on Physical Fitness and Health reflect the continuation of this advocacy. The low levels of funding reflect the lip-service which sadly often accompanies such efforts.

Community organization strategy

As the work of early health behaviourists became fully understood, and the implications of healthful behaviours in general to the readiness to incorporate any individual health message became clear, health programmes to induce the individual to be health conscious and/or health ready, became the rule and the educational medium therefore became the message. Insofar

as the promotion of health requires individual action o behalf of the self, the individual needs to have a reason care. Motivational techniques, helping the individual understand the value of his or her own actions and, the more fundamentally to value the benefits of positive actio on his or her own behalf, became central to health promotic programmes. Extension of these principles into action involve community organization around health issues, on the premi that the organization of the community – in and of itself – wa 'healthful' behaviour and would help individuals in the con munity to value their health and therefore act on their ow behalf to promote and protect their own health. Such pro rammes around the world have taken many different form In the US they are embodied by the health programmes of th Office of Economic Opportunity during the revolutionar post-Kennedy era of health care. Federally-funded neighbou hood health centres in the US were often offshoots of othe community action programmes. Others were directly funde as health centres but included their own programmes o community organization and concepts of community contre and governance, justified by the rhetoric of health and relyin heavily upon community-indigenous health workers, couplin the basic principles of good communication with a strategy a fundamental as more and new jobs. Pride, security, a sense o relevance and a hope for future become the ingredients fo health.

RISK REDUCTION PROGRAMMES

Screening strategies

The second major programmatic thrust for health promotio employs physical manipulation and technology as instructiv tools to stimulate healthful behaviour. The screening chest X ray became the virtual symbol for public health during th 1940s and 50s – the era for conquering the tuberculosis past However, with the advent of antimycobacterial therapy an major strides toward conquest of tuberculosis, the system wa left with a powerful and symbolic tool, and a public sensitize to the 'healing powers' of a screening system. The tuberculosi societies became tuberculosis and respiratory disease activities lung associations succeeded tuberculosis associations; an public programmes for control of tuberculosis were redirecte toward control of chest diseases, notably disability from chronic lung disease and emphysema. Smoking became th enemy, as its clear linkage to cancer and cardiovascular diseas became apparent and surgeon generals and ministers o health world-wide lent their policy credentials to the epidemio logical wisdom. Thus, smoking-cessation programmes pre date the 'risk-factor' terminology, and health life-style an health promotion jargon, yet were destined to become th mainstay of both.

Extension of the technology and philosophy of tuberculosi screening to general screening for other diseases was easil understood by the generation of tuberculosis screenees. Wit the technology of automated blood chemistries came the er of multiphasic screening. Here again, for public health prog ramming purposes, the early detection of the disease wa perhaps less important than the visible demonstration tha

est and heart and blood were associated with possible
ease states and that one should be concerned about such
tters. The costs of health care and illness have become
ogressively publically borne around the world by various
grees of socialization of health care from universal entitle-
nt – for example, the national health service in Great
itain or provincial health services in Canada – to specialized
vernmental support for special categories – such as the
or and elderly under Medicaid and Medicare in the US. As
tial estimates of costs were supplanted by realistic experience
orders of magnitude greater, one would have expected an
gressive search for activities which would reduce the burden
illness. Screening programmes – such as the early periodic
reening, detection, and treatment programmes of Medicaid
PSDT) – became viewed as legitimate public expenditure
ternatives and seized upon in lieu of expenditures for direct
re. However, the emphasis upon screening in these pro-
ammes was on 'traditional' preventive medicine. Their cost
s justified on the basis of the logic of 'outreach' – that is,
cruitment into early medical treatment. Funding for the
alth education and case management corollaries necessary
translate the programme into effective behaviour change
s paradoxically not been forthcoming. The EPSDT
reening has fallen short of its potential as a health promotion
ol.

sk factor analysis

igh costs with low yields, high levels of client confusion and
necessary referral, and disappointing levels of effectiveness
a health education tool have rendered the 'shotgun'
pproach to screening *passé* in the 1970s. Replacing it, is the
ore scientific application of epidemiological principles to
e screening of otherwise healthy individuals, applying tests
ith high sensitivity and specificity – that is, high predictive
lue (see Volume 3), and with high likelihood that a positive
nding would result in a meaningful intervention. A natural
tension of this logic addresses those variables demonstrated
idemiologically to be associated with various disease
ates – the so-called risk factors. Risk-factor analysis or
alth hazard appraisal, are described in detail elsewhere in
is text. Public programmes to include systematic assess-
ents of risk and prescriptive approaches, relying heavily on
lf-help, have been encouraged by national policies in the US
rived from the Surgeon General's report, *Healthy People*
979). However, only very limited funds for programme
evelopment were made available as grants-in-aid in the early
980s and with the new federalism, these, too, have not been
ntinued.

The extension of the concept of personal risk-factor
duction as an integral part of policy-making and community
rogramming is only in its infancy. A major step forward,
owever, was taken when this approach was included in a
ational effort in the US to develop model standards for
ommunity preventive health services under Congressional
andate (Department of Health, Education and Welfare
979). In this effort, the model of risk recognition and
duction was extended to encourage community-wide efforts
recognize patterns of behaviour in populations which
might place the overall population at risk, as a key to needed
public programme development.

THE RESEARCH AND DEMONSTRATION STRATEGY

A public policy of investment of resources in the sharpening
of the epidemiological focus of the expenditure for public
health represents the third implementation thrust. The high
costs of curative medicine coupled with demands for medical
rigorousness have resulted in the recent addition of modest
public funding to the longer standing private research interests
in health promotion, though here the corporate interests in
controlling costs of medical benefits had made the first move
to fund 'basic' research projects in health promotion. Research
is now underway to validate the association between individual
behaviours and disease states, exploring, for example, correlates between dietary patterns and cancer, smoking patterns
and lung disease, drugs and accidents, and alcohol and high-
density lipoproteins. Similar public investments have recently
been made in documenting the effectiveness of behavioural
interventions in lowering the rates of diseases in those at-risk
populations, though again only after pioneering private efforts
at such programmes; for example, in the occupational setting.
Best known and perhaps most controversial of the public
programmes is the already mentioned MRFIT programme in
which thousands of patients have been enrolled into behaviour
modification schemes to address risk factors – notably
smoking, nutrition, and exercise patterns – to reduce the risk
of multiple adverse health outcomes – notably the associated
cardiovascular disease states. This project is described elsewhere in this text as are many other scientific efforts to
document the validity of health promotion assertions.
Many in the public health community had looked to this
ambitious undertaking to provide the definitive scientific
direction needed to ensure the health promotion revolution its
legitimate place in health policy. For a series of complex
reasons, the preliminary results of the project have been
disappointing. A tough evaluative challenge was built in from
the beginning because of the 'soft' nature, both of inputs and
endpoints. And an evolving set of external and uncontrollable
concurrent stimuli in health conscious America resulted in
unexpected improvements in the control population which
weakened the predictive power of the ambitious design.

THE CHALLENGE AHEAD

Health promotion should not remain an arena bolstered as
much by faith as by science and practised as much by default
as design. Just as the great sanitary reforms which launched
public health coupled the science of reducing the infectious
environment with the aesthetics of putrid odours and dead
salmon in the Thames, so it is reasonable that the second
public health revolution of health promotion and prevention
of chronic diseases also had to begin with a mixture of popular
and scientific agendas riding as much on a desire for physical
fitness and beauty as it may upon the epidemiological evidence
linking specific behaviours with specific health outcomes. Yet
to use this ambiguity as an excuse not to incorporate health
promotion programming and logic into public policy is to fail

to recognize two fundamental truths of public health policy – first, that science serves the public and not the other way around; and second, that science policy is itself an inexact science.

Explicit and rigorous policy-making for action programmes in health promotion is overdue. Such policies are justified already on the basis of what is presently known about cost-effective means of promoting health, and are urgently needed to enhance the application of current knowledge and the development of needed extensions of what we know. The establishment of clear policy at national and local levels – and the prerequisite justifications for those policies – can focus attention upon wastefulness of the present lack of application of rigorous decision-making. The results of present policy are far too often the allocation of resources to high-cost options with less proven and far less promise of social benefit.

The resulting programmes in health promotion will vary widely from country to country, and community to community. Especially in a field as incomplete in its science and as dependent upon culture and values, this variety is appropriate, as long as those governing such activities are clear about the policies and programmes they create and base them upon the science, embark on reasonable, affordable, rigorous evaluations, and then learn from them. Of particular importance are programmes directed at behaviour change among those factors of life-style which are already known (or highly suspected) to increase the risk of one or more major illnesses, which are under the individual's control, and for which tools for intervention (to reduce the risk) with some degree of documented effectiveness are available.

No less important is the need for a set of science policies world-wide which incorporates the same spirit. The promise offered by the concept of health promotion is applicable, not only in the efforts of the affluent to live longer, but to the people of the entire developed and developing world to live in better health. A substantial investment of development resources is needed into research which can improve our understanding of cause and effect relationships between environment, behaviours, and well-being, and which can therefore strengthen our grasp of cost-effective methods of intervention.

The job of the health worker is to promote the evolution of science and in the absence of perfect certainty to apply the available principles thoughtfully and creatively. Public policy which does any less is a disservice to the public it serves. And in the area of health promotion, a burdened, sick, troubled, and over-taxed society expects effective and affordable action, not simply pious words, to help to move it toward the vision of health for all.

REFERENCES

Barefoot doctor's manual. The American translation of the official Chinese paramedical manual. (1979). Running Press, Philadelphia.

Brandt, E. N. (1981). Block grants and the resurgence of federalism. *Public Health Rep.* **96**, 495.

Committee on the Costs of Medical Care (1932). *Medical care for the American people: The final report of the Committee on the Costs of Medical Care—Adopted October 31, 1932.* University of Chicago Press.

Department of Health and Human Services (1980). *Promoting health, preventing disease: objectives for the nation.* US Government Printing Office, Washington, DC.

Department of Health, Education and Welfare (1979). *Model standards for community prevention health services: a report to the US Congress from the Secretary of Health, Education and Welfare.* Department of Health, Education and Welfare, Center for Disease Control, Washington, DC.

Flexner, A. (1910). *Medical education in the United States and Canada. A report to the Carnegie Foundation for the Advancement of Teaching. Bulletin No. 4.* Updyke, Boston.

Lalonde, M. (1974). *A new perspective on the health of Canadians, a working document.* Tri-Graphic Printing, Ottowa.

Surgeon General (1979). *Healthy People: the Surgeon General's Report on health promotion and disease prevention.* (US Public Health Service Pub. No. 79-55071.) US Government Printing Office, Washington, DC.

FURTHER READING

Advisory Commission on Intergovernmental Relations (1977). *The Partnership for Health Act: Lessons from a pioneering block grant; The intergovernmental grant system: an assessment and proposed policies.* Publication No. A-56. ACIR, Washington, DC.

Advisory Commission on Intergovernmental Relations (1978). *Summary and concluding observations. The intergovernmental grant system: an assessment and proposed policies.* Publication No. A-62. ACIR, Washington, DC.

American Public Health Association (1940). An official declaration of attitude . . . on desireable standard minimum functions and suitable organization of health activities. *Am. J. Public Health* **30**, 1099.

American Public Health Association (1951). The local health department – services and responsibilities: an official statement of the American Public Health Association adopted November 1950. *Am. J. Public Health* **41**, 302.

American Public Health Association (1980). Local decision-making in prevention oriented health services. Policy statement. *Am. J. Public Health* **70**, 303.

Bergner, L. (1982). *The role of state and local health departments in health promotion and disease prevention.* (Unpublished Report.) Institute of Medicine, Washington, DC.

Breslow, L. (1978). Prospects for improving health through reducing risk factors. *Prev. Med.,* **7**, 449.

Canadian Task Force on the Periodic Health Examination (1979). The periodic health examination. *Can. Med. Assoc. J.* **121**, 3.

Chadwick, E. (1842). *Report on an Inquiry into the Sanitary Condition of the Labouring Population of Great Britain—1842,* as cited in Rosen, G. (1958). *A history of public health.* MD Publications, New York.

DeFriese, G.H., Hetherington, J.S., Brooks, E.F. *et al.* (1981). The program implications of administrative relationships between local health departments and state and local government. *Am. J. Public Health* **71**, 1109.

Department of Health and Human Services (1980*a*). *Health education—risk reduction grant program, FY 1980.* Bureau of Health Education, Atlanta, GA.

Department of Health and Human Services (1980*b*). *Health United States: 1980, with prevention profile.* (US Public Health Service Pub. No. 81-1232) US Department of Health and Human Services, Hyattsville, MD.

Doll, R. (1978). Prevention: some future perspectives. *Prev. Med.* **7**, 486.

ull, H.B. (1978). Progress in prevention of infectious disease. *Prev. Med.* **4**, 459.

alk, I.S. (1983). Some lessons from the fifty years since the CCM final report, 1932. *J. Public Health Policy* **4**, 135.

ielding, J.E. (1977). Health promotion – some notions in search of a constituency. *Am. J. Public Health* **67**, 1082.

Graduate Medical Education National Advisory Committee (1980). *Report. Volume 1, summary report.* US Government Printing Office, Washington, DC.

Health and Welfare Canada and Statistics Canada (1982). *The Health of Canadians. Report of the Canada Health Survey.* Health and Welfare, Ottawa.

Hjermann, I., Velve Byre, K., Holme, I. *et al.* (1981). Effect of diet and smoking intervention on the incidence of coronary heart disease: report from the Oslo Study Group of a randomized trial in healthy men. *Lancet* **ii**, 1303.

Holme, I. (1982). On the separation of intervention effects of diet and antismoking advice on the incidence of major coronary events in coronary high risk men: the Oslo study. *J. Oslo City Hosp.* **32**, 31.

Klos, D.M. and Rosenstock, I.M. (1982). Some lessons from the North Karelia Project. *Am. J. Public Health,* **72**, 53.

McAlister, A., Puska, P., Salonen, J.T. *et al.* (1982). Theory and action for health promotion: illustrations from the North Karelia Project. *Am. J. Public Health* **72**, 43.

Milio, N. (1981). *Promoting health through public policy.* Davis, Philadelphia.

Miller, C.A., Gilbert, G., Warren, D.G. *et al.* (1977). Statutory authorization for the work of local health departments. *Am. J. Public Health* **67**, 940.

Miller, C.A. and Moos, M. (1981). *Local health departments: fifteen case studies.* American Public Health Association, Washington, DC.

Multiple Risk Factor Intervention Trial Group (1976). Multiple Risk Factor Intervention Trial (MRFIT). A national study of primary prevention of coronary heart disease. *JAMA* **23**, 235.

Multiple Risk Factor Intervention Trial Group (1977). Statistical design considerations in the NHLI Multiple Risk Factor Intervention Trial (MRFIT). *J. Chronic Dis.* **30**, 261.

Multiple Risk Factor Intervention Trial Research Group (1982). Multiple Risk Factor Intervention Trial. Risk factor changes and mortality results. *JAMA* **248**, 1465.

National Public Health Program Reporting System (1980). *Public health agencies 1980. A report on their expenditures and activities.* Association of State and Territorial Health Officials, Suite 403, 962 Wayne Ave., Silver Spring, Md.

Nightingale, E.O., Cureton, M., Kalmer, V. *et al.* (1978). *Perspectives on health promotion and disease prevention in the United States, revised.* National Academy of Sciences, Washington, DC.

Office of Health Information and Promotion (1980). *Promoting health. A source book.* Office of Health Information and Promotion, Washington, DC.

Pickett, G. (1980). The future of health departments: the government presence. *Ann. Rev. Public Health* **1**, 297.

Puska, P. and Mustaniemi, H. (1975). Incidence and presentation of myocardial infarction in North Karelia, Finland. *Acta Med. Scand.* **197**, 211.

Robbins, A. (1975). The threat of national health insurance to preventive programs. *N. Engl. J. Med.* **293**, 503.

Rogers, P.J., Eaton, E.K., and Bruhn, J.G. (1981). Is health promotion cost effective? *Prev. Med.* **10**, 324.

Shattuck, L. (1850; reprinted 1948). *Report of the Sanitary Commission of Massachusetts, 1850.* Harvard University Press, Cambridge, MA.

Silver, G.A. (1978). *Child health, America's future.* Aspen System, Germantown, MD.

Somers, A.R. (ed.) (1976). *Promoting health: consumer education and national policy.* Aspen Systems Corporation, Germantown, MD.

Terris, M. (1976). The epidemiologic revolution, national health insurance and the role of health departments. *Am. J. Public Health* **66**, 1155.

Terris, M. (1983). *The complex tasks of the second epidemiologic revolution: the Joseph W. Mountin Lecture. J. Public Health Policy* **4**, 8.

Tilson, H. (1982). Standards – a model for the nation. *Am. J. Public Health* **72**, 1223.

University of North Carolina (1981). *The role of the health department in health promotion, a conference report. Health Services Research Center, Chapel Hill, NC.* University of North Carolina, Chapel Hill.

Veterans Administration Cooperative Study Group on Antihypertensive Agents (1967). Effects of treatment on morbidity in hypertension: Results in patients with diastolic blood pressure averaging 115 through 129 mm Hg. *JAMA* **202**, 1028.

Veterans Administration Cooperative Study Group on Antihypertensive Agents (1970). Effects of treatment on morbidity in hypertension: results in patients with diastolic blood pressure averaging 90 through 114 mm Hg. *JAMA* **312**, 1143.

Wagner, E.H. (1982). The North Karelia Project. What it tells us about the prevention of cardiovascular disease. *Am. J. Public Health* **72**, 51.

Wagner, E.H., Berry, W.L., Schoenback, V.J. *et al.* (1982). An assessment of health hazard/health risk appraisal. *Am. J. Public Health* **72**, 347.

Weiler, P., Bogges, J., Eastman, E. *et al.* (1982). The implementation of model standards in local health departments. *Am. J. Public Health* **72**, 1230.

World Health Organization (1976). Health services in Europe – 1. Administration and preventive services. *WHO Chron.* **30**, 407.

Disease control and health promotion

Governmental and legislative control and direction of health services – two models

3 Governmental and legislative control and direction of health services: United Kingdom

Clifford Graham*

INTRODUCTION

In observing developments over the almost 40 years life of the National Health Service in the UK, the outside observer is likely to note the apparent absence of clearly defined measures for the control and direction of health services by Government and Parliament. This could be interpreted as a demonstration of the real difficulty of exercising such control and direction. The Department of Health and Social Security (DHSS), which is charged with exercising this general responsibility on behalf of Government and Parliament, essentially must rely on persuasion and exhortation in dealing with all the many other central government departments with an indirect interest in health services; and its direct operations with the National Health Service (NHS) are based on an agency relationship not a chain of command. But this apparent absence of control and direction could also be explained by reference to the fact that, after the early years of centralization required to establish the NHS, it has been the will of recent Governments and Parliaments that responsibility for the control and direction of health services should be devolved to the local administrative unit most closely involved in the actual delivery of services. In England, with effect from 1 April 1982, this responsibility falls on the District Health Authorities (DHAs) working within general guidelines produced by the DHSS and Regional Health Authorities (RHAs).

In the final analysis, it may simply be that health is too complex and local an issue to be generalized about or subjected to central control and direction. But, so long as Parliament pays the piper, in meeting almost all the massive costs of the NHS through general taxation, the Government will continue to have to call the tune; at least in terms of the general strategy to be adopted towards the provision of health services if not the operational activities required for day to day direction, management and control.

THE CONSTITUTIONAL FRAMEWORK IN ENGLAND

The planning, management, and delivery of health services in England depends on an agency relationship between the Secretary of State for Social Services (Minister) and the DHSS on the one hand, operating at the national level, and on the other hand the NHS, operating sub-nationally through 14 RHAs and 192 DHAs. It is the duty of the Minister to 'promote the establishment . . . of a comprehensive health service designed to secure improvement in the physical and mental health of the people of England . . . and the prevention, diagnosis and treatment of illness, and for that purpose to provide or secure the effective provision of services' (National Health Services Act 1977).

The Minister has wide general *powers* to provide health services, and specific *duties* to provide services, including hospital and other accommodation; medical, dental, nursing, and ambulance services; facilities for the care of expectant and nursing mothers and young children; facilities for the prevention of illness; other facilities required for the diagnosis and treatment of illness; and facilities for family planning. But the Minister's specific duties to provide services are qualified 'to such extent as he considers necessary to meet all reasonable requirements'.

The Minister's responsibilities are for providing services and facilities, not for providing diagnosis and treatment etc. It is for the patient's doctor (or other professionals with clinical responsibility) and not the Minister to decide whether and what treatment is appropriate. For services provided by general medical, dental, and ophthalmic practitioners and the pharmaceutical service the Minister's duty is to 'make arrangements' with practitioners who are responsible for providing services as independent contractors. An illustration of the organization and management of the NHS and DHSS is given in Fig. 13.1.

ORGANIZATION AND MANAGEMENT

The NHS from 1948 to 1973

Until 1 April 1974, the health service in England was organized in three separate parts:

1. *Hospital and specialist services,* managed by hospital authorities responsible to the Minister of Health. England was divided into 14 hospital regions each with its own Regional Hospital Board. The Hospital Boards were required to set up Hospital Management Committees (about 200 in all) to manage local groups of hospitals. The undergraduate and postgraduate teaching hospitals, however, were managed by their own Boards of Governors which were also directly responsible to the Minister.

*This chapter contains the views of the author alone: it should not be read as an expression of the views of the Department of Health and Social Security.

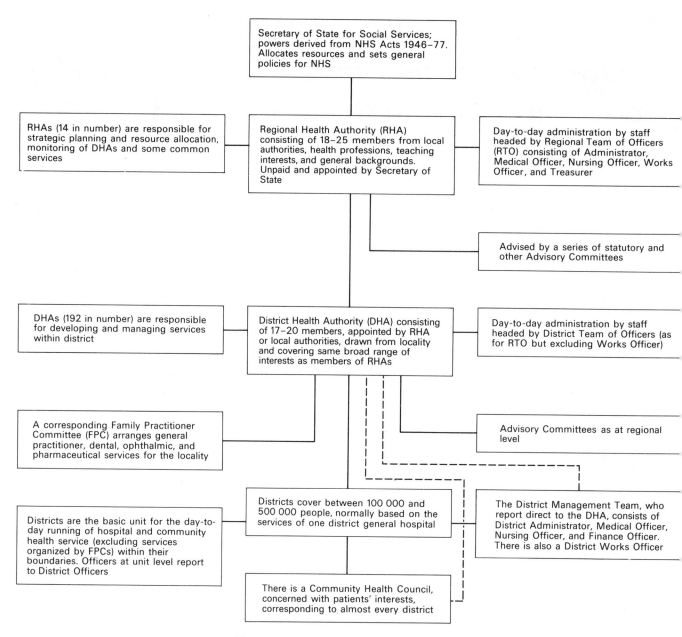

Fig. 13.1. Structure of the NHS and DHSS.

2. *The family doctor service and the general dental, pharmaceutical, and ophthalmic services,* provided by independent practitioners in contract to some 130 Executive Councils which were responsible to the Minister for making arrangements for these services within the Council's area.

3. *Local authorities,* 180 in all (reduced in 1965 by London Government reorganization), which in addition to general responsibilities for public health such as sewage, refuse disposal, port health, and food hygiene, had a wide range of specific health responsibilities, including health centres, ambulance services, family planning, immunization, health visiting, home nursing, and midwifery. Local authorities were also responsible for school medical and dental services.

The functions of these distinct organizations were often interdependent, if not actually overlapping. For example, for maternity services, the hospital authorities, the local health authority and the family doctor service all had responsibilities for the care of mothers and their babies. And yet the three services were each concerned with different local populations; they were separately financed, separately planned and developed according to different assessments of priorities.

here was no single authority responsible for providing the population of a given area with the right combination of comprehensive health services.

The constitutional framework in England between 1974 and 1982

reorganization of the health service which would bring all these separate services under one management was discussed over many years. Green Papers on the reorganization of the health service in England and Wales were published by the Labour Government in 1968. These were followed by further Green Papers in 1970. Consultative documents for England and Wales appeared in 1971 and finally the Conservative Government published White Papers for England and Wales in August 1972 containing proposals for the organization of the health service in England which subsequently formed the basis of the National Health Service Reorganization Act 1973 (now consolidated in the NHS Act 1977). This reorganization came into effect on 1 April 1974.

The main feature of the 1974 reorganization was the unified control of the health services at three levels – central Department, Regional Health Authority (RHA), and Area Health Authority (AHA). The Secretary of State for Social Services remained accountable to Parliament not only for the broad development of health services in England but also for their detailed functioning. However, differences in the need for health services over the country and in the existing level of provision call for local variety and flexibility in their management, and a degree of local knowledge which a central government department could not possess. Responsibility for managing the health services was delegated, therefore, as much as possible to local bodies but in such a way that the Secretary of State remained fully accountable to Parliament for their operation. Accordingly RHAs and AHAs were accountable for the performance of the functions delegated to them to the Secretary of State, who had powers to direct them on the functions which they might exercise on his or her behalf and on the manner in which they carried out these functions.

The formal structure was hierarchical but the management arrangements relied on consensus rather than direction even where formally there was a line management structure. This was reflected both in the NHS management team approach (doctor, nurse, administrator, treasurer, and works officer), and in the way that the DHSS settled national health policies. Such policies were invariably the subject of consultation both with the health authorities and other bodies including those representing the health care professions, and were normally issued as guidance to be interpreted in the light of local needs and circumstances.

THE DEPARTMENT OF HEALTH AND SOCIAL SECURITY

The Department is headed by the Secretary of State for Social Services, aided in respect of health service responsibilities by a Minister of State for Health and two Joint Parliamentary Under Secretaries of State (usually drawn from both the House of Commons and the House of Lords). Five groups of administrative Divisions within the DHSS have functions related to the NHS, as follows:

1. *The Services Development Group,* responsible for the development of national policies and priorities.
2. *The Regional Group,* responsible for the operation of the health services by health authorities, the arrangements for allocating resources to health authorities, medical supplies and industries, and medical exports.
3. *The NHS Personnel Group,* responsible for staffing policies, and pay and conditions, including the operation of family practitioner services, and the education and training of nurses, midwives, and health visitors.
4. *The Finance Group,* responsible for the overall administration of financial resources including accounting and control systems.
5. *The Administration and Support Group,* including headquarters establishment and personnel, statistics, management services, computers and research, and liaison with the media.

The staff of the DHSS includes members of the main professional groups serving in the NHS.

The functions of these five groups of Divisions include those related to the NHS, services provided direct to the public and a number of other functions not mainly related to the NHS. The main functions and services provided under these headings are:

1. NHS-related functions
   Development and explanation of policy
   Allocation of resources
   Monitoring and control
   e.g. – Financial controls (including audit)
        – Quality controls (including Health Advisory Service)
        – Information including statistics
        – Planning system
   Provision of central services for NHS
   e.g. – Building development and guidance
        – Central pay negotiations
        – Procurement
        – Advisory functions such as NHS computing; technical advice; personnel development
        – Management services
   Research and development
2. Provision of services to public
   Special hospitals
   Disablement services
3. Functions not related exclusively to the NHS
   Public health
   Medicines legislation
   International relations
   Industries and exports
   Control of abortion and inspection of private abortion clinics
   Work on smoking and health including voluntary and statutory agreements with the tobacco industry

CONTROL AND DIRECTION OF HEALTH SERVICES IN THEORY

The NHS is one of the largest users of the nation's resources. At present it spends some £12 000 millions a year in England, and receives about 88 per cent of its money from general taxation. About 9 per cent comes from the health element in the national insurance contribution, and the rest mainly from charges to patients. Therefore, the main method of control and direction lies in the allocation of resources and the monitoring of expenditure.

Allocation

Resources are distributed between hospital and community health services, Family Practitioner Services, and central services. About 70 per cent of the NHS's total money is spent on the hospital and community health services, through cash limited budgets administered by RHAs and DHAs. This has recently grown in real terms by about 1.5 per cent a year. The Family Practitioner Services – i.e. family doctors, general dental, and ophthalmic practitioners, and the drugs and appliances they prescribe – use about 20 per cent of the NHS's money for current services. They are funded so that they can meet the needs of patients as they arise. Current spending on these services has grown in real terms by 2.3 per cent a year on average. The remainder of NHS current spending is on a small group of services provided centrally. These include, support for the Health Education Council and for training of some health and personal social services staff, central grants to voluntary bodies, the provision of some welfare milk, the special hospitals at Broadmoor and elsewhere, wheelchairs, and other aids for disabled people, and the public health laboratory services.

Distribution of resources to health authorities

Present policy for public health care accepts that the most appropriate unit for direct administration of health services is a local one, the DHA. The most recent reorganization is intended to make local management stronger and more efficient. The main employers of NHS staff are the RHAs and DHAs, and to a large extent they are free to decide what mix of manpower and other resources they should use to produce the services they seek to provide, within the overall constraint of their cash limits.

The current approach to national control and direction of NHS resources seeks to balance the decentralization in decision-making by systematic monitoring, using the chain of accountability from the DHA through the RHA to the DHSS, Ministers, Government, and Parliament. It also seeks to help RHAs and DHAs improve their use of resources in various specific ways.

Once cash limits have been set for current and capital expenditure on hospital and community health services, this money is allocated by the DHSS to RHAs. Allocations are determined on the basis of a formula which broadly follows the recommendations of the Resource Allocation Working Party (RAWP) (1976). It is intended to ensure that each year's 'new' money is distributed to those parts of England whi are short of services or where the population is growing, so to secure as far as possible equal opportunity of access health care for people at equal risk. The RAWP formu means that RHAs receive different proportionate increases their cash allocations. RHAs are then responsible for t allocation of funds to DHAs, and for monitoring their use. allocating funds, RHAs and DHAs are expected to ta account of the need to remedy local shortages of services a to implement Government priorities, such as improvi services for the elderly, mentally ill and mentally handicappe and expanding community care. Where a hospital has bee built, the RHA is expected to take account of the need provide new services, manpower, and other running costs.

In addition the DHSS gives RHAs, and RHAs give DHA planning guidelines which include specific resource assum tions one year ahead *and* very broad long-term resour assumptions as a basis for strategic planning.

The money allocated to DHAs becomes their cash-limite budget, Districts in turn allocate funds to the differe services and budget holders, and this in practice determin the level of 'funded establishment' (the level to which tr budget holder for any particular function or department ca afford to recruit). It ensures, broadly speaking, that levels c staffing in each authority are within its revenue capabilitie and that future budgets are not over committed in advance b unplanned recruitment. The system also means that the fir responsibility for ensuring that services are provided and sta deployed as efficiently as possible lies with health authoriti and, within them, with managers at all levels.

Monitoring

RHAs and the DHSS have a responsibility to ensure that th resources distributed to DHAs are used effectively and i accordance with Government priorities. Spending is moni tored in a number of ways:

1. There is a fully developed *financial control system* a DHA, RHA, and DHSS levels to ensure that cash limits ar observed. The DHSS determines the RHAs' cash limits and the RHAs and DHAs are subject to their strict discipline, nov based on statute through the Health Services Act 1980.

2. During the course of the financial year, the DHS! monitors RHA spending – and RHAs monitor DH/ spending – on a cash basis through a *financial informatior system* which in turn enables the DHSS to supply informatior required by HM Treasury's financial information system.

3. DHAs are responsible for producing *strategic plan* fitting within outline RHA strategies, which look ahea about 10 years and deal with major shifts in resources an services. Examples of strategic decisions are building new acute hospitals to replace old ones and/or providing new services, and reshaping services for the elderly or mentally il or handicapped so that large isolated long-stay hospitals are gradually replaced by small local units and domiciliary and day care. Changes such as these require long-term planning to build and close hospitals and to recruit, train, and redeploy staff.

4. The RHA is responsible for pulling the DHA plans ¿ether into a *regional strategic plan*, and ensuring that this serves national priorities and is compatible with the ¡ancial, staff, and capital resources likely to be available. It ¡st also be reasonably flexible so that it can be modified if ¿ource expectations change. DHA plans may need to be ¿dified when they are brought together in this way. The ¿SS then examines RHA plans to ensure that they observe ¿tional priorities and are feasible in terms of the resources ¿ely to be available to the RHA: it considers not only overall ¿ancial constraints, but also key manpower constraints, ¿. the shortage of geriatricians. Strategic plans are discussed ¿h the RHAs, and may be modified as a result.

5. In the shorter term, DHAs are responsible for ¿oducing *operational programmes* to implement their ¿ategy, looking ahead firmly for one year and tentatively for ¿second. These short-term programmes are monitored by the ¿SS to ensure that they fulfil the strategy and are actually ¿plemented.

6. DHAs and RHAs also monitor what services are ¿ovided in order to identify deficiencies, as a starting point ¿r preparing their plans. The Department has developed a ¿mprehensive system of monitoring the *development of ¿rvices* historically looking at trends over a long period. This ¿onitoring is based on national activity and manpower ¿atistics and the health authority accounts and hospital ¿sting returns. These are drawn together to provide an ¿erall picture of how services have developed and resources ¿ve been used.

The DHSS also carries out *manpower planning*, of a ¿rategic kind, principally for doctors and for other groups of ¿aff where the NHS is a major employer. The DHSS sets the ¿rget level of intake into medical schools. It can also ¿directly influence the teaching capacity for nurses taking ¿asic nurse training courses through the central funding of ¿egional Nurse Training Committees, which administer the ¿nding of the salaries of tutors and certain running costs of ¿hools of nursing. Training for occupational therapists is ¿nded centrally but for other professional groups the main ¿le of DHSS is to provide a national overview to help local ¿ecision makers. The DHSS exercises a number of other ¿rategic controls over staff. New consultant posts (which are ¿id for by RHAs on the basis of their assessment of the ¿vailability of the resources to support them) cannot be ¿stablished without DHSS approval; and the DHSS also ¿xercises close control over the number and distribution of ¿aining posts. Where there is a national shortage new posts ¿re rationed on a basis of need. There are also direct controls ¿ver certain top management posts.

There are other specific ways in which the DHSS and ¿egions seek to direct, control and improve the use of ¿esources:

1. At the *national* level, both the Health Advisory Service, ¿hich advises on long-stay services and services for children, ¿nd the Development Team for the Mentally Handicapped, ¿rovide regular reports on services they have visited which are ¿opied to the appropriate RHA(s) and are available within the

DHSS. Staffing levels are also monitored on a regular basis by statutory auditors, who identify high-cost areas by comparison with costs in other authorities, and through periodic examination of costs under specific heads of expenditure. Through this process both excessive staffing and excessive or unwarranted use of overtime are drawn to the attention of NHS Chief Officers, and to the RHA and DHA formally by way of an Audit Report in the worst cases. The Department also promulgates good practices in the use of resources in many ways, e.g. by encouraging cost consciousness in clinical services, and by providing direct advice to the NHS.

2. *Within regions*, RHAs are responsible for ensuring that suitable information is available for line managers to set and monitor manpower levels. Where comparisons suggest that more economic and efficient use of resources may be possible the authority in question is responsible for ensuring that managers take appropriate action. RHAs provide management services such as operational research and 'organization and method (O & M)' studies. Several RHAs also issue guidelines on staffing levels (or other indicators) which managers can use in planning or reviewing their use and development of manpower locally. For example, several RHAs (e.g. Trent) have devised formulae to assess staffing requirements in particular areas, and the South East Thames RHA manpower information system produces routine manpower reports for each constituent authority, and the region follows up such matters as abnormally high overtime levels or exceptionally high proportions of staff employed in higher grades.

Alongside the services provided by the NHS are those provided by local authority social services departments. For groups such as the elderly, the disabled, the mentally ill, and the mentally handicapped, effective care requires joint planning of health and social services. To encourage provision of services across administrative barriers health authorities have since 1976–77 been given special allocations by DHSS to use on projects planned and funded jointly with local authorities. From a modest beginning of £8 million in 1976–77 the money available for 'joint finance' projects had risen to £85 million in 1982–83.

The planning and resource allocation processes of the NHS and DHSS were designed to operate on the basis of the agency relationship described above, in which most of the responsibilities are devolved to health authorities but with the chain of accountability stretching back through the Minister to Parliament and the people. These processes therefore form a most important part of the organization of the NHS and DHSS and secure the Government and legislative control and direction of health services required by Parliament.

In terms of organization and management these requirements have been summarized as follows:

1. An essential feature of the management arrangements which the Minister requires the NHS to adopt is a system of control in which performance is monitored against plans and budgets.

2. Planning systems are seen as a principal means of achieving a clear line of responsibility for the whole NHS from the Minister down to and within DHAs, with corres-

ponding accountability from DHAs back to the Ministers through the DHSS.

3. The NHS planning system is intended to provide the main management control to be exercised by the Minister and health authorities in undertaking the functions covered by the NHS legislation.

Thus the planning process provides the main means by which the requirements of the law are made explicit and can be monitored in accordance with the law.

The resource allocation process has a clear relationship to, and a very considerable influence on, the organization of the NHS and DHSS, and their planning processes. In particular, the resource allocation process provides:

1. A realistic framework in which planning options can be considered and a balance of priorities agreed.

2. A need-related baseline, showing the share of the available resource which should be consumed by a given population.

3. An important first stage in planning the provision of services for defined populations.

4. An organizational tool for the monitoring of performance.

Accordingly, the DHSS has been operating a comprehensive planning process since 1974, drawing on a Programme Budget devised by the DHSS Finance Division and a balance of care model devised by the DHSS Operational Research Service. The NHS has been operating a complementary planning process since 1976 (DHSS 1976a), and both the NHS and DHSS introduced in 1976 an improved method of resource allocation based on the recommendations contained in the Report of the Resource Allocation Working Party (1976).

But this very improvement of the planning and resource allocation processes only served to illustrate the apparent deficiencies in existing information systems in England. For example:

1. Too much information was collected and processed overall but not enough was collected on morbidity, patient flows, specialty costing, and out-patient activity.

2. Information collected for central planning purposes was not clearly related to the operational needs of the NHS: this led to duplication of information; and, more important, it encouraged local planners to ignore centrally produced information.

3. Existing systems were not flexible enough to accommodate the inevitable changes that could be foreseen; either in terms of fundamental changes in the balance of care in England, e.g. from care in institutions to support in the community; or in terms of international requirements, e.g. the need to accommodate the Ninth International Classification of Diseases.

4. Existing systems did not provide for compatibility between the main sets of activity, finance, and manpower statistics collected centrally and locally. For example, ways had to be found of relating these separate sets of, sometimes conflicting, statistics which in addition do not cover the same period of time.

5. The presentation of data needed to be much improv[ed] especially if it was to be used by non-scientific planners a[nd] policy makers. At a meeting of the Royal Statistical Soci[ety] some time ago a Professor at the London Business Sch[ool] laid the blame for this on the producers of data!

In England, therefore, the DHSS has recently embarked [on] a review of existing information systems and services in or[der] to identify areas with potential for change in the context [of] the improved systems for the management, planning, a[nd] resource allocation processes of the NHS and DHSS ([see] below).

The reorganized NHS and DHSS were designed to oper[ate] and interact with one another by means of a clearly-defin[ed] monitoring relationship to supplement the organization[al,] planning, and resource allocation relationships. In Engla[nd] the DHSS and NHS are still in the process of sorting out th[ese] ideas but it is clear that there are many aspects to this relatio[n]ship. For example:

1. The planning relationship, in which the DHSS attemp[ts] to monitor the overall performance of the NHS against th[e] agreed plans.

2. The client group and service relationship, in which t[he] DHSS attempts to monitor the performance of the NHS [in] respect of a particular health care programme, e.g. servic[es] for the mentally ill (DHSS 1971) and the mentally hand[i]capped (DHSS 1975).

3. The financial relationship, in which the DHSS attemp[ts] to monitor the performance of the NHS in terms of accoun[ts,] cost statements, and audit.

4. The organization and management relationship, [in] which the DHSS attempts to monitor the performance of t[he] NHS organization as a whole in terms of the existing legisl[a]tion.

5. The health relationship, in which the DHSS attempts [to] monitor the effects of all these measures on the levels [of] health observed in the community at large.

It also requires a systematic process of review, for examp[le] addressing itself to questions along the following lines:

1. Has adequate account been taken of national polici[es] and priorities as set out in the national guidelines?

2. To what extent do regional plans, taken togethe[r,] produce an acceptable national strategy, and how far is th[is] consistent with central government guidelines?

3. How far do NHS policies need amendment, and ho[w] far should central government press RHAs to amend the[ir] plans?

4. Are RHAs planning to move towards financial an[d] service equality between their DHAs?

5. Are RHA plans likely to be capable of achievemen[t] within financial, manpower, and other constraints within th[e] planning timescale?

6. Is there consistency between the proposals in the RH[A] plans and the known RHA capital programme and the likel[y] national availability of capital?

And, in each case the answers must be looked at from sever[al] different points of view, as follows:

1. National aggregate answer.
2. National range of variation, i.e. the range of variations tween RHAs.
3. For each of the RHAs, a regional aggregate answer.
4. For each RHA, an illustrative indication of the extremes variation.

Each answer should be related to three time points, now, dway through the strategic planning period (5–7 years ead), and the end of the planning period (10–15 years ead). This enables the DHSS to reconstruct its national licies, priorities, and resource assumptions on a more listic basis; and enables the Minister to set revised national jectives as necessary for the NHS.

ONTROL AND DIRECTION OF HEALTH SERVICES IN RACTICE

what has actually been achieved in practice? Over the past cade, successive Governments have set broad objectives for e NHS. A number of key documents have set out these jectives (DHSS 1971, 1975, 1976b, 1977, 1981). The main jectives of the hospital and community health services in cent years have been to:

1. Expand services sufficiently to keep pace with the creasing numbers of old and very old people, and to meet e demands placed on the NHS since 1978 due to the rising rthrate.
2. Develop services generally, to make use of new chnology (e.g. dialysis, hip replacement), and to reduce aiting times.
3. Reduce perinatal mortality and morbidity.
4. Improve standards of care for the mentally ill, mentally andicapped, and long-stay patients, and to care for patients the community rather than in hospital whenever possible.
5. Develop and extend preventive measures to decrease the cidence of disease (for example immunization and cervical ytology).
6. Level up services in deprived regions and districts.
7. Improve efficiency and obtain better value for money.

response, the NHS has many achievements to show for its erformance since the 1974 reorganization:

1. With the assumption of community health responsibili-es, RHAs have greatly improved the integration of hospital nd community services. There has also been much progress f integrating health services with personal social services, articularly in the case of the elderly, mentally ill, and nentally handicapped.
2. Services for the elderly, mentally ill, and mentally andicapped have been improved. In hospitals the urse:patient ratios have risen, and the balance of care has hifted towards local provision. Day and domiciliary care ave also been increased, e.g. home nursing has risen by about our per cent per annum since 1976 and day hospital attendances y about three per cent a year.
3. There has been a substantial increase in the level of ctivity in the acute sector; more than enough to keep pace vith the increasing number of old people, but still not enough

to make full use of new treatments such as hip replacement and renal dialysis.
4. Resources have been redeployed to relatively deprived regions; the most deprived region is now 6 per cent below its revenue target, while in 1977–78 the most deprived region was 11 per cent below target; and the best-off region is 12 per cent above target compared with 15 per cent above in 1977–78.
5. The new cash limits system has been introduced successfully.
6. Unit costs have in general steadied or fallen, whereas previously they were rising rapidly, in acute and maternity services. This has been achieved in the face of a rising number of elderly treated in acute hospitals.

There are, however, still serious weaknesses in the service. In particular:

1. There are still major deficiencies in care of the elderly and mentally handicapped, and long waiting lists for some specialties in some places.
2. There is still some mismatch between capital developments and the ability to finance their running costs, though this is partly due to the fact that hospitals planned in the early 1970s when growth was expected to be twice the post-1975 level, are still coming on stream.
3. The planning dialogue between the NHS and the DHSS has been devoted mainly to longer-term strategies, and there has not been enough emphasis on what should be achieved in the short term, and whether short-term plans have in fact been implemented.
4. Systematic planning and monitoring has been concerned with deployment of resources between services – by client group, the balance of care, geographical distribution – and less with efficiency; there has been a lot of work on efficiency, but it has been ad hoc.
5. The information systems have been inadequate in certain respects, such as the difficulty in relating financial and manpower information to information about activity or output, and the lateness and inaccuracy of some returns.
6. There has been an excessively long chain of command, which results in duplication of effort and diffusion of responsibility; this is being remedied from 1982–83 by the reorganization of the health services structure.

In recognition of these difficulties, the DHSS is both stepping up existing efforts to encourage efficient management and resource use in the NHS and is developing new initiatives.

Apart from the general channels of control and direction identified above, these impressive results have been achieved by the other means of general advice and exhortation through which the DHSS is able to help promote efficient ways of working in the NHS. These include:
1. Publication of building and engineering standards and cost allowances for health authorities, and advice on operating and maintenance costs.
2. Advice on catering and domestic service matters.
3. Publication of papers and reports produced by the Joint Manpower Planning and Information Working Group (MAPLIN); joint conferences at King's Fund, NHS Training Centre etc.

4. Advice, by visits of medical officers to general practitioners, on better practice organization and premises, and improved co-operation with other primary health care workers.

5. Information about central promotion and development of transferable computer systems and information technology, intended to produce economies and greater efficiency.

6. Provision of national data for use in incentive bonus schemes for maintenance craftsmen and some groups of ancillary staff.

7. Advice to the professions on ways of achieving the most efficient use of available skills.

8. Reports of working parties, research groups etc., dealing with better use of resources in many fields.

These long standing and regular ways of advising the NHS are now augmented by several new initiatives designed to help the NHS cope with the problems which still need solving.

New management structure

The establishment of a simpler and tighter management structure from April 1982, is the most important of these new initiatives. This in itself should provide a greater degree of control. The main changes in the reorganization involve:

1. Replacing the 90 Area Health Authorities comprising 199 districts with a single structure comprising 192 District Health Authorities. The number of chief officer teams has fallen from 251 to 193, reducing duplication and referral 'up the line'. Authority members are now better placed to answer for the local working of the NHS.

2. Shortening the 'chain of command' by removing the sector management level and introducing strong unit management. Management skills are focused where they are needed – in running hospital and community health services. Local problems will be settled locally. A more flexible system of pay and grading allows authorities to grade managers according to the degree of personal management responsibility in the post.

3. Altering the arrangements for providing professional advice to NHS authorities and managers, thus freeing professionals from non-essential routine and ensuring that their expertise can be used to best effect.

Regional reviews and the planning system

The maximum delegation of responsibility to health authorities must be accompanied by systematic monitoring to ensure that DHAs are properly accountable through RHAs to the Minister and to Parliament. The planning system – seen as an essential tool for monitoring the performance of health authorities in meeting Ministers' broad policy objectives and strategies for the NHS since the 1974 reorganization – has been refined considerably since it was introduced in 1976. The Government has now introduced annual Regional Reviews to strengthen the monitoring of strategic planning and to broaden it to include an assessment of overall performance. Starting in 1982, Ministers are leading a Departmental review of the long-term plans, objectives, and effectiveness of each region with

the Chairman and Chief officers of RHAs. Each Region Review will aim to:

1. Ensure that each region is using the resources allocat to it in accordance with the Government's policies, to agr with the Chairman on the progress and development whi the regions will aim to achieve in the ensuing year, and review progress against previously agreed plans and objective

2. Assess the performance of RHAs and DHAs in usi manpower and other resources effectively. Ministers will ho RHAs to account for the ways in which resources are used their regions and RHAs will in turn hold their constitue DHAs to account.

Performance indicators

A DHSS Group was set up in 1981 to explore which indicato at RHA and DHA level could be used to help assess perfo mance, with particular emphasis on the efficiency with whi resources are used. The Group proposed a range of indicato including cost per case and average length of stay, whi could be used in annual review meetings between the DHS and RHAs, and the RHAs and DHAs. Indicators drawing the work have been developed in one region and were intr duced into regional reviews in autumn 1982.

Rayner reviews

Following the success of the scrutinies of particular function operations or activities of government departments carrie out under the auspices of Lord Rayner since the prese Government took office in 1979, it is proposed to app similar techniques to the NHS. Routine administrative a managerial functions, systems and processes will be subjecte to intensive investigation starting from the initial justificatio for the continued existence of the system or function a continuing with a detailed examination of the cost-effectivene of the way in which it is carried out. Scrutinies will b conducted by senior NHS officials, perhaps operating joint with DHSS officials, and reporting direct to the appropria RHA Chairman who will in turn report to the Minister. Th advice and support of Lord Rayner and the DHSS will b made available to those responsible for conducting th scrutinies.

The NHS information system

This is undergoing fundamental review under the directio of a Steering Group chaired by Mrs E. Körner (vice-Chairma of South Western RHA). The review began in 1980. Most o the work is being undertaken by a series of working group The main objective of the review is to provide informatio which is useful to local management, including linking wher possible information on activity or output with informatio on financial and manpower resources, so that the resourc cost of activities is known. There will be a common core o information so that DHAs can be compared and informatio aggregated at Regional and National level. It is hoped tha information used locally will be more accurate and will b provided more quickly. The computerization of manpowe ata together with the implementation of the Körner Group's recommendations should have a marked effect on the provision of statistics.

NHS procurement

The Government set up the NHS Supply Council to develop policies and to introduce arrangements which would enable health authorities to make the best use of their resources. To that end the Council has already put proposals to RHAs on how the NHS supplies services should be organized in future; has urged health authorities to introduce computer-based information systems to improve their procurement decisions; has advised health authorities on the application to the NHS of the Government's policy for using public purchasing to improve the competitiveness of UK suppliers; and supported the introduction of a quality assurance scheme designed to help the NHS to purchase goods manufactured to an acceptable standard. Each of these initiatives is subject to continuing surveillance.

The Council is now focusing more on specific areas where improved value for money can be achieved. These include the identification of new purchasing arrangements which will result in savings; the development of a means of monitoring the effectiveness of the Council's policies; a review of training for supplies staff and a review of storage and distribution arrangements.

Land sales

The Government has introduced greater flexibility into the rules governing the disposal of land and property by the NHS in order to increase the efficiency and effectiveness of their estate management and to speed up the process and produce a greater return on sales for the benefit of the Exchequer and individual health authorities.

PROMOTING MORE COST-EFFECTIVE PRACTICE IN THE NATIONAL HEALTH SERVICE

Clinical practice and procedure

The DHSS, the Medical Research Council (MRC), the Royal Colleges (professional medical associations concerned with maintenance of standards), the NHS, and Universities carry out a significant programme of evaluation and research into the cost-effectiveness of clinical procedures, both of existing and new technology. According to the American 'Office of Technology Assessment' Britain actually leads the world in per caput number of clinical trials. To an increasing extent economic evaluation is built into many of these. Examples of such research sponsored by DHSS include: the breast cancer screening trials, co-ordinated at the Institute of Cancer Research; evaluation of cardiac transplantation at Papworth and Harefield Hospitals; and the multi-centre study of the cost-effectiveness of diagnostic radiology co-ordinated at the Welsh National School of Medicine. In the psychiatric field the Department sponsored the recent survey of Electric Convulsive Therapy (ECT), based at the Royal College of

Psychiatrists, which uncovered failings in some ECT departments, requiring changes in practice.

Although Britain has led the way with clinical trials, research into the economic consequences of clinical practice has been hampered by the comparative crudeness of available costing data. To help to remedy this, a method of specialty costing has been developed recently, and tested successfully in seven hospitals. An attempt is also being made to develop a practical method of patient, or disease, costing within the Financial Information Project based in the West Midlands.

It has often been said that clinicians in Britain (and, indeed, in other countries) are given few incentives to economize. Providing clinicians with better cost information alone may not lead to significant improvements in resource allocation. The DHSS is now sponsoring, via the King's Fund, a series of trials of clinical budgeting for consultants and their clinical teams. These will allow clinical managers to assume financial responsibility for the considerable resources of which they dispose.

International comparisons

It is well-known that England devotes a lower proportion of national income to health expenditure than most other industrialized countries. At present the share in this country is about 6 per cent (including private as well as public spending), compared with shares which are typically in the range 7–10 per cent in the major European and North American countries. But such aggregate comparisons say little about the comparative standards of health care between countries, as allowance needs to be made for other factors such as differences in relative costs and in the efficiency with which health services are organized.

There are a number of reasons for thinking that the NHS provides relatively good value for money. For example, as a national organization it can achieve economies in the purchase of drugs and other supplies; the building of new hospitals is planned and organized so as to avoid any duplications of expensive facilities; the strength of the primary care system, and in particular the 'gatekeeper' role of the GP, probably reduces the extent of any unnecessary hospitalization; the administrative costs of financing the NHS are very low because of the absence of insurance and reimbursement arrangements; in contrast to the more open-ended financing mechanisms commonly found elsewhere, the cash limits system provides a continuing incentive for service managers to seek efficiency savings; and the method of paying doctors and other professionals mainly by salary or capitation payments minimizes incentives for the over-provision of services such as laboratory tests and X-rays.

The impact of these various factors on standards of health care and on the health status of the population cannot easily be assessed. It is, however, worth noting that according to conventional indicators of health such as mortality rates, there is little difference between England and other leading industrialized countries, despite our lower level of health spending. For example, life expectancy at birth is somewhat lower in England than in Sweden, the Netherlands and

Denmark, but broadly the same as in France and Canada, and higher than in West Germany, Australia, and the US.

CONCLUSION

Although in theory the legislature has not chosen to provide itself with too many direct and explicit measures for the direction and control of health services in England, in practice the NHS is under reasonably tight governmental control without recourse to detailed legislation. But there can be no doubt that, if the NHS were seen to be getting out of control, Parliament would take urgent steps to arm itself with the necessary means of direction and control as it did recently in the case of cash limits (Health Services Act 1980). At present this characteristically English system operates on the basis of an unwritten constitution and relies heavily on general advice and exhortation; coupled with a carefully

conceived structure for the organization and management of health services and well-ordered systems for the planning, funding, and monitoring of the delivery of services. This reflects the general constitutional approach in England and the workings of the English democracy. But the apparent reluctance of Government and Parliament to be drawn into the development and implementation of more detailed measures of direction and control could also reflect the clear understanding of all concerned that the delivery of health services in England is far too complex a matter to be directed and controlled through legislative means. The complexity of these issues is reflected in the model presented in Fig. 13.2.

This suggests that, although attempts are being made through the delivery of health services, to affect the health status of the population in England, at present health status cannot be defined too well, e.g. Section 1(1) NHS Act 1977 (which repeats the 1946 legislation); and so far no usable

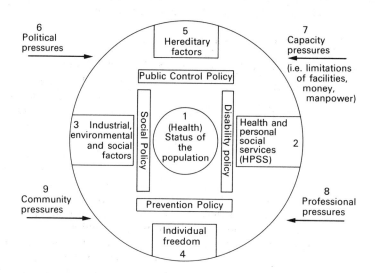

1   **Health status** – includes direct measures such as prevalence and incidence of a particular disease, or disability, functional levels of individuals or population groups, and behaviour and attitude towards health-related activities; and indirect or proxy measures such as marital status, use of health services, risk factors, and outcome from particular services or programmes

2   **HPSS** – covers the full range of policies and services as at present developed by DHSS and delivered by NHS and local authorities

3   **Industrial, environmental, and social factors** – includes health consequences flowing from policies developed by industry (presence or absence of factories), environment (the living and working environment of the population), employment (increases in unemployment and leisure), education (falling school population, redundant buildings, health education, and prevention) and Home Office (mentally disordered offenders, children, fire precautions)

4   **Individual freedom** – covers all individual aspects of human behaviour at which the prevention policy is directed, plus wider health and social issues controlled by the individual in his or her chosen environment

5   **Hereditary factors** – embrace both the inescapable consequences of human inheritance and possible control concepts, such as screening, cloning, euthanasia, abortion, etc.

6   **Political pressures** – the expressed demands of national and local politicians within the general political process as it effects the HPSS. This includes pressure from the trade unions

7   **Capacity pressures** – the limitations on change presented by the physical features and location of the HPSS estate, the money allocated to or assumed to be available for HPSS, and the manpower actually or potentially available for employment or use within the HPSS

8   **Professional pressures** – the expressed demands of the national and local professionals engaged in delivering the HPSS, within both the NHS and local government

9   **Community pressures** – the organized (Community Health Council, Parliamentary Commissioner for Administration, i.e. the Ombudsman), and spontaneous ('Campaign Against the Cuts') expression of community reaction to the existing pattern of services, or proposals for change, in the HPSS

Fig. 13.2. Limited model to assist the development of a strategy for the HPSS before the twenty-first century.

ndicators to this end have been devised, collected, or displayed. Instead, improvements in health status have been attempted by devising policies for health services, without assessing first the full significance of hereditary, industrial, environmental, and social factors, and individual freedom. In retrospect these latter sets of factors, which are in the main outside the control of the DHSS, might be judged to have a much bigger impact on health status than DHSS policies. In any event, these factors need to be taken more fully into account in devising and implementing health service policies. This could suggest a broader central strategy for health services and related activities, not only to take account of all the different factors affecting the health status of the population but also of the pressures for or against change from politicians, the professions and the community and of the capacity for change in the existing system, facilities, money, and manpower.

But the real key to success in determining approaches to the direction and control of health services in England, as describe above, lies in the careful blending of the essential interests in pursuit of a clearly defined and accepted goal. In England we have chosen to blend the contributions of the statistician, economist, and operational researcher; the doctor, the nurse, and the social worker; the treasurer and administrator; and the epidemiologist. Equally important is the blend of general disciplines: the political and policy making requirement, the academic approach, the professional discipline and the administrative action. But an overriding and invaluable requirement is a clearly stated and accepted general objective, strongly backed by central government and set against a reasonably tight deadline. There are many possible permutations in deciding on the provision of the academic approach and the professional discipline, depending upon the country and health care system in question and the desired objectives, but to make this contribution relevant and effective it must be related to the political and policy making requirement and its implementation must be secured through administrative action. In short, for any such method to be sensibly developed and successfully applied there must be multi-professional teamwork at all levels.

REFERENCES

Department of Health and Social Security (1971). *Better services for the mentally ill.* Cmnd. 4683. HMSO, London.

Department of Health and Social Security (1975). *Better services for the mentally handicapped.* Cmnd 6233. HMSO, London.

Department of Health and Social Security (1976a). *The National Health Service planning system.* HMSO, London.

Department of Health and Social Security. (1976b). *Priorities for health and personal social services in England—A consultative document.* HMSO, London.

Department of Health and Social Security (1977). *The way forward: priorities in the health and social services.* HMSO, London.

Department of Health and Social Security. (1981). *Care in action: a handbook of policies and priorities for the health and personal social services in England.* HMSO, London.

Resource Allocation Working Party (1976). *Sharing resources for health in England.* HMSO, London.

14 Governmental and legislative control and direction of health services: United States

Philip R. Lee

INTRODUCTION

Consideration of governmental and legislative control and direction of health services in the US requires an examination of the health care system and the political context within which health care policies are established. It also demands an understanding of the respective roles of government and the private sector in the planning, provision, financing, and regulation of health care. It is the purpose of this chapter to provide the context for understanding the evolution of health care policies in the US, particularly the role of federalism in those policies.

People in the US may obtain health care from a wide variety of providers, agencies, programmes, and institutions. Governmental policies and programmes play a major role in the planning, regulation, and financing of health care. The major function of governmental policy is to support services in the private sector, particularly those provided by physicians, hospitals, and nursing homes. Health workers total approximately seven million, including more than 1.5 million nurses, 450 000 physicians (Califano 1981), and more than five million workers in 150 other health service and support categories. More than six million of these people are engaged directly in providing health care services. There are approximately 7000 hospitals in the country, including non-profit community hospitals, public and proprietary hospitals admitting approximately 38 million patients and providing over 273 million days of in-patient care annually. Over 18 000 nursing homes provide care for more than 1.4 million patients, most of them elderly. There are a variety of different arrangements for ambulatory medical care including: solo practitioners and small partnerships; large and small multi-specialty and single specialty group practices, including health maintenance organizations (HMOs); community health centres, mental health centres, and public health clinics, usually subsidized by government funds; hospital out-patient clinics; emergency rooms; adult day-care centres; and a host of other arrangements.

The complicated system of health services in the US is composed of a large private sector, increasingly dependent on public subsidy or direct financing; multiple federal, state, and local government programmes and agencies; thousands of independent sector (non-profit) institutions; and over 223 million consumers threading their way through the maze. In 1969, the Secretary of Health, Education, and Welfare

Robert Finch summed up the problem faced by federal policymakers:

The tremendous proliferation of federal assistance programs over the years has resulted in a tangled net of programs which threaten to negate entirely the basic reason for most of the programs: the delivery of service. The overwhelming need today is to improve the delivery systems: to find the means of sorting out the overlapping programs and cutting through the array of technical and administrative requirements to insure that the intended services reach the intended recipients effectively and economically (Roemer *et al.* 1975).

Notwithstanding the variety of providers, the extensive array of personal health services available, and the variety of financing mechanisms, there remain basically four separate systems of health care in the US: (i) the system serving the urban and suburban upper and middle class, which is based on non-profit community and university hospitals, and private practitioners, and paid for largely by private health insurance, Medicare (for the elderly), and individuals 'out-of-pocket'; (ii) the system serving the urban poor, which is based on public hospitals, hospital out-patient clinics, emergency rooms, and community clinics, and financed largely by public funds, including Medicare, Medicaid, and local tax funds, as well as by 'out-of-pocket' payments by individuals; (iii) the system operated by the federal government serving members of the armed forces and their beneficiaries; and (iv) the system of hospitals and out-patient clinics operated by the federal government to serve veterans of the armed forces who either have service-connected disabilities or who cannot afford private care (Torrens 1980). These latter two systems are financed entirely with federal tax funds, while services for the poor are financed largely by federal, state, and local tax funds.

In 1983, with over $300 billion dollars spent annually and this vast array of programmes and providers, there remained millions of people with limited access to personal health care in the US. These are largely the working poor and those with chronic illness who do not have adequate third party insurance coverage, public or private. Although Medicare and Medicaid dramatically improved access to care of the elderly and the poor after 1965, in recent years federal, state, and local cutbacks, particularly in Medicaid, have raised doubts about the future.

Despite the many problems existing in the health care

stem, it is evident that medicine has made important contri-
utions to the health of Americans during the past 20 years.
Many factors are involved in this improvement: a dramatic
reduction in poverty between 1960 and 1978; marked changes
in behaviour related to cigarette smoking, diet, and exercise;
reduction in many environmental and occupational health
hazards; and greater access to medical care. Enactment of
Medicare and Medicaid in 1965 opened the door to more
adequate health care for millions of the aged and poor.

Improvements in health status are related to the sharp
decline in infant mortality that has occurred since the mid-
1960s, certainly due in part to Medicaid financing of care for
the poor. Declines in mortality among adults also have been
significant. Although Medicare's objectives were concerned
primarily with reducing the financial burden of health care
and assuring the elderly access to care, recent studies indicate
dramatic improvements in the health of the elderly since the
implementation of Medicare (Friedman 1976; US Department of Health and Human Services 1981; Davis 1982).
During the period from 1955 to 1967, mortality rates of aged
males increased slightly, while they declined for aged females
at an annual rate of 1 per cent. In the period from 1968 to
1977, after the enactment of Medicare, death rates for elderly
males declined at an annual rate of 1.5 per cent and for
elderly females at a rate of 2.3 per cent (US Department of
Health and Human Services 1981). These mortality declines
have been examined, and it appears that they are related to
the advent of Medicare (Drake 1978). It is also interesting to
note that declines in mortality for elderly men and women in
Canada and Europe exceeded those in the US between 1955
and 1967, but declines in the US exceeded those of Canada
and Europe between 1968 and 1977.

A number of special health programmes, such as neighbourhood health centres and maternal and infant care
projects, which were targeted to high-risk populations,
particularly poor women and their children, also contributed
to declining mortality rates among the poor. Neonatal intensive care units established in hospitals throughout the country
have played an important role in reducing infant mortality.
Intensive care units for coronary heart disease patients also
have proliferated, but their relationship to declining heart
disease mortality has not been clearly established. The federal
government, in co-operation with state and local governments, professional organizations, and community groups,
has launched a massive effort to provide appropriate care for
the 25 million or more people of all income groups with
hypertension. The results to date appear to be impressive,
with far more people receiving effective dietary and drug
treatment and an accelerated decline in mortality rates for
hypertension, which appears to be related to this national
effort. Other large-scale federal efforts, such as support for
family planning and immunization programmes, have also
contributed to improvements in health status. Growing
knowledge of the behavioural, socio-cultural, and environmental determinants of health has led policymakers in the
past 15 years to pay greater attention to the potential of
programmes for health promotion and disease prevention, in
part to affect people's health, in part because it is hoped they
can help stem the rapidly rising costs of medical care.

A POLITICAL FRAMEWORK FOR HEALTH POLICY: THE FEDERAL SYSTEM AND THE ROLE OF GOVERNMENT

Federalism is the term commonly used to describe the relationship between the US government and the 50 states. As
originally used in the US, federalism was a legal concept,
emphasizing the constitutional division of authority and
function between the national government and the states. The
concept, however, had its roots not in the US, but in ancient
Greece and in even earlier times (Hale and Palley 1981).

Federalism represents a form of governance different from
that in a unitary state, where regional and local authority
derive legally from the central government, and a confedera-
tion, in which the national government has limited authority
and does not reach individual citizens directly (Reagan and
Sanzone 1981). Federalism initially stressed the independence
of each level of government from the other and incorporated
the idea that some functions, such as foreign policy, were the
exclusive province of the central government, while others,
such as education and police protection, were the responsibility of regional units – state and local government. Both
public health and medical care were long thought to be
primarily the responsibility of state and local government and
the private sector, and responsibility for payment for health
services rested with the individual. Although the concept of
separation of functions continues today, there is greater inter-
dependence among federal, state, and local governments,
particularly with respect to such major national issues as
income maintenance (e.g. unemployment insurance), health
care, housing, transportation, and education. There is also a
growing public role in financing health care and other social
services.

Government plays a major part in planning, directing, and
financing health services in the US. Some pertinent facts
illustrate the importance of government: public programmes
pay approximately 40 per cent of the nation's personal health
care bill; most physicians and other health care personnel are
trained at public expense; almost 65 per cent of all health
research and development funds are provided by the government; and most non-profit community and university
hospitals have been built or modernized with government
subsidies. The bulk of governmental expenditures are federal,
with state and local government contributing significant but
much smaller amounts.

The enactment of Medicare and Medicaid in 1965 as
amendments to the Social Security Act represented a watershed in the role of federal and state governments in financing
and regulating personal health care. Since then, public suport
has risen from 21.6 per cent of total personal health care
expenditure to almost 40 per cent. Medicare and Medicaid
represent the largest, most important, and most expensive
federal health programme. In addition, hundreds of other
federal and state programmes affect health care. These range
from federal grants that support biomedical research in
university health science centres to local health planning
projects in communities throughout the country. Well over
100 separate federal programmes provide support for
research, training, services, or construction of health
facilities.

Although US government policies have evolved over a 200 year period, most of those affecting health services have developed since the enactment of Social Security in 1935. Many federal health programmes evolved because of failures in the private sector to provide necessary support, for example biomedical research; others arose because results of the 'free market' were grossly inequitable, for example hospital construction; and some programmes, such as Medicare and Medicaid, developed because health care was so costly that many could not afford the private option. Some federal health programmes, such as biomedical research, benefit virtually everyone, while others, such as the Indian Health Service, reach only a small but needy segment of the population. Some programmes, such as poliomyelitis immunization and health manpower development, have been effective in achieving their goals; others, such as health planning, have failed to realize even limited objectives; still others, like Medicare, have reached some goals, albeit at much higher cost than originally anticipated.

Health policies and programmes of the US government have evolved piecemeal, usually in response to needs that were not being met by the private sector or by state and local governments. The result has been a proliferation of categorical programmes that are administered by more than a dozen government departments. Over the years new programmes have been added, old ones redirected, and numerous efforts made to integrate and co-ordinate services. The functions of the public and private sectors have become increasingly interrelated, and roles are often blurred. The primary function of most government programmes has been to support or strengthen the private sector (e.g. through support of non-profit community hospital construction and reimbursement of private sector providers such as hospitals, nursing homes, and physicians) and not to develop a strong system of publicly provided health care (e.g. city and county hospitals).

It is not surprising, in view of the wide range of federal health policies, that the score card is a mixed one. The most serious problems now relate to the growing costs of health care, the variable quality of care, and the emphasis on acute and institutional care. The benefits of governmental interventions are many, particularly declining mortality rates, increased access to care, and improved quality of care.

The political context in which US health policy is debated, developed, and implemented has greatly influenced its scope and effectiveness. Most federal laws designed to affect the health of the American people, their access to health care, and the resources available for such care, reflect the public's faith in the ideology of pluralism, the strength of special interests, and the primary role accorded the private sector (Cater and Lee 1972; Alford 1975; Estes 1979). Ginzberg (1977) identified four power centres in the health care industry that influence the nature of health care and the role of government: (i) physicians; (ii) large insurance organizations; (iii) hospitals; and (iv) a highly diversified group of participants in profit-making activities within the health care arena. These groups are major actors, with governmental executives and congressional committee members, in what Cater (1972) describes as 'a new form of federalism'. He notes:

In the politics of modern America, a new form of federalism ha emerged, more relevant to the distribution of power than the ol The old federalism which ordered power according to geograph hegemonies – national, state, and local – no longer adequate describes the governing arrangement. New subgovernment arrangements have grown up, by which much of the pressir domestic business is ordered.

Health has become one of the largest and most powerf sub-governments, and the growing influence of the powe centres identified by Ginzberg (1977) is evident in goveri mental policies at the federal, state, and local levels. Medica and Medicaid policies reflect the powerful influence c physicians and hospitals, as well as their allies in the healt insurance industry. In enacting Medicare, Congress ensure that the law did not affect the physician–patient relationshir including the physician's method of billing the patient. Th system of physician reimbursement adopted by Medicare highly inflationary because it provides incentives t physicians to raise prices and to provide ancillary service: such as laboratory tests, electrocardiograms, and X-ray: Hospital reimbursement is based on costs incurred i providing care, creating strong incentives to provide mor and more services. In spite of the impact of the rising costs c the Medicare programme on the Social Security trust func Social Security taxes (on employers and employees), and th elderly, Congress has steadfastly refused to alter Medicare methods of payment to physicians and hospitals.

AN HISTORICAL FRAMEWORK: THE DEVELOPMENT O HEALTH POLICY FROM 1798 TO 1982

The evolution of health policy: dual federalism and th role of the private sector

The slow emergence of public policies and programmes relate to health and health care in the US has generally followed th pattern of other industrialized countries, particularly those i western Europe (Lee and Silver 1972). At least three stages i the process have been identified:

1. Private charity, individual contract between user an provider, and public apathy or indifference.
2. The public provision of necessary health services tha are not provided by voluntary effort and private contract.
3. The substitution of public services and financing fo private, voluntary, and charitable effort.

The changing and emerging role of government at the federal state, and local levels in health and health care evolved a changes were occurring in the health care system (Torren 1980).

With the major changes in health care that have occurre over the past 200 years, particularly the changes in the past 50 years, has come a transformation in the role of government During the early years of the republic, the federal governmen played a limited role in health care activities, which wer largely within the jurisdiction of the states and the privat sector. Private charity shouldered the responsibility of car for the poor. The federal role in providing health care bega in 1798, when Congress passed the Act for the Relief o ck and Disabled Seamen, which imposed a 20 cent per onth tax on seamen's wages for their medical care. The deral government later provided direct medical care for erchant seamen through clinics and hospitals in port cities, policy that continues to this day. The federal government so played a limited role in imposing quarantines on ships tering US ports, in order to prevent epidemics (Lee and ver 1972). It did little or nothing, however, about the read of communicable diseases within the US.

In the eighteenth and nineteenth centuries, and early in the entieth century, the major disease burdens in the US, as in urope, were infectious diseases. Tuberculosis, pneumonia, onchitis, and gastrointestinal infections were the major llers. As the sanitary revolution progressed in the nineteenth ntury, as social and economic conditions advanced, as trition improved, and as reproductive behaviour modified, e burden of acute infection declined. National health licies during the nineteenth century were limited to the position of quarantines to stop epidemics and the provision medical care to merchant seamen and members of the med forces.

The states, within the federal system, have always played a le in protecting the health of the public. Indeed, the health f every citizen is protected under the authority of state law Miller et al. 1977). States first exercised their public health thority through committees or commissions. The first state ealth department was established by Louisiana in 1855, and Massachusetts followed in 1869. Gradually other states llowed suit.

The most significant role played by state health depart-ents in personal health care was in the establishment of state ental hospitals. These first developed as a result of a reform ovement in the mid-nineteenth century led by Dorothea ix. Over the next century, state mental institutions evolved to isolated facilities for custodial care of the chronically entally ill. The development of these asylums reinforced the igma attached to mental illness and placed the care of the verely mentally ill outside the mainstream of medicine for ore than a century (Foley 1975).

Local health departments were established in some large ties even before state departments of health. Later, local ealth departments were set up in rural areas, particularly in e South, to counteract hookworm, malaria, and other fectious diseases that were widespread in the nineteenth and rly twentieth centuries. Originally, the emphasis of local ealth departments in the cities was on environmental sanita-on and epidemic diseases (Miller et al. 1981).

Hospitals began to emerge in the nineteenth century from mshouses that provided shelter for the poor. Hospital onsorship at the local level was either public (local govern-ent) or through a variety of religious, fraternal, or other ommunity groups. Thus the non-profit, community hospital as born in the eighteenth century. And these hospitals, ther than the local public hospital, were to gradually ecome the primary locus of care. The relationship of doctors American hospitals differed from that in many European ountries. Physicians provided voluntary service to care for e sick poor in order to earn the privilege of caring for their aying patients in the hospital (Silver 1976). Charity was the

major source of care for the poor. Publically provided or supported services also began to grow in the nineteenth century. Gradually, the public sector assumed responsibility for indigent care.

The Civil War brought about a dramatic change in the role of the federal government. Not only did the federal govern-ment engage in a war to preserve the union, but it began to expand its role in other ways that were to alter forever the nature of federalism in the US. The changing federal role that began with the Civil War was reflected in congressional passage of the first programme of federal aid to the states. In 1862, Congress passed the Morrill Act, which granted federal lands to each state. The profits from the sale of these lands supported public institutions of higher education, known as land grant colleges (Hale and Palley 1981). Toward the end of the nineteenth century, the federal government began to provide cash grants to states for the establishment of agricul-tural experiment stations. Although the federal role was expanding, the change had little impact on health care. One step was made, however, in the late 1870s when the Surgeon General of the Marine Hospital Service (later to become the US Public Health Service) was given congressional authoriza-tion to impose quarantines within the US. This was the first time that the federal government assumed a public health responsibility in an area where the states had previously held jurisdiction.

The next major change in the role of the federal govern-ment in health was in the regulation of foods and drugs. This occurred because of public outcry about adulteration and misbranding of foods. Initially, it was money, not health, that was the primary concern. After 20 years of debate, Congress enacted the Federal Food and Drug Act in 1906 to regulate the adulteration and misbranding of food and drugs. The law was designed primarily to protect the pocketbook of the consumer, not the consumer's health. It represented a major change in the role of the federal government, which assumed a responsibility previously exercised exclusively by the states. The legislation had some impact on fraudulent practices but far less than was hoped by its advocates. It was not until 1938, following the death of a number of children due to the use of elixir of suphonamide, that health protection became a real issue. The result of this disaster was the Food, Drug and Cosmetic Act of 1938, which required drug manu-facturers to demonstrate the safety of drugs before marketing. This was a further extension of the federal role and one consistent with the major changes in the role of the federal government that occurred during the depression of the 1930s. Following this, little change was made in drug regulation law until the Thalidomide disaster of the early 1960s. Amend-ments in the Food, Drug and Cosmetic Act in 1962 enhanced the law by specifying that drugs be effective, as well as safe. Advertising was also strictly regulated and more effective provisions included the removal of unsafe drugs from the market.

Although the federal role in health policy was limited until the 1960s, major changes occurred during the 1930s. Federal-ism in the US evolved from a pattern of dual federalism, with a limited role in domestic affairs for the federal government, to co-operative federalism, with a strong federal role in the

1930s. The Great Depression in the US brought action by the federal government to save the banks, support small business, provide direct public employment, stimulate public works, regulate banks and business, restore consumer confidence, and provide Social Security in old age. The role of the federal government was transformed in the period of a few years.

The evolution of health policy: from dual federalism to co-operative federalism

The Social Security Act of 1935 was, without doubt, the most significant domestic social programme ever enacted by Congress. This marked the real beginning of co-operative federalism. This act established the principle of federal aid to the states for public health and welfare assistance. It provided federal grants to states for maternal and child health and crippled children's services (Title V) and public health (Title VI). It also provided for cash assistance grants to the aged, the blind, and destitute families with dependent children. This cash assistance programme provided the basis for the current federal/state programme of medical care for the poor, first, as Medical Assistance for the Aged in 1960 and then as Medicaid (Title XIX of the Social Security Act) in 1965. Both programmes linked eligibility for medical care to eligibility for cash assistance. More important, however, the Social Security Act of 1935 established the Old Age, Survivors' and Disability Insurance (OASDI) programmes that were to provide the philosophical and fiscal basis for Medicare, a direct programme of federal health insurance for the aged, also enacted in 1965 (Title XVIII of the Social Security Act).

Federal concern for maternal and child health, particularly for the poor, was reflected in a temporary programme instituted during the Second World War to pay for the maternity care of wives of Army and Navy enlisted men. This means-tested programme successfully demonstrated the capacity of the federal government to administer a national health insurance programme. With the rapid demobilization after the war and opposition by organized medicine, the programme was terminated, but it was often cited by advocates of national health insurance, particularly those who accorded first priority to mothers and infants.

The introduction of the scientific method into medical research at the turn of the century and its gradual acceptance had a profound effect on national health policy and health care. The first clear impact of the growing importance of research was the establishment of the National Institutes of Health (NIH) in 1930, followed by the enactment of the National Cancer Act of 1937, and the establishment of the National Cancer Institute within the framework of NIH. There followed multiple legislative enactments after the Second World War that created the present-day institutes, primarily focused on broad classes of disease, such as heart disease, cancer, arthritis, neurological diseases, and blindness. In the 15 years immediately after the Second World War, NIH grew from a small government laboratory to the most significant biomedical research institute in the world. NIH became the principal supporter of biomedical research, surpassing industry. Indeed, federal support for biomedical research was then one of the few areas of health policy activity, because the

federal government avoided involvement in medical care for the civilian population and it did little to support the education of health professionals in the 1950s and 1960s. The influence of organized medicine was a critical factor in limiting the federal role during this period. The growth of specialization and sub-specialization, which accompanied the rapid advance in biomedical research and the application of technological advances, has been of major importance in the quality, effectiveness, and cost of care.

After the Second World War, it was evident that many of America's hospitals were woefully inadequate, and the Hill–Burton federal-state programme of hospital planning and construction was launched. This was a major federal initiative. Its initial purpose was to provide funds to states to survey hospital bed supply and develop plans to overcome the hospital shortage, particularly in rural areas. The Hill–Burton Act was amended numerous times as its initial goals were met. This legislation provided the stimulus for a massive hospital construction programme, with federal and state subsidies primarily for community, non-profit, voluntary hospitals. Public hospitals, supported largely by local tax funds to provide care for the poor, received little or no federal support until the needs of private institutions were met. The programme was a model of federal-state–private sector co-operation and a prime example of co-operative federalism. It was the major force – until enactment of Medicare and Medicaid – behind modernization of America's voluntary (non-profit) community hospital system.

During this same period, repeated attempts by President Harry S. Truman to have Congress enact a programme of national health insurance, funded through federal taxes, were thwarted, largely due to the efforts of the American Medical Association (AMA). No progress was made in extending the federal role into medical care financing.

By 1953, when the Department of Health, Education, and Welfare (now the Department of Health and Human Services) was created, the federal government's role in the nation's health care system, although limited, was firmly established. This role was designed primarily to support programmes and services in the private sector. Biomedical research, research training, and hospital construction were the major pathways for federal support. Traditional public health programmes such as those for venereal disease control, tuberculosis control, and maternal and child health, were supported at minimal levels through categorical grants to the states. Federal support for medical care was restricted to military personnel, veterans, merchant seamen, and native Americans (Indians) until 1960, when enactment of the Kerr–Mills law authorized limited federal grants to states for medical assistance for the aged. This programme proved short-lived but it highlighted the need for a far broader federal effort in medical care for the poor and the aged.

The transformation of health policies: from co-operative federalism to creative federalism (1961–69)

A number of major federal health policy developments took place between 1961 and 1969, during the presidencies of John F. Kennedy and Lyndon B. Johnson. Although federal upport was extended directly to universities, hospitals, and non-profit institutes conducting research, most federal aid in health was channelled through the states. The term 'creative federalism' was applied to policies developed during the Johnson presidency that extended the traditional federal-state relationship to include direct federal support for local governments (cities and counties), non-profit organizations, and private businesses and corporations to carry out health, education, training, social services, and community development programmes (Reagan and Sanzone 1981).

The primary means used to forward the goals of creative federalism were grants-in-aid. Over 200 grant programmes were enacted during the five years of the Johnson presidency. Among the many programmes initiated, only Medicare was directly administered by the federal government. Among the more important new laws enacted during the Johnson presidency were the Health Professions Educational Assistance Act (1963), which opened the door for direct federal aid to medical, dental, pharmacy, and other professional schools, as well as to students in these schools; the Maternal and Child Health and Mental Retardation Planning Amendments (1963), which initiated comprehensive maternal and infant care projects and centres serving the mentally retarded; the Civil Rights Act (1964), which barred racial discrimination, including segregated schools and hospitals; the Economic Opportunity Act (1964), which provided authority and funds to establish neighbourhood health centres serving low-income populations; the Social Security Amendments (1965), particularly Medicare and Medicaid, which financed medical care for the aged and the poor receiving cash assistance; the Heart Disease, Cancer and Stroke Act (1965), which launched a national attack on the major killers through regional medical programmes; the Comprehensive Health Planning and Public Health Service Amendments (1966); and the Partnership for Health Act (1967), which re-established the principle of block grants for state public health services (reversing a 30-year trend of categorical federal grants in health). This legislation created the first nationwide health planning system, which was dramatically changed in the 1970s to focus on regulation of health care as well as health planning.

The programmes of the Johnson presidency had a profound effect on inter-governmental relationships, the concept of federalism, and federal expenditures for domestic social programmes. Grant-in-aid programmes alone (this excludes Social Security and Medicare) grew from $7 billion, at the beginning of the Kennedy–Johnson presidencies in 1961, to $24 billion in 1970, at the end of that era. In the next decade the impact was to be even more dramatic, as federal grant-in-aid expenditures for these programmes grew to $82.9 billion in 1980. 'Grants-in-aid', note Reagan and Sanzone 1981), 'constitute a major social invention of our time and are the prototypical, although not statistically dominant (they now constitute over 20 per cent of domestic federal outlays) form of federal domestic involvement'.

Not only did the programme of the Johnson presidency have a profound effect on the nature and scope of the federal role in domestic social programmes, they also had an impact on health care itself. Federal funds for biomedical research

and training, health manpower development, hospital construction, health care financing, and a variety of categorical programmes were primarily designed to improve access to health care and, secondarily, to improve its quality. Fundamentally, the Kennedy–Johnson presidencies (1961–69) were a period where the agenda was one of equity (Lewis 1982).

Health policy in an era of limited resources: from creative federalism to new federalism and an expanded role for the private sector

During the 1970s, President Richard M. Nixon coined the term 'new federalism' to describe his efforts to move away from the categorical programmes of the Johnson years toward general revenue sharing – transferring federal revenues to state and local governments with as few federal strings as possible – and, later, block grants – grants to state and local governments for broad general purposes – which fall between the 'no-strings-attached' approach of general revenue sharing and the detailed restrictions characterized by categorical grants. During the Nixon and Ford presidencies (1969–77), continuing conflict raged between the executive branch and the Congress with respect to domestic social policy, including the new federalism strategy originally advocated by President Nixon. Congress strongly favoured categorical grants and was opposed to both revenue sharing and block grants. This period also experienced an erosion of trust between federal middle-management and congressional committees and subcommittees (Walker 1981).

President Nixon also differed sharply with President Johnson in his explicit support for private rather than public efforts to solve the nation's health problems. On this fundamental issue the Nixon administration made its position clear:

Preference for action in the private sector is based on the fundamentals of our political economy – capitalistic, pluralistic and competitive – as well as upon the desire to strengthen the capability of our private institutions in their effort to provide health services, to finance such services, and to produce the resources that will be needed in the years ahead (Richardson 1971).

Although the Nixon administration attempted to implement its policies of new federalism across a broad front, progress was made primarily in the fields of community development, manpower training, and social services. Categorical grant programmes in health continued to expand despite attempts by the Nixon and Ford administrations to transfer programme authority and responsibility to the states. During the period from 1965 to 1970, over 75 major pieces of health legislation were enacted by Congress, indicating continued support for the categorical approach by the federal government (US Department of Health, Education, and Welfare 1976).

Although a host of categorical health programmes proliferated in the 1960s and 1970s, the expansion of two programmes – Medicare and Medicaid – dwarfed the others. Their growth was due largely to the rapidly rising costs of medical care in the 1970s. The federal government basically bought into a system that had few cost constraining elements, and the staggering expenditures had profound effects on health policy.

The federal government's response to soaring medical care costs (and thus governmental expenditures) took a variety of forms. Federal subsidies of hospitals and other health facility construction were ended and replaced by planning and regulatory mechanisms designed to limit their growth. In the mid-1970s health manpower policies focused on specialty and geographical maldistribution of physicians rather than physician shortage, and by the late 1970s, concern was expressed about an oversupply of physicians and other health professionals (Lee *et al.* 1976). Direct subsidies to expand enrolment in health professions schools were cut back and then eliminated. Funding for biomedical research began to decline in real dollar terms when an abortive 'war on cancer' launched by President Nixon appeared to produce few concrete results and when Medicare and Medicaid pre-empted most federal health dollars.

More important than the constraints placed on resources allocated for health care were regulations instituted to slow the growth of medical care costs. Two direct actions were taken by the federal government, first, a limit on federal and state payments to hospitals and physicians under Medicare and Medicaid (included in the 1972 Social Security amendments) and, second, a period of wage and price control applied to the economy generally and continued for health care providers in the early 1970s. After wage and price controls on hospitals and physicians were lifted in 1974, costs rose rapidly.

Another regulatory initiative was designed to control costs through limiting the utilization of hospital care by Medicare and Medicaid beneficiaries. Although the original Medicare and Medicaid legislation required hospital utilization review committees, these appeared to have little effect on hospital utilization or costs. In 1972, amendments to the Social Security Act (Public Law 92-103) required the establishment of Professional Standards Review Organizations (PSROs) to review the quality and appropriateness of hospital services provided to beneficiaries of Medicare, Medicaid, and maternal and child health and crippled children programmes (paid for under authority of Title V of the Social Security Act). These organizations are composed of groups of physicians who review hospital records in order to determine if length of stay and services provided are appropriate. Results of these efforts have been mixed. In only a few areas where PSROs are in operation is there evidence that cost increases have been restrained, and in these areas it is not clear that the PSRO has been a critical factor.

An attempt was also made to control costs through major changes in the organization of health care. Efforts were made to stimulate the growth of group practice prepayment plans, which provide comprehensive services for a fixed annual fee. These capitation-based prepayment organizations were defined in federal legislation enacted in 1973 as health maintenance organizations, or HMOs. Studies have demonstrated that HMOs provide comprehensive care at significantly less cost than fee-for-service providers, primarily because of lower rates of hospitalization (Luft 1980). Predictably, the federal stimulus for development of HMOs ran up against strong resistance from organized medicine. Nevertheless, the programme successfully enhanced professional and public awareness of HMOs and assisted in the development of a number of small pre-paid group practices. However, the impact on costs at the national level was minimal by the early 1980s.

An additional regulatory initiative enacted during President Nixon's second term was the National Health Planning and Resource Development Act of 1974 (Public Law 93-641). This law incorporated some of the planning principles from the Partnership for Health Act of 1967 and the Heart Disease, Cancer and Stroke Act of 1965, both of which were terminated with the enactment of Public Law 93-641. In addition to the health planning responsibility assigned to State Health Planning and Development Agencies (SHPDAs), and local health planning agencies, Health Systems Agencies (HSAs), the law required that health care facilities obtain prior approval from the state for any expansion, in the form of a Certificate of Need (CON).

The National Health Planning and Development Act was enacted when decentralization of government authority and new federalism were primary strategies for achieving national objectives and when the role of special interests, such as organized medicine, was expanding at both federal and state levels. State and local health planning agencies created by the law resisted efforts to impose what they considered to be too much federal direction and regulation. With few exceptions local health planning agencies (Health Systems Agencies were not part of local government, but rather non-profit private agencies strongly influenced by health care providers particularly physicians and hospitals represented on their boards of directors. With their broad and ambiguous mandates, with pressure to do something about the rising costs of health care, and with their inexperienced staffs and limited resources, it is not surprising that local health planning agencies did not attach a high priority to planning for health promotion and disease prevention.

The role of local and state health planning agencies in the development of health promotion and disease prevention programmes was further limited by the regulatory role that they were required to play, particularly the approval (or disapproval) of the Certificate of Need required for new hospital and nursing home construction. It was this regulatory role, even though it apparently had little impact on total investments by hospitals (Salkever and Bice 1976), that later led to efforts to limit the authority of health planning agencies.

Although it is commonly thought that the new federalism advocated by President Ronald Reagan was a dramatic departure from past policies and trends, the roots of these policies were first evident in the comprehensive Health Planning and Public Health Service amendments enacted in 1966 during the presidency of Lyndon Johnson. They were increasingly evident in both the policy initiatives and the budgetary decisions of President Nixon and President Ford. Not only were the new federalism policies of Presidents Nixon and Ford similar to those later advocated by President Reagan but their fiscal and monetary policies also were designed to reduce the growth of federal spending and programme responsibility.

In the Carter years (1977–81) there were few new health

policy initiatives. The Carter administration tried, without success, to get Congress to enact hospital cost containment legislation. The special interests – particularly hospitals and physicians – prevailed. They were able to convince Congress that a voluntary effort would work more effectively. The rising costs of health care did moderate during the debate in Congress, but when mandatory controls were discontinued, health care costs shot up at a record rate. The picture in the late 1970s was one of frustration with the efforts to control costs. Concern about access was a secondary consideration.

In 1979, when the legislative authority for health planning was renewed, two conflicting congressional attitudes led to a three-year extension of the health planning programme with severe restrictions or elimination of some health planning authority. In the 1979 legislative hearings, an anti-regulatory, pro-competitive sentiment surfaced that was to grow in the 1980s (Budetti 1981). While the anti-regulatory sentiment prevailed in some areas, there was also a continuing move toward decentralization of existing planning and regulatory programmes, in order to provide state and local authorities with increasing responsibility. Congress was not anxious to spend more money on medical care, and the pro-competitive approach was promoted as a more effective means of cost containment than continued expansion of regulatory cost controls.

Since it is inherently difficult to make specific changes in health planning and regulatory processes that increase beneficial competition, these new provisions simply added impossible goals to the already lofty purposes identified for health planning – improving access and assuring quality of care while controlling costs. These pro-competitive, anti-regulatory, and pro-decentralization forces found full expression two years later with the enactment of the Omnibus Budget Reconciliation Act of 1981 and with efforts in 1982 to eliminate federal support for local health planning.

The Reagan administration accelerated the degree and pace of change in policy that had been developing since the early years of the Nixon presidency. Three major shifts in federal policy advanced by the Reagan administration that have directly affected health care are, first, significant reduction in federal expenditures for domestic social programmes; second, decentralization of programme authority and responsibility to the states, particularly through block grants; and third, de-regulation and greater emphasis on market forces and competition to address the problem of continuing increases in the costs of medical care. A fourth policy development of major importance, the Economic Recovery Tax Act, will have direct and indirect effects on health care – first, by reducing the fiscal capacity of the federal government to fund programmes and, second, by providing possible incentives for private philanthropy. These latter will be mediated largely through philanthropic contributions to independent sector institutions, but they cannot begin to compensate for federal revenue losses. The effects of the policy shifts are difficult to gauge, in part because of severe problems in the economy generally.

An important consequence of the block grants enacted by Congress at the urging of the Reagan administration is that the wide discretion that they provide the individual states fosters great inequities among the states. This, in turn, makes it impossible to assure uniform benefits for the same target population (for example, the aged) across jurisdictions or to maintain accountability with so many varying state approaches (Estes 1979). Because the most disadvantaged are heavily dependent on state-determined benefits, they are extremely vulnerable in this period of economic flux. These policies also have increased pressure on state and local governments to underwrite programme costs at the same time that many states, cities, and counties are under great pressure to curb expenditures.

Although the Reagan administration strongly favours de-regulation and the stimulation of competitive market forces, this has had little impact except in the health planning area. Indeed, in the Medicare programme regulations to limit hospital reimbursement and physician fees have increased.

Congress currently is considering a number of pro-competition proposals related to Medicare, Medicaid, and private health insurance. By early 1984, none of these had been enacted. Although proposals differ in detail, several elements characterize this approach. These are: (i) changes in tax treatment, for employers, employees, or both, regarding employer contributions to health insurance plans; (ii) establishment of incentives or requirements for employers to offer employees multiple choice of health insurance plans subject to certain limitations with respect to coverage of services and cost sharing, including catastrophic benefits and preventive care; and (iii) establishment of Medicare and Medicaid voucher systems under which elderly, disabled, blind, and persons eligible for Aid to Families with Dependent Children would receive a fixed value voucher that could be used toward the purchase of a qualified health insurance plan.

Although President Reagan's new federalism and pro-competition/de-regulation policies have attracted attention, it is the dramatic reduction in federal fiscal capacity due to tax cuts and high interest rates that has had the most significant effect on health services. While the federal government debates cost containment strategies, a number of states have moved to restrict expenditures for Medicaid beneficiaries because of the continued impact of the rising costs of medical care and Medicaid expenditures at the state and federal levels. Several states have enacted dramatic policy changes that restrict patients' freedom to choose providers, reduce levels of hospital and physician reimbursement, and shift the burden of care for large numbers of poor back to local government. The fiscal crisis – recession, reduced government revenue growth, and record high interest rates – will have a profound effect on health policy at all levels of government.

The politics of limited resources began to dominate the American political scene in the 1970s, and this continues into the 1980s, with little prospect of change in the near future. Controlling costs is critical at the federal and state levels. To date, policy efforts have focused more on limiting expenditures in Medicare and Medicaid than on addressing the root causes of the problem – the rising costs of medical care. The two alternative strategies – regulation and competition – have been used half-heartedly and often simultaneously.

THE FUTURE OF HEALTH POLICY: PLURALISTIC, BUREAUCRATIC, OR RADICAL CHANGE

In examining the health policy developments from 1965 to 1980, one of the nation's ablest health policy scholars, Lewis (1982), notes:

The period of the 1960s and the 1970s was the age of special-interest liberalism. What we did was denigrate government and public service to the point where we regarded them as just another special interest instead of the essential broad framework for the processes of choice and effective decisions in the public interest. It is very easy to be smart when there is a lot of money, but it is not so easy to be smart when money is tight, especially when there is no solid political framework for choice.

It is the lack of a solid political framework for choice that represents the most important barrier to addressing the issue of health care costs, their impact on government expenditures, patients' access to care, and equity. To achieve equity, some of the liberties currently accorded physicians, dentists, pharmacists, hospitals, nursing homes, and other health professionals and institutions will have to be restrained.

Pluralism is a prime characteristic of the US health care system, and it also characterizes the process by which domestic social policy decisions are made. As Lewis notes, 'Pluralism has come to mean a system of government where everybody is in charge, and nobody is in charge' (Lewis 1982). In this pluralistic system of interest group influence, government has become only another actor at the bargaining table.

Another astute analyst of health care politics, Alford (1975), has described three models or theories of the causes of existing arrangements in health care: (i) the pluralist or market perspective; (ii) the bureaucratic or planning perspective; and (iii) the institutional or class perspective. Much of the description and analysis of health care policies has been based on either the pluralist or the bureaucratic perspective. While the pluralists hold that the present system is appropriate for our time and society, the bureaucrats see a more rational planned system in which resources are effectively coordinated (as opposed to the fragmentation accepted by the pluralists) and more appropriately allocated. Perceiving the primary obstacle to rational planning and resource allocation as the professional monopoly of physicians over medical education and practice, bureaucratic reformers would basically adjust the existing system to achieve agreed upon goals, such as equity of access and cost containment.

There has been relatively little research in the US examining the class basis of health policies. Those who hold that the defects in health care are deeply rooted in the structure of a class society would radically alter the present health care system, creating a national health service, with decentralization of administration and community control over health care institutions and health professionals. Those who view the defects in health care as having a class basis do not believe that tinkering with the health care system can achieve the desired outcomes. They call for major structural changes in society.

Policy developments of the coming decades will depend on which of these views of health care politics – pluralist, bureaucratic, or class – predominates. To date, the pluralist have played the most influential role in health care politic and policies.

REFERENCES

Alford, R.R. (1975). *Health care politics; ideological and interest group barriers to reform.* University of Chicago Press.

Budetti, P. (1981). Congressional perspectives on health planning and cost containment: lessons from the 1979 debate and amendments. *J. Health Human Res. Admin.* **4**, 10.

Califano, J.A. Jr (1981). *Governing America, an insider's report from the White House and the Cabinet.* Simon and Schuster, New York.

Cater, D. (1972). An overview. In *Politics of health* (ed. D. Cater and P.R. Lee) p. 1. Medcom Press, New York.

Cater, D. and Lee, P.R. (eds.) (1972). *Politics of health.* Medcom Press, New York.

Davis, K. (1982). Medicare reconsidered. Paper presented at Duke University Medical Center, Seventh Private Sector Conference on the Financial Support of Health Care of the Indigent, Durham, North Carolina.

Drake, D.F. (1978). Does money spent on health care really improve U.S. health status? *Hospitals* **52**, 63.

Estes, C.L. (1979). *The aging enterprise.* Jossey-Bass, San Francisco.

Foley, H.A. (1975). *Community mental health legislation.* Lexington Books, Lexington.

Friedman, B. (1976). Mortality, disability, and the normative economics of Medicare. In *The role of health insurance in the health services sector* (ed. R.N. Rossett) p. 365. National Bureau of Economic Research, New York.

Ginzberg, E. (ed.) (1977). *Regionalization and health policy.* US Government Printing Office, Washington, DC.

Hale, G.E. and Palley, M.L. (1981). *The politics of federal grants.* Congressional Quarterly Press, Washington, DC.

Lee, P.R. *et al.* (1976). *Primary care in a specialized world.* Ballinger, Cambridge.

Lee, P.R. and Silver, G.A. (1972). Health planning – a view from the top with specific reference to the USA. In *International medical care* (ed. J. Fry and W.A.J. Farndale) p. 284. Medical and Technical Publishing, Oxford.

Lewis, I.J. (1982). Evolution of federal policy on access to health care, 1965–80. Presentation to New York Academy of Medicine.

Luft, H.S. (1980). *Health maintenance organizations: dimensions of performance.* Wiley Interscience, New York.

Miller, C.A., Moos, M., Kotch, J.B. *et al.* (1981). Role of local health departments in the delivery of ambulatory care. In *Role of state and local governments in relation to personal health services* (ed. S.C. Jain). Reprinted from the *Am. J. Public Health* Vol. 71.

Miller, C.A., Brooks, E.F., DeFriese, G.H. *et al.* (1977). Statutory authorizations for the work of local health departments. *Am. J. Public Health* **67**, 940.

Reagan, M.D. and Sanzone, J.G. (1981). *The new federalism.* Oxford University Press, New York.

Richardson, E.L. (1971). *Towards a comprehensive health policy in the 1970s.* Department of Health, Education, and Welfare, Washington, DC.

Roemer, R., Kramer, C., and Frink, J. (1975). *Planning urban health services: from jungle to system.* Springer, New York.

Salkever, D.S. and Bice, T.W. (1976). The impact of certificate-of-need controls on hospital investment. *Milbank Mem. Fund Q.* **54**, 185.

Silver, G.A. (1976). *A spy in the house of medicine.* Aspen Systems Corporation, Germantown.

Torrens, P.R. (1980). Overview of the health services system. In *Introduction to health services* (ed. S.J. Williams and P.R. Torrens) p. 3. Wiley, New York.

US Department of Health and Human Services (1981). *Health United States.* DHHS Publication No. PHS82-1232. US Government Printing Office, Washington, DC.

US Department of Health, Education, and Welfare (1976). *Health in America: 1776–1976.* DHEW Publication No. (HRA)76-616. US Government Printing Office, Washington, DC.

Walker, D. (1981). *Toward a functioning federalism.* Winthrop, Cambridge.

15 Health through social policy

Ellie Scrivens

INTRODUCTION

The link between policies described as social is that they all seek to improve and maintain the welfare of individuals and of society as a whole. As such, social policies reflect societal values, since they promote behaviours and consumptions that are considered to be 'good' for both the individual and society. To achieve a well-ordered society in which all individuals can obtain the maximum benefits from life, some adjustment of what appears to be the natural social order has to be made. People are born with different physical abilities, talents, and intellects. At different times of their lives they require protection from others who may inflict harm upon them through a variety of actions ranging from polluting the atmosphere to depriving them of the liberty to freely participate in society. The role of governments is to organize the disruption of the natural social ordering according to selected criteria for redistribution of resources and to protect its citizens from their own actions and from the actions of others which may put their welfare at risk.

Social policy is associated with the organization and provision of facilities and services commonly referred to as social services. The precise definition of a social service is fraught with difficulty but in general they are services which are considered basic to social and physical life, such as housing, income maintenance, education, social welfare, and community development programmes. There are numerous effects of social services upon a society and its members, many of which are upheld as conscious goals of social policy (Wilding 1976).

Wilding (1976) has identified a number of objectives of welfare or social services. The most obvious is the promotion of individual and social welfare by enhancing the life of those who are in some way disadvantaged, relative to other members of society. In doing so, social services also reduce anxiety and concerns about the future which may prey upon the minds of people. No one can predict when sickness or physical disability will strike, nor in the modern industrial world can one be assured of continued employment and income from work.

A second associated objective is that social services can provide compensation for the personal costs associated with such events as illness, unemployment, or disability. 'Our growing inability to identify and correct cause and effect in the world of social and technological change is thus one reason for the historical emergence of social welfare institutions in the West' (Titmuss 1968). Social policies have enabled the burden of social and individual misfortune to be shared by all members of society.

A third aim, which is becoming increasingly important, is the promotion of social integration and harmony, to prevent the division of communities into aggressive and prejudiced groupings, and to encourage individuals to be concerned about their neighbours and the world in which they live.

Social services redistribute resources between members of society and the majority do so on the basis of disadvantage or need. The precise organization of the means of allocating resources result in different schemes of redistribution. This can be horizontal across society, for example, from people with no children to people with children through the medium of child benefits, State-supported schools, and State-funded schemes of health care for children. Or vertically from people with large incomes to people with small incomes, or from the young to the old, through progressive tax systems with benefits allocated to dependent groups.

Because social policies have to be funded from tax revenue or other methods of persuading the general public to give up money, the policy-makers have to be sensitive to the wishes of the electorate and to dominant societal values. Traditionally, income maintenance provisions have been subservient to what is popularly known as the work ethic, resulting in pressure to maintain the amount of money given at less than the lowest level of wages. Social policies also have to balance the demands of freedom and security. Freedom to think and to act in one's personal interest can often conflict with both demands for national and personal security and the protection of the weakest and dependent workers of society. The balance is determined by political acceptability and political ideologies. These are predicated upon notions of equity, or fairness in the treatment of individuals plus beliefs about the most efficient and effective methods of achieving goals such as increased production and national efficiency. Societal values change over time, often in accordance with knowledge of factors associated with social problems. The development of social indicators has done much to influence both the direction of social policy and thoughts on preventing social problems, as the following sections of this chapter demonstrate.

Much evidence has now been accumulated to demonstrate that the factors which create human suffering and distress also affect the health and physical functioning of individuals. At its very basic level, deprivation of the basic necessities of life such as food or shelter will cause great distress and ultimately will kill. Poor housing and malnutrition will cause serious developmental retardation in children and can have a profound effect upon their physical health in childhood and adulthood. In addition deprivation is felt by some to have serious effects upon the human spirit. The motivation to succeed, compete, and participate in society is diminished.

The curious circular relationship between health and welfare is of such complexity that in many areas of social policy, arguments related to health are taken for granted. Any policy which has an impact upon individual or societal well-being can be described as social. There are, however, some which can be described as more 'social' than others in that they attempt to affect directly the welfare of members of society by meeting needs which are basic to physical and social life. Many of these aspects of life have been demonstrated to have an impact upon health and are discussed elsewhere (see Chapter 8, on war, disaster and social disorder; Volume 4, Section 3, the needs of special client groups, and Volume 3, Chapter 23, on alcoholism). Here are examined the most obvious social policies: social security; housing; education; social welfare; community development; and employment policies. A brief review of the main issues relating to each area is given, with reference to policies implemented in different western countries. The problems of particular client groups, such as the disabled, are not considered here, though for all of these policy areas special provisions are often required within the context of the general policy approach.

SOCIAL SECURITY

Incomes policies are designed primarily to help people who are unable to earn or whose income is too low to support themselves and their dependants. Lack of income is due to a number of causes such as loss or interruption of work through unemployment, disablement, maternity, retirement, or sickness. Insufficient earnings result from low wage levels or families being too large in relation to earnings.

Nineteenth century social provisions met only the basic needs of those with no income through the 'poor law' schemes and private charity, ensuring individuals obtained the minimum requirements of life, mainly through in-kind allocations. Monetary transfers were later developments, often the result of increasing numbers of claimants who placed great demands upon the limited administrative systems of the 'in-kind services'. Frequently it proved administratively cheaper and less complex to allocate money and allow people to meet their basic needs themselves. These poor-law-based transfer schemes of both cash and kind, commonly referred to as public or social assistance, are characterized by a dependence upon an investigation of means and an assessment of needs for determining the amount and nature of the allocation. As such, receipt of public assistance developed and continues to have world-wide associations with charity and a belief in the inadequacy of the recipient, creating feelings of shame and stigma.

The development of approaches to income maintenance based upon social insurance heralded dramatic innovations. Social insurance schemes, into which persons pay regular contributions provide income when earnings are lost through sickness, unemployment or retirement. On their introduction,

large sections of the population were moved both from dependence upon public assistance and, because contributions had been paid, from the associated stigma. Decisions on eligibility were automatic because they were based on formal rules rather than the discretion of the administrators of the service.

A review of different national experiences demonstrates that many differences in rationale, emphasis, and ideas for policy development can result in very different systems of provision. The first social insurance plan, introduced in 1881 in Germany, was an accident programme. It was compulsory, administratively centralized, subsidized by the State and limited to industrial manual workers. In contrast, Britain, a country with greater industrial development but a poor system of central administration (partly due to a distrust of State intervention in the lives of its citizens), created a national system of unemployment insurance and a scheme of health insurance limited to manual workers in 1911. And Sweden introduced a contributory social insurance scheme covering the whole population in 1913. This provided only insurance and did not aim for wider goals such as redistribution. In the rest of Europe, similar schemes were introduced, though administration was by semi-public funds, reducing the level of State intervention.

Politics, culture, national ideologies, and the extent of administrative structure have all influenced the way in which income maintenance policies developed in different countries. Coherent income maintenance policies have never been given priority by any country and as a consequence, most national programmes have developed in an *ad-hoc* fashion, responding to needs as they arise. Supplementary insurance programmes have tended to develop out of the initial schemes to provide care for independent groups such as the disabled, sick, widowed, and orphaned. The progress in covering these other groups has been disjointed and uncoordinated, and, in general, has resulted in a two-tier income maintenance system, of insurance schemes and public assistance. This is most apparent in the US, where for example, pensioners obtain adequate levels of income from their insurance schemes whereas the uninsured remain wholly dependent upon public assistance. In Europe, including Britain, the contribution rules have resulted in some claimants receiving very low levels of income which have to be added to by means-tested 'supplementary benefit'.

There are complex problems associated with the definition of an adequate level of income. Most public assistance programmes are based upon minimum, subsistence income levels which are calculated according to specific criteria. The subsistence levels tend to rise with the costs of living associated with the various criteria, while other income levels including those from insurance schemes fall below them. In many countries wages are not linked to costs of living and fall below this subsistence level or 'poverty line' and some individuals in work find that they would be better off out of work. Such a situation is considered anathema in the western world and attempts have been made to supplement low incomes through a variety of schemes. Britain has introduced a wage supplement, known as Family Income Supplement for low-paid workers with dependent children.

One of the results of the *ad hoc* development of income maintenance policies has been the proliferation of means tested public assistance schemes. Concentrating resources on those in specific need is often felt to be a more economic use of resources than universal increases in benefits. Because these schemes have grown in different ways and to meet different needs, potential recipients are often eligible for a host of different benefits, each subject to its own unique means test. The result is that the receipt of one benefit increases income to such a level that the amount of another benefit received is reduced or even discontinued. In addition, small amounts of earnings can push income levels over the eligibility level, thereby making it not worthwhile to seek employment, however limited. This phenomenon, known as the poverty trap, has made receipt of benefits so complex that public agencies in most countries (often social work agencies), take responsibility for guiding clients through the minefield of entitlement calculations in order to maximize their income. Interactive computer systems are being developed to help clients to welfare rights assessments.

For many of the insurance schemes, the benefits received are considered to be income and therefore are taxed. In addition, State schemes are not run on an actuarial basis. The income from the contributions does not provide the benefits. These are often dynamized to match price increases, which means that the pool of money from contributions is often less than the amount paid out. Contributions for many people are a form of taxation which cannot be increased because of the need to maintain personal income levels. Governments therefore, have to subsidize the insurance schemes from tax revenue. In consequence, governments are effectively paying out benefits with one hand and drawing back taxes on the benefits with the other, which is administratively inefficient.

Another major objective of income maintenance schemes is to achieve a form of horizontal equity, by redistributing income from those without children or other dependants to those with dependants. Children are future contributors to society and, it is argued, society should bear the cost of their upbringing. In Europe, family allowances or child-benefit programmes have been developed to ensure that families have enough money to support children adequately and to share the costs of child-support with parents.

New developments in income maintenance 'technology' have been proposed to overcome the variety of inadequacies of the present system, such as the idea of negative income tax (NIT). In this system, if a person's income exceeds a certain minimum level, he or she pays a proportion of it in tax, but if income falls below the minimum level he or she would receive a payment proportional to the shortfall between actual income and the minimum level. An adaptation of this is a social dividend scheme which guarantees a minimum weekly income to everyone and all earnings are taxed. Another variation, tax credits, was proposed in 1972 in Britain, though never implemented. Credits would be calculated for each family or lone individual. Where credits amounted to less than the tax due on income there would be a net payment of tax; where the credit exceeded the tax liability there would be a net payment from the State (Polanyi and Polanyi 1973, 1974). Sweden has also considered negative income tax as an alternative to its present system of provision.

The introduction of a negative income tax scheme would produce simplification of and economies in administration (Polanyi and Polanyi 1973, 1974). Those in receipt of benefits would not pay taxes and would receive automatically, benefits of a guaranteed level. In Britain the tax credits scheme was rejected because the problems of implementing the scheme appeared too great. The proposed scheme only covered those who were currently earning wages and, thus, excluded those on public assistance, who would derive most benefit from the scheme. To keep the scheme administratively simple it was felt necessary to have only one level of tax and one level of credits irrespective of income. Tax credits large enough to raise the poor over the poverty line would therefore have to be awarded to everyone, which would benefit the rich and the poor equally and so not reduce income differentials. Universal allocations of tax credits would also be very costly. A progressive tax rate would be the only solution, but this would not have achieved the desired simplification of the administration of the tax system. The ultimate flaw of any negative income tax system is that it subsidizes low incomes and does not therefore place pressure on employers to pay better wages. In fact, it could be argued that it would encourage employers to pay wages at below subsistence levels in the knowledge that employees would be helped by the State.

Germany and Britain have both decided to improve untaxed child benefits and eliminate tax exemptions for children, thereby increasing the income of all families but removing the advantages of tax exemptions to the highly paid. This helps to alleviate some of the immediate problems of the low paid and families with no earnings but does not fully achieve the objective of guaranteed levels of income, as of right, for all members of society.

EDUCATION

Education is an important facet of welfare in society, enabling children to grow into informed literate adults who can actively and intelligently participate in society. It generally absorbs the highest percentage of public expenditure after social security. The rationale for government intervention is that education can help individuals to cope with the difficulties of modern life, and trains them to become experts in certain technological areas which contribute to the functioning of society.

A wide variety of organizational systems for schooling have developed in different countries which it is not necessary to discuss here. There are, however, a number of fundamental questions to which any policy has to address itself. Education can achieve a number of goals: it can give children a minimum level of learning; it can enable society to have a mixed balance of scientists, artists and technocrats which are necessary for industrial development; and finally, and most importantly, it can reinforce religious, secular or societal values in future generations.

Education policies have to balance the promotion of individual freedom of thought and societal values. 'Drawing a line between providing for the common social values on the one hand, and indoctrination inhibiting freedom of thought and belief on the other is another of those vague boundaries that it is easier to mention than to define' (Friedman 1963). Social stability requires that children are well integrated into mmunity life, aspiring to common goals and values, and minimizing racial and class tensions which can lead to social disruption. The differentiation of a community into different groups which are prejudiced against others can lead to discrimination and inequalities felt to constitute social disorder. On the other hand, to indoctrinate children with a particular view of life, especially in societies with mixed nationalities can lead to a loss of cultural continuity and a breakdown of inherited traditions which are also felt to be important for individual and community development.

Schooling in most countries is provided through a mixture of privately and State-funded schools. The Labour party in Britain has argued that this results in a social division between the rich and the poor and they introduced policies to remove subsidies to private schooling. Britain also had a system of State schooling (up to the 1970s) which attempted to meet the educational needs of different children by providing academic and technical training in different schools from the age of 11 years onwards. The result was that the more academically able children were segregated from their less able peers, a phenomenon felt by some to be socially divisive. Policies for comprehensive or integrated schooling were introduced to prevent the separation of children into different groups on the basis of academic ability, which are being questioned by the present (1984), Conservative Government.

The area of education exemplifies a major policy problem. How can poorer members of society be helped to compete equally with those who are better off, whilst at the same time allowing freedom to parents and children to choose the value systems and organizations in which children will be educated.

A number of policy models exist using State-provided schools, private schools or a combination of the two. Alternatively there could be a free market in education, leaving any decisions concerning the quality and the amount of schooling within the education sector. A different approach is to introduce legislation to make formal education compulsory for children within a specified age range. For low-income parents, however, who could not afford education, a supplementary system of free education would have to exist. A third option is the combination of compulsory but free-market education with consumer subsidies in the form of cash grants. A fourth solution is based on vouchers.

There are two schools of thought concerning vouchers – one supports unrestricted vouchers and the other restricted. Unrestricted vouchers effectively give cash grants to parents which would allow them money to spend on the education of their choice for their children. Richer parents could top up the value of the voucher if they so wished and purchase a greater amount of and/or more expensive education. The voucher allows low-income families to choose the school to which they wish to send their children, from any schools that are within this price range. Because the voucher has a set value, the parents cannot spend less than the voucher value on education (La Noue 1972).

Restricted vouchers cannot be topped up by rich parents. The objective of restricted vouchers is not to give parents a minimum amount of money to spend but to promote equal access to educational establishments of the family's choice. Parents could compete equally with each other for the schooling of their choice. Bad schools would have few pupils and would be forced to improve their teaching or close down.

Education voucher schemes have been tried in the US – one of the most well-known being conducted in Alum Rock in California (Wolf 1974). The parents of each school-aged child received a voucher valued at the cost of the child's schooling for twelve months. The voucher was handed over to the school of the parents' choice, and the school then redeemed the value of the voucher from the local education authority, leaving the school free to spend the money as it chose. The proponents of this scheme identify a number of advantages. Schools should be able to respond easily and quickly to the demands for meeting particular and different needs. More importantly, interested parents can get together to support a school and get more involved in their children's education.

The critics point out that there are a number of unproven and possibly erroneous assumptions in this argument. One assumption is that parents are as concerned as the government to give their children a good education. It also assumes that schools will respond to parents' demands for education.

The Alum Rock scheme is described as a 'regulated compensatory model' to safeguard against segregation and discrimination. Because supplementation of the voucher value is prohibited, low-income families have their vouchers revalued upwardly to make them worth more. The increased value of the vouchers makes the child from a poor family more desirable to the school because he or she brings more income to the school than children from richer families. The funds follow the child to a school of his or her parents' choice rather than going to a particular school or district. A further elaboration of this scheme, a taxable voucher has been proposed. If progressive taxation rates were applied to the voucher, the wealthy would have a reduced net benefit from the voucher.

UNEMPLOYMENT

Levels of unemployment are growing in the western economies and are causing concern to economic and social policy makers. Not only is there a decrease in production, but there is a loss of spending power amongst the unemployed. A recent phenomenon causing great concern to governments is the increase in youth unemployment. Social policy makers have emphasized the damaging effects of boredom not only because the individual's health and general well-being may be affected, but also because it may lead to social disruption. 'Is there not a danger that young people may undermine the stability of institutions, question the permanence of values, the continuation of the existing social and economic order?' (Montilibert 1979).

For a variety of different reasons therefore, unemployment is seen as a social problem and attempts have been made to reduce levels of unemployment. There are, however, a number of different views about the nature of unemployment, its causes and its cures. It is almost universally accepted that any country will permanently have some minimum level of unemployment which is allowed for in calculations of 'full employment' levels. The British White Paper on Employment Policy of 1944 accepted that 3 per cent of the working population would be unemployed at any one time though for individuals the situation would be temporary whilst they sought new jobs. Such unemployment is referred to as frictional, and is an unavoidable aspect of the functioning of industrial economies. Indeed, it may be acceptable to an innovative society – provided that provisions are made to retrain those affected by technological developments. Unemployment which is generated by decreases in the demand for particular commodities, however, tends to have much more devastating effects for both the individual and a nation. Unemployment is longer-term for individuals because in the main those who became unemployed have skills which are becoming increasingly redundant.

Criticisms of existing social policies in relation to unemployment have been many. Schools are blamed for inappropriately equipping children for the job market; women are blamed for not freeing jobs for men and youngsters; and the unemployed are accused of a reluctance to move in order to look for jobs. Blame has been liberally apportioned to many factors but relatively little progress has been made in policy development to arrest the growth of unemployment. The most progress is in the area of combating youth unemployment where governments have devised measures to help school leavers to find employment.

Essentially there are only three existing approaches to reduce unemployment. The first is to stimulate economic activity, though the best means of achieving this has not yet become clear. The second is to adjust the supply of and demand for skilled labour by introducing educational and vocational guidance services better suited to equip workers for the modern job market – this of course pre-supposes that new jobs will be available. Training and apprenticeship systems and retraining schemes are being developed. These, however, are dependent upon systems which will yield accurate knowledge and forecasting of labour market trends and these are not yet well developed. Various countries have adopted different approaches to introducing retraining and training courses. Belgium has established new centres and pays allowances to students whilst training. In the UK emphasis has been placed upon training unskilled workers through government-sponsored courses. Ireland has increased the amount of funds awarded to vocational training centres. France has also extended the number of places available on training courses but has in addition introduced a number of innovatory fiscal policies to encourage employment, such as payment by the State of employers' social security contributions.

A major policy problem has been to decide whether jobs and training are better promoted through the private or public sector. Britain has tended to emphasize the role of the State in retraining and manpower planning, whereas France, for example, has tended to encourage private industry through government grants to take responsibility for training and job creation.

The third approach is to create jobs in both economic and non-economic sectors, and to protect and change existing working conditions. A host of measures were introduced in approximately 1977 in most European countries. Belgium, France, and the UK have made it possible for people to retire before the customary retirement age; France and West Germany have introduced legislation to restrict immigration;

Italy, France, and the UK have created schemes to subsid firms to create jobs for young people; and Belgium and the U have introduced community work for unemployed youngste

Many of the jobs, such as temporary work schemes Britain, are 'artificially' created and do not result from demand for increased supply of labour. They are tempora social expedients which enable people, particularly the you to gain experience in employment rather than actually creati bona fide employment. The underlying philosophy of su programmes is that it is preferable to use an otherw unemployed workforce to undertake socially useful tasks th to merely subsidize the essential needs of the unemployed. T jobs so created often include cleaning and repairing pub monuments and other public works, helping the elderly and handicapped, and providing auxiliary support in education a health care systems.

No country has yet developed a co-ordinated comprehensi plan of action to combat rising levels of unemployment. T main emphasis of policies appears to be upon increasing a adjusting the level of skills in a population to the range qualifications required by the job market, thus enabling tho who wish to work to do so. This approach does assume th jobs are available for those who are properly trained which yet to be proven correct. Alternative proposals include forcib reducing employment levels by measures such as loweri retirement age, raising school leaving age, reducing the leng of the working week and increasing holidays. A more extrer view claims that if employment were given less social value, t stresses of unemployment and the consequent devaluation the individual would be minimized. Leisure should promoted rather than the artificial creation of jobs which ha little intrinsic worth.

HOUSING

There are two broad approaches that governments can ado towards intervention in the provision of housing. The fir described as comprehensive, is aimed at planning a controlling the total volume of building within the nation economy. The second is directed towards bolstering the priva housing market to supplement any shortfall that might occ if private builders were left to determine the volume of hou building. Comprehensive policies therefore attempt calculate and meet the housing needs of a nation where supplementary policies rely on private industry to provide f most of the population and merely concentrate on ensuri that any deficit is made up by the government. The physic destruction of the Second World War was a major incentive f European countries to develop housing policies. Many we faced with the urgent necessity of rebuilding their towns. Ev neutral countries such as Sweden had fallen behind in hou construction during the war and had to make up the shorta which had occurred (Marshall 1975).

Comprehensive planning was adopted by a number European governments such as France, Germany, a Sweden, but all developed very different policies towards hou building. In Sweden and Norway home construction is th responsibility of semi-public bodies which cover a variety terest groups, from semi-public utility companies to housing associations. The majority are non-profit organizations in receipt of large government subsidies. The government, which controls the allocation of the major part of resources used for construction, gave preference to the builders who worked for non-profit housing organizations and reduced speculative private ventures. In addition, the timing, volume, and location of all residential accommodation is determined by the government. France, in keeping with her national aversion to overt state intervention has almost no direct government building programmes, though the government maintains its traditional tutelary function in this field and has influence over the construction industry. France has tended towards a system of independent housing co-operatives which construct semi-public units of housing, the most well known being the *Habitations à Loyer Modéré* (HLMs), financed through government subsidies.

Whether a government adopts a comprehensive or a supplementary policy for housing, it also has to decide whether housing provided from public funds is intended to meet the needs of the low-income groups. Britain and the US, which both adopted supplementary housing programmes, have trodden very different paths in tackling this question. Public housing in Britain was never intended to be a part of the public assistance programme for low-income families. Eligibility for housing is not means tested, though because of the relative scarcity of public housing, priority for housing is determined by criteria of need such as homelessness or having dependant children. The amount of rent paid, however, is related to the income of the tenant; rent and rate rebate provisions are now firmly entrenched.

Housing is the one area of British social policy which has demonstrated a complete ideological divide between past governments. Conservative governments have been committed to the ideal of private property ownership and have introduced policies to promote home ownership by selling off public housing to tenants. Labour governments have viewed public housing as the most appropriate solution to shortages and have been committed to public ownership as a means of controlling the welfare of their tenants.

In contrast, public housing programmes in the US have developed into assistance for low-income families. The depression of the 1930s created the impetus for public housing programmes. Post-war policies required housing programmes to offer accommodation at reduced rents to low-income families. As many poor families moved into these houses, the better-off families moved elsewhere and by association it is claimed the projects become stigmatized as housing for the poor, a highly unsatisfactory situation that may lead to 'ghetto' developments and a disintegration of local communities.

In Europe, the post-war housing shortages threatened to force up home prices and rents so sharply that large proportions of the population were in imminent danger of being thrust into great economic hardship. Rent controls were introduced in many countries, limiting the amount of rent that landlords could charge, whether public or private. One effect of rent controls is that families tend to stay in accommodation because with fixed rents and rising incomes they are increasingly better off. A traditional assumption underlying housing policies is that enlarging the total stock of housing will ultimately benefit the entire population. Even if the immediate beneficiaries are those who can afford to rent or purchase new homes, an increase in the number of accommodation units available will release housing for the less well off. Thus all housing policies are dependent upon tenants moving on as their incomes rise and their children grow up, thereby freeing accommodation for those newly in 'need', such as newly-weds and those with young children and low incomes. When tenant populations become static, the fluidity of the housing market decreases and the desired redistribution of accommodation does not occur.

There are in general too few houses to meet needs. Houses are fixed and cannot be moved when vacant whilst occupants are increasingly mobile. Homes take a long time to build and therefore the supply of and demand for homes is difficult to match. Poor-quality housing can have serious physical and mental effects on health and so governments often attempt to control not only the supply but also the quality of housing. However, unlike, for example, air pollution, it is not possible to set international standards for housing. 'There are no absolute standards for housing, and it is impossible to develop such standards. For one thing, the specific requirements which need to be met in order to safeguard health and to assure a given standard of comfort will be determined according to local customs and local states and social conscience.' (International Labour Office 1948).

Though the requirements for housing may differ from nation to nation, certain types of design have a harmful effect upon populations. A popular form of public housing during the two decades after the Second World War was high-rise apartment blocks. In the later 1950s and the 1960s US housing officials became aware that high-rise apartments were associated with social problems. In Europe this has not been so readily accepted though the popularity of tall apartment blocks has greatly declined. Greater concern has been shown in Europe over the ugliness of many buildings constructed in the 1960s and the resulting unattractive environment in which communities have been forced to live. Concern has also been generated about the size of new housing developments. Often planners were so keen to house populations that the dynamics of local communities were forgotten. France and Britain, during the 1960s produced a large number of suburban towns which developed many social problems including boredom, loneliness, violence, and discontent among their tenants. In recognition of this, France limited all housing projects in 1973 to a maximum of 2000 units in all communities over 50 000 people.

The alternative to subsidizing housing construction is to subsidize the consumers of housing. In Europe, where rapidly increasing costs of housing have their most serious impact upon low-income families, housing policies have tended to concentrate on those in greatest need. Since 1967 Sweden has moved towards a policy of replacing the interest rate subsidy to housing starts with a housing allowance specially directed towards low-income families. France has similarly introduced housing allowances to integrate low-income families with richer families in the HLMs. The allowances make up the difference between the charged rent and a fair rent calculated from the income level of the family.

In Britain, help is given to individuals and families in receipt of public assistance, the amount of rent payed being incorporated into the calculation of benefit received. A universal housing allowance, along the lines of a negative income tax, which would be subject to taxation was considered in 1977 and rejected as administratively too complex.

A final option is the introduction of a housing voucher. This has been experimented with in Australia to fund low-income housing consumers (Katz and Jackson 1978). Vouchers to be spent specifically on housing act as a form of housing allowance similar to that found in France, but allow great flexibility for consumers to purchase forms of housing other than public-assisted housing.

Community development and participation

Increased urbanization is experienced by all post-industrial societies. The problems of urban dwelling, such as over-crowding, physical decay and poor housing are experienced throughout the western world. Since the mid-1960s techno-logical change has created economically depressed and deprived areas to appear in both inner cities and in some more rural areas highly dependent upon specialized local industries such as mining or car production.

During the 1960s there was a growing international realization that policy makers were not dealing solely with individual delinquents, clients, or patients, but with local communities and the neighbourhood environment in which they lived. The development of social indicators exposed the problems associated with deprived environments. British social policy prescriptions became dominated by thoughts of community policies and neighbourhood development plans in an attempt to revitalize demoralized and decaying communities. Calls were made for educational priority areas in primary school education to concentrate resources on deprived communities (the Plowden report – Department of Education and Science 1967), comprehensive attacks on poor housing (Department of the Environment, 1965), the concentration of resources on areas of special need (Seebohm Report – DHSS 1968), and the redistribution of health services resources to areas of need (DHSS 1976).

'Neighbourhood', 'priority area' and 'community' have become well worn in the vocabulary of debate about social policies. Thus it was that town planners (who had been talking about neighbour-hoods and communities since the days of their founding fathers who tried to build Utopias in the eighteenth and nineteenth centuries) met the social policy makers coming from the opposite direction (people now rediscovering the community and the spatial aspects of the problems they had for so long contended with in a spatial fashion) (Donnison 1980).

Britain has tried a number of policy approaches to revitalizing communities the most notable of which were the Community Development Projects (CDPs) of the 1970s. These are described by Donnison (1980) as twelve Home Office funded projects, employing people with experience of social planning and research, and social work based in a variety of types of deprived neighbourhoods. The main aim of these projects was to study the needs of these areas and to assist the local public services to

devise more effective social programmes. In addition the p jects were intended to enable local people to enter into lo decision-making, to become more aware of their perso abilities and the resources within their communities, and innovate improvements in their environments and their soc lives.

The CDP workers did manage to emulate other urb development schemes by introducing nursery schools, host for the homeless, and other such well-tried remedies. Howeve they did not succeed in motivating the local people into acti or changing their deprived environments. The neighbourhoo were suffering from economic decay mainly due to the decli of certain industries which formed the *raison d'etre* of t communities.

The present popular theories postulate that the revitalizatio of communities can be achieved through participation by th members – a currently used phrase is self-determination which will increase personal and neighbourhood self-esteem. appears, however, that the ability to encourage participation a function of the organization of local government processe

Decision-making in the US is pluralistic, shared by a wi range of boards, commissions, and agencies. The local counc are highly political and rarely reach policy decisions until t large number of local interest groups have fought and wo battles on issues amongst themselves. The policy-making pr cess therefore tends to be very open, with public hearings allow community members to express their opinions. One co sequence of this, or perhaps one of the factors which cause this form of decision-making, is that private interests tend dominate policy decisions. The collective or public good oft takes a back seat compared to the wishes of powerful pressu groups. In European countries, collectivist approaches policies have been more apparent, and these are reflected in t decision-making structure.

In Britain, local government is carried out by committees elected members. The councils take responsibility for almost a the functions of local government, including the majority social policy-making, with the notable exceptions of t National Health Service (NHS) and the income maintenanc systems. Public consultation is limited and usually occurs whe pressure groups, given prior warning of decisions, demand a open hearing. Sweden has a similar system of local governme with executive functions carried out by a cabinet of counc members who are selected by the council to steer its work Unlike Britain, the full time administrative posts are filled on partizan basis, and therefore reflect to some degree the politic constitution of the council. In Sweden, however, nearly a local policy conflicts are dealt with by official and expe decision-makers and tend to be dominated by technic considerations rather than local pressure groups which ar almost absent in Swedish local policies.

Sweden and West Germany for example, are now faced wit growing demands from the local population for increase participation. In contrast the Netherlands has already achieve a very high level of community participation which has bee actively pursued by the Government. Community workers ar employed by central government to encourage the develop ment of local interest groups.

The British answer to eliminating pockets of deprivatio

as been to call for increased personal and community self-
determination. The population, however, seems so accus-
tomed to passive receipt of collective decision-making by local
government, it is difficult to motivate. Though community
action can identify needs which are not obvious to political
institutions and can encourage an understanding of the
community structure in its members, many commentators now
believe that such action will do relatively little to help individual
citizens improve their personal conditions. Research by
Donnison and Sota (Donnison 1980) has shown that manual
workers who live in areas where there has been investment and
industrial development are less likely to become unemployed,
more likely to have a car, and more likely to live in areas with
plenty of public housing. Not surprisingly, economic
prosperity and urban growth generally benefit everyone but
especially manual and unskilled workers. 'Growth, prosperity,
for vulnerable people, and a movement towards greater
equality can, therefore be achieved together' (Donnison 1980).
Donnison, however, issues the following note of caution –
untramelled economic growth will not necessarily achieve
automatic improvement in conditions for everyone. Social
policies are required to achieve an equitable distribution of
resources and to protect the more vulnerable groups of
society.

Economic growth in the present world recession seems highly
unlikely. The search for ways of improving the redistribution
of societal resources between members of society must
continue. The idea of 'spatial' policies, however, does indicate
that the limited social services objectives of social policy are not
enough on their own. Regional and area dimensions to redistribution and self-determination are required. New 'techniques'
for local government need to be developed. Population
referenda are one solution – others may be possible.

SOCIAL CARE

All western nations have evolved systems of social care to help
resolve problems faced by individuals in coping with the
pressures and strains of modern life (Brown 1974). At its most
simplistic, social care is deemed necessary for people who
cannot look after themselves for some reason or lack the
essential social support provided by families and local communities. The need for social care comes from many different
causes. Children require care if their parents do not provide a
standard of care deemed necessary by society. The frail elderly,
the disabled, and the mentally ill and handicapped often cannot
survive in an environment designed for self-sufficient individuals. One-parent families and families living on poverty line
incomes often find the struggle to make ends meet, and coping
with the stresses of the way of life imposed upon them, a great
strain. The unemployed can face boredom and feelings of
inadequacy generated in a society where work is a highly valued
activity. For some people, life-changes such as marriage,
divorce, bereavement, or retirement can prove traumatic
experiences through which care and support is required. If the
social structure of family and community life is inadequate to
provide support, help must come from other sources.

The causes of such human suffering are disparate and often
unconnected, but they all reflect an inadequate functioning of
human support systems. In the past the need for social care was
felt to be the product of individual failing, and policy
emphasized the need for treatment and control. Social inadequacy often results in poverty, and the traditional response was
to meet the immediate needs of life, shelter, food, and
clothing, by placing people in institutions. As research into the
causes of social inadequacy and dependency has progressed, it
has become apparent that factors external to the individual can
contribute to a breakdown in social functioning. This has
created a change in the way in which social problems are
viewed and treated.

A classic example is the treatment of parental child abuse.
Relationships between non-accidental injury to infants by
parents and having too many children too closely spaced has
been observed. Baby battering is more common amongst
(teenage) mothers with premature babies. The attitude of
policy makers is now one of helping families to overcome the
problems which cause a breakdown of 'normal' parent–child
relationships rather than punishing the parents for their
abnormal behaviour (Court 1973).

The importance attached to interpersonal relationships,
especially, within the family is reflected in many policies of
social care. The prevention of breakdown of and the
promotion of ties within the family are actively pursued, and
reflect the current world-wide trend of decreasing the amount
of institutional care which is provided. Where possible,
children from inadequate (however defined) homes, are
placed in environments where surrogate parental care is
available if their parents find coping with them too difficult.
This may be an institution but the preference expressed in many
recent policy decisions is for foster care where children can
experience a near normal family life.

The needs for social care are politically highly controversial
because they are tied so firmly to the basic values of a society.
The post-war emphasis on the family as the fundamental unit
of society has tended to focus policies on the problems of
preventing family and community disintegration. A British
report on personal social services (DHSS 1968) identified two
approaches to the prevention of human suffering and family
breakup. First there should be services orientated to meeting
the specific needs of individuals who are at risk of suffering.
These services should help in two ways. First by enabling people
to make the best of life in the face of their particular disabilities
or difficulties: offering support in crises; preventing isolation
and boredom; and ultimately rehabilitation or adjustment to
circumstances which cannot be changed. This includes: the
provision of aids, recreation centres, day care, domiciliary
services and physical therapy to the disabled and the elderly;
advice and support to single-parent families and families with
special problems; and ensuring that income allowances and
other provisions which are available to such people are received
and used.

The second approach is for more general community wide
policies, as discussed in the previous section, to enable communities to develop in ways which will promote the desired
social values and encourage all members of a community to be
interested in the welfare of their neighbours and their physical
and social environment. Integration of people into their local
communities and participation in the world around them are

believed to be the only means of creating social harmony, and hence destroying social tensions which create violence and the breakdown of interpersonal relationships, leading to disintegration of families and individual isolation.

The services designed to meet specific needs have moved from an emphasis on treatment towards prevention, attempting to identify those at risk of falling into situations which will create stress and suffering. Because of the breakdown of the essential community support systems, the role of 'filling the gap' that now exists and attempting to recreate communities has fallen to formal organizations, who employ social workers trained specifically to undertake the tasks. In Britain the majority of social workers are employed in local government departments which also provide many other forms of social care such as meals-on-wheels, home helps, day centres, residential care, aids for the disabled, and advice on how and where to get financial and other forms of help. Some social workers (probation officers) are employed to help people found guilty of criminal behaviour and a relatively small number are employed by voluntary organizations. Because social workers are employed by local government they have been described as 'agents of social control', whose main purpose is to maintain social order and to perpetuate certain social values. In contrast, in many European countries social workers are more frequently employed by non-profit, independent organizations which are felt to reflect community ideals and values more than those of the government and the national policy makers.

As with housing policies, social welfare policies have tended to concentrate upon the poor because they suffer from the most serious effects of social problems. A major division of opinion has occurred between social policies in relation to the causes of social problems. In Britain, there is a tendency to assume that the socially inadequate drift down the income groups. Their problems cause their poverty rather than poverty causes their problems. Thus, any preventive social care should be directed, not at the poor but at anyone who is at risk of falling into specified social difficulties. The Seebohm report (DHSS 1968) outlined a scheme for social welfare services which would be accessible by and useful to all members of society. All individuals are at risk of stress caused by life changes such as marriage, childbirth, divorce, and retirement. As a consequence these services should help all those who suffer from life-changes, and identify those people who are especially at risk. Income maintenance provisions, handled by central government are kept completely separate from the social welfare services (Hill and Laing 1979).

In contrast, many European countries, for example France and Belgium, have adopted the view that poverty causes social problems. The semi-public funds which deal with social insurance and the public assistance offices employ social workers who offer advice and help to clients at the same time that they receive financial aid. Much advice is given concerning budgeting and the purchase of necessary commodities and goods. In France, the socio-medical aspects of care are so tied into the social welfare system that, for example, the receipt of maternity and family allowances are contingent upon mothers receiving ante- and postnatal checkups.

CONCLUSION

Owing to the deteriorating world-wide economic situation many countries are facing difficulties in achieving wide social objectives. Policies are tending to concentrate on deprived selected groups in the population such as the elderly, the disabled, and the disorganized family. The main groups at risk of poor health and low quality of life are those who have low incomes and live in poor environments and those who have little chance to improve their situation on their own.

The twentieth century has seen a dramatic change in attitudes towards the poor and the disadvantaged. Many social problems experienced by these groups are now believed to be caused by factors external to the individual though the precise causes of a large number of social problems and diseases are unknown. In general, evidence of external factors affecting individual behaviour is very limited and social policies tend to place responsibility for changing behaviour damaging to health and welfare upon the individual. Evidence does indicate a relationship between certain social problems, for example child abuse as described above, and external factors. In such cases policies have tended to move towards amelioration of the effects of social factors which place the individual at risk of developing behaviours which may be destructive to himself or to others. To use a more health-related example, policies towards cigarette smoking are now broadening from health education and include punitive fiscal measures to deter people from buying cigarettes and towards finding ways of producing cigarettes less harmful to health by reducing, for example, the tar content.

A social service provided to meet a particular need or to prevent a specific problem, should be used by all those for whom it is intended. Services which are provided for every member of the population and used by all, are most desirable because no individual can be identified as different or stigmatized by receiving what may appear to be charity. To provide services universally is very expensive and can conflict seriously with the view that the individual should be free to choose the nature and the form of the service he or she receives. To ensure that the worst-off in any context receive an adequate amount of help requires that the services are provided at a level high enough to achieve the objectives of the provision. For example, universal flat-rate monetary benefits which are high enough to achieve an acceptable standard of living for those with no income of their own would cost a government an enormous amount of money. A negative income tax could overcome this, but raises great difficulties, one of the most significant being that those who earn an amount which is equal to or just above the minimum amount would feel they were working for no reason.

Because governments have only limited resources available to them to spend on social services, a selective approach concentrating resources on those people and families identified as disadvantaged is preferred. This, however, can and does lead to problems of stigmatization. In addition, selective services which provide for specific needs tend to lead to a proliferation of services and monetary benefits. People who are disadvantaged in one area of life often tend to be disadvantaged in

any other areas of life and therefore are eligible for help
om many services. The complexity of the welfare system in
any countries means that people with low incomes have to
pe with a bewildering array of often competing services for
hich they might be eligible. It is hardly surprising that many,
ho feel distress at asking for help, abandon the search for
mproving their income and personal situations.

Poverty and deprivation go hand in hand with poor environ-
ental conditions and health behaviours, and with a seeming
ability to continue the struggle for improvement in personal
d social conditions. 'A way of life in poverty induces social
d psychological traits which are characteristics of oppression
d one dimension is the lower valuation of life' (Blaxter 1981).

High value is placed upon the maintenance of personal
dependence and self-esteem in western social policies.
owerlessness and dependency are felt to have detrimental
fects upon individual morale and ultimately upon health.
esearch evidence has demonstrated the importance of
sychological independence for the continued physical and
ental health of the elderly, the unemployed, and the poor.
he dramatic growth of social work since the Second World
/ar has been associated with a belief in the need to provide
upport and to encourage self-determination for those who
ave fallen foul of life. The role of the social worker is to
ncourage individuals to overcome the disadvantages of their
articular problems and to cope with behavioural responses to
fe's stresses and strains.

Opinions are divided as to the most effective solutions to
ocial problems which have a damaging effect on welfare and
ealth. Three differing views can be identified, and are outlined
elow.

1. The first view, which emphasizes the crucial importance of
esources, leads to three ideas about how improved control of
esources should be achieved.

i) The first is based upon an argument that the poor are ill
because they are deprived relative to other members of
society. As a consequence, inequality of any form will lead to
ill health, and reduced levels of well-being. In its extreme
form, it is argued that if every member of society were given
the same resources and the same opportunities the only
remaining diseases are exposure to infections and environmental hazards. Control over resources being equal, social
policies would then only be concerned with ensuring that
each member of society was as well protected from such
hazards as possible, by providing services for all.

ii) A less extreme version of this view calls not for total
equality in terms of distribution of resources but a fairer
and more equitable distribution, to reduce though not to
eradicate, relative deprivation. The proponents of this view
can be divided into a number of factions. First there are
those who believe that it is simply economic poverty which
causes people to live in poor environments and to be
exposed to greater environmental and occupational
hazards.

Considerable evidence exists to demonstrate that prolonged illness is associated with low income (Butler et al.
1981). It is possible, therefore, to hypothesize that low
income leads to inadequate living conditions which in turn

cause chronic health conditions. It is equally plausible that
chronic health conditions lead to reduced working ability
which in turn leads to low income (Butler et al. 1981). A
circular process probably exists in which all conditions seek
to exacerbate the effect of each other. Chronic illness leads
to low income which results in a lowering of living standards which can exacerbate many chronic health conditions. One explanation therefore is that if chronically-ill
people had higher incomes they would be able to improve
their living conditions themselves and thus reduce their
exposure to environments conducive to ill health.

(iii) A concomitant of this view is that certain groups, especia-
ally the poor, are, because of their deprived states, isolated
from other members of society. Social policy should attempt
to integrate society's groups and prevent social division
which can only lead to conflict and friction. Much of the
conflict thus generated is caused by a feeling of inferiority
and inadequacy created by having less.

2. Another belief is that each individual should experience
certain levels of, for example, housing, nutrition, and education, in order to achieve a level of personal well-being which will
allow him or her to appreciate life to the full. Where people are
in danger of falling below a desired level in any of those aspects
of life, services should be available to prevent this from
happening. The result is a policy emphasis upon social and
physical environments and minimum levels of provision in
certain aspects of life, which are considered to have a
significant impact upon the welfare and the health of individuals. Where these aspects of life have achieved a connotation
of special 'value' individuals should be able to demand
resources, as a right, to help meet his or her 'need' or make up
the deficiency he or she is experiencing.

Social policy in Britain has been influenced by observations
that there are deprived geographical areas in which poor
housing, environmental conditions, and poor levels of social
services combine together. A succession of reports have called
for improvements in these areas and hence the removal of
many of the factors which are thought to relate to poverty
and ill health.

3. A further view credits the problems of the poor as lying
with themselves – if they made more effort to find better
work, budgeted better, followed better health behaviours –
then their situations would improve. The inability to cope
adequately with life may be due to failings in the individual or
due to the irreversible effects of the environment in which
adults have lived all their lives. Opinion is divided as to
whether this inability to cope is due to personality or a series
of damaging experiences to which each following generation
are exposed. Support for the latter view is based on ideas of
transmitted deprivation in which it is thought that children
born into disadvantaged homes and environments will experience the same health risks as their parents and continue the
habits and problems of their parents. The object of policy is
to break the 'cycle of disadvantage' by protecting children
from the detrimental effects of their environment.

The discussion up to now has concentrated upon the effects
of poverty upon individual health, a view which has found relatively little sympathy with policy makers. Policies have tended

to focus upon social problems, which though often concentrated among the poor have attempted to view these not as problems of poverty, but as problems open to any individual who develops certain characteristics. Stress can have effects on general welfare and health. Epidemiological and social studies have demonstrated a relationship between ill health and events such as moving home, financial worries, unemployment, and bereavement.

Social policy in the western world has adopted two approaches to the prevention of social problems. The first approach, rather than attempting to identify particular population groups such as those of social classes IV and V who may be at higher risk of social problems, identifies all individuals as being potentially 'at risk' of various social difficulties. These policies are general, aiming to provide community-wide approaches conducive to individual and community well-being. The second approach is specific, focusing upon individuals at high risk of social breakdown or social distress. Predictors of high risk are sought to enable those responsible for social welfare to intervene and to arrest the social degeneration of the individual.

It is obvious that welfare and health are interrelated. At present there are many theories and little understanding or evidence to help indicate which theory is the most appropriate. Economic constraints are forcing policy makers to concentrate on poverty and client groups with tangible problems such as the disabled and the elderly. How best to resolve, even these limited problems is one of the great issues of our time, and as yet, little evidence is available to help us.

REFERENCES

Blaxter, M. (1981). *The health of children. DSRC/DHSS studies in deprivation and disadvantage.* Heinemann, London.

Brown, M. (1974). *Introduction to social administration in Britain.* Hutchinson, London.

Butler, L.H., Newacheck, P.W., Piontowski, D.L., Harper, A.K., and Franks, P.E. (1981). *Low income and illness. An analysis of national health policy and the poor.* School of Medicine, University of California, San Fransisco.

Court, J. (1973). Some reflections on non-accidental injury young children. *Soc. Work Ser.* **3**, 6.

DHSS (1968). *Report of the Committee on Local Authority and Allied Personal Social Services (the Seebohm report)* Cmnd 3708, HMSO, London.

DHSS (1976). *Sharing resources for health in England.* Report of the Resource Allocation Working Party. HMSO, London.

Department of Education and Science (1967). *Children and the primary schools (Plowden Report).* HMSO, London.

Department of the Environment (1965). Housing in Greater London. Cmnd 2605. HMSO, London.

Donnison, D. (1980). Urban development and social policies. In *Health, wealth and housing* (ed. R.A.B. Leaper) p. 51. Blackwell, Oxford.

Friedman, M. (1963). *Capitalism and freedom (the role of government in education).* Chicago University Press.

Hill, M. and Laing, P. (1979). *Social work and money.* Allen and Unwin, London.

International Labour Office Housing and Employment (1948). Cited in Bish, R.L., and Noure, H.O. (1975). *Urban economics and policy analysis.* McGraw Hill, Maidenhead.

Katz, A.J. and Jackson, W.S. (1978). The Australian housing allowance voucher experiment. A venture in social policy development. *Soc. Econ. Admin.* **12** (3), 197.

La Noue, G.R. (1972). *Educational vouchers—concepts and controversies.* Teachers College Press, Columbia University, New York.

Marshall, T. (1975). *Social policy.* Hutchinson, London.

Montilibert, C. (1979). *Youth and employment in Europe.* Council of Europe, Strasbourg.

Polanyi, G., and Polanyi, P. (1973). Tax credits: a reverse income tax. *National Westminster Bank Q. Rev.* February.

Polanyi, G. and Polyani, P. (1974). Tax credits: a missed opportunity. *National Westminster Bank Q. Rev.* February.

Titmuss, R. (1968). *Commitment to welfare.* Allen and Unwin, London.

Wilding, P. (1976). Richard Titmuss and social welfare. *Soc. Econ. Admin.* **10** (3), 144.

Wolf, A. (1974). Educated by voucher. *New Soc.* **4**, 12.

Disease control and health promotion

The provision and finance of health care services – two models

16 The finance and provision of health care in the United Kingdom

Alan Maynard

ECONOMICS, HEALTH, AND HEALTH CARE: SCARCITY AND CHOICE

The economic approach

Economics is concerned with the process of informing choice in a world of scarcity. Economists seek to identify and evaluate the costs and benefits of alternative ways of achieving given ends (or goals) such that decision makers, be they individual members of the public, bureaucrats or politicians, are informed in an explicit analytical framework about the nature of their choices. The existence of scarcity makes choice unavoidable. The role of economics is to inform the choices that must be made by measuring and attaching values to alternative means of achieving desired policy goals.

Health and health care problems are all around us regardless of the society in which we live. Economists have a particular way of analysing these problems, usually in an 'ends-means' framework with an emphasis on the alternative means of achieving preferred policy ends. This 'view of the world' or 'tool-kit' is based on three assumptions about the way in which the world operates: the ubiquitous nature of scarcity, the inevitability of all resources having alternative uses, and the existence of differing preferences amongst the individuals who make up society.

In most countries individuals are dying because of inadequate resources to finance, for example, renal dialysis and transplantation. More children could be kept alive if resources to finance bone marrow transplants were available. In less developed countries infant mortality rates are sometimes ten times those in the UK. Every day our neighbours and friends may be faced with having to wait in pain or discomfort for hernia and hip replacements. Clearly much more could be done by health care services in all countries to improve the quantity and quality of life: more quality adjusted life years could be produced if only we had resources to finance their creation.

However, scarcity is ubiquitous and unavoidable. Individuals, groups, and societies all face the same problem: their means (resources) are limited and the ends (expenditure possibilities) are infinite. The combination of finite means and infinite ends is all pervasive through time and across societies.

Thus decision makers are obliged to ration this finite supply amongst competing demanders: who will get access to renal dialysis facilities and who will receive a transplant? Such difficult questions arise inevitably everywhere because of scarcity. It is impossible to offer all the treatment we would like to. We have to ration, hopefully in a way which maximizes the benefit of the scarce resources which are used up.

The inevitability of scarcity does not prevent decision makers from adopting macro-economic policies which deliberately leave resources unused: the goal of such policies which generate unemployment is the preferred policy goal of the mitigation of inflation. Nor does it prevent waste and inefficiency in a world of scarcity: if decision makers do not have the right incentives to minimize costs and maximize benefits, they will probably use resources inefficiently. Whilst unemployment, whether the result of deliberate government policy or not, makes resources relatively more scarce, technological advances may make them relatively less scarce. However, even in Japan it is unlikely that the fruits of rapid economic growth will remove scarcity. Furthermore, the most scarce resource of all, a person's own time, becomes more valuable as productivity increases.

This increase in the value of an individual's time arises from the second economic constant: all resources have alternative uses. A decision to play squash means that an individual gives up time which could be used in work-related or alternative leisure activities: wages or the benefits of less preferred leisure activities are foregone. A decision to finance the training and employment of more community physicians means that such resources cannot be used to improve services for, say, the mentally ill, to build Trident missiles, to finance Falkland 'adventures', to mitigate poverty in the Third World, or to construct new roads. The employment of more health economists means that society gives up the services of doctors, nurses, soldiers, footballers, and other labour. If society wants more hospitals, it has to forgo the benefits of more schools, houses and motorways. A decision to buy a whole-body CAT scanner, implying £500 000 of capital expenditure and £50 000 of current expenditure, automatically deprives other users of these scarce resources.

It is a depressing but unavoidable fact of life that every decision to use resources involves an opportunity cost. A decision to buy A means that B, the most favoured alternative, is given up: the value of this most favoured alternative (B) is the opportunity cost (what you give up) of the preferred allocation (on A). There is no such thing as a free lunch: my provision of food and drink to you at zero price involves at least 'own-time' opportunity costs for you. Always, a decision to choose one alternative means that you give up another. Only if scarcity is abolished will opportunity costs be zero and this is unlikely to occur in this or the next century.

The third facet of economic life is that people have differing tastes and preferences. Some people prefer more of one good or service than another. Not only do individuals have different degrees of willingness to pay for goods and services, they also have differing abilities to pay. Thus people's preferences differ: some prefer guns to butter and others butter to guns. Furthermore, people's capacity to buy guns and butter vary. In some societies this has led to the production and distribution of some goods and services collectively with expressed preferences for allocation on the basis of 'need'. An example of such a decision in the UK is the National Health Service (NHS).

However, the channelling of decision-making through institutions of collective choice such as government, may not lead to outcomes consistent with avowed tastes of society. There is a difference between the definition of collective provision of health care (the objective or end of policy) and the establishment of means to achieve this end.

It is commonplace for individuals and societies to act at variance from avowed objectives. The familiar declaration that 'health is the most important thing in my life' is often contradicted by behaviour. Everday individuals adopt patterns of behaviour which are harmful to their health: they choose poor diets with too little bran and too much tobacco and alcohol, they fail to take adequate exercise, and they work too hard. All these decisions imply that at the time a low value was placed on the long-term costs: people prefer pleasure or satisfaction now to costs in the future or, in economic jargon, individuals have a high rate of preference for benefits now and discount future costs.

Thus the main characteristics of the world from an economic point of view are that resources are scarce and choices have to be made about how to allocate (ration) these scarce resources amongst competing demands. All such choices have opportunity costs. The values of these alternatives differ between different individuals and groups, and stated preferences may be different from those inherent in behaviour. The central economic problem which emerges from these characteristics is how to allocate resources so that they satisfy human wants in the best possible way.

Economic efficiency

Economic efficiency is a term which is often used and often ill-understood. The efficient use of resources implies that two criteria are met. First, efficiency implies that goods and services are provided at least cost, sometimes termed technical efficiency. Secondly, efficiency implies that the goods and services provided are those most highly valued (preferred) by society, i.e. the benefits derived from the use of scarce resources are maximized. These characteristics of efficiency demand that benefits should be identified, quantified, and maximized. Opportunity costs should be quantified and minimized, and the most highly-valued by society. Social

valuations may take place in a market, in which consumption implies value equal to (or proxied by) price, or in a system of public choice with politicians defining priorities and, by so doing, implying values for the services provided by, for instance, the NHS.

This economic perspective can be compared to its rivals which tend to be romantic or monotechnic. The romantic refuses to believe in the existence of scarcity and denies the inevitability of the need to choose. Such people blame the unions, the US or the USSR, political leaders, the price of oil, socialism or the idleness of capitalists or trade unions. Occasionally they behave in a paternalistic manner, asserting the primacy of their preferences, in so doing subverting the preferences of others, by telling people 'what is needed' and what is 'useless'. These people insist that we 'should spend more on . . .' and this position ensures naïve analyses of policy options and inefficient use of resources because it ignores opportunity costs.

The monotechnic view of the world emphasizes the narrow perspectives and interests of particular groups. Such groups tend to ignore scarcity, opportunity costs, and the manifest large differences in people' tastes. The Admiral wants the best frigate possible even though surface vessels are vulnerable to air attack. The aviation expert wants the fastest plane possible even though Concorde may not be cost-effective. The doctor wants the best diagnostic and therapeutic resources that are available even though their benefits may be unclear and their opportunity costs high.

These preferences may seem sensible to the technical experts but they may be inefficient from the social point of view. The production of the most electronically-sophisticated frigate either deprives the navy of other ships which might be 'better buys' or it deprives society of other, potentially more valuable, goods and services. The production of supersonic transport (e.g. Concorde), whilst producing a technologically superb machine, led to the provision of a service which lost money. As a consequence, resources, which could, for example produce care for the elderly and handicapped, are used to subsidize businessmen who fly on Concorde at a price less than cost. The doctor who gets the best in diagnosis and therapy either reduces the supply of equipment to his fellow physicians who could perhaps use such resources more efficiently, or uses scarce resources which might give greater benefit to society outside the health-care industry.

In these circumstances, where monotechnic preferences rule supreme, the advice of the experts would seem to offer an incomplete and poor guide to public policy. The desire of the doctor for the best whole-body CAT or NMR scanner available is understandable but irresponsible: such bids for scarce resources often offer little evidence about the benefits of such scanners relative to alternative diagnostic techniques, and tend to ignore or underplay the claims of other resource users (opportunity costs).

From this perspective the health economist is providing two fundamental challenges to doctors. First, to demonstrate that in a world of scarce resources they are providing care for their patients at least cost to society, and that this care is that which gives the most benefit to their patients, i.e. doctors must demonstrate that the cost of therapy or diagnosis are min-

zed and the benefit maximized. Secondly, doctors have to
e the fact that the quantity and quality of the services they
ovide will be affected by the preferences of patients, and
 preferences of the patients' 'guardian angels', with all its
ects, the State. Public preferences, expressed either in the
rket place or by the State, will divert resources from or to
al dialysis, heart transplantation, cosmetic surgery, and all
er types of medical work. Such decisions, which are unavoid-
le in the presence of scarcity, will affect relative scarcity but
l not remove the basic problem facing all decision makers:
w to ration finite scarce resources amongst infinite coming activities and to choose who will die, and who will live
d with what degree of pain and disability.

The ubiquitous nature of scarcity and choice offers the
onomist the role of 'bargain maker'. The bad accountant is
ncerned with the minimization of costs regardless of benefits.
e bad doctor is concerned with the maximization of benefits
gardless of opportunity costs. The economists' training
rces him or her to bridge this gap: ideally those choices with
 best benefit–cost ratios should be chosen and this is only
ssible if information about costs and benefits are available
d can be evaluated in an explicit analytical framework.
ch analyses can be used to provide the relevant information
r decision making: the costs and benefits at the margin of
re, that is they inform the decision-maker of the costs and
nefits of one more unit of care and identify the relevant
ationships between different ways of achieving given goals.
us the marginal perspective enables efficient decisions to be
ade about how to allocate incremental resources: scarce
ditional resources are allocated to those activities which
ve the most benefits or to use an American colloquialism
e 'the biggest bang for the buck'.

This chapter will seek to discuss the nature of goal setting
d policy making in the context of the NHS in the UK.
though the institutions in the UK are different from those
 the US, Canada, Australia or elsewhere, the nature of
onomic analysis is the same: resources are scarce everywhere
d all decision-makers are obliged to demonstrate that they
e the scarce resources at their disposal in an efficient
anner.

HE PRINCIPLES OF THE NHS: ENDS AND MEANS

entifying the policy goals

ne precise definition of the goals of policy, in health care or
 any other sector of the economy, is often absent from the
nunciations of politicians, bureaucrats, professionals, and
hers. Such behaviour is perhaps not surprising (if you do
ot define goals you cannot be shown to have failed to have
et them!), but it makes policy analysis very difficult.

Also it is commonplace to see no clear identification of the
eans of achieving policy goals even if they are defined.
ather it is usual that institutions (the British NHS, the
merican Medicare system, or the Australian Medibank) are
eated with all too little rigorous appraisal of the nature of
ese policies and their merits relative to alternatives.

The principles of much public and private endeavour in
alth care in Britain and abroad lead to lack of clarity in

defining policy 'ends' (goals) and 'means' (ways of achieving
goals), and reluctance to evaluate the success, or lack of it, of
programmes in achieving their goals. This implicit maxim in
much public and private activity must be questioned.

However, this does not lead to the easy acquisition of
suitable answers. What is the NHS seeking to achieve? Are
the goals of NHS policy explicit and constant between the
organizational tiers of the Service? What are the means by
which the goals of the NHS are to be achieved? What are the
alternative policies which could be used to achieve the goals
of the Service, and what are their relative attributes in terms
of costs and benefits? Such questions can be asked at the
macro, whole system level or at the micro-service level, e.g.
what are the goals of caring policies for patients with
duodenal ulcers? (e.g. healing). What are the alternative ways
of achieving these goals? (e.g. no treatment, antacids, surgery
or cimetidine). What are the costs (full opportunity costs) and
benefits (in relation to the goal of treatment) of the alternatives
and which procedure gives you the best healing rate (however
measured) at the lowest cost?

It is all too usual for decision makers not to formulate these
questions, let alone seek to answer them. The ends and means
of the NHS which are set out here are not derived from the
pronouncements of the Service's founding fathers. Rather
they are culled from their statements and subsequent ones by
policy makers and politicians: policy objectives are inferred
rather than declared. Inevitably such definitions of objectives
and policy may be disputed. However, they seem to be consistent with the statements of policy makers and they are not set
out here to provide a framework for subsequent analysis.

The nature of the policy goals

The principal element in the arguments of the architects of
the NHS was that access to health care should be made more
equal and, all too ill-defined notions of distributional justice
served. Thus the writer (Willink) of the 1944 White Paper of
the Coalition (Churchill) Government stated that:

the Government . . . want to ensure that in the future every man,
woman and child can rely on getting . . . the best medical and other
facilities available; that their getting them shall not depend on
whether they can pay for them or on any other factor irrelevant to
real need (Ministry of Health, 1944)

The 1946 Labour Government Bill stated that no limits were
imposed on:

availability e.g. limitations based on financial means, age, sex,
employment or vocation, area of residence or insurance qualification (Cmnd 6761 (HMSO 1946)).

This notion of equality of access to health care based on
the principle of need rather than willingness and ability to pay
is fundamental to the NHS. It can be elaborated in a variety
of ways. The objective of equality has a geographical dimension: it implies that regardless of the person's place of residence
in the UK he or she should have an equal capacity in relation to
need to consume health care. A second dimension of this objective is that there should be equal access to health care regardless
of social or family background: the distribution of health care

(inputs) and of health status (outputs) between different social groups (measured by sociological notions of social class or, better still, by measures of income) should not exhibit inequalities except in relation to need in the case of inputs (health care).

The economics of the policy goals of the NHS: inputs and outputs

The publicly-stated objective of the NHS implies that citizens should only get more health care if their need was greater. However, this objective is perhaps interpreted in too simple a manner. Implicit in the notion of equality is the assumption that citizens will benefit from health care. If this assumption is accepted for the moment, it is clear that health care is the means to the end of improved health status. If British policy makers wish to maximize the output of the NHS budget, in terms, for instance, of the number of quality-adjusted man years (QUALS) that are produced, the objectives of the NHS can be re-defined as the allocation of health care resources in relation to equality in the production of health: scarce health care resources will be allocated in relation to their capacity to improve health status, regardless of whether patients come from social class I (rich) or social class V (poor), and regardless of their willingness and ability to pay for health care.

This is an economic elaboration of the statement in the 1944 White Paper. It shifts the emphasis to outcomes and their distribution in relation to benefit criteria. It contrasts with the emphasis on inputs (often measured crudely in terms of health care expenditure). Equality in the distribution of inputs (health care) may not maximize the output (improved health status) of the NHS: the marginal (additional) £x spent on the poor could perhaps improve the health status of the rich more if they were given access to care. Such an outcome is an empirical issue and only further research will determine whether such clashes between input and output equality goals might arise.

If a marginal unit of health care was more productive, however measured, in providing better health for the rich than the poor, this might open up a new debate where some adherents to the socialist ideology might advocate positive discrimination in favour of the poor even though this prevented the maximization of the output of the health care budget.

Because of our ignorance about input and output linkages in health production, in particular the absence of knowledge about whether one more (marginal) unit of health care, education, better nutrition, income redistribution or whatever other input increases health status outcomes the most, the discussion of policy tends to be narrow (related to one input, health care) and input dominated.

Thus the NHS was designed in relation to collectivist or socialist goals of equality of access to health care and health. Often the distinction between the input and the output is not clear: health care is one input which may generate the socially desired goal of improvements in health status (outcome). The ultimate objective of public policy is the maximization of outcomes and a more equal distribution of such outcomes amongst socio-economic groups or classes.

The means for achieving NHS goals

The goal of equalizing access to health care in Britain pursued in a State-financed and largely State-owned system which the following means are usually identified as be necessary to achieve the goals of policy:

1. Allocation: citizens get access to care on the basis need or their capacity to benefit from the consumption resources. The overall objective of the NHS is to maximize benefits (in terms of improved health status) which can derived from budget.

2. Finance: consumers pay through the general tax syst and pay nothing (or nominal sums) at the point of consum tion, i.e. there are no price barriers to consumption.

3. Ownership: public ownership of the means of productio

4. Budget distribution: central control over budgets a some physical direction of resources (capital and labour).

5. Remuneration: the pay and conditions of labour will mediated by State countervailing monopsony (sole buy powers which will affect the impact of market forces.

The discussion of the ends and means of the NHS and market counterpart is set out in greater detail in Culyer et (1982) and McLachlan and Maynard (1982).

THE PRACTICE OF THE NHS

Using as a framework the ends and means set out in t preceding section, the practice of the NHS will now be co pared with its principles.

Health and health care

Perhaps the most influential report about British social poli this century was written by William Beveridge in 194 Beveridge's primary concern was the reform of incon maintenance policies. However, he saw that this was only o element in social progress:

Social insurance fully developed may provide income security; it an attack on Want. But Want is one of the five giants on the road reconstruction and in some ways it is the easiest to attack. T others are Disease, Ignorance, Squalor and Idleness (Beveri 1942 p. 6).

In setting out his plan to reform social insurance Beverid; assumed that this policy would be underpinned, *inter alia,* comprehensive health and rehabilitation services. Althou; he advocated comprehensive insurance rather than a NH: his discussion emphasized the need for an active consideratic of preventive policies and an awareness that health care wa not the only factor that affected health. This awareness reiterated in the White Papers of the Coalition and Labo Governments in the 1944–46 period.

Despite this early awareness of the interaction of incon redistribution, education, housing, health care, and oth social policies, the NHS has operated in isolation of othe social services and the exact nature of the interactions betwee the component parts of the Welfare State remain poor! explored. Little is known about the costs and benefits o alternative policies: is an additional £1 million spent on heal

e a 'better buy' than the same expenditure on education as
means of improving health status?

There is evidence which indicates that the marginal product
health care in terms of its capacity to improve health is
atively low. For instance Newhouse and Friedlander (1980)
laced the usual 'success' measures of mortality and
rbidity with physiological measures (diastolic blood
ssure, serum cholesterol concentration, electrocardiogram
normalities, abnormal X-rays, prescience of varicose veins,
d a peridontal index). Controlling for age, sex, race,
ucation and income, and using a large US data set they
ncluded:

hough additional education and income were associated with
er abnormal chest X-rays and less peridontal disease, the
ysiological measures were little affected by additional medical
ources. The results are consistent with the view that what the
ividual does (or does not) do for himself affects health more
n do additional medical resources (Newhouse and Friedlander
30 p. 200).

The micro-evidence (e.g. as in Newhouse and Friedlander's
dy) raises questions similar to those of McKeown (1977,
79). Using historical data for the UK, McKeown argues
at the cause of the modern rise of population is reduced
ortality and this was generated by better nutrition (associated
th greater affluence) and public health measures. The
ntribution of health care, McKeown argues had been
ited.

Results such as these are controversial and require careful
aboration with new research. Unfortunately, despite the
clarations of the architects of the NHS and similar periodic
terations of such sentiments since the 1940s (e.g. the
oposed Joint Approach to Social Policy of the 1970s), the
alth care system has remained isolated from the other
rvices which affect health status. The practice of the NHS,
e practice elsewhere in the world, has been compartment-
zed and is at variance with statements of principle.

llocation on the basis of need

ather than allocate health care, as in a market, on the basis
willingness and ability to pay, the NHS seeks to allocate
sources on the basis of need. Need is an ambiguous concept
Williams (1978) emphasized. Fundamentally the question
hich has to be answered is which party, the patient and
her beneficiaries, the doctor, the politicians, or the electorate
large, shall determine need. Once this question is resolved,
e 'how to define need' question can be tackled.

The economist would approach these issues in steps.
etaining benefits in terms of outcomes, the first step is to
valuate the benefits of competing therapies. This requires
reful clinical evaluation by doctors and others intent on
eking out the medical, psychological, and sociological
aracteristics or effectiveness of the alternative ways of
iagnosing and treating ill health.

The identification of the clinical attributes of medical
ctivity has to be followed by an economic appraisal of the
lternatives: therapy A may be twice as effective as therapy B
ut it may be four times as expensive.

This economic evaluation has to be followed by some

mechanism of social choice. The market rations demands
according to willingness and ability to pay, i.e. patient preferences exhibited independently or via his or her agent, the
doctor, determines which services are provided. In the NHS
there is collective decision making at the macro-level (choice
between different sectors): the politicians decide the total
budget and express preferences about priorities. At the micro-
level (choice between different therapies) the doctor determines
the allocation of resources. Unfortunately neither method of
allocating scarce health care resources (the market or the
State) seems to be efficient. In the first place the medical
profession has failed to evaluate its practices in an efficient
manner. Cochrane (1972) took up the pre-war advocacy by
Bradford Hill of randomized controlled trials (RCTs). It was
emphasized that observational studies and quasi-experimental
methods generate biased estimates of the relationship between
inputs and outputs. Such biases could be avoided only by
using prospective RCTs which are difficult to design and
execute, raise ethical issues, and are expensive to finance.
Cochrane has asserted that the majority of medical therapies
in use have not been evaluated scientifically and their efficacy
can, as a consequence, be questioned. Those who have evaluated established medical practices carefully (e.g. Bunker *et
al.* 1977), have charted the histories of expensive therapies
adopted after little or poor evaluation and then discovered to
be expensive errors (e.g. gastric freezing).

This failure by doctors, to evaluate the structure, process
and outcome of health care (Donabedian 1980), has ensured
that resources are used inefficiently. However, this is not
surprising: the doctor is poorly trained and has all too little
incentive to search out the cost-effective means of improving
his or her patients' health status. Weed (1981) criticizes the
training of doctors in the following way:

Present licensing procedures and medical school curriculums grew
out of what 'professionals' in the past identified as desirable; they do
not reflect what was proved to be possible in meeting very well
defined goals. Because the system has been so poorly defined over
the years, there has been no way to relate outputs of the system to
inputs; conjectures piled on conjectures have hardened into curriculums and licensing laws. Reviewing some of these conjectures in
terms of the tasks of medicine, we can now see how far off the
track the medical establishment has strayed. There is no evidence
that keeping medical students in a passive mode for the first two
years of medical school is accomplishing the basic objectives of
education. Students are stuffed with the facts of basic science, but
the behaviour of a scientist escapes them, as shown by their
inadequacy in keeping medical data over long periods and by their
failure to use feedback systematically. One might even argue that
superficial efforts in their basic scientific education do more to
prevent their reaching the original objectives than to help them to
achieve them; there is no question that time and money are diverted
from acquiring other needed skills. (Weed 1981 p. 306)

The failures of the existing system of medical education
lead to the production of doctors who are unscientific and
casual in their evaluative work. Thus it is unsurprising to find
(Der Simonian *et al.* 1982) that 48 per cent of clinical trial
articles in the *British Medical Journal* and 54 per cent of such
articles in the *Lancet* in the period July–December 1979 failed
to meet 11 criteria for reporting the design and analysis of

their work. The approach to the design, execution, and reporting of clinical trials leaves much to be desired.

Where trials are carried out, all too often the cost aspects of the diagnosis or treatment are not investigated. The economist is equipped to determine the opportunity cost of alternative policies and is not interested merely in public expenditure (e.g. the costs to the NHS) outlays alone. The objective of economic analysis is to determine the opportunity costs of the programme to society as a whole, i.e. the individual and his family, the NHS, and all other public (e.g. local authority social services) and private providers of care. The techniques of the economic appraisal of health care have been elaborated in many places (e.g. Drummond 1980, 1981) but taken up all too rarely.

The reluctance of doctors to use scientific techniques of clinical and economic evaluation to assess the costs and benefits of their work is unsurprising given the lack of incentives inherent in the NHS and other health care systems: the doctor may not gain by doing evaluative work and is unlikely to lose out if he or she omits to do it or fails to apply the results produced by more industrious colleagues (McLachlan and Maynard 1982).

The cost of the NHS is met neither by the provider nor by the patient. The patient, within the limitations of his or her knowledge about medicine, can make demands on the NHS and the costs of these demands are met by the taxpayer. Usually the patient delegates this role to his or her agent, the expert, the doctor. The doctor then makes demand decisions on behalf of his or her patients but again does not bear the costs, the taxpayer meets the bill. In insurance systems the incentives are the same, only instead the insurer meets the bill. This 'moral hazard' may lead to over-consumption and waste: the incentives to be frugal and efficient in the use of scarce resources is absent because a third party (the taxpayer) pays the bill and the decision maker (whether patient or doctor) has no economic incentive to avoid waste.

If waste occurs (i.e. resources are used inefficiently) and it is agreed that the doctor is the decision-maker who decides who will get what care, then the costs of this inefficiency must be laid at the doors of the medical profession. To the economist they are acting in an unsurprising way consistent with incentives. However, this pattern of activity means that patients are getting inefficient care, financed by resources which could give more benefits to other patients, i.e. the opportunity costs (benefits foregone) may exceed the value of the services provided when resources are used inefficiently. In effect the inefficiency of one doctor deprives other patients of resources from which they can benefit, surely an unethical mode of practice?

Resources are allocated in the NHS by doctors who, as in other health care systems, have all too little idea of the nature of the benefits of the services they are providing and the opportunity costs they are imposing on patients who cannot get access to care. Their ethic is individual: to look at the individual patient rather than social opportunity costs. Doctors also have little knowledge of the costs of the care they provide. Ideally, if resources are to be used in an economically efficient manner, doctors should know the costs and benefits at the margin of the services they provide. Until they

evaluate scientifically these aspects of their practice, they will be unable to determine optimal standards of practice and demonstrate that they are using societies scarce resources efficiently and ethically.

The NHS principle of allocation according to need, expressed in terms of benefit potentials, is practised very imperfectly. The medical profession has failed to train doctors adequately and as a result their evaluative work, standard setting, and performance have been unsatisfactory. The policy makers in the NHS have failed to create incentives for doctors to work efficiently: they have tended to maintain the perverse incentives whose nature is similar to those in other health care systems and which, as they do elsewhere, generate inefficiency and a discrepancy between principle and practice. Until more is known about benefits and costs in health care it will not be possible to demonstrate that the NHS meets the need in the most efficient manner possible.

Price barriers to consumption

The abolition of the price barrier to consumption was seen as a means of reducing the divergence in health care consumption between social or income groups. Thus it was believed that such barriers affected utilization rates and that these effects were more pronounced amongst poor groups. The poor, who generally have health status characteristics (mortality and morbidity) worse than those of the rich, were thus dissuaded by prices from consuming health care. These conclusions are theoretical statements and the evidence available seems to indicate that the behaviour of people in health-care markets is consistent with the predictions of theory (Cairns and Snell 1978; Maynard 1979; Newhouse et al. (1981), i.e. demand is responsive to price change.

However, the abolition of the price barrier to consumption does not mean that health-care consumption is free to the patient. There remain significant opportunity costs which have to be paid by the consumer of the services of the NHS. The manual worker at a chocolate factory who is ill has to take time off work to consult the doctor (wages are forgone), he has to travel to the doctor's surgery (travel costs are incurred), and drug prescriptions can only be made up with further time and cost to the worker. The academic at the university on the other hand will not generally forgo wages when consulting a doctor and will have a car which will reduce the monetary and time-cost of travel. These time-costs may affect utilization and the differential in these costs may produce differences in health-care consumption patterns: in the simple preceding example the academic would, other things being equal, consume more than the manual worker.

The effects of such time-costs may be mitigated or accentuated by the location decisions of health-care planners. The location of hospitals in 'green field' sites away from city centres where the poor may be concentrated may affect utilization patterns. Planning decisions need to take into account these costs in a careful appraisal of the social costs and benefits of alternative investment decisions.

Language, attitudes, and education may also affect utilization. Health-care professionals are typically middle-class and communicate using complex sentence structures and words. Many people from low-income groups are poorly educated

d do not fully comprehend middle-class language. The poor
ay regard this as a barrier to consumption, and this
ovides another explanation of the lower utilization rates of
e poor in health care systems.

The effects of these non-price barriers to consumption have
en poorly investigated. Simply hypothesizing is possible but
e interaction of prices, time costs, education, language, and
her factors is likely to be complex and requires much more
reful investigation. If the poor are disadvantaged by
rriers such as these, and if policy makers wish to increase
eir utilization, 'positive' discrimination may be necessary,
her directly or indirectly through linked social security
nefits (e.g. maternity grants linked to antenatal care), and
ay require radical innovations such as paying poor people
consume care.

anning and control

formed American analysts of the NHS seem to believe that
e Service is controlled tightly and planned in detail (e.g. see
odman 1980). In fact, controls are lax and planning is
ticeable by its relative absence. The Department of Health
d Social Security (DHSS) has no capacity to control in
tail the working of the NHS. There is no 'head office'.
stead it operates within the framework of administrative
thorities (regions and districts), responsible to a government
partment (DHSS) which has no developed capacity to
aluate or plan the NHS. The potential to control and plan
s not been developed.

A major attribute of the NHS is that it is 'cash limited', i.e.
any accounting period most of the expenditure, the majority
its budget, of the NHS is fixed by decisions made by
liticians in Whitehall. The Family Practitioner Committees
PCs) finance provision of primary care by GPs (primary
re physicians), dentists, pharmacists, and opticians. These
oducers are self-employed and the expenditure they induce
demand-determined: this has tended to be an increasing
rtion of the total NHS budget in recent years and is equal
rrently to about 20 per cent of total health care expenditure.

The remaining 80 per cent of the budget is largely spent by
e Regional and District Health Authorities. The budget in
ngland is divided amongst 14 regions and, since April 1982,
ese regions have allocated resources to the local units,
stricts, each serving a population of about 250 000. The
ganization of the regions and the districts is curious, with
ur management structures, one each for the financial
nction (the treasurer), the administrative function, the
edical function, and the nursing function. Cross-disciplinary
anning is not facilitated by this structure and there is no
ear identification of the *primus inter pares*, i.e. the boss!

The allocation of the budget to the regions and districts has
ly recently been placed on a sensible basis. Until the 1970s
e budget allocation formula can be approximated as
llows:

dget (1963) = Budget (1962) + inflation proofing + a little real
owth money + an allowance for any scandals (usually in the
ental illness sector) revealed in the media!

his *ad hoc* process, allocation to the noisiest rather than to
e neediest, did not affect in any significant way the inequal-

ities in the financial capacity of the regions to provide health
care. As a consequence the geographical inequality in provision
of health care, which the NHS was created to remedy, was
rediscovered in the late 1960s and became a much discussed
policy issue (see e.g. Cooper and Culyer 1970, 1971, 1972;
Maynard 1971).

This debate led to the evolution of the budget allocation
formula of the Resourse Allocation Working Party (referred
to as RAWP) (Department of Health and Social Security
1976b; Maynard and Ludbrook 1980b) for England. Separate
formulae were created for Wales, Scotland, and Ulster. These
formulae all contained similar elements; in particular, financial
capacity to provide health care was distributed in relation to
need, which was proxied by population, weighted by specific
Standardized Mortality Rates (SMRs were used in the absence
of good morbidity data). However, the inequality in the
allocation of the funds between the constituent parts of the
UK (England, Wales, Scotland, and Ulster) means that intra-
UK inequality is maintained: presumably one price of the
political union!

The effect of the RAWP formula in England has been to
reduce regional inequalities. Resources have been shifted out
of the London areas towards the north. The majority of this
movement has been funded by differentials in growth monies,
that is, real budget cuts amongst the 'losing' regions have been
rare. Whilst this has made redistribution easier politically, it
has run into difficulties in the 1980s when growth monies are
minimal and, as a consequence, the 'losing' regions face
budget cuts. The opposition to these cuts, in the heartlands of
Conservative political support, may make vigorous implementation of RAWP somewhat difficult.

Another difficulty of the policy is that it has not been
evaluated effectively. The 'growth monies' acquired by the
'deprived' northern regions have been spent but how is not
too clear. Whether expenditure has gone to renewing ancient
acute care facilities or, as advised by Whitehall, been spent on
priority areas, the mentally ill and handicapped, the elderly
and the chronic sick, is unclear. The lack of monitoring of the
use of RAWP monies is in the grand (and bad) tradition of
health services policy: a good policy is a new policy and if a
new policy throws money at the policy problem it must be
effective! Earlier the distinction between structure, process,
and outcome was emphasized and the RAWP policy requires
careful evaluation within this framework.

The development and implementation of the RAWP
formula came nearly 30 years after the creation of the NHS.
In intent and design it was admirable, although its effectiveness at the service level is unclear. However, it was an unusual
innovation in that much of what the NHS does is unplanned.

It was not until the late 1970s that the Department of
Health (DHSS) obliged regions to prepare service plans on a
five- and ten-year rolling basis. This exercise went into a limbo
induced by expenditure constraints until 1982 when the Secretary of State decided to monitor the performance of regions
and to establish a system of 'performance indicators'.
Monitoring, performance indicators, and planning require
information about process and outcome but this information
is absent. The curious four-sector management structure
(treasurer, administrator, nurse, and doctor) has led to the

poor information systems which are functionally rather than specialty organized. Much of the routine data that are available could be used for planning but require reorganization and manipulation, activities which cannot be financed out of inadequate administrative budgets which the politicians are seeking to cut as demonstrations of the effectiveness of their wars on bureaucracy!

Another bold attempt to plan the NHS was the statement about priorities in 1976 (DHSS 1976a). This document advocated the shifting of resources out of acute into the deprived priorities sectors. The output of the acute sector was to be maintained by greater efficiency. Whether such greater efficiency was forthcoming is not clear because of the poor information and evaluation but the sector has refused to decline in size. The services for the elderly, the mentally ill, the physically and mentally handicapped, and the chronic sick have tended to be improved with development (extra) monies. Again the cash limits of the 1980s are putting novel pressures on the planners: the opportunity costs of service developments are becoming clearer as expansion can only be met out of contraction elsewhere.

Planning and control in health care as in any economic sector is difficult to design and execute. Planning in the NHS is characterized by limited efforts to design and execute policies which might make it possible to achieve the ultimate NHS goal of equality, or intermediate goals related to process (e.g. an adequate level of provision for the mentally ill). There are limited incentives to plan and limited incentives for decision makers to use resources efficiently or strive after the attainment of equity goals. With such discrepancies between principles and practice, it is hardly surprising that inequalities in health and health care in the 1980s are still apparently quite large.

THE FAILURE OF THE NHS: INEQUALITY MAY HAVE BEEN RETAINED

This section will present an overview of the data which indicate that the primary goal of the NHS, equality in health, has not been attained. Following on from the previous section it is argued that this outcome is inevitable because of the feeble manipulation of the policies required to achieve this goal. It is to be emphasized that the inequitable outcomes indicated in the UK are similar to those in other European countries where inadequate attempts have been made to

achieve the collective goal of equality in health (Mayna 1981; Maynard and Ludbrook 1981).

Inequalities in health care

The objective of allocating health care resources in relation need requires that the scarce health care is allocated to the who could benefit most from its use, regardless of willingn and ability to pay. To determine benefit it is necessary to ha information about the link between inputs (health care a other items) and output (health status). Ideally we would li data which gives details of variations in access to inputs differing health status, and information on how each inp contributes towards the creation of health.

This is crudely summarized in Fig. 16.1. The individua health stock is determined by a variety of factors, includi genetic inheritance. The consumption of education provid you with information and new tastes which may induce y to avoid (or love?) dangerous habits such as 'wine, oth persons(!) and song'. More education may enhance yo personal income and enable you to indulge more generou in such habits. Sound housing may shelter your recove from your excesses as you are ministered to (or not!) by yo domestic partner, who gives 'family time' to assist yo recovery. These and other inputs affect your health capi stock over your life-cycle and determine the production of t desired outcome health, proxied in Fig. 16.1 by healthy day

Whilst this analytical framework gives many insights in the process of health creation (see Grossman 1972; Muurin 1982) its testing requires life-cycle (longitudinal) data s which are noticeable by their absence. Consequently little known about the relative productivity at the margin of t various inputs which create health, however measured. In t discussion of inequality in the NHS it is assumed that diffe ences in the consumption of health care do lead to differenc in health status and that to mitigate the latter, the form must be corrected. This assumption of a precise input–outp link will be maintained in the following discussion of heal care inequalities. Evidence which causes this association to questioned, may imply that health-care inequalities, as cau of health inequalities, may be less important and may requi that resources are shifted out of health care into inputs who health-creating characteristics are superior.

Although geographical inequalities in the financial capaci of regions to provide health care were 'rediscovered' in t

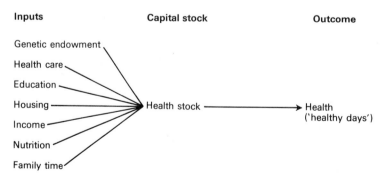

Fig. 16.1. The production of health.

e 1960s, it was not until the late 1970s that the individual nsumption of health care was subjected to analysis (Le and, 1978; 1982). Le Grand used General Household rvey data for 1972 and found that health-care consumption tween social classes did not favour the rich. However, if ese data were weighted by need (reports of acute illness), a w social class profile emerged which showed more expend-re on the rich (professional) than the poor. These data are own in Table 16.1, and indicate that substantial inequalities NHS health-care consumption seem to exist.

ble 16.1. *Public expenditure on health care by socio-onomic group. All persons, England and Wales, 1972*

cio-economic group	Expenditure per person percentage of mean	Expenditure per person reporting illness percentage of mean
ofessional, employers, d managers	94	120
ermediate and ior non-manual	104	114
illed manual	92	97
mi and unskilled nual	114	85
ean (£) = 100	18.1	103.2

Source: Le Grand (1982), p. 26

equalities in health

espite the creation of the Welfare State in the 1940s signifi-nt inequalities remain in income, education, housing, and ealth care. For income and health care, the evidence seems suggest that relative inequalities have changed little over e last 30 years. This is not surprising given the incentives herent in the institutional structures created in the 1940s and e lack of evaluation of social policies until the late 1970s. As consequence it would not be surprising if inequalities in rms of inputs had led to little change in relative inequalities health. The current conventional wisdom is that this is so: lative inequalities in health have changed little since the eation of the NHS.

Some evidence to substantiate this conclusion are presented Tables 16.2 and 16.3. The data for male SMRs in Table 16.2 ggest that the relative position of the poor (Social Class V) in ach period, 1949–52, 1959–63, and 1970–72, has worsened nd that of the rich improved. It seems from these data that the

able 16.2. *Male standardized mortality ratios: by social lass, England and Wales*

ocial ass	(1) 1949–52 (age 20–64)	(2) 1959–63 (age 15–64)	(3) 1970–72 (age 16–64)
	86	76	77
	92	81	81
I	101	100	104
v	104	103	113
	118	143	137

Table 16.3. *Neonatal (post-neonatal) death rate per 1000 live births by social class Scotland 1950–77*

Social class	1950	1960	1970	1977
I	20.0 (5.9	13.0 (2.7)	9.2 (3.0)	6.7 (2.5)
II	16.5 (7.7)	17.2 (4.3)	8.8 (3.1)	8.9 (3.7)
III	22.7 (14.3)	17.1 (7.2)	12.3 (6.3)	10.2 (4.0)
IV	24.9 (18.9)	20.7 (10.2)	14.3 (7.9)	10.8 (4.5)
V	28.5 (25.1)	21.0 (12.8)	18.8 (13.0)	14.5 (7.0)

Source: Register General Scotland Annual Report (1977) Pt. 1. Mortality Statistics, HMSO (1978), Table F1.4, p. 371.

relative chances of survival of the poor are no better than in the 1940s.

The Scottish data in Table 16.3 indicate that neonatal (and post-neonatal data in brackets in the table) continue to exhibit sharp social class profiles and, if a very crude indicator of difference is used, as in the final line of the table, it seems that class differences in survival rates have widened. This widening has taken place when absolute rates have declined, thus for Social Class V the rate of neonatal mortality was halved in the 1950–70 period.

So if attention is concentrated on mortality data (few morbidity data of any accuracy are available) and social class measures are used it seems that although health has improved, the differences between social groups have remained remark-ably stable.

This outcome may be the product of the none too radical structures of the Welfare State. Alternatively it may in part or in whole be a statistical artefact. Social class may be a poor indicator of social and economic well-being. Over the period since 1948 the size of Social Class V has fallen (to about 6 per cent of the population) as people's skill levels rose and their social class changed. The data in Tables 16.2 and 16.3 are concerned with social status at death (Table 16.2) and of the father (Table 16.3). Such cross-sectional measures ignore life-cycle changes and social mobility (upwards and downwards) that may complicate the interpretation of the data in these tables: the ill (regardless of their social class origin) may be destined to die in Social Class V. Stern (1982) has argued that social mobility biases data such as that in Table 16.2 and makes current conclusions about health inequality incomplete.

Conclusion: inequalities remain

Until the 1970s economic growth fuelled increased finance of the services provided by the Welfare State and increased inputs were believed, without much evidence, to be achieving better outcomes, absolutely and relatively. The recent harsher economic climate has led to a long overdue appraisal of distributional outcomes (summarized in DHSS 1980; and Townsend and Davidson 1982). This appraisal has been accompanied by a 'rediscovery' of the obvious fact that health care is only one input which may affect health status.

The conventional wisdom is that substantial inequalities exist in the consumption of health care and in health, as proxied by mortality rates. This position is unlikely to be completely wrong, although the statistical artefact problem raised by Stern (1982) must make us cautious. It seems that although the NHS has provided more care and that the effects of economic growth (even at Britain's pedestrian rate) and the Welfare State have improved the quantity if not the quality of life, significant inequalities in health care consumption and health status remain. Britain remains an unequal society.

THE NHS: DOING BETTER IN THE FUTURE

If British society wishes to pursue the goal of the NHS, greater equality in health, what policy initiatives might be adopted?

The policy debate in all countries is very similar: the alternatives seem to be the 'rolling back' of State involvement (this is called 'competition' in the US and 'privatization' in the UK) and the refinement of the clumsy attempts made to regulate health care markets by the State. (This is called 'regulation' in the US and in the UK it is associated with the reform of the NHS.) Both parties see health-care markets as inefficient, although the emphasis of distributional issues is clearly different with the pro-competition lobby tending to minimize its importance and believing in the 'hidden hand of the market' as the means to resolve equity issues. Such a position seems optimistic but the issues are complex (McLachlan and Maynard 1982).

Privatizing the NHS

A much-discussed policy in the UK is the 'privatization' of the NHS. This option is pressed by those of the market ideology (e.g. Seldon 1980) who believe that a competitive health-care market could provide health care more efficiently than the 'bureaucratic' NHS. To make the market work in a competitive manner would require the abolition of many powerful interest groups which have monopoly powers. As Friedman (1962) has shown the abolition of professional licensure (the capacity of the medical profession to influence the price, quantity, and quality of health care) would permit the use of cheaper substitute inputs (cheaper nurses instead of expensive doctors) and the creation of information about the quality and price of competing practitioners. Such radical reforms seem unlikely as they would be opposed by strong professional interests. Without such reforms, the competitive market would be an inefficient user of resources (Maynard 1983).

Although the private sector in the UK has expanded in the recent past, its role is minute: its activities amount to less than 2 per cent of NHS income and 2 per cent of the NHS bed stock. Furthermore, in 1982 it exhibited severe economic problems: the British United Provident Association, the largest UK private insurer, made an operating loss in 1982 and is about to raise premiums substantially. As argued elsewhere (Maynard and Ludbrook 1980; Maynard 1982), the problems faced by BUPA and the rest of the private sector are similar to those faced by the NHS. Existing possibilities for the privatization of the NHS are unlikely to remedy any of the fundamental problems of efficiency or equity in the health-care market.

Reforming the NHS

The Priorities document and the RAWP formula (DHSS 1976a, 1976b) were pioneering developments in the evolution the NHS. Such policies will have to be evaluated and develop in the future. However, the fundamental challenge facing t NHS is the development of a set of incentives appropriate f the pursuit of policy goals. This thesis will be elaborated here the exclusion of other material because its primacy is such th if it is not developed, other policy innovations, however wi and clearly articulated, are unlikely to be effective.

The existence of scarcity obliges all decision-make whether academics, doctors, or admirals, to make choic Efficiency requires that the decision maker has informati about the costs and benefits at the margin of alternati choices: which treatments will improve health status the m at least cost? In fact, as has been shown above, the doctor trained poorly and tends not to have at his disposal the inf mation necessary to make efficient decisions.

One approach to this problem is to induce the medic profession to train its students more thoroughly and impro training over the doctor's life-cycle. It is peculiar that cons tants who make decisions and, on average, commit abo £500 000 of scarce resources per year should not be trained economic and management skills. In the medical mark place it is common to find the primary decision-maker, t doctor, ignorant of the cost of the services he provides. A executive in Shell who did not know the cost of his oil wou fare ill in the market place!

However, even in some Utopia where the costs and benefi of alternatives are known, the incentives to use this informati and strive after efficient practise would be absent. W should a doctor give up inefficient habits if the opportuni costs to him or her of such practices are low?

A variety of incentive mechanisms can be developed increase the opportunity costs of inefficiency. Informati can be used by the profession to determine practice standar and systems of peer review and medical audit can be develop to ensure some conformity with these standards. Howeve decision-makers using such mechanisms may tend to ado conservative norms and enforce them gently.

The economist would favour the use of financial rewar to induce efficient behaviour although the efficiency of su devices would have to be evaluated with care. The objecti of this type of innovation would be to make the doctor, or t ward team, the budget holder to whom is given a share in a surpluses of revenue over expenditure. The allocation of su surpluses, rewards for efficiency in an ideal environmen would give an incentive to doctors to minimize costs a maximize benefits. In their struggle to behave in this fashi the doctor and other health-care professionals would induced to evaluate practice and identify the link betwe health-care inputs and health outcomes.

The evaluation of such budgeting arrangements is not eas In the US, Health Maintenance Organizations (HMOs) off incentives for efficient practice (Luft 1981) and appear have some attractive attributes: such organizations could set up to provide NHS primary care in inner cities. In the U careful experimentation is required with clear definition goals and long-term evaluation of outcomes.

As argued elsewhere the problems of health care systems everywhere are very similar (Maynard and Ludbrook 1980, 1981; McLachlan and Maynard 1982). Until appropriate incentive mechanisms are devised, all systems, both public and private, will continue to use scarce resources inefficiently and are unlikely to achieve the goals of policy.

The reformation of the incentives in the NHS might induce efficient practise in health care. Major initiatives are also needed in evaluating the links between inputs and the output of health (Fig. 16.1). Currently many people prefer prevention to cure but little is known about the efficiency of competing policies of prevention. The rhetoric and the advocates need to be replaced by scientific evaluation of the options even though this is difficult due to the long nature of the 'pay-off' period: reducing tobacco consumption generates benefits in ? years.

One important research activity in health care is the provision of incentives which induce efficient behaviour in producers and consumers: the identification and adoption of efficient methods of treating illness and less harmful patterns of consumption. The research priority in health is the unravelling of the inputs–output link. Such complex tasks require multidisciplinary work by doctors, sociologists, psychologists, and economists. Until these tasks are carried out more vigorously the process of groping towards the goals of the NHS may produce all too little success.

OVERVIEW: AN ECONOMIC APPROACH TO THE NHS

The problems faced by the NHS are considerable. There is evidence of inefficiency in the use of resources. The inefficient use of resources in the treatment of one patient deprives other patients of care which might save their lives or improve its quality by reducing pain and discomfort. Inefficiency is thus prevalent and unethical. Despite clear policy goals concerning the distribution of health care and health, the NHS has performed in a disappointing fashion with substantial inequalities surviving over 30 years of the Welfare State. Thus, future NHS policy makers may have to discriminate in favour of disadvantaged groups (by treating people unequally) and follow the objectives of the NHS (to treat people in equal need equally).

In order to analyse these defects in the NHS, and very similar defects in the health care system of other western nations, it is useful to apply the economists' 'tool-kit' as such analysis will provide useful insights into a variety of problems. In a world of scarce resources where all decisions impose opportunity costs, it is necessary to identify the costs and benefits of alternative ways of allocating society's resources. Information about costs and benefits will enable decision makers to determine the efficiency and equity characteristics of the way health care is provided. The NHS has objectives which are specified poorly but the evidence seems to be that the principles and practice of the NHS are at variance and the quality goal of the Service has not been achieved with any great success. In order that the Service be seen to achieve its objectives more clearly, new incentives have to be devised and implemented to induce efficiency amongst decision makers, usually doctors, and the nature of the links between the inputs

(health care, education, income, and other policies) and output (health) must be explored in a robust conceptual framework which is capable of testing scientifically.

Thus the research priorities in health care are the systematic analysis of the behaviour of health-care decision-makers so that we can identify new incentives which can be used to alter behaviour at the margin, and the careful evaluation of the costs and benefits of alternative health-care therapies and alternative ways of improving the health status of the community. The potential role of economics in this work is considerable: economics offers a systematic and explicit framework for the analysis of behaviour and the evaluation of policy options (Drummond 1980, 1981) and is an essential ingredient of any endeavour which seeks to improve public health. The fruitful combination of economical, sociological, statistical, psychological, and epidemiological skills is a difficult task. However, its challenges are unavoidable if the considerable inefficiency and inequalities which exist in the British health care system, and all other health care systems, are to be mitigated.

REFERENCES

Beveridge, W. (1942). *Social insurance and allied services.* Cmnd 6404. HMSO, London.

Bradford Hill, A. (1977). *A short textbook of medical statistics.* Hodder and Stoughton, London.

Bunker, J.P., Barnes, B.A., and Mosteller, F. (1977). *The costs, benefits and risks of surgery.* Oxford University Press, New York.

Cairns, J. and Snell, M. (1978). Prices and the demand for health care. In *Economic aspects of health services* (ed. A.J. Culyer and K. Wright) p. 95. Martin Robertson, London.

Cochrane, A.L. (1972). *Efficiency and effectiveness: random reflections on health services.* Nuffield Provincial Hospitals Trust, London.

Cooper, M.H. and Culyer, A.J. (1970). An economic assessment of some aspects of the operation of the National Health Service. In *Health services financing.* Appendix A. British Medical Association, London.

Cooper, M.H. and Culyer, A.J. (1971). An economic survey of the nature and intent of the British National Health Service. *Soc. Sci. Med.* **5**, 9.

Cooper, M.H. and Culyer, A.J. (1972). Equality in the National Health Service: intentions, performance and problems in evaluation. In *The economics of medical care* (ed. M. Hauser) p. 47. Allen and Unwin, London.

Culyer, A.J., Maynard, A., and Williams, A. (1982). Alternative systems of health care provision: an essay on motes and beams. In *A new approach to the economics of health care* (ed. M. Olsen) p. 131. American Enterprise Institute, Washington, DC.

Department of Health and Social Security (1976*a*). *Priorities for health and personal social services in England.* HMSO, London.

Department of Health and Social Security (1976*b*). *Sharing resources for health in England: the report of the Resource Allocation Working Party.* HMSO, London.

Department of Health and Social Security (1980). *Inequalities in health,* (The Black Report). DHSS, London.

Der Simonian, R., Charette, J., McPeek, B., *et al.* (1982) Reporting on methods in clinical trials. *N. Engl. J. Med.* **306**, 1332.

Donabedian, A. (1980). *The definition of quality and approaches to its assessment.* Health Administration Press, Ann Arbor, Michigan.

Drummond, M. (1980). *Principles of economic appraisal in health care.* Oxford University Press.

Drummond, M. (1981). *Studies in economic appraisal in health care.* Oxford University Press.

Friedman, M. (1962). *Capitalism and freedom.* University of Chicago Press.

Goodman, J. (1980). *National health care in Great Britain: lessons for the USA.* Fisher Institute, Dallas.

Grossman, M. (1972). *The demand for health.* National Bureau of Economic Research, New York.

Le Grand, J. (1978). The distribution of public expenditure: the case of health care. *Economica* **45**, 125.

Le Grand, J. (1982). *Strategy for equality.* Allen and Unwin, London.

Luft, H. (1981). *Health maintenance organization: dimensions of performance.* Wiley, New York.

Maynard, A. (1971). Inequalities in psychiatric care. *Soc. Sci. Med.* **6**, 221.

Maynard, A. (1979). Health care and the price mechanism. In *Pricing the social services* (ed. K. Judge) p. 86. Macmillan, London.

Maynard, A. (1981). The inefficiency and inequalities in the health care systems of Western Europe. *Soc. Pol. Admin.* **15**, 145.

Maynard, A. (1982). The regulation of public health and private health care markets. In *The public/private mix for health: the relevance and effects of change* (ed. G. McLachlan and A. Maynard) p. 473. Nuffield Provincial Hospitals Trust, London.

Maynard, A. (1983). Privatising the National Health Service. *Lloyds Bank Rev.* **148**, 28.

Maynard, A. and Ludbrook, A. (1980*a*). Applying the resource allocation formulae to the constituent parts of the U.K. *Lancet* **i**, 85.

Maynard, A. and Ludbrook, A. (1980*b*). Budget allocation in the NHS. *J. Soc. Pol.* **9**, 3.

Maynard, A. and Ludbrook, A. (1980*c*). Whats wrong with the NHS? *Lloyds Bank Rev.* October 27.

Maynard, A. and Ludbrook (1981). Thirty years of fruitless endeavour: an analysis of government intervention in health care markets. In *Health, economics and health economics.* (ed. J. v der Gaag and M. Perlman) p. 45. North Holland, Amsterdam.

McLachlan, G. and Maynard, A. (eds.) (1982). *The public/private mix for health: the relevance and effects of change.* Nuffield Provincial Hospitals Trust, London.

McKeown, T. (1977). *The modern rise of population.* Edward Arnold, London.

McKeown, T. (1979). *The role of medicine,* 2nd edn. Blackwell Oxford.

Ministry of Health (1944). *A national health service* Cmnd. 650 HMSO, London.

Muurinen, J. (1982). The demand for health: a generalised Grossman model. *J. Health Econ.* May, 5.

Newhouse, J.P. and Friedlander, L.J. (1980). The relationship between medical resources and measures of health: some additional evidence. *J. Human Res.* **15**, 200.

Newhouse, J.P., Manning, W.G., Morris, C.N. *et al.* (1981). Some interim results from a controlled trial of cost sharing in health insurance. Rand Corporation, Health Insurance Experiment Series, R-2847-M-MS, Santa Monica.

Seldon, A. (1980). *The litmus papers.* Centre for Policy Studies London.

Stern, J. (1982). *Social mobility and the interpretation of social class mortality differences.* Centre for Labour Economics London School of Economics, Discussion Paper 123.

Townsend, P. and Davidson, N. (1982). *Inequalities in health: the Black Report.* Penguin, London.

Weed, L.L. (1981). Physicians of the future. *N. Engl. J. Med.* **30** 903.

Williams, A. (1978). Need: an economic exegesis. In *Economic aspects of health services.* (ed. A.J. Culyer and K. Wright) p. 3 Martin Robertson, Oxford.

7 The application of economics to problems of public health and the delivery of medical services

Joseph P. Newhouse

INTRODUCTION

Can economics help solve or ameliorate problems in public health and medicine? Should students of public health concern themselves with economics? Economics applies to problems of medicine and public health at two levels. It can help explain what actually happens; this part of economics is known as positive economics. Economics also is concerned with what should happen; this part is known as normative economics and tends to be more controversial. In this chapter we discuss some of the relatively non-controversial parts of normative economics, as well as some propositions in positive economics.

Fundamentally, both positive and normative economics are the study of scarce resources. Although physicians, public health practitioners, and patients sometimes prefer not to admit it, personal medical services use scarce – often quite scarce – resources. Public health measures are often less costly per person than personal services, but none the less use scarce resources. Especially in less developed countries, resources for even public health measures may be a large burden. As a result, economics is highly relevant both to problems of public health and the delivery of personal medical services.

Some physicians and public health professionals appear to fear economics and argue that it is actually inimical to public health and to patients (Loewy 1980; Wolfe 1974). To an economist this seems rather like saying physics is inimical to public health because its knowledge can be used to produce weapons. Such fears arise from a misunderstanding of economics, which starts from the premise that resources – meaning goods and services – are scarce. Given this premise, economics is concerned that: (i) the greatest medical benefit be derived from a given quantity of resources devoted to producing 'health';* and (ii) if more resources are added to public health or medicine, that such resources *not* be capable of producing still greater benefits elsewhere, i.e. that the

resources not be diverted from more highly valued uses. Of course, hidden in these two concerns are a host of problems, especially those of how benefits are to be computed and what health is. For the most part we shall have to ignore these problems in this chapter.

Sometimes the notion that resources are scarce is challenged on the grounds that additional income in wealthy countries is buying rather frivolous goods; that is, we have all we 'need,' and therefore more could be devoted to medical care with no meaningful sacrifice (Loewy 1980). Even if such were the case in wealthy countries (and of course the person consuming the frivolous good may not think it at all frivolous!). One has only to recall the grinding poverty of parts of the less-developed world to realize that not everyone does satisfy all their wants. Realistically all wants could not be satisfied, given the volume of goods and services that the world now produces.

The scarcity of resources for satisfying people's wants creates three questions that any economy must solve: what goods and services will be produced; how those goods and services will be produced; and who will consume the goods and services.

Each question admits of alternative answers. In response to the first question, for example, a society could spend more on medical care and less on other goods and services, or vice versa. And in response to the second, a society could produce medical care with more physicians and fewer nurses, or more nurses and fewer physicians. In response to the third question, a greater or lesser share of medical care could be allocated to the well (e.g. preventive measures) rather than to the sick, or, within the category of the sick, the society could allocate more services to individuals with one disease and fewer to individuals with another. In short, precisely because resources are scarce, every society must collectively or individually choose how best to use them; economics is the study of those choices.

Unfortunately, in a chapter such as this, one can neither systematically explain economics, nor comprehensively demonstrate its applicability to health and medical care. The most that can be hoped for is to interest the reader in

*This formulation overlooks the problem of a good that may produce enjoyment or thrills but is inimical to health (e.g. alcohol consumption). In such cases all benefits must be valued, not just medical benefits or costs.

pursuing the study of economics further. Those who want amplification of the economics described here should refer to any one of the dozens of introductory economics textbooks. Those who wish more on the application of economic principles to medical care should refer to a number of texts on the economics of health or medical care (Fuchs 1974; Newhouse 1978; Cullis and West 1979; Feldstein 1979; Eastaugh 1982).

This chapter has three goals. First, the reader should become acquainted with how economists reason; second, the reader should obtain some notion of the kinds of problems for which economics is suitable; third, the reader should be better able to spot a few common errors. We will begin by treating some seemingly dry issues in the analysis of cost. Perhaps because cost is sometimes perceived as a subject best left to accountants, many analysts err in their treatment of cost. This introductory section, then, can be regarded as treating some basic issues in measuring cost that are relevant to both positive and normative economics. Rather than systematically present the abstract theory of cost, this section will be organized in the form of rules or tips for the practitioner who may be undertaking some analysis of cost. After this discussion of cost measurement, we will take up some issues in behaviour. An appendix gives a thumbnail description of the economics of American personal medical care services.

ANALYSES OF COSTS

Use marginal cost, shun average cost

Frequently individuals wish to estimate the cost of a public health project or a personal medical service. Often the suspicion that the funds could be more productively employed in some other endeavour motivates such a study. Unfortunately, an all too common method employed to calculate cost will produce a value that is irrelevant for ascertaining the correctness of the suspicion.

Figure 17.1 shows a typical cost curve for some service. The first unit of the service is often relatively expensive because some fixed costs must be incurred merely to produce anything. Perhaps a machine must be purchased, which, once in place, can produce several units of service relatively cheaply; perhaps a person must be hired who, once hired, can provide one or several units of service at the same price. In

such cases the cost per unit will decline as more units are pr duced. As Fig. 17.1 is drawn, after the first unit, the cost purchasing any additional units is the same (about 7). This unlikely to be the case in practice, but to assume it w simplify understanding the general principle involved.

A depressingly frequent procedure at this point is to calc late the average cost of the product or service, multiply th value by the number of units by which production mig change, and announce the result as 'the cost of the servic (By average cost is meant the total cost of the service divid by the number of units produced; i.e. the cost per unit. Fig. 17.1 the average cost of OA units is 10, and of OB un is 8.)

Costs calculated in this fashion should only be used make decisions in two special cases: first, when there are fixed costs *and* the cost of producing each unit (including t first one) is the same, or second, when one is interested in m producing any units at all; i.e. complete shut down.

Because these two conditions are rarely satisfied, ev approximately, the average cost figure is seldom helpf Unless the conditions hold, the average cost figure does n answer the relevant question; that is, how many resources a given decrease in production would release (or require expansion is at issue). Suppose one is now producing X uni and is contemplating producing D units fewer. The co figure one wants is the difference between the cost producing X units and the cost of producing $X - D$ units; th is precisely the additional resources one will have if t proposed change is made. This difference in total cost called the marginal cost of decreasing production by D unit given that one was already producing X units. If fixed cos are large and D is small, the marginal cost will be much le than the average cost. There are other cases, however, whe marginal cost can exceed average cost; there is no necessar relationship between the two (but the mathematically incline can verify that marginal cost must equal average cost at t minimum value of average cost).

To illustrate an application of this principle, we turn to t debate over how much waste is caused by the duplication medical facilities in the US. For a variety of reasons, princ pally the extensive insurance coverage of hospital service many argue that there is excessive capital devoted to hospit. services in the US.* Anecdotes abound about two hospita across the street that each have the same equipment whe they could reduce costs by sharing facilities.

Because of the alleged duplication, regulatory measures reduce the amount of capital in hospitals have been imple mented. For example, (US) Certificate of Need legislatio requires hospitals to seek approval from a planning agenc for projects whose cost exceeds a certain threshold figure. A part of the effort to plan hospital facilities better, guidelin were issued by the US Department of Health and Huma Services for consolidating hospital facilities. The guidelin usually specified the minimum utilization for certain pieces c

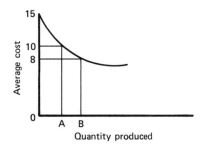

Fig. 17.1. Average or unit cost as a function of quantity produced. With a fixed cost to produce any unit and constant cost per unit, average cost falls at a decreasing rate as the quantity produced increases.

*The same premise would also imply that there is excessive labo employed in the hospital sector, but this charge is heard less often. Not however, the figures on beds in the Appendix; on a comparative basis, th US has fewer beds per person than other developed countries.

apital equipment and in addition made recommendations oncerning overall hospital size. For example, some of the apital equipment covered by the guidelines included: (i) comuted axial tomography (CAT) units, for which the standard as that at least 2500 procedures per year should be erformed; (ii) cardiac catheterization units, for which a ninimum annual caseload of 200 was specified; (iii) megaoltage-radiation-therapy units, for which the minimum nnual caseload was 300 cases, with somewhat fewer being ermissible in rural areas; and (iv) hospital beds, for which he guidelines held that four beds per 1000 population was a esirable maximum.

How serious is the problem of duplicated facilities? Some vho argue that there are too many facilities really mean that here are too many services delivered. And there can be little oubt that reducing the number of facilities would reduce the umber of services delivered. If beds do not exist, they will ot be filled! But the rhetoric surrounding the issue of dupliated facilities sometimes seems to imply that monies can be aved without affecting the quantity of services delivered. For xample, one presumes the two hospitals across the street vould continue to treat the same volume of patients if they ad an agreement to share facilities. Thus, if equipment is eally duplicative instead of excessive, one can take the urrent volume of care being delivered as a datum and ask ow much could be saved in delivering that volume of care if acilities were consolidated. Framed this way, the question ecomes a straightforward exercise in cost analysis. If one ospital is delivering X units of service and another hospital is elivering Y units, how much would it cost for just one of hem to deliver $X + Y$ units?

Schwartz and Joskow (1980) have estimated an upper ound on how much could be saved if the government guideines for the four types of equipment described above had een strictly adhered to in 1978, and the volume of services elivered did not change. Their best estimate of the maximum avings is $1000 million, less than 2 per cent of actual hospital xpenditure in that year. In fact, this upper bound is very oose. The true savings would almost certainly be much less han $1000 million, and could well be negative, because the chwartz and Joskow estimate does not include the direct osts of any regulation that would be necessary to implement onsolidation activities (e.g. salaries of regulators, data ollection costs, costs of litigation), nor does it include any dditional costs of travel imposed on patients if facilities were onsolidated.

The savings are relatively small, because in some cases most acilities already satisfy the guideline (cardiac catheterization, negavoltage-radiation therapy). Consolidating CAT scanners aves little because marginal costs are not very different from verage costs. (Another way economists make this point is to ay that economies of scale are exhausted rather quickly. conomies of scale are the region in Fig. 17.1 over which verage costs are declining. If marginal and average costs are imilar, the additional cost of treating all the cases at a newly nlarged facility will approximate the savings from closing a econd facility.)

By contrast, reducing beds by closing rooms, wards, or vings of a hospital saves little because the marginal cost is

much less than the average cost. As Schwartz and Joskow point out, reducing beds would save some housekeeping and maintenance staff, but those items amount to only about 5 per cent of total hospital expenditure, so the total costs at the hospital where the rooms are closed are little changed. Meanwhile, by assumption the same number of patients are being treated so expenditure on their behalf for such services as ancillary facilities, food, supplies, and materials would continue. The nation's hospital bill would thus be little affected. Marginal cost more closely approximates average cost (and the savings are potentially greater) if entire hospitals are closed, but even here Schwartz and Joskow estimate that closing 7 per cent of all hospital beds will save only about 1 per cent of total hospital expenditure (provided the same volume of patients continues to be cared for). The additional costs incurred from treating patients in the remaining facilities will offset much of the savings from closing some facilities.

Laboratory tests provide another example of a case in which marginal cost is frequently much less than average cost. Once the laboratory has set up equipment to perform a certain test, it can often perform many tests of that type relatively cheaply. As a result, the widely expressed concern about excessive testing's adding to cost seems somewhat misplaced. Although there is some marginal cost for the additional tests, that cost is typically not nearly as large as the amount billed for the tests. Thus, the true cost saving to society from eliminating a few tests is much less than would be implied by the charges for the tests. Put another way, if tests were reduced by 10–20 per cent, the cost of setting up the test would still be incurred. In effect, the charges for remaining tests would then rise, because the set-up costs would have to be recovered on a smaller number of tests.

Use real costs, not allocated costs

In the same spirit as the use of marginal cost in cost analyses is the use of real or actual costs. It may seem patently obvious that any cost analysis must use actual costs, but in fact many costs analyses fail to do so. Instead they include as part of cost some portion of allocated or overhead costs. Allocated costs are usually fixed costs that are averaged over a number of units. For example, the hospital administrator's salary is frequently 'stepped down' (i.e. allocated over other departments of the hospital). If one wishes to calculate the savings from closing a wing, the administrator's salary will not be saved, but it may appear in the stepped-down 'costs' of operating the wing that are kept on the hospital's books. Another way to put this point is that any organization's cost figures are kept for certain purposes. (In the case of the American hospital a major purpose if for insurance plans that reimburse costs (Danzon 1982).) Those purposes may not, and often do not, require the hospital to reflect the real resource costs from changing the scale of operations. An analyst simply must look behind the cost figures on the books rather than accept them at face value.

Cross subsidies in the hospital (Harris 1979) create another opportunity for individuals not to use real costs and reach misleading conclusions. For example, many argue that medical care expenditures could be substantially reduced if there were less use of the emergency room for non-emergency services. To support this claim, they usually cite the high price (relative to an office visit) that emergency rooms charge for their services. But this argument fails to recognize the cross-subsidy between the true medical emergency and the non-emergency case. In the US all users typically pay the same basic charge for emergency room services (say $60 per visit). As a result, those who use the emergency room as a walk-in clinic effectively subsidize those who are the true medical emergencies.

Another way to make this point is to consider the situation where users of the emergency room who were not true emergency cases ceased to use that facility. Usually it is advocated that they should use some new type of free-standing facility that would be open around the clock (Bliss 1982). By how much would the total costs of medical care change if such a facility were constructed and if, in fact, it treated the non-emergency cases now using the emergency rooms? The present emergency room's costs would change only by the amount of costs that the non-emergency cases impose on it. Precisely because of the cross subsidy, that amount is substantially less than the amount the non-emergency cases are currently being charged. Instead of lowering the total costs of the medical care system, building a free-standing facility may well add to them, because then there would be in fact two facilities providing what one was providing before. This indeed may be a case of creating duplicate facilities!

Include all costs, not just monetary costs to the decision-maker

Sometimes those calculating the cost of a project do not account for all the costs (nor all the benefits). Frequently non-monetary costs or costs that do not appear on the decision-maker's budget are ignored. An example comes from certain studies that calculate the cost savings from consolidating facilities. Typically such studies only include the direct costs at the institutions being consolidated, and ignore other costs.

We have already mentioned one example of a cost that is often ignored by such studies – the additional cost of patient (and maybe physician) travel when facilities are merged. If there were substantial savings in direct costs from consolidating, one would then have to ascertain whether accounting for additional travel costs might offset the savings. But frequently those estimating the savings from having hospitals of the optimum size do not account for travel costs. (For a critical review of the literature on the measurement of hospital cost, see Berki (1972).)

Many have noted that less political resistance from the community is encountered when planning bodies seek to close a wing of a hospital than when such bodies seek to close the entire hospital. The existence of travel costs may help explain this phenomenon. If only a wing is closed, travel costs are likely to change much less than if the entire facility is closed. (Religious or ethnic preferences may also be at play.)

Travel costs, except for the time involved, are relatively easy to value. Other costs, such as waiting times for an appointment, may not be. Reducing the capacity of a clinic may save some operating costs, but it is likely to force some users of the clinic to wait longer for an appointment. The cost of such waiting cannot readily be measured, but it is certainly a real cost.

Should an institution consider costs not on its books? It is clear that it must account for those costs it bears directly because to survive financially it must over the long run at least break even (taking account of any endowment income or gifts). Subject to this constraint, however, it is a reasonable goal for a non-profit or eleemosynary entity to maximize the benefits it delivers to the community (Taylor and Newhouse 1970). If it is to do so, it must consider costs that do not necessarily appear in its books. Because many American hospitals and public health activities are non-profit making, the injunction to include all costs and benefits seems appropriate.

The treatment of depreciation

Depreciation illustrates both omission of certain costs and failure to use real costs. Depreciation, of course, is simply the amount of a capital asset that is used up in the process of producing services. Sometimes this amount can be 'replaced' by ordinary maintenance of the asset (repair of a machine, painting a room), but at other times it becomes uneconomic to incur repair costs; it is cheaper to purchase a new asset (e.g. buy a new machine). Depreciation is an actual cost of production, but it is frequently not treated correctly in analysing cost. All too often it is completely omitted; only operating and no capital costs are counted. At other times it is included but at some assumed value that may bear little relationship to the true depreciation cost (i.e. to the true amount of capital used in production). Probably the most common method for calculating depreciation is to assume some lifetime for the asset (e.g. 30 years) and then assume that the asset is used up at a uniform rate over that lifetime. (This is called straight-line depreciation.) The depreciation carried on the books for one year of production is then the cost of the asset divided by its assumed lifetime.

Two mistakes can be made in this procedure. The most significant is that the depreciation on the books will value the asset at its cost when purchased, not the amount it would take to buy the asset today (the jargon for this is that the asset is valued at historical cost rather than replacement cost). Given recent experience with inflation, if the asset is at all long lived, its cost when purchased may be far below the cost it would take to replace the asset. As a result, depreciation using historical cost can result in a severe underestimate of the true economic cost of production. The less significant problem is that the assumed lifetime may be incorrect; the actual wear and tear on the asset may make its lifetime more or less than that used in the calculation.

The problem becomes even more complicated if a new machine comes on the market that has the capabilities of the old machine but costs less, a frequent occurrence in medicine. In that case the market value of the old machine will fall – a current example is provided by older computers – and historical cost may overstate the true depreciation being ncurred; in effect, the machine that is wearing out is no longer very valuable because it could be replaced for less. For this reason the use of historical cost does not always understate true depreciation.

Although depreciation is an important aspect of cost, it is not the only part of capital cost. The correct capital costs to include in an analysis are depreciation plus foregone interest on the funds tied up in the asset.

Discount costs (and benefits) from different time periods

Frequently one is interested in evaluating projects whose costs or benefits extend over a considerable period of time. Preventive care of all types is an example; costs are incurred at the time the preventive service is delivered, but benefits continue to accrue for many years into the future.

When comparing costs and benefits, the figures must be put in the same year of account. This means more than simply adjusting for inflation. The fundamental concept one must work with is discounting, which is quite important and widely applicable.

The idea behind discounting is that a dollar today is more valuable than a dollar in the future, provided one can take the dollar today and invest it in a productive fashion. The simplest case to think about is one in which one purchases some sort of riskless, interest-bearing financial instrument (such as a government bond). After one year the bond will return one's original principal plus interest. If one were to continue to invest one's principal at some interest rate r, after n years one would have $(1 + r)^n$ dollars for every dollar that one had originally invested. (Note that r, here, is a decimal fraction and not a percentage interest rate.)

Suppose that one can invest in some sort of project that will require no operating costs (i.e. the only costs are a one-time investment at the beginning of the project). The project will pay back a certain amount in the future. If one is comparing the payback to one's investment, each year of payback must be deflated by $(1 + r)^n$, where n equals the number of years that one must wait for the return. Although discounting as just explained may appear to require the existence of some sort of financial instrument as an alternative investment, in fact this is not the case. Fundamentally, the discount rate reflects the availability of projects that yield larger returns in the future than the investment required in the present (what economists call the social return to capital). If one invests in a project whose discounted (social) returns do not equal (social) costs, one will generally be foregoing an investment that would have yielded higher returns. (Recall that economics is concerned with the channelling of resources to their most highly valued uses.)

Another way to state the principle of discounting is that it makes dollars received or spent at different times commensurate. For example, a dollar received in exactly one year is worth $1/(1 + r)$ dollars today because if one invests $1/(1 + r)$ dollars today, one will have exactly one dollar in one year. ($1/(1 + r)$ is called the present value of the dollar to be received in the future.) Similarly a dollar that will be spent or received in two years is worth $1/(1 + r)^2$ today, and one spent or received in three years is worth $1/(1 + r)^3$. Thus, if a project

yields one dollar in one year and another dollar in three years, the benefits in today's dollars is $1/(1 + r) + 1/(1 + r)^3$.

One immediate implication of discounting is that at any reasonable size of r, dollars that are to be spent or received far in the future do not count for very much. For example, if r were 10 per cent, and if we were considering the value today of a dollar that was to be received 50 years from now, the value is $1/(1.1)^{50}$, which is less than one cent. Thus, decisions should not be dominated by events that occur many years in the future unless these events represent truly enormous benefits or costs, but over an intermediate term the choice of projects might be quite sensitive to the discount rate.

So much for theory. In reality we must choose an actual discount rate. As any reading of a newspaper's financial page will reveal, there are many different interest rates. Which, if any, is the appropriate rate to use to discount in our problem? Economists have never agreed on the answer to this question, but one defensible value is 10 per cent (see Shishko 1975). Other analysts tend to use lower rates; few use a rate below 4 per cent. These values do not include any adjustment for inflation; that is, they assume any future costs or benefits have been deflated by the assumed inflation rate; i.e. that costs and benefits are in constant dollars. (Alternatively, one can add an assumed inflation rate to the discount rate and use current dollars.)

Up to this point, we have assumed that any project being evaluated had monetary costs and benefits. But this assumption is often incorrect in the case of public health projects. Benefits, for example, might accrue in the form of improved health status. Suppose, for example, that decreased morbidity will come about in the future as a result of some investment in preventive health today. Should one discount future morbidity reductions just like one discounts dollars? Another way to put this question is to ask whether saving one sick day next year is worth more than saving one sick day ten years from now?

Although virtually all economists agree that monetary benefits and costs should be discounted, discounting non-monetary benefits or costs is more controversial. None the less, a powerful argument can be made that they should be discounted (Keeler and Cretin 1983). At first blush it may seem that the rationale for discounting that was presented above would not apply. Clearly if the future benefits are in dollars, some sort of a financial instrument such as a bond is an alternative and it is appropriate to compare the yield on the project under consideration with the yield on the bond. But what if the future benefits are fewer sick days?

In fact, the rationale presented above for discounting can be extended to cover the case of non-monetary benefits (or costs) if money can be spent in such a way as to obtain the non-monetary benefit (e.g. to reduce sick days). Suppose, for example, that one could, by spending x today, save a sick day next year. If it will still cost x (in today's dollars) to save a sick day in ten years, one need only invest $1/(1 + r)^{10}$ today to have enough resources in ten years to save the sick day then. In effect, healthy days ten years from now are cheaper to produce than healthy days next year because one can invest the money in the interim in some productive project. (The rule must be modified if the real cost of producing the benefit, e.g. reducing sick days, changes over time; none the less, the principle of discounting would still apply.)

The only exception to discounting occurs if dollars cannot at all affect the benefit. For example, one might be choosing between, say, one programme that will save one sick day in one year or an alternative one that will save two sick days three years hence. If sick days could not be affected by any expenditure of dollars, discounting is no longer relevant; one simply must choose the outcome one prefers, and market interest rates have nothing to do with the decision. But sick days (and in general almost any non-monetary cost or benefit) can certainly be altered by spending additional resources either now or in the future (e.g. investing more resources in building safer highways). Thus, the exceptional case in which the non-monetary benefits cannot be affected by expenditure will be extremely rare. Almost always it will be correct to discount non-pecuniary as well as pecuniary benefits and costs.

ANALYSES OF BEHAVIOUR

The foregoing secton might be regarded as a somewhat mechanical exercise in cost acounting, partly because the material was mainly presented in the form of rules for treating cost when making decisions. Of course, the reasoning about how costs should be treated could be turned around to generate hypotheses about how individuals or firms behave; for example, one might test whether firms or individuals acted as if they minimized costs.

The generation and testing of hypotheses is the more usual fare in economics, because, as a social science, economics is vitally concerned with explaining behaviour. Explanation occurs at two levels. First, economists seek to explain the choices of individuals under given conditions. Second, they seek to explain how the choices of a group of individuals may interact in such a way as to change the original conditions confronting that group of individuals, which in turn may alter the original choices of some or all of the group. Both these points can be illustrated by considering how physicians in the US locate their practices.

Choice under given conditions: the physician's choice of location

Economics is in a large part the study of choice, and it usually assumes that the chooser acts as if something is being maximized or minimized given certain constraints. If consumers are making choices, the usual assumption is that they act as if they are maximizing their utility (or welfare), subject to (at least) their incomes and the prices they face. If business firms are making choices, it is usually assumed that they maximize profits. We will begin with an example concerning physicians' choice of practice location, and we will assume that in so doing physicians act as if they are maximizing their utility.

What affects a physician's utility in various locations? We shall assume it is the fee that he or she can earn as well as the attractiveness of each location. (If fees are fixed by some third party, we will assume that physicians evaluate each location on the basis of the income that can be earned there,

as well as its attractiveness.) Suppose two locations a equally attractive to a new physician, but one location offe higher fees or income. We assume that the physician w choose to enter the location with the higher fee or incom Similarly, if two locations offer the same income, but one more attractive than the other, we assume the physician w choose the more attractive location. Finally, we assume that two locations have the same number of physicians, th location with a greater demand for physician services wi other things equal, have higher fees or incomes. All this ca be summarized by assuming that physicians value locatio with more demand per physician, as well as more amenities.

Choice under changing conditions: physician locatio continued

As just described, the choice of the individual physician straightforward, even boring. More interesting is the patter of location that is produced by a group of physicians, all c whom choose in this fashion. (As we shall see later, it is no necessary that all physicians choose this way, but it wi simplify the exposition to make that assumption.) In such case a characteristic pattern of physician location wi develop.

It is perhaps easiest to understand the characteristic patter if we begin with a concrete example. Consider a specialty tha has negligible competition with other specialties (perhap neurosurgery). Again suppose, to keep things simple, that a locations are equally attractive. The first neurosurgeon will g to the location of highest demand, which will usually be th largest city. Although epidemiological and socio-economi factors have some effect on demand per person, most of th variation among cities in the demand for physician service comes about simply from variation in population. We als make the readily supportable assumption that demand fall with the distance that the patient must travel (Phelps an Newhouse 1974). For if all prospective patients were willin to travel to the one physician no matter where he or she wer located, then there would be no advantage to locating in th largest city. Assuming the first neurosurgeon locates in th largest city, the second neurosurgeon will examine th demand for his services at each location. Because he mus split the market in the largest city with the first neurosurgeon the second neurosurgeon will generally locate in the secon largest city (provided it is more than half the size of the larges city). The third neurosurgeon will consider the demand fo his services in each city given the location of the first an second neurosurgeons, and so forth. Out of this will emerge pattern of served and unserved cities; the number of citie served will depend upon the number of neurosurgeons.

The process can be shown using Fig. 17.2. That figur shows three cities, of three, two, and one million populatio respectively, that are equidistant from one another. Assum that the cities are equally attractive and that demand pe resident is the same. The first neurosurgeon locates in the cit of three million and the second in the city of two million Where will the third locate? If he splits the demand in the cit of three million with one other neurosurgeon, they will eac face demand from approximately 1.5 million patients plu

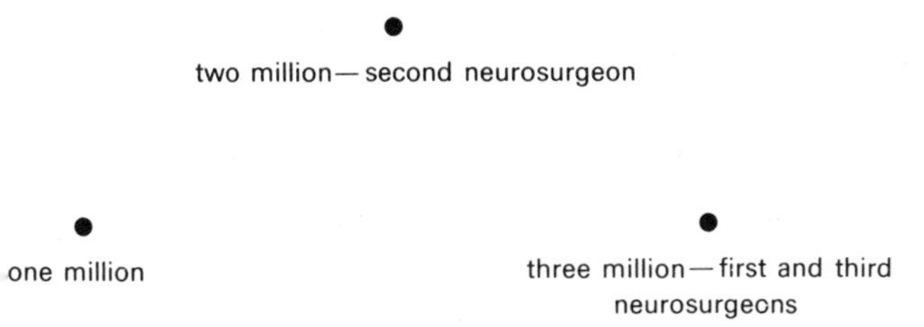

two million—second neurosurgeon

one million

three million—first and third neurosurgeons

Fig. 17.2. Three hypothetical cities and the location of three neurosurgeons. With three physicians two locate in the city of three million and one in the city of two million.

ny patients travelling to them from the city of one million. Because he will split the demand in the city of two million with the second neurosurgeon, he will face a demand from only around one million patients (plus travelling patients) if he locates in either of the other two cities. So the third neurosurgeon will locate in the city of three million. The fourth neurosurgeon is nearly indifferent among all three cities, because he will encounter the demands of about one million patients in each. The fifth neurosurgeon will locate in one of the two cities that the fourth neurosurgeon did not choose, and the sixth will locate in the city that the fifth did not choose. From this point on, as neurosurgeons grow in multiples of six, each city will gain neurosurgeons at the same proportionate rate (e.g. if there were 12 neurosurgeons in total, each city would have twice as many as when there were six).

Several testable hypotheses can be drawn out of this example. First, if locations are similar in both amenities and demand per person, there will be a critical town size. Cities and towns that are larger than the critical town size will have a member of a given specialty present, and those that are smaller will not. In the above example, if there are two neurosurgeons, the critical town size is two million. Clearly the critical town size will be smaller, the larger the number of specialists in a given specialty. As a result, we should expect to find general surgeons in smaller communities than neurosurgeons.

Moreover, as a given specialty grows over time, the critical town size will fall. Hence, we should expect specialists to diffuse into smaller communities as their numbers grow. As the diffusion occurs, groups of smaller towns, not all of which possessed a specialist of a given genre, should gain specialists at a more rapid rate than groups of larger towns, all of which had specialists of that genre.

We have made some unrealistic assumptions in deriving these implications, but relaxing most of them does not change the predictions in any fundamental way. First, suppose that not all towns are equally attractive. In that case, some physicians should be willing to accept a lower (real) fee or a lower (real) income to live in a more attractive area. (A physician in an attractive area would have to give up something or all physicians would locate in the most attractive area.) More attractive areas will therefore have more physicians and a smaller demand per physician. Second, suppose that not all cities have the same per person demand. Then cities with greater per person demand are just like larger

cities. For both these reasons, there will be some randomness around the critical town size. We can say that, as a town's population increases, the likelihood of a given type of physician's being present should increase. But some towns with a physician may be smaller than other towns that are still without one.

Table 17.1 confirms all these hypotheses. It shows the percentage of towns of a given size that had a board-certified specialist in 1960 and 1977. (These data come from a 23 state sample of the US; see Schwartz *et al.* (1980) for further details.) Inspection of the data will show that all three hypotheses are borne out. Within a given specialty, larger towns are more likely to have a board-certified specialist present. Second, larger specialties are more likely to have members present in smaller towns. Third, as their numbers have grown, board-certified specialists have diffused into steadily smaller towns. Fourth, as Table 17.2 shows, smaller towns have been gaining specialists at a faster (percentage) rate than larger towns. (Formal tests of significance confirm that larger towns are more likely to have a specialist present and that specialists are growing at a more rapid percentage rate in smaller town size intervals.)

Table 17.1. *Percentage of communities with board-certified specialists in 1960, 1970, and 1977*

Specialty	Population of towns in thousands						
	2.5–5	5–10	10–20	20–30	30–50	50–200	>200
Internal medicine							
1960	2	11	25	65	85	90	100
1970	2	9	32	75	92	95	100
1977	9	23	51	92	98	95	100
Surgery							
1960	5	19	58	82	95	100	100
1970	10	25	66	92	100	100	100
1977	14	38	71	98	100	100	100
Paediatrics							
1960	1	6	22	68	88	100	100
1970	1	7	30	73	93	97	100
1977	3	14	43	82	98	100	100
Obstetrics/gynaecology							
1960	0	3	12	46	88	95	100
1970	1	4	30	75	93	100	100
1977	4	11	44	87	98	100	100
Radiology							
1960	3	12	44	77	88	98	100
1970	4	16	56	85	98	100	100
1977	9	28	63	89	100	100	100
Urology							
1960	0	1	9	37	58	93	100
1970	0	1	11	40	78	100	100
1977	1	5	26	74	98	100	100
Dermatology							
1960	0	1	1	9	33	83	97
1970	0	1	5	10	59	92	97
1977	1	1	7	39	76	95	100
Neurosurgery							
1960	0	0	1	4	8	40	100
1970	0	0	1	2	14	43	94
1977	0	1	2	5	27	74	97
Family practice							
1977	37	56	68	79	90	92	100
Number of towns in each population range, 1970	621	361	185	52	59	37	33

Table 17.2. *Ratio of specialists per person in 1977 to specialists per person in 1960**

Specialty	Population of towns in thousands						
	2.5–5	5–10	10–20	20–30	30–50	50–200	>200
Internal medicine	5.1	2.7	2.8	2.3	2.7	2.6	2.5
General surgery	3.4	2.4	1.7	1.7	1.7	1.6	1.5
Paediatrics	3.6	2.6	2.6	1.9	2.0	1.9	2.0
Obstetrics/gynaecology	–	4.4	5.4	4.0	2.7	2.3	2.0
Radiology	3.0	2.8	2.0	1.8	2.0	2.0	2.3
Urology	–	2.5	3.0	2.4	2.3	1.7	1.7

*Obstetric and urology in the 2500 to 5000 range are omitted because there were one and zero specialists, respectively, in 1960; the actual value for obstetrics is 25.4.

Thus, these data are consistent with a simple economic model of physician location. The reader is warned, however, that the model does need elaboration to explain some phenomena; in particular, the assumption of no competition among specialties needs to be relaxed in order to explain why some types of physicians, such as internists, are disproportionately located in metropolitan areas while others, such as general practitioners (GPs), are disproportionately located in small towns. (The interested reader is referred to Newhouse *et al.* (1982*a,b,c*) for further discussion.)

Not everyone believes that the simple economic model can explain physician location behaviour. In particular, the premises of US public policy (based at least in part on the analyses of a number of economists) assume that physicians choose their location solely on the basis of tastes or preferences with little or no regard for economic considerations. Because physicians are said to prefer to live in larger towns, it is assumed that physicians are maldistributed (too many in large cities) and that public intervention is required to ensure sufficient physicians at certain locations (including rural areas).*

One can understand how such notions originated. Economic theory suggests that physicians will earn about the same amount in each location although they will earn somewhat less in attractive locations. If physicians did not earn approximately the same amount, some physicians would enter locations where they could earn more. Precisely because the individual physician will earn about the same amount in any location, individual preferences about the non-monetary attributes of any location are likely to seem paramount in that person's choice.

In addition to casual introspection about what was 'important', two pieces of data supported the thesis that physicians were not subject to the usual economic constraints in their choice of location. First, physician population ratios markedly favour metropolitan areas. If physicians located so as to even out demand, it did not seem possible that demand could be so much higher in metropolitan areas. Indeed, it appeared that physicians were 'thumbing their noses' at non-metropolitan areas.

The fallacy in this comparison is the implied assumption that non-metropolitan residents seek their care from non-

**See the quotations cited in Newhouse *et al.* (1982*a*), as support for this assertion.*

metropolitan physicians. In fact, for many non-metropolitan residents the closest physician is located in a metropolitan area. Non-metropolitan residents who use a metropolitan physician should be taken out of the denominator of the non-metropolitan ratio and placed in the denominator of the metropolitan ratio. When this is done, the gap between the two ratios substantially closes.

Second, throughout the 1960s and into the early 1970s, the physician/population ratio in the US grew in metropolitan areas but did not change very much in non-metropolitan areas. Although additional physicians were being trained, they all appeared to be going to metropolitan areas, contrary to the prediction of the simple economic model just described.

But these comparisons of growth rates in metropolitan and non-metropolitan areas failed to recognize the distinction among specialties. Not all categories of physicians were growing equally. In fact, the GP, who for good economic reasons was disproportionately located in small towns, was dying out; the number of GPs was falling in absolute terms. The number of specialists, however, was increasing sufficiently so that the overall physician/population ratio was increasing. But the critical town size for the specialist was larger than for the GP. Thus, specialists were moving into non-metropolitan areas, but their increased numbers there did no more than roughly offset the fall in the number of GPs. New specialists were, of course, continuing to increase in number in cities, which accounted for the increase in the physician population ratio there.

Of importance for policy purposes, this change in specialty composition has now reversed itself. During the 1970s family practitioner programmes came into being (stimulated by government subsidies), and the category of general and family practitioner is now growing. There is both theoretical and some empirical reason to think that the certified family practitioner with three years of postgraduate training does not locate in the same way as the GP with but one year of postgraduate training; specifically, the family practitioner is more likely to locate in larger cities than the GP. Nevertheless, the two types of physicians probably locate in a sufficiently similar manner that, unlike the 1960s, the total physician/population ratio will increase fastest in small towns in the 1980s.

Does the economic model mean there is no room for government intervention, particularly on behalf of underserved groups? The answer is emphatically no. The economic model of physician location does not imply that no groups in the population are underserved by some normative criteria. It only suggests that physicians locate in accordance with the demand for their services. If some groups are underserved, it suggests that those groups' demands for care are not great enough to attract physicians to serve them. But the public may very well want to assure some access to care for those groups, and a logical vehicle for doing so is a public programme. Such intervention could take the form of insurance programmes to increase the demand of such groups for services, or alternatively could take the form of public delivery of services to such groups. The latter method will be relatively more advantageous, the more geographically concentrated are the disadvantaged groups. (This assumes continued private delivery of services to most of the population.)

The whole does not necessarily equal the sum of its parts

A decade ago the paucity of physicians in rural areas was seen as an important policy problem. Because it was thought that physicians located solely in response to their preferences for non-monetary attributes, attention focused on the determinants of those preferences. The hope was to identify certain traits or attributes of physicians who were likely to locate in rural areas. The implication was that if one wished to increase the number of physicians locating in rural areas, one might change the mix of medical school admittees in favour of students who had such traits.

A number of studies were carried out that compared characteristics of physicians who located in rural areas with those of physicians who located in metropolitan areas. A common finding was that physicians who were reared in rural areas were much more likely to locate their practice in rural areas. Assuming there is an overriding goal to have more physicians in rural areas, can such a finding be used as a basis for discriminating in medical school admissions in favour of students reared in rural areas?

The economic model warns us to be careful in drawing the inference that such discrimination will change the outcome. The problem can be illustrated by considering a possibly extreme case. To define such a case, we assume that there are some physicians who do not care about location at all, but are only interested in maximizing the fees (or income) that they receive, while others have strong location preferences. Thus, we now relax the assumption that all physicians value locations similarly.

The model described in the preceding section showed that there was a critical town size; physicians were unlikely to be present in towns smaller than that size, and were likely to have similar patient loads in towns above that size. Consider again the example of three towns of three, two and one million, and suppose that there are six physicians for these three towns. Suppose further that two of the physicians feel strongly about location; one wishes to be in the city of three million and the other in the city of two million. Perhaps they were reared in those cities. The other four physicians do not particularly care which city they practise in. According to the model, the two who care will each go to the city they desire; two of the other four will be in the largest city; one of the other four will be the second physician in the city of two million, and the sixth will locate in the city of one million.

Even though some physicians had strong location preferences, the overall distribution of physicians was the same as that when no physician cared about location. Moreover, if one carried out a study of physician location and place of rearing, one would have found a correlation between the two variables, yet the number of physicians in each town was unaffected by this correlation.

Now suppose an 'enlightened' policymaker knew about the correlation and, using it as a rationale, had discriminated in the medical school admission process. Specifically, the policymaker had admitted an individual from the 'small' town of one million in lieu of one of the six who was admitted. We will assume, for the sake of argument, that this person strongly desires to practice in that town. Even in this case the overall distribution of physicians still would not be changed, as one can verify by working through the example.

Of course, this example may be a special case. The strong location preferences of some physicians have no effect at all on the ultimate location because there are enough physicians who do not care about location to arbitrage the market. If the policymaker continued to increase the number of physicians from rural backgrounds (e.g. if he or she admitted a second person who strongly desired to practise in the town of one million), it is likely to decrease the number of physicians who do not care and increase the number who want to locate in rural areas. At some point there may well be more physicians in rural areas than there would have been without the discrimination. But the increase will not be nearly as great as might be thought by looking at the likelihood that, within a given cohort of physicians, a physician from a rural background will locate in a rural area. The fallacy of assuming that the response can be predicted by looking at the correlation between background and location is called the fallacy of composition.

The fallacy of composition occurs frequently among non-economists. It comes from assuming that individuals, when making future decisions, will face the same constraints and incentives as they did when they were studied. But if enough individuals make a certain kind of choice, the constraints will change. In the example of the three cities, one physician who strongly preferred the city of one million could be accommodated without affecting the relative income of any of the physicians. But if a substantial number of individuals strongly prefer the city of one million (perhaps because of changed admission policies), the relative incomes that can be earned in different locations will change; physicians practising in small towns will start to earn relatively less, and some who otherwise would have located in small towns will choose to locate instead in large cities.

Another example of the fallacy of composition may serve to fix the idea. Consider the demand for fine wine. Consumers with higher incomes spend a much larger fraction of their incomes on fine wine than the less fortunate. Suppose we observe the consumption of wine by those with incomes of $50 000 per year and those with incomes of $20 000 per year. Suppose the consumption of those with $50 000 incomes is three times the amount of those with $20 000 incomes. Now suppose the economy will grow in real terms around 3.7 per cent per year. Those now making $20 000 will after 25 years be making $50 000 per year (in constant dollars). Can we predict that their consumption of fine wine will triple?

Unfortunately, there is a limit on how much fine wine can be produced in a year; there are only a limited number of vintners who can produce truly fine wine. As incomes rise, the demand for fine wine will increase, but because the supply cannot increase very much, the price will rise. This will serve to reduce the demand at each income level; in fact, if the supply of fine wine cannot be increased at all, the consumption of today's $20 000 income families may scarcely increase at all, even when they are earning $50 000 (provided the income of all other families increases proportionately). In effect, the constraints facing consumers, namely the relative price of wine, will change, and their choices will change. Rather than the consumption of wine, the incomes of vineyard owners will rise.

Consumers (patients) respond to changes in the constraints they face

We have already seen one example of individuals' responding to changes in the constraints that they face, namely physicians altering their location choice in response to changes in demand at various locations. The behaviour of patients seeking medical care services provides another example. In general, consumers who are maximizing their utility will demand less of a good whose price has risen. Some have maintained that this general principle of 'downward sloping demand' does not apply to medical care. The rationale for this claim varies; sometimes it is asserted that medical care is not a pleasant experience; therefore, a person seeks care only when he or she is sick. At other times it is argued that physicians are trained to treat problems in a particular manner and that this manner is independent of the price facing the consumer, and that consumer ignorance fosters the irrelevance of price to physician decision-making.

The view that the number of medical care services received is independent of price has now been demonstrated to be wrong. Newhouse et al. (1981) randomized 7706 individuals to 16 different health insurance plans that varied the cost of care that they faced: 25 per cent received all medical services free, another 14 per cent had 25 per cent co-insurance (they paid 25 per cent of any expenditure), 5 per cent had 50 per cent co-insurance, and 15 per cent had 95 per cent co-insurance. Those with co-insurance had an upper limit on their expenditure of $1000, or 5, 10, or 15 per cent of income, whichever was less. (Families were randomized in roughly equal proportions to the three percentage of income limits.) Another 17 per cent of the families had a plan that approximated a $150 per person per year deductible; in this plan the cost sharing applied only to out-patient services; in-patient services were free. The remainder of the sample received their care from a prepaid group practice.

The 75 per cent of the sample in the fee-for-service system showed marked disparities in utilization among the various plans. Roughly speaking, those enrolled in the free-care plan utilized about 50 per cent more services (measured in dollars) than those in the least generous plan (the plan with 95 per cent co-insurance); other plans were intermediate between these two. Out-patient services and hospital admissions for adults accounted for most of the differences among plans. Neither cost per visit nor cost per hospital stay appeared to vary by plan, nor was there any apparent effect of insurance on hospital admission rates for children. The percentage of individuals seeing a physician one or more times during the year varied from about 70 per cent in the least generous plan to about 85 per cent in the free-care plan. This increase in the fraction of patients seeing a physician accounted for somewhat less than half of the difference among plans in the use of ambulatory services, with the remaining difference accounted for by those who made one or more visits.

These data firmly refute the notion that patients seek care irrespective of economic incentives. The responsiveness of hospital admission rates also suggests that the physician may take account of the insurance plan. (The physician may also have ignored plan; hospital admissions could have risen simply because the physician hospitalized a given percentage of all patients with a certain condition, and more individuals bestirred themselves to visit the physician as the co-insurance rate fell.)

The degree to which health is affected by the additional services that free care induces is not yet clear. But some have argued not only that free ambulatory care improves health, but that in the case of the poor it actually saves money relative to the situation in which only hospital care is well covered (Roemer et al. 1975). Their argument is that if the poor must pay for ambulatory care, they will put off seeing the physician when they have symptoms. Subsequently, their disease may require hospitalization. (Others have also argued that cost sharing for ambulatory services and not for in-patient services may induce the physician to treat some patients on an in-patient basis who could be treated on an out-patient basis.)

The results from the experimental plan that imposes cost sharing only for ambulatory services do not support the hypothesis that free care saves money. Hospital admission rates for adults in this plan were below those in the free plan, and there were no detectable differences between the response of the poor and the middle class. Total expenditures on medical services were significantly lower than in the free care plan. Although reduced coverage of out-patient services may lead to deferred care-seeking behaviour and less appropriate use of the hospital, the reduced use of ambulatory services that it engenders apparently leads the physician to see less illness that he or she wishes to hospitalize. The reduced rate of office visits and hospitalization, of course, may have inimical effects on health status; those effects remain to be determined.

In sum, the price of services – one of the constraints facing patients – does affect behaviour. Whether its effect is for good or ill in terms of health status is not yet known.

Health care spending across countries

Various countries spend quite different amounts on medical services, both in absolute levels and as a fraction of their gross national product (GNP). Is there any simple explanation for this diverse behaviour?

Figure 17.3 shows that, as of the early 1970s, almost all the variation among developed countries in per caput spending for medical services could be explained by variation in per caput income. Not surprisingly, the wealthier countries spent more. But they also spent a higher percentage of their income on medical care than did the less well-off countries. The same finding holds if one expands the sample to include less developed countries (Kleiman 1974). The remarkable finding

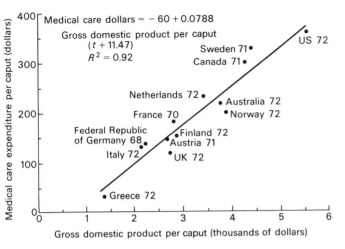

Fig. 17.3. Health care expenditure across developed countries as a function of income. Wealthier countries spend a higher fraction of their income on health care. (Source: Newhouse 1977.)

that the share of GNP devoted to medical care rises as a country's GNP rises causes one to question the traditional view of medical care as a necessity.

Economists define a necessity as a good or service upon which one spends a smaller share of income as income rises. Conversely, they define a luxury as a good that comprises a larger share of income as income rises. Thus, fine wines are a luxury; potatoes are a necessity. The results just cited seem to imply that medical care is a luxury rather than a necessity, which certainly conflicts with many views about the character of personal medical services. But remember that the monies in question are the additional monies spent by countries such as the US and the Federal Republic of Germany relative to those spent by the UK and Italy. Such monies could well be purchasing discretionary services.

If this conclusion appears jarring, consider the behaviour of medical care expenditures within one country across time. In most developed countries the percentage of the GNP devoted to medical care has risen over time. Such an increase is consistent with the hypothesis that the additional medical care spending (including the implementation of new technologies such as artificial hip replacement) that countries undertook as their real incomes rose was discretionary. Even such life-saving technologies as renal dialysis appear to have a discretionary component; the rate of dialysis in the US is approximately double that of the UK, with virtually all the difference concentrated in the over-45 year age group.

One reason that the finding of medical care as discretionary may strike us as strange is that the relationship between medical care spending and the income of households within a country at any point in time does not fit the same pattern. Indeed, low-income households may even spend a higher absolute amount on medical care than more fortunate households. The relationship between income and spending within a country at one point in time has doubtlessly influenced our thinking of medical care as a necessity.

There are at least two explanations for the different relationship between medical care and income within a country compared with across countries. First, income of households is influenced by health status (Grossman and Benham 1974; Berkowitz and Johnson 1974; Luft 1975; Parsons 1982). For example, individuals who are disabled tend to have low incomes but spend relatively much on medical care. Causality in this case does not run from income to spending on medical care, but rather both are influenced by a third factor. Second, in most developed countries there is relatively little use of out of pocket payments at the time of use. For this reason we should not expect a strong relationship within a country between household income and medical care use.

Neither of these explanations applies to variation observed across countries. The variation in health status between countries that are more or less wealthy is much less than across individuals within a country. There is little reason to think, for example, that the UK has a markedly higher rate of disability than the Federal Republic of Germany. Second, although insurance (or public production) shields individuals from the full cost of medical services, the country must face the full costs. For example, if the UK as a country allocates resources to the National Health Service (NHS), it forgoes the use of those resources for other purposes. Such is not the case for the individual household using the NHS.

The additional spending of the higher income countries could represent more medical services or higher prices for the same services. It is difficult to say how much of the difference should be attributed to each factor. But in so far as one can compare incomes of physicians, nothing striking emerges. Table 17.3 shows the average salary of a physician in five countries compared to the average salary of a manufacturing worker in those same countries in the early 1970s. There is no

Table 17.3. *Ratio of average earnings of a physician to average earnings, selected developed countries*

Country	Year	Average physician income	Average compensation, employed person	Ratio
Canada	1972	n.a.	n.a.	5.30*
France	1973	Fr 129 500	Fr 26 433 †	4.90
Federal Republic of Germany	1971	DM 115 580	DM 17 720‡	6.52
UK	1972	£6794	£1367	4.97
US	1971	$42 700§	$9030‖	4.72

Sources: *International health costs and expenditures* (ed. Teh-wei Hu) United States Government Printing Office, Washington, DC (1976). (DHEW Publication No. NIH 76-1067. Pp. 83, 154, 260. And *Annual abstract of statistics, 1974*, No. III. Central Statistical Office. HMSO, London (1974).

*Ratio of average total incomes assessed for tax purposes to average income.

†Data on wage per employed calculated from *Europa yearbook, 1975. A world survey*, Vol. I. Europa Publications, London. Pp. 649, 656. The 1972 unemployment rate of 2.37 per cent was applied to 1973 labour force data to derive an estimate of 21 343 000 employed.

‡Reinhardt's figure comes from the *Gesellschaft für Sozialen Fortschritt e.V.* 'Der Wander der Stellung des Artzes im Einkommenagefüge'. United Nations data show a figure of DM 17 436.

§Median income.

‖Excludes self-employed businessmen, professionals, and farmers.

obvious relationship between this ratio and the country's level of income. Data in Maxwell (1981, Table 4-7) also support this point. Thus, it seems likely that much of the expenditure difference across countries represents real differences in the amount of services consumed.

What are the characteristics of the additional services consumed in the wealthier countries? What, for example, is the rate of coronary artery bypass operations in various countries? What are visit rates for individuals with such non-threatening chronic problems as acne and hay-fever that can none the less cause discomfort? What are visit rates for more serious conditions such as hypertension? Do physicians in wealthier countries tend to perform more ancillary procedures or more complete workups? If so, are their diagnoses more often right?

Some evidence comparing the US and UK is available. Office visits are shorter in the UK, but there are many more home visits. Furthermore, American physicians make greater use of ancillary procedures (Mechanic 1971; Marsh et al. 1976; Robinson 1977). It may well be that longer visits and the (possible) greater certainty of diagnosis from more use of tests provide real benefits, but that such benefits are discretionary. Thus, these data seem consistent with a finding that real spending rises disproportionately with income, but the only safe conclusion is that rather little is known in this important area.

CONCLUSION

Economists have only been applying the tools of modern economic theory and econometrics to problems in the delivery of medical services for about two decades. Compared to what was understood in the early 1960s, much has been learned. But, as in any field of science, there is no lack of questions that remain to be investigated.

APPENDIX: the American medical care delivery system: some descriptive and comparative notes

Organization

Most Americans receive physician and dental care from private physicians and dentists who are reimbursed on a fee-for-service basis. A small number (around 5 per cent) receive their medical care from Health Maintenance Organizations (HMO); the distinguishing feature of an HMO is that the provider and insurer are combined. Typically the HMO charges a certain amount per time period in return for agreeing to provide all necessary services. Some persons, primarily indigent patients, receive both in-patient and out-patient care from hospitals run by local government, while veterans are eligible for care in a system of hospitals operated by the federal government.

The bulk of Americans in the fee-for-service system will be treated by the same physician in and out of the hospital. Of course, specialist consultants may be called in to advise or treat in complex cases. Americans have direct access to both specialists and GPs.

Short-term general hospitals in the US are mostly voluntary (private, not for profit), although 21 per cent of short-term general beds are operated by state and local governments. Of the private beds, 11 per cent are operated by for-profit hospitals. The situation is reversed in the case of nursing homes; 68 per cent of the residents are in homes operated for profit. Drugs and durable medical equipment are generally supplied on a for-profit basis.

Flow of funds

Table A.1 shows the distribution of personal health expenditures in the US in 1981; those expenditures comprised 9.8 per cent of the GNP in that year. The majority of the personal health care dollar is spent in institutions, with hospital care alone accounting for nearly half the total. Approximately a third of all physician expenditure is for services rendered in the hospital, and hospital and physician services together make up over two-thirds of the total.

Coverage of services

Americans have both public and private insurance coverage. The two major public programmes are the Medicare and Medicaid programmes, both of which have been in effect since July 1966. Medicare covers almost all of those aged over 65 years, and in addition covers those under 65 unable to work because of a disability, and all those with end-stage renal disease. Medicare consists of Part A, which covers hospital services, and Part B, which covers physician services. Part A contains a deductible equal to the average cost of one hospital day (in 1982, $260). After the deductible is met, Medicare fully covers all other hospital expenses for the first 60 days of a stay. Thereafter there is a co-payment per day of one-fourth the deductible amount from the 61st to the 90th days. After the 90th day there are no benefits unless the insured is out of the hospital for six months, although everyone eligible does have a lifetime reserve of 60 days. Each lifetime reserve day has a copayment per day of one-half the deductible amount.

Part A benefits are financed by a payroll tax on employers and employees. Hospitals have traditionally been reimbursed on the basis of Medicare's share of reasonable costs. Recently, limits on Medicare hospital reimbursement have been

Table A.1. *Personal health care expenditure, United States, 1981*

	Dollars (in thousand millions)	Percentage
Hospital care	118.0	46.3
Physicians' services (including in-patient)	54.8	21.5
Dentists' services	17.3	6.8
Other professional services (e.g. chiropractors, optometrists, private duty nurses)	6.4	2.5
Drugs and medical sundries	21.4	8.4
Eyeglasses and appliances	5.7	2.2
Nursing home care	24.2	9.5
Other health services (e.g. industrial, school)	7.2	2.8
Total personal health care	255.0	100.0

Source: Gibson, R. M. and Waldo, D. R. (1982). National health expenditure, 1981. *Health Care Financing Rev.* September.

proposed; these limits would vary as a function of the diagnosis. If implemented, these changes would be a marked change in the method of reimbursement of hospitals.

Part B covers physician services in and out of the hospital. It has an annual per person deductible (in 1982 $75), followed by 20 per cent co-insurance, and is financed by premiums and general revenues. Payment is based on a fee schedule that is a function of usual, customary, and reasonable charges. The physician may, if he or she chooses, bill an amount greater than the fee schedules, but then payment of the Medicare benefit will be made to the beneficiary; the physician is at risk to collect the entire fee from the patient; somewhat over half the physicians now extra bill (do not accept assignment). Most eligibles elect to pay the premium for Part B coverage.

Although Medicare is a uniform federal programme, Medicaid is a state-run programme with federal matching funds. States determine eligibility; generally certain of the poor are eligible. Those with very large medical expenses in relation to their incomes are also eligible. States also determine whether certain services (e.g. dental) will be covered, but hospital and physician services must be covered in every state. Traditionally no co-payments were allowed for any covered service, but in recent years states have been allowed to introduce co-payments. Frequency limits (e.g. a maximum of two visits per month) may also be used. Physicians are reimbursed on the basis of a fee schedule, which is typically below what Medicare or private insurance pays. In most states, hospitals are reimbursed similarly to Medicare. In general, the generosity of the Medicaid programme varies considerably by state. Most Medicaid dollars go to a few states.

As is apparent from Tables A.1 and A.2, the bulk of Medicaid dollars go for nursing home care (among the aged), whereas most Medicare dollars go for acute hospital care (among the aged also). This pattern arises because Medicare does not cover most long-term care services.

Table A.2 shows that coverage is quite differential by service. Almost all hospital services are covered; in-patient physician services are also well covered, although this is not apparent from the table. Coverage for dental services, drugs, and eyeglasses and appliances is much less, but has been growing rapidly in recent years (not shown in the table).

Table A.2. *Selected sources of funds for selected services, United States, 1981*

Service	% Out-of-pocket	% Private insurance	% Medicare	% Medicaid
Hospital	10.8	33.4	26.6	9.1
Physicians' services (including in-patient)	38.0	34.7	17.5	4.9
Dentists' services	71.1	24.9	0	3.5
Drugs and medical Sundries	79.9	11.2	0	7.5
Eyeglasses and appliances	82.5	5.3	8.8	0*
Nursing home care	42.6	0.8	1.7	49.6

Source: Gibson, R.M. and Waldo, D.R. (1982). National health expenditures, 1981. *Health Care Financing Rev.* September.
*Figure given is suspicious.

Summary figures on medical resources and utilization

Although many American observers believe the US has too many hospital beds and is overly dependent upon the hospital, in fact its beds per thousand and bed-days per thousand are well below other developed countries (Table A.3). The difference occurs in shorter lengths of stay; discharge rates are not as dissimilar. Although the US has fewer beds per thousand, it tends to have about an average number of physicians per thousand for a developed country. But the great bulk of those physicians, 86 per cent, are specialists. The US has a higher proportion of specialists than any other country shown in the table and probably has the highest proportion in the world. Unlike physicians, about 90 per cent of dentists are general practitioners. In 1979, the US population averaged about four visits to the physician per person per year (excluding telephone consultations), and 75 per cent saw the physician. There were 1.7 dental visits per person in 1979 and 50 per cent of the population saw the dentist. There were 1.3 million nursing home residents in 1977, of whom 86 per cent were over 65 years of age and 35 per cent over 85 years. Approximately 25 per cent of all women over 85 years are now in nursing homes. Expenditure on nursing homes is the fastest growing component of the medical dollars; in constant dollars it has grown by more than a factor of 10 in the two decades from 1960 to 1980.

Table A.3. *Medical resources*

Country	Hospital beds per 10 000*	Discharges per 10 000	Days of hospitalization per caput	Physicians per 10 000	Per cent of physicians who are GPs	Dentists per 10 000
USA	65.6	1712	1.8	16.7	14	5.0
Australia	123.9	1900	2.4	15.2	40	3.0
Canada	92.0	1717	2.7	16.4	34	3.5
France	102.4	1613	3.4	14.6	62	4.8
Federal Republic of Germany	118.0	1616	3.6	19.2	54	5.1
Italy	104.9	1661	3.0	18.0	40	NA
Netherlands	101.4	1028	2.3	15.0	23	3.0
Sweden	152.4	1811	4.7	17.1	–	8.6
Switzerland	113.9	NA	NA	18.6	19	6.1
UK	89.3	1151	2.7	11.9	37	3.2

Source: Maxwell, R.J. (1982). *Health and wealth.* Heath, Lexington. Tables 4-5 and 4-14. Years are various between 1971 and 1975. By 1980 the US figure for physicians/10 000 was 20.2.

REFERENCES

Berki, S.E. (1972). *Hospital economics.* Heath, Lexington.

Berkowitz, M. and Johnson, W.G. (1974). Health and labor force participation. *J. Human Res.* **9**, 117.

Bliss, H.A. (1982). Primary care in the emergency room: high in cost and low in quality. *N. Engl. J. Med.* **306**, 998.

Cullis, J.G. and West, P.A. (1979). *The economics of health: an introduction.* New York University Press.

Danzon, P.M. (1982). The effects of reimbursement policies. *J. Health Econ.* **1**, 29.

Eastaugh, S. (1982). *Medical economics and health finance.* Auburn House, Boston.

Fein, R. (1971). Testimony. In *United States Congress, 'Health Care Crisis in America, 1971. Hearings before the Subcommittee on Health of the Committee on Labor and Public Welfare'.* United States Senate, 22 and 23 February 1971, Part 1. United States Government Printing Office, Washington, DC.

Feldstein, P. (1979). *Health care economics.* Wiley, New York.

Fuchs, V.R. (1974). *Who shall live? Health, economics, and social choice.* Basic Books, New York.

Grossman, M. and Benham, L. (1974). Health, hours, and wages. In *The economics of health and medical care* (ed. M. Perlman) p. 205. Wiley, New York.

Harris, J.E. (1979). Pricing rules for hospitals. *Bell J. Econ.* **10**, 224.

Keeler, E.B. and Cretin, S. (1983). The discounting of life saving and other non-monetary effects. *Management Sci.* **29**(3), 300.

Kleiman, E. (1974). The determinants of national outlay on health. In *The economics of health and medical care* (ed. M. Perlman) p. 66. Wiley, New York.

Loewy, E. (1980). Cost should not be a factor in medical care. *N. Engl. J. Med.* **302**, 697.

Luft, H. (1975). The impact of poor health on earnings. *Rev. Econ. Stat.* **57**, 43.

Marsh, G.N., Wallace, R.B., and Whewell, J. (1976). Anglo-American contrasts in general practice. *Br. Med. J.* **ii**, 1321.

Maxwell, R.J. (1981). *Health and wealth.* Heath, Lexington.

Mechanic, D. (1972). General medical practice: some comparisons between the work of primary care physicians in the United States and England and Wales. *Med. Care* **10**, 402.

Newhouse, J.P. (1978). *The economics of medical care: a polic[y] perspective.* Addison-Wesley, Reading, Mass.

Newhouse, J.P., Williams, A.P., Bennett, B., and Schwartz, W.B. (1982*a*). *Does the geographic distribution of physicians reflec[t] market failure?* The Rand Corporation, Santa Monica, (Pub[l]. No. R-2734-KFF).

Newhouse, J.P., Williams, A.P., Bennett, B., and Schwartz, W.B. (1982*b*). Where have all the doctors gone? *JAM[A]* **247**, 2392.

Newhouse, J.P., Williams, A.P., Bennett, B., and Schwartz, W.B. (1982*c*). Does the geographical distribution of physicians reflec[t] market failure? *Bell J. Econ.* **3**, 493.

Newhouse, J.P., Manning, W.G., Morris, C.N. *et al.* (1981). Some interim results from a controlled trial of cost sharing in health insurance. *N. Engl. J. Med.* **305**, 1501.

Parsons, D.D. (1982). The male labour force decision: health reported health, and economic incentives. *Economica* **49**, 81.

Phelps, C.E. and Newhouse, J.P. (1974). Coinsurance, the price of time, and the demand for medical services. *Rev. Econ. Stat.* **56**, 334.

Robinson, D. (1977). Primary medical practice in the United Kingdom and the United States. *N. Engl. J. Med.* **217**, 188.

Roemer, M.I., Hopkins, C.E., Carr, L. and Gartside, F. (1975). Copayments for ambulatory care: penny-wise and pound-foolish. *Med. Care* **13**, 457.

Schwartz, W.B., Newhouse, J.P., Bennett, B. and Williams, A.P., Jr (1980). The changing geographic distribution of board-certified physicians. *N. Engl. J. Med.* **303**, 1032.

Schwartz, W.B. and Joskow, P.L. (1980). Duplicated hospital facilities: how much can we save by consolidating them? *N. Engl. J. Med.* **303**, 1449.

Shishko, R. (1975). *Choosing the discount rate for defense decision-making.* The Rand Corporation, Santa Monica. (Publ. No. R-1953-RC.)

Taylor, V.D. and Newhouse, J.P. (1970). *Improving budgeting procedures and outpatient operations in nonprofit hospitals.* The Rand Corporation, Santa Monica. (Publ. No. RM-6057-1.)

Wolfe, S. (1974). Conservative economics: a menace to health planning in the United States. *Int. J. Health Serv.* **4**, 319.

18 Education and modification of behaviour

S. Leonard Syme

INTRODUCTION

The way we behave as individuals affects both the occurrence of disease and the outcome of treatment. A wide variety of behaviours have been shown by research during the last 30 years to contribute to the aetiology of many diseases and conditions. In the case of coronary heart disease, for example, risk factors have been reported to include cigarette smoking, physical activity patterns, hard-driving competitive behaviour and diet (not only what people eat – saturated fat, salt, and perhaps fibre, alcohol, and coffee – but also how much they eat). As behavioural risk factors have been identified, intervention programmes have been developed to modify or eliminate them. The rationale for these intervention programmes is that if a behaviour increases the risk of disease, it should be changed to lower that risk. In addition to changing old behaviours, many treatment and control programmes require also that people begin for the first time to initiate new behaviours such as taking medications, beginning substantial dietary changes or beginning exercise programmes.

These behavioural approaches to disease contrast with activities that emphasize doing something 'to' people. While some diseases and conditions can perhaps best be treated by injection, surgery or other non-behavioural manipulations, most chronic diseases and conditions of concern today cannot. Chronic diseases such as cancer, diseases of the cardiovascular system, cirrhosis, chronic respiratory disease, and injuries caused by accidents and other forms of violence, to a greater or lesser degree, are caused by particular behaviours and hopefully can be prevented or treated by behaviour change. For example, it has been estimated that both one-fifth of the morbidity and of the years of life lost between the ages of one and 70 may be attributed to just two behaviours: cigarette smoking and excessive use of alcohol.

When direct, non-behavioural, interventions are possible, they often are not effective or efficient in the long run. Thus, while a dietary deficiency can be treated by the continuing injection of missing nutrients, it is probably more useful to teach better eating habits to persons with such a deficiency. To insure successful behavioural change, not only must people be 'dealt with', but increasingly we must also involve people as active partners rather than as passive recipients.

Behaviour modification is necessary both in the treatment and in the prevention of disease. In treatment, we ask that people recognize the need for medical help, that they seek such help in timely fashion, that they listen to advice given and, finally, that they follow that advice. Without co-operation of patients, treatment plans have little value. With regard to the control of disease, treatment programmes must be continued either permanently, or, at least, for long periods of time. The prevention of disease similarly involves the active compliance and co-operation of people. They must become aware of health hazards associated with particular behaviours, accept that this information is personally relevant, and be willing to change that behaviour in the interest of some future gain.

There are two things that we have learned in efforts to modify people's behaviour: (i) it can be done and (ii) it is not easy. In this chapter these issues will be examined by emphasizing some of the difficulties typically encountered in effecting behaviour changes and some of the approaches that should be considered in overcoming these difficulties will be reviewed. To do this, two cases will be reviewed in some detail. One case, hypertension, involves a condition that is not as yet easily prevented and that requires a programme of behaviour change for treatment and control. The second case, cigarette smoking, is very difficult to treat and requires instead an aggressive programme of prevention to achieve results. Both cases pose different interesting problems that must be dealt with in programmes to modify behaviour. Both cases also illustrate the ineffectiveness of the 'usual' approach to education and behaviour modification which have, in the past, included developing the facts about hazardous behaviour, educating people about risks, informing professionals of the need to take action and providing convenient services for people. A review of these cases will be helpful in developing a better understanding of the challenges we face in this important area.

THE CASE OF HYPERTENSION

Magnitude of the problem

Hypertension is a condition that leads to a variety of serious complications and diseases; the complications of even mild hypertension involve progression to moderate and severe hypertension, coronary heart disease, strokes, and congestive heart failure. Mortality rises with progressive increases in systolic or diastolic blood pressures, even at blood pressure levels previously considered acceptable (Paul 1978). In addition to its seriousness, hypertension also is a very widespread condition. While it is always difficult to measure the prevalence of such conditions with accuracy because of differences in definition and peculiarities of population sampling, virtually every estimate of the prevalence of hypertension in the US reports that the number of hypertensives is about 23 million persons, yielding a prevalence rate in the adult population of about 20 per cent (Gordon 1964; Roberts 1975). With a condition of such magnitude and importance, a programme of primary prevention should be a first priority. Unfortunately, the risk factors for hypertension are still unclear (Syme and Torfs 1978) and it is difficult to urge people to make significant changes in their life-style when the efficacy of those interventions still is being debated. While prevention ultimately must be our priority, preventive programmes must await the development of more definitive information about hypertension risk factors. In the meantime, emphasis must be given to the treatment and control of hypertension among those millions who now have the condition.

The treatment challenge

Hypertension is a chronic condition requiring lifetime treatment. There are two major issues in the long-term treatment of hypertension. One is to select an appropriate treatment plan for individual patients and the second is to insure that patients adhere to it. Of course, these issues have applicability to many other diseases as well. However, there are some special features associated with hypertension treatment that must be noted. The first is that most persons with moderately elevated blood pressure experience no symptoms and no discomfort. Treatment for hypertension therefore requires that patients be convinced to embark upon a long-term course of drug treatment even though they feel well. Further, it is virtually certain that initiation of treatment will not make these patients feel better; indeed, in many cases, they will feel worse. Nor can it be said with certainty that treatment will prevent the development of other diseases; while a substantial proportion of untreated hypertensives may develop serious complications, this is essentially a statistical or probablistic estimate of what may happen in the future. If patients discontinue treatment for a day or two, it is unlikely that they will immediately fall ill or die.

During the 1960s, the two major problems posed by hypertension in the US were that few people knew they had it, and even if they knew, most either were not under treatment or were being treated inadequately. In a nationwide survey conducted between 1960 and 1962 by the National Health Survey, it was found that 43 per cent of adults in the US diagnosed as having hypertension were previously unaware of it (Gordon 1964). In a survey conducted in the state of Georgia in 1962, 41 per cent were unaware of their hypertension (Wilber 1967). In Chicago in 1967, a study of 23 000 persons revealed that 59 per cent of those with hypertension were not aware of it (Schoenberger *et al.* 1972).

This situation has changed dramatically in recent years. In 1974, the Hypertension Detection and Follow-up Program (1977) found in a nationwide study of the US that only 25 per cent of adults with hypertension were unaware of it. This is a

substantial improvement in awareness. In 1979, we complete a survey of a random sample of 1000 people living in selecte areas of Alameda County, California. Areas selected fo study were those with high percentages of black residents an those in which incomes were low since these areas were expec ted to have high prevalence rates of hypertension. In the past these areas also contained high proportions of hypertensiv patients who were unaware of their condition. In our survey we found that of all hypertensive patients, only 30 per cen were now unaware of their condition.

Nevertheless, while we have succeeded in increasing th awareness of hypertensive patients regarding their condition we continue to observe a high level of uncontrolle hypertension in the community. In our study in Alameda County, for example, 361 hypertensive patients were found i the community of 1000 households. Of those already awar of their condition, 74 per cent were under the care o physicians; of this group, less than half (44 per cent) had thei blood pressure under control. Thus, of all the hypertensiv patients in the study community, only 23 per cent had controlled blood pressure.

Our local experience is comparable to the national picture in the US. Blood pressure control findings of a nationwid survey conducted by the Health and Nutrition Examination Survey from 1971 to 1974 (Roberts 1975) are virtually identi cal to the findings of the National Health Survey conducted nationally between 1960 and 1962 (Gordon 1964). The bloo pressure distributions in the country in these two time period are almost identical, and the prevalence of hypertension during this 14-year interval remains about the same. Therefore, even though there have been improvements in the US during this 14-year period in patient awareness and in treatment methods, no reduction has been observed in the prevalence of hypertension, nor importantly, in the percent age of patients able to control their blood pressure.

Therefore, in spite of our success in alerting persons to their high blood pressure, the prevalence of uncontrolled hypertension remains high. There are many reasons for this. One of the more important reasons is that patients fail to follow the physician's advice. We recently completed a survey of 880 physicians who practise in and around Alameda County, California. In this survey, we asked physicians how they diagnosed and treated hypertension and what major problems they had in the management of hypertensive patients. Of the total studied, 441 physicians regularly treated hypertensive patients, and the major treatment problem they reported was that of patient adherence to recommendations. Specifically, 40 per cent of the physicians reported that patients did not adhere to the recommended follow-up schedule, 15 per cent said that patients did not adhere to recommended medication prescriptions, and 27 per cent reported that patients did not adhere to other treatment recommendations. It should be noted that these figures may underestimate the magnitude of the problem, since patients who discontinued treatment entirely were probably not included by the physicians.

We are confronted with a medical condition that is clearly of great importance and seriousness and for which good treatment is available; a condition that has been brought to patients' attention and for which medical help is being sought; and yet a condition that has not been brought under control, in large part, owing to the failure of patients to follow medical advice. Why do patients fail to follow advice given to them by physicians? This is a complex and difficult question that cannot be answered simply. To guide us in studying problems in patient adherence, there exists a 'health belief model' (Becker 1976) that may provide a useful conceptual framework for characterizing patient behaviour. Briefly, this model proposes that people are more likely to take preventive medical action and follow medical advice (i) if they perceive the illness or condition as being serious; (ii) if they feel personally susceptible to becoming ill if they fail to take appropriate action; (iii) if they feel that the proposed programme of medical treatment is likely to be effective; and (iv) if the number of difficulties they experience in following advice is within reasonable limits.

When this model is applied to patients with mild hypertension, it is perhaps not surprising that so many are not under adequate medical care. First, high blood pressure is not generally regarded as an overly serious condition. In a survey of 3181 adults living in the US conducted by the Harris Poll in 1973 for the National Heart and Lung Institute (Harris et al. 1973), only six of every ten persons felt that high blood pressure was serious, a level of concern equal to that for diabetes and kidney trouble. This contrasts with the seriousness seen for other diseases such as cancer (94 per cent), stroke (90 per cent), and heart conditions (83 per cent). Among those between the ages of 17 and 35 years, only 48 per cent felt that high blood pressure was a serious condition. When asked whether high blood pressure caused other illnesses or symptoms, 42 per cent said no. Clearly, a substantial proportion of the population does not view high blood pressure as a serious condition and probably would not feel personally susceptible to suffering serious consequences if their high blood pressure were not treated.

When hypertension is viewed as a serious problem, there is a question as to the perceived effectiveness of available treatment. In the Harris survey, a surprising 65 per cent of the national sample of adults felt that the term 'hypertension' referred to bad nerves, nervous conditions, too much tension and pressure, over-anxiety, over-activity, or over-excitement. Therefore, it may not be unusual for people to feel that hypertension might better be treated by 'relaxing' and 'taking it easy' than by taking physician-prescribed medications or engaging in difficult dietary or other changes in life-style.

Even if patients view their hypertension as a serious problem that should be treated with appropriate medication, they often encounter a number of difficulties in complying. First, most persons with high blood pressure are asymptomatic. As Sackett (1976) has noted in his comprehensive review of 40 studies on this topic, asymptomatic patients are only 60 per cent as co-operative in following therapeutic regimens as are symptomatic patients. Second, many antihypertensive medications have side-effects. Smith and associates have reported that 69 per cent of subjects on hypertension therapy experienced side-effects (Smith 1978). While most of these side-effects are relatively minor, they can be bothersome. The list of reported side-effects included nasal stuffiness (34 per cent), lethargy and drowsiness (37 per cent), mental depression (20 per cent), sleep disturbance (20 per cent), gastrointestinal disturbance (21 per cent), postural faintness (14 per cent), and sexual impotence (20 per cent). These side-effects are of special consequence because they occur among persons who were originally symptom free and apparently in good health. When such side-effects appear, the 'benefits' perceived by persons receiving drug treatment for mild hypertension may be modest indeed.

One of the problems in interpreting this high frequency of side-effects is that even placebo-treated patients claim to experience them. In the study reported by Smith and colleagues, half of the patients were randomized to a placebo group. As expected, they also reported a substantial number of drug side-effects; however, the frequency of each side-effect reported was only half that reported among those on active drugs.

In addition, hypertensive patients need to take drugs over a very long period. For this to occur it is helpful if one of two conditions exists: (i) patients feel better as they continue to take the drug or (ii) patients realize clearly that failure to take the drug will immediately result in unpleasant consequences. Neither condition exists in hypertension treatment: patients do not feel better, and their failure to take drugs as prescribed rarely results in immediate pain or other crises.

It has been suggested that one way to improve patient adherence to medical advice is to recommend non-pharmacological treatment. An advantage of this approach is avoidance of the side-effects of medication. A disadvantage is that non-pharmacological treatment may not be as effective as drugs are in controlling blood pressure, especially in the very high blood pressure range. However, since 70 per cent of hypertensive patients have borderline or mild essential hypertension, non-pharmacological approaches to treatment must be seriously considered. Of all the alternatives to drugs that are available, weight loss and sodium restriction appear to have the greatest empirical support. As our experience grows, it may be that physical exercise, biofeedback, meditation, and relaxation will also prove effective in controlling blood pressure. While these approaches avoid the side-effects of drug treatment, they hardly can be considered simple or easy alternatives. Patients find it difficult to lose weight and to substantially reduce sodium intake, especially when these reductions must be maintained over a long period. Therefore, the gains of non-drug treatment may be lost.

Interaction between physician and patient

How, then, can patient adherence be improved? One of the most effective and practical approaches to achieving this goal may be through more effective and appropriate communication between physician and patient. Let us examine this issue closely. Most physician–patient interactions in the treatment of hypertension involve the gradual adjustment and change of medications over time to maximize blood pressure reductions and to minimize drug side-effects. From the physician's viewpoint, this gradual development of a treatment plan is essential, given the different circumstances of each patient and the wide variety of drug choices available.

From the patient's standpoint, however, this often is a troublesome situation. Many patients expect the physician to make a diagnosis and to prescribe appropriate treatment 'once and for all'. If patients experience unpleasant side-effects or if their blood pressure does not respond as expected, the physician may alter the drug prescription. Patients may see this change as evidence that the first prescription was an error and that the error is now being corrected. Should the prescription be changed once again at a subsequent visit, patients may question the competence of the physician.

Thus, while the physician almost certainly must adjust drug prescriptions and dosages, this adjustment may be seen by the patient as a reflection of uncertainty on the part of the physician, if not an indication of outright error. In fact, many patients have a magical conception of the physician and are not prepared to accept the possibility that he does not know exactly which drug to prescribe to solve the problem 'once and for all'. It is difficult for the patient to follow the physician's advice over long periods when confidence is thus weakened. It is especially difficult to follow that advice when the drugs prescribed involve side-effects and do no apparent good.

To improve patient adherence it is essential that physicians give the patient a realistic description of the long-term treatment outlook. This description should include reference to the fact that physician and patient are embarking on a treatment programme in which mutual co-operation is essential. Patients must be helped to realize that the physician does not know everything. They must be invited to share in the treatment process as an informed and responsible partner.

This often is easier said than done. In many medical encounters, patients invest physicians with enormous god-like power and authority and cannot tolerate physician confessions of ordinary humanity. In effect, patients take on a child-like, dependent role in relation to the power of the physician. This is problematic because successful behaviour change requires that patients assume adult responsibility themselves for their health. The physicians may provide advice and aids but these essentially are only adjunctive. The decision to change behaviour must be the patient's and the physician only can help to support that decision. Nevertheless, since patients must go to physicians for help, and since physicians are powerful and expert, many patients find it difficult to take upon themselves such personal responsibility in that setting.

We recently had a revealing experience in attempting to influence a low-income group of hypertensive patients to follow medical advice. These patients had for years been a problem for the physicians practising in a community clinic which the patients attended. We randomly divided these patients into three groups: one to visit physicians at regular intervals, one to meet in the clinic in groups led by a nurse and a health educator, and one to be visited in their homes by a community health worker. Those in the home group did far better in following the treatment programme. Note that the community health workers achieved excellent results even though they knew very little about hypertension and its treatment and even though they were instructed not to give medical or treatment advice when they visited the homes. Our interpretation of what happened was that the workers, in visiting homes repeatedly, forcefully suggested to patients that (i) the Blood Pressure staff cared about them and (ii) their blood pressure problem was important and serious. In spite of this caring and communication of seriousness, the workers withheld specific advice or help. In this circumstance, patients were forced to take upon themselves responsibility for obtaining help. And they did.

An alternative approach

Since hypertensive patients must follow a treatment plan over a long period, it is essential that they accept responsibility for their behaviour. An authority figure can only provide facts, advice, guidance, support, and reinforcement. This acceptance of responsibility is adult behaviour. As long as patients view the physician as a parent figure, they behave as children. This may be a useful role for some patients, but it is not for most, and it is certainly not useful when we expect patients to follow advice for a long time.

It may be that as long as patients regard physicians as parental figures, they cannot help but take on the child role. It may be that no matter how unparental physicians are, many patients will continue to invest them with parentlike qualities. If this is so, we must begin to consider alternatives to the traditional physician–patient situation, especially since treatment must be continued for a lifetime. A new pattern may be required in which the physician makes the diagnosis and develops a treatment plan but in which other health professionals or friends are involved in helping the patient effect long-term behaviour change. These others would act as peers and as support groups but not as parent figures, a model already existing in Alcoholics Anonymous, Overeaters Anonymous, and Gamblers Anonymous. In these self-help groups, no professional staff exists, no formal leadership exists, and all support comes from peers. There is no question that these self-help groups have been very effective in helping many people make long-term difficult changes in behaviour and it is possible that this model may have relevance for the other medical conditions.

Alderman *et al.* (1980) have summarized the results of a major hypertension education project sponsored by the National Heart, Lung and Blood Institute. In that project, 11 separate studies were organized to test various strategies for improving compliance of patients with high blood pressure. A few conclusions emerged as common findings from all 11 studies. Three of these findings were: (i) self-monitoring of blood pressure improves patient adherence to physician recommendations; (ii) patients follow advice more faithfully when they have support and encouragement from at least one other significant friend or helper; and (iii) adherence is much better when patients are actively rather than passively involved in setting treatment or behaviour change goals.

Before proceeding further with consideration of these issues, let us review another difficult behaviour change problem which provides another perspective on this issue.

THE CASE OF CIGARETTE SMOKING

Magnitude of the problem

Cigarette smoking is an unhealthy behaviour that remains remarkably resistant to modification. It is a widespread problem around the world, the health hazards associated with it are clear and, while progress has been made, it remains a most difficult behaviour to change. The disease risks associated with cigarette smoking are clear and undisputed. Cigarette smoking increases the risk of morbidity and mortality for a wide variety of diseases (Schuman 1979) and there is evidence that smoking cessation is associated with a lowering of disease risk (Adams 1979). The adverse health effects of cigarette smoking are particularly acute for women (and especially pregnant women), for teenagers, and for workers exposed to toxic occupational agents. It may also be that the side-stream smoke of smokers affects the health of those around them, but the evidence on this point is not yet settled (Hirayama 1981; Garfinkel 1981; Trichopoulos *et al.* 1981; Hammond 1981; *British Medical Journal* 1981). These facts are based on an exhaustive and accumulating body of evidence that may be unique in the history of research in health and disease.

Not only is smoking a serious health hazard, like hypertension it too affects an enormous number of people. While the prevalence of cigarette smoking in several countries has declined in recent years, a very substantial number of people still smoke a large quantity of cigarettes. For example, the percentage of adult men and women who smoked regularly in 1978 in the US was 38 per cent and 30 per cent respectively (NIH 1980). Among young male adults 20–24 years old, over 40 per cent smoked in 1978 while approximately 30 per cent of young women smoked. Among teenage girls, 26 per cent age 17–18 years and 12 per cent age 15–16 years smoked. For teenage boys, the comparable figures are 11 per cent and 19 per cent (NIH 1980). In 1978 an estimated 54 million men and women in the US smoked 615 billion cigarettes. Thus, even though major declines have been observed in smoking prevalence, a very substantial number of people still begin and continue to smoke. Indeed, some have speculated that those who have quit were 'easy cases' and that those now smoking are more 'hard core'. Friedman *et al.* (1979) have shown that, compared to current smokers, those who quit smoking are lighter smokers (that is, they smoke fewer cigarettes, they smoke for shorter periods of time, and inhale less). In spite of declines in smoking, therefore, this behaviour continues to be of great significance and magnitude and is probably the single most preventable cause of disease known today.

Cigarette cessation programmes

The major problem posed by cigarette smoking is that so few smokers have been able successfully to give up and to maintain cessation once it has been achieved. An enormous number of programmes have been established since the early 1960s to help people give up smoking. The range and variety of techniques and approaches that have been developed to help people to quit are also enormous (Pechacek 1979). Three general conclusions can be reached about these efforts: (i) no one technique or approach is superior to any other; (ii) most people who join cessation programmes do not stop smoking; (iii) of those who do stop, most do not remain off cigarettes for any substantial period of time.

Hunt and Matarazzo (1973) have studied cigarette cessation relapse rates among smoking cessation clinic participants who had stopped at the end of treatment. They demonstrated that the proportion of participants remaining abstinent fell to about 25 per cent three to six months later and remained fairly stable after that time. This trend was observed also by Evans and Lane (1980). Even less gratifying are data showing a long-term abstinence rate of 18 per cent among 559 participants surveyed five years after attending smoking cessation clinics (West *et al.* 1977). In addition to the fact that cessation rates are relatively low, Schwartz and others (Schwartz 1969; Schwartz and Rider 1975; Wilson 1979) have suggested that no one cessation technique stands out as particularly more effective than any other.

These statistics regarding cessation rates stand in stark contrast to other findings indicating that most smokers want to give up the habit. Most smokers acknowledge, at some level, the health hazards associated with smoking and most wish that there was a simple and painless way to give up (Horn 1960; Wilson 1979). In recent years, there has been a decline in smoking in several countries. While about 32–35 per cent of the adult population now smoke cigarettes in the US, about 40 per cent smoked in 1964. Among teenagers, 29 per cent smoked cigarettes in 1977 and this figure had dropped in 1981 to 21 per cent. Clearly, however, there is a long way to go to substantially reduce the prevalence of smoking and present indications are that previous approaches to this problem are not likely to be effective or efficient (US DHEW 1982). For example, if the estimated 54 million adult smokers in the US were to enrol in organized cessation smoking clinics with 30 participants in each clinic, well over 1.5 million clinics would be needed to treat all of these smokers (US DHEW 1982). Since the success rate of these clinics likely would be modest, an enormous investment of time, money, and energy would be required for a substantial period of time before any sizeable reduction in the number of smokers would be noted. However, even as this reduction was being achieved, new smokers would be entering the smoking population at an unaffected rate since cessation clinics are not aimed at the prevention of smoking. Therefore, while it is useful to support cigarette smoking cessation clinics for those who may benefit from them, they cannot be viewed as an overall solution to the problem and they must be regarded as only one component of an integrated programme.

Smoking as a social behaviour

It is possible that one of the difficulties we have had in dealing successfully with smoking is that we have viewed it almost entirely as a problem of the individual. It is true that cigarette smoking is an individual behaviour: individuals begin to smoke, they become regular smokers, and they give up smoking. However, this individual behaviour occurs in a social and cultural context. To discourage the initiation of smoking and encourage the cessation of smoking once established, we perhaps ought to consider both the individual and social dimensions of the behaviour. To date, most attention on smoking has been focused on the individual – his or her motivations and perceptions, need for information, and disease risks. It would be useful to review some of the ways in which social and cultural forces influence the initiation of the establishment of smoking behaviour in order to suggest ways in which these forces might be used to intervene and prevent smoking.

The fact that smoking is a social and cultural phenomenon is forcefully brought to our attention by the systematic patterning of this behaviour. Smoking regularly occurs more or less frequently among certain groups in the population suggesting that this behaviour is neither random nor idiosyncratic. It further suggests that there are social forces at work influencing individuals in these groups to smoke. Even though the number of smokers in these various groups may have changed over the years, the patterns of difference remain remarkably constant (National Clearing House for Smoking and Health 1976). Men smoke more than women, and men and women in the age group 25–44 years smoke more frequently than those in other age groups. The prevalence of smoking decreases among older groups and, especially among men, the proportion of 'former smokers' increases with age. In the US, the prevalence of smoking is higher among blacks than among whites in both sexes, and higher among those with less education than among those with more education; smoking cessation has occurred more rapidly among the better educated. With regard to income, men in the highest income category smoke the least while the opposite is true for women; in the highest income category, more women smoke. A similar pattern is seen for occupation: white-collar male workers smoke less than blue-collar workers and those currently unemployed smoke the most. The sex difference in smoking virtually disappears among professional, managerial, and sales workers. The highest prevalence of smoking is seen among those divorced and separated.

Dekker (1975) has identified several components of the social and cultural environment that influence smoking behaviour. These components include the cultural associations between smoking and relaxation, adulthood, sexual attractiveness and emancipation; the socio-economic structure of tobacco production, processing, distribution, and legislation; explicit advertising on the part of the tobacco industry based on cultural values that favour smoking; implicit advertising by such influential persons as film stars, television personalities, teachers, and doctors; and the influence of parents, siblings, peers, and other significant persons. These components of the social environment influence the initiation, maintenance, and cessation of cigarette smoking behaviour.

Teenage smoking: social influences

With regard to the initiation of smoking, it seems reasonable to focus most attention on the teenage years since most smoking begins at that time. During these years, teenagers are attempting to: (i) disentangle from the influence of an identification with parents; (ii) establish stronger links with their peers; and (iii) establish a sharper and more independent self-identity. It has been suggested that smoking is initiated at this time because it is a symbolic vehicle for many of these efforts.

Two important factors that affect the initiation of smoking among teenagers are peer influence and the media. With regard to peer influence, almost 90 per cent of teenage smokers acknowledge that at least one of their four best friends smoke on a regular basis while only 33 per cent of non-smokers claim a smoker among their best friends (Green 1975). Further, even though some of the friends of teenagers who are smokers do not smoke, they have experimented with smoking far more often than have the friends of non-smokers. In brief, the teenage smokers and their friends share a life pattern that includes smoking.

Teenage smoking seems influenced by the smoking of parents and older siblings. Compared to non-smoking parents, parents who smoke are more likely to have children who smoke (Dekker 1975). Teenagers with two parents who smoke are more than twice as likely to smoke as those with no parents smoking. A teenager with an older sibling who smokes is far more likely to become a smoker (Green 1975).

For many teenagers, smoking appears to constitute a 'rite of passage' into adulthood (Williams and Shor 1979). Smoking helps teenagers feel more mature because smoking is an adult behaviour forbidden to children. In this connection, it is interesting to note that the initiation of teenage smoking seems to be triggered by transitional life changes such as graduation from high school or college, changes in residence, and absence of a parent (Bergin and Wake 1974). Teenage smoking also is a means to defy adult authority. Teenagers who smoke are more likely to chafe under restrictions imposed by adults in control (Green 1975). They are much less likely to report that they turn to their parents for advice.

The association between smoking and the characteristics of teenage life is not inevitable and permanent. This connection can be changed if the environment is changed and recent evidence suggests that such changes are now taking place. As noted previously, daily cigarette use among teenagers in the US has declined from 29 per cent to 21 per cent between 1977 and 1980 (Johnstone and Bachman 1980). Among those teenagers smoking a half-pack or more a day, use has fallen from 19 per cent to 14 per cent. These reductions in smoking may be accelerating; there has been a 4 per cent drop in teenage smoking during 1980. While regular teenage smoking is now disapproved by 71 per cent of teenagers, this change seems to be occurring more among boys than girls. For the first time, girls caught up with boys in 1977 in regular cigarette smoking.

It is possible that these changes in teenage smoking are due to a change in the social support of smoking among teenagers. Williams and Shor (1979) describe the previous support systems as an 'interwoven fabric of social definitions, beliefs, attitudes, customs, norms and laws that define smoking as normal, expected, appropriate, socially acceptable, socially respectable and an implicit fundamental right'. There is now a decrease in peer acceptance of teenage

moking. In 1975, 55 per cent of high school seniors in the US
elt their friends would disapprove of their smoking a pack of
igarettes a day; in 1980, 74 per cent felt that way (Johnston
nd Bachman 1980). In 1976, 37 per cent of these seniors said
hat most or all of their friends smoked cigarettes; in 1980,
nly 23 per cent said this. In addition, 95 per cent of the
eniors feel their parents would disapprove of their smoking.

Teenage smoking and the media

The media have an important influence on the initiation of
moking among teenagers. Johnson and his colleagues
ttribute this change in teenagers' attitudes to an increasing
concern with health (Johnston and Bachman 1980). In 1975,
1 per cent of high school seniors in the US felt the regular
use of cigarettes was harmful to health. In 1980, 64 per cent
had this view. In part, this increase in negative beliefs about
moking is due to 20 years of media campaigns and
educational programmes about the harmful health effects of
moking. The media have challenged the 'glamorous' image
of smoking behaviour – not only by explicit advertising but
also through the implicit values portrayed. For example,
many television teenage heroes now are non-smokers. While
such examples may still be a minority, they stand in dramatic
contrast to the situation that existed in the cinema during the
1940s and 1950s which portrayed a desirable and glamorous
image of smoking in the media. Gerbner et al. (1981) recently
reported that only 11 per cent of television males and 2 per
cent of television females (major characters) now smoke in
US television prime time. While there is less smoking in
situation comedies, there is more in crime and adventure
programmes and even more in serious drama (including
movies) but even here only 13 per cent of men and 4 per cent
of women smoke. The impression that television characters
now smoke a great deal is unwarranted and probably is
derived from older movies.

In spite of recent changes, the media continue to show
attractive people smoking and to emphasize the pleasures
associated with this behaviour (Evans et al. 1979). While this
portrayal is changing, it still is pervasive and one can hardly
spend a day without being exposed to the message that
smoking is fun, glamorous, and exciting. It should be noted,
however, that it is not clear whether such explicit advertising
influences the initiation of cigarette smoking. Considerable
research has been done on this topic but the results are
equivocal. McGuiness and Cowling (1975) have suggested
that media advertising was an important factor in the increase
of smoking in the US since 1900. Whiteside (1974) notes that
from 1922 to 1952 in the US, cigarette sales increased 63 per
cent while the population grew only 54 per cent and he argues
that media advertising was a major influence in building this
market. Others have noted that the influence of media is
more to shift brand preferences rather than to initiate
smoking behaviour. Empirical support for these various
contentions is neither consistent nor convincing (Kozlowski
1979).

The difficulty of using the media to influence behaviour is
shown by the recent cancellation of the Brooke Shields anti-
smoking advertisements. In dropping the advertisements, the
US government indicated that Ms Shields was not a credible
symbol for an anti-smoking campaign because she previously
had participated in a seductive advertising campaign for jeans
and was seen more as a sex-symbol than as an influential role
model. One might have argued that Ms Shields' previous
exposure made her an ideal candidate for the anti-smoking
campaign. The American Lung Association raised this point
and accused the government of bowing to pressure from the
tobacco industry who feared that Ms Shields' campaign
would be too effective.

Educating the public about the hazards of smoking

During the 1960s and 1970s, various regulations and prohibitions were instituted in the US regarding cigarette advertising
(Doron 1979). In 1964, the first Surgeon-Generl's Report was
published officially noting the health hazards of smoking; in
1965, health warning labels were required on all cigarette
packages; in 1967 public funds were made available to film
anti-smoking commercials for television; in 1971, health
warnings were required in all cigarette advertising and, also in
1971, all television and radio advertising for cigarettes was
prohibited.

While the release of the Surgeon-General's Report and the
controversy that surrounded it was followed by an immediate
reduction of about 4 per cent in the total consumption of
cigarettes, the labelling acts had no significant effect. There
has been considerable speculation regarding the lack of
impact of warning labels. The 1981 Staff Report published by
the Federal Trade Commission (FTC) has reported that 50
million Americans still do not know that cigarette smoking
can cause heart disease and 20 per cent of the population still
do not know that smoking can cause cancer. The FTC claims
that much of the blame for this rests with the warning labels
on packages and in advertising, both of which have become
so 'worn out' that fewer than 3 per cent of all adults exposed
bother to read them. Thus, while many people know that
smoking 'affects' health, a sizeable proportion do not appear
to have a clear or exact view of the precise nature of the
danger.

Doron (1979) has suggested that the banning of television
and radio advertising actually benefited the tobacco industry
by reducing the aggressive and very expensive competition
among tobacco companies. With these savings, the
companies were able to focus their energies on more direct
marketing techniques such as displays and promotions at the
point of sale, and advertising in other media has increased
dramatically. Perhaps even more important to the tobacco
industry, the anti-smoking advertisements on radio and
television have been stopped. If advertising had created a
favourable milieu of acceptability for cigarette smoking, and
if anti-smoking advertisements effectively countered that
image, the best thing that could happen from the industry's
point of view was that the anti-smoking campaign be
stopped. The new advertising campaigns now launched in
other contexts have no countering anti-smoking messages.
According to Doron, the net balance of influence clearly
favours the tobacco industry.

The prohibition or regulation of smoking are possible

strategies to prevent the initiation of smoking. Given the cultural perception of smoking as acceptable and legitimate behaviour, however, these strategies are not likely to be easily implemented. More realistic is the idea that people should become better informed about the hazards of smoking so that they will act in their own self-interest. As noted earlier, this approach does not work very well. Health education campaigns usually occur in sporadic and isolated contexts, they rarely take into account that smoking is part of an accepted and valued way of life, and they assume implicitly that health is the most important priority for people – an assumption rarely supported by empirical evidence (Gray and Daube 1980).

While it is true that individuals begin to smoke for individual reasons, it is also true that the social situation is an important factor in influencing these individual decisions to smoke. It is not enough to educate the individual to the dangers inherent in smoking if the social context within which the smoker finds him or herself makes smoking more attractive than not smoking. Often, social pressures are more powerful than even the most determined and informed rationality.

Most people in the US know that smoking is harmful to health. In a recent government survey of adults in the US, 90 per cent agreed with the statement: 'Smoking cigarettes is harmful to health'. In another government survey of teenagers (12–18 years of age), 92 per cent agreed with the statement: 'Cigarette smoking can harm the health of teenagers' (Fishbein 1977). This awareness on the part of the American public is a relatively recent phenomenon. The Gallup poll in 1958 reported that 40 per cent of the population believed that smoking was harmful to health while another Gallup poll in 1974 showed this proportion to be 80 per cent. With this doubling in awareness over the 15-year period, there was only a very modest decline in the number of smokers in the US population. In 1958, 55 per cent of the population did not smoke; in 1974, 60 per cent did not. The Gallup data indicate not only that people know about the health hazards of smoking but that many of them have tried to do something about it. In 1974, half of the current smokers studied had actually tried to give up smoking at some prior time.

Discrepancy between behaviour and attitudes

From one point of view, those who have attempted to inform the public about smoking and its consequences for health, have succeeded. People in overwhelming proportions know about the dangers of smoking and increasing numbers of the smoking population want to give up the habit; in fact, a great many have actually tried to do so. In spite of this, many people nevertheless continue to smoke. There are at least three reasons for this discrepancy between behaviour and attitudes. One reason is that smoking is biologically and/or psychologically addictive. Green (1975) refers to a 'rationalization factor' suggesting that people who begin to smoke suffer from the illusions: (i) that cigarettes do not produce dependence; and (ii) that giving up will be easy. If you believe that smoking causes disease only after many years

of smoking and if you also believe that you will be a 'short term' smoker – that you can give up any time you want – the health consequences of smoking will not deter you from beginning. In fact, smoking is dependence-producing and all the evidence suggests that giving up is extraordinarily difficult.

A second reason for people to continue smoking is that it is seen as a pleasurable, relaxing, and helpful behaviour. In interviews we are now conducting in the San Francisco area, smokers report that smoking helps them relax, concentrate, work, sleep, and stay awake. Many report that smoking and smoking behaviour (finding a match, opening the package, extracting a cigarette from the package, lighting up, inhaling) provide important time for thinking when talking with associates. Still others report that they could not talk on the telephone, drink coffee, or end a meal without a cigarette. Cigarettes often are referred to as a dependable 'best friend' through both happy and difficult times.

A third reason for people smoking when 'they know better' is to be found in the social situation. Cigarette smoking is perceived as sociable behaviour. It is viewed as a way of establishing links with other people and of being 'one of the group'. This motivation is one of the major reasons people begin to smoke in the first place and it continues to be a factor in maintaining the behaviour. One of the most difficult accomplishments for people who are trying to give up smoking is to attend a cocktail party or other social event without their cigarettes. Even imagining themselves at such a gathering without a cigarette in hand is cause for anxiety.

Cigarettes are advertised everywhere, many people still smoke them and they are easily accessible at all times. This social circumstance provides a climate that encourages smoking, and that makes it easy and convenient. As such, smoking is acceptable behaviour that is supported by social institutions.

While at first glance the behaviour of smokers seems irrational 'when they clearly know better', the situation is in fact more complex. Our society is organized to encourage the initiation of smoking and to encourage the maintenance of this behaviour. As the social climate becomes less supportive of smoking, the attitude-behaviour inconsistency will become more uncomfortable for smokers and their behaviour will become 'more rational'.

Thus, it is not useful to view this problem simply as that of the individual smoker since that approach ignores the very strong social and cultural pressures that act upon and support the individual. The data suggest that we have already done an excellent job in educating individual smokers; we now need to focus attention on the social context in which the smoker lives (Leventhal and Cleary 1980).

Factors affecting cessation of smoking

The factors that encourage cessation of smoking are different from those that influence people to start smoking or from those that help maintain smoking once started. For cessation to be successful, the negative aspects of smoking must outweigh the positive benefits. Most cessation efforts are unsuccessful because they do not provide enough anti-moking support over the broad range of dimensions that onstitute the behaviour. Thus, if people smoke for ociability, to feel mature, to relax, or because of physical ddiction, a smoking cessation effort based primarily on ealth hazards will probably not succeed. All the evidence rom smoking-cessation programmes that focus on only one imension suggests that this approach is not likely to be uccessful to any significant extent.

Schwartz and Dubitsky (1968) have suggested that three actors are necessary to maximize success in smoking essation: (i) methods must be both acceptable to smokers nd effective in helping them give up; (ii) a combination of emographic, social, psychological, and environmental nfluences must be supportive of individual efforts to quit; nd (iii) the total environment must be conducive to ehaviour change by favouring smoking cessation, accepting he health dangers of cigarettes, favourable mass media dvertising, and governmental involvement in the anti-moking movement.

Clearly, such changes are now taking place. Evidence of uch changes are all about us in airplanes, offices, estaurants, and private homes. In a recent issue of the *San Francisco Chronicle,* for example, an article on 'dating clubs' n the area emphasized that several clubs now make smoking tatus one of the primary criteria for compatibility. One lating club manager noted: 'Aside from the usual criteria – nonesty, a sense of humor, spontaneity, openness, and good ooks – smoking is a very important consideration. If some-ne has just quit, for example, they are going to want to go ut with a non-smoker and a heavy smoker would probably prefer to date another smoker, so he doesn't feel pressured not to smoke.' As the issue of smoking becomes more mportant in daily life and as more anti-smoking messages ecome obvious, the likelihood increases that individuals will want to give up smoking and that they will succeed.

Much progress remains to be made, however. Cigarettes and cigarette smoking are an important part of mainstream everyday life. In many groups in society, smoking is still considered 'normal' and typical. An interesting illustration of this is provided by the latest guidelines from the US Internal Revenue Service. Permissible medical and dental deductions include meals and lodging provided by a centre during treatment for alcoholism and drug addiction. Deductions not permitted include such items as dancing lessons, household help, cosmetics, and 'programmes to stop smoking'. It is clear in what context smoking-cessation programmes are regarded.

An approach to prevention

Individuals decide to begin smoking cigarettes and individuals decide to give up. Since smoking is hazardous to health and since most smokers know this, their behaviour may be regarded as nonsensical, irrational, or defiant. With justification, we can be critical of smokers' decisions to begin smoking and of their inability to give up. On the other hand, this view of smoking ignores a social environment that implicitly induces people to start and continue smoking. These societal pressures, supports, and rewards are of importance in understanding individual behaviour. Without taking these pressures into account, we easily can 'blame the victim'. While it is true that only individuals can begin and stop smoking, it also is true that the tobacco industry has gone to extraordinary lengths to create an atmosphere where smoking is still an attractive and desirable behaviour. Surely the individual smoker must be informed and helped? But this assistance will be substantially weakened unless action also is taken at the societal level. We gain little by helping some people to give up smoking while an equal number of people are newly entering the smoking population.

Whether a person uses cigarettes or not depends on a special kind of personal choice – a choice influenced by how much the social milieu encourages or discourages the behaviour. We must learn more about the ways in which various social pressures affect behaviour and of the ways in which these pressures can be used in more constructive ways. We must better understand and neutralize the many forces generated by cigarette companies to encourage cigarette consumption. Included here are such matters as public advertising (the image that cigarette smoking is associated with the 'good life') and the lobbying in opposition to legisla-tion and other governmental action that would restrict the manufacture, sale or use of cigarettes. In addition, public policy still reflects smoking as a normal behaviour. Efforts to inform the individual smoker of the undesirability of smoking will be of little value unless action is also taken at the societal level.

To counteract the many societal pressures and inducements favouring smoking, a variety of public programmes are necessary. Some of the actions that could be included in such programmes are the following (Syme and Alcalay 1982):

1. Continue to increase public awareness of the health con-sequences of smoking. Although the results of individual health education programmes have not been significantly effective in persuading people not to start smoking or to stop smoking, the sum of years and years of continuous exposure to pro-smoking information has created a social milieu in which smoking is a normal part of life. Exposure to information on the health consequences of smoking is required as a necessary and constant warning for adults and for new generations.

2. Create an atmosphere in which it is realized that smoking is not the normal or majority behaviour. The increasing number of constraints on smoking behaviour (e.g. special sections for smokers in public places, increasing the rights of non-smokers) provides specific barriers against smoking and serves as a pervasive reminder about the hazards of smoking.

3. Influence public policy. This recommendation is directed mainly toward informing government, politicians, and organizations about health issues, policy objectives, and critical analysis of tobacco industry activities.

4. Increase anti-smoking advertisements. Although it is frustrating to counteract the enormous amount of smoking advertisement with very limited resources, it is necessary to maintain and increase anti-smoking advertisements. Positive anti-smoking advertisements should include the portrayal of

positive images of non-smokers and of the success of non-smoking programmes. Especially useful are frequent reminders that the majority of teenagers and adults are non-smokers.

Cigarette smoking is dangerous to health and most people know this. Nevertheless, we have had great difficulty in helping people to give up once they have begun to smoke. In this circumstance, prevention programmes are more reasonable than treatment programmes. To effectively prevent this behaviour, it must be recognized that individuals live in a social and cultural setting that importantly influences behaviour. Prevention programmes, therefore, must operate both at the individual and environmental level.

CONCLUSION

Statement of the problem

The treatment and prevention of many diseases of concern today require that people in one way or another change behaviour. We ask that people begin to do new things they have not previously done, to stop doing things they have been doing for years, to do more of some things and less of other things. Increasingly, these behaviour changes are the key and essential ingredient in both treatment and prevention programmes. It makes little difference that a drug is available for treatment if people will not take it; it is of little use to identify a hazardous behaviour if people will not change it. As our fund of useful information increases regarding treatment and prevention, the gap between what we want people to do and what they are willing to do becomes more important and potentially more frustrating.

While estimates of the magnitude of this problem vary, there is no doubt that a substantial gap exists. For example, averaging results over many studies of medications, Sackett (1976) suggests that 50 per cent of patients do not take prescribed medications in accordance with instructions. Some 20–40 per cent of recommended immunizations are not obtained. Crude averages from many studies show that scheduled appointments for treatment are missed 20–50 per cent of the time (Kirscht and Rosenstock 1979). When changes in habitual behaviour are recommended, as in dietary restrictions, cessation of smoking, and increases in physical activity, there is even greater non-compliance. As noted earlier, programmes designed to deal with smoking are considered effective if more than a third of entrants have reduced their smoking at the end of six months; large percentages drop out of weight control programmes; and dietary restrictions are often observed primarily in the breach. It should be noted, of course, that wide variability exists in the results of studies depending on the population under study, the type of recommendation, the treatment setting and so on.

Factors influencing adherence to advice

Haynes (1976) has reviewed 185 original research reports dealing with factors that influence the likelihood of people following expert suggestions. His review summarizes the findings for the following such factors: demographic characteristics of patients; features of the disease, the regimen,

and therapeutic source; aspects of patient–physician interaction; and socio-behavioural characteristics of patients. He concludes that only a small number of variables have demonstrated a consistent relationship with patient adherence. Among those factors (all associated with lower rates of compliance) are: a 'psychiatric' diagnosis; the complexity, duration and amount of change involved in the regimen itself; inconvenience associated with treatment; inadequate supervision by professionals; patient dissatisfaction; 'inappropriate' health beliefs'; non-compliance with other regimens; and family instability. Factors that did not yield consistent relationships with adherence across different situations and regimens included demographic factors, personality characteristics, knowledge, health status, social norms, and patient provider interactions. Other reviewers have noted that few associations are found between adherence and such social characteristics of patients such as age, sex and education (Becker and Maiman 1975; Kasl 1975).

Especially interesting in this connection is the consistent finding that information is not an important factor influencing patient behaviour. With regard to hypertension, Kirscht and Rosenstock (1977) found that knowledge about high blood pressure was unrelated to taking medications or following dietary advice. Similarly, Sackett et al. (1975) also found that hypertension knowledge did not predict adherence. In our own study of hypertension in a low-income community in California, we found very high levels of knowledge regarding hypertension and its treatment but found also that this knowledge had little relation to whether or not people had controlled blood pressures.

While none of these factors have been shown consistently to be associated with behaviour change, it would be inappropriate to conclude that they are unimportant. A more useful view would be that these factors are necessary but not sufficient (Tagliacozzo and Ima 1970; Becker et al. 1972; Kirscht and Rosenstock 1977). No one would argue, for example, that information and knowledge are irrelevant and unimportant in behaviour change. People certainly should be made aware of the facts regarding hazardous and unhealthy behaviours. By itself, however, such information is not likely to result in behaviour change. The crucial issue is to ensure that information, favourable treatment settings, appropriate practitioner attitudes and other important ingredients are made available together.

A recommendation

In our detailed review of cigarette smoking and hypertension, two of these crucial ingredients were emphasized. First, whatever else occurs, patients must be motivated to change behaviour. This motivation can come only from within the person. It is suggested that the way we traditionally organize care and information settings makes it more difficult for people to take responsibility for their behaviour. By requiring that people come to experts for help, we subtly and perhaps inevitably induce people to rely on these experts rather than on themselves. To the extent that this occurs, no amount of information or techniques or other inducements will yield important improvements in patient adherence. We therefore must devise alternative methods of assisting people where such dependance is less likely.

The second crucial element is that the environment be carefully considered in intervention programmes. It makes little sense to request that people change their behaviour when everything else in the social, cultural, and physical environment conspires against such change. Not only does such environmental pressure work against persons attempting such changes, also continuously produces new patients even as we successfully deal with old ones. Clearly, this is a self-defeating and unproductive activity that is unfair to all parties involved.

As our knowledge and technology grows concerning the causes of disease and of ways that diseases can be prevented and treated, it increasingly is important that we seriously and systematically attend to the non-technological element in treatment and prevention programmes. We cannot induce people to change their ways simply by force of logic, information, statistics, or pressure; instead, we must provide such assistance in social contexts that are supportive and in ways that do not interfere with people taking active responsibility for their health. All the evidence is that people are intelligent, thoughtful and sensitive and that they surely will act in their own best interest. Our challenge is to encourage this to happen.

REFERENCES

Adams, E.E. (1979). Mortality. In *Smoking and health,* p. 36. DHEW, PHS, NIH, Washington, DC.

Alderman, M., Green, L.W., and Flynn, B.S. (1980). Hypertension control programs in occupational settings. *Public Health Reports* **95**, 158.

Becker, M.H. (1976). Sociobehavioural determinants of compliance. In *Compliance with therapeutic regimens* (ed. D.L. Sackett and R.B. Haynes) p. 40. Johns Hopkins University Press, Baltimore.

Becker, M.H., Drachman, R.H., and Kirscht, J.P. (1972). Motivations as predictors of health behavior. *Health Services Reports* **87**, 852.

Becker, M.H. and Maiman, L.A. (1975). Sociobehavioral determinants of compliance with health and medical care recommendations. *Med. Care* **31**, 10.

Bergin, J.E. and Wake, F.R. (1974). *Report to the Department of National Health and Welfare on Canadian research on psychosocial aspects of cigarette smoking: 1960–1972.* Canadian Department National Health Welfare, Ottawa.

British Medical Journal (1981). Letters to Editor. *Br. Med. J.* **282**, 915, 985, 1393, 1464.

Dekker, E. (1975). Youth culture and influences on the smoking behavior of young people. In *Smoking and health,* p. 381. DHEW, PHS, NIH, Washington, DC.

Doron, G. (1979). *The smoking paradox.* Abt, Cambridge, Mass.

Evans, R.E., Henderson, A., Hill, N.A., and Raines, P. (1979). Smoking in children and adolescents: psychosocial determinants and prevention strategies. In *Smoking and health,* p. 5. DHEW, PHS, NIH, Washington, DC.

Evans, D. and Lane, D.S. (1980). Long-term outcome of smoking cessation workshops. *Am. J. Public Health* **70**, 725.

Fishbein, M. (1977). Consumer beliefs and behaviour with respect to cigarette smoking: a critical analysis of the public literature. In *Federal Trade Commission Report to Congress: Pursuant to the Public Health Cigarette Smoking Act,* p. xxx. Washington, DC.

Friedman, G.D., Siegelaub, A.B., Dales, L.G., and Seltzer, C.C. (1979). Characteristics predictive of coronary heart disease in ex-smokers before they stopped smoking: comparison with persistent smokers and non-smokers. *J. Chronic Dis.* **32**, 175.

Garfinkel, L.A. (1981). Time trends in lung cancer mortality among nonsmokers and a note on passive smoking. *J. Natl Cancer Inst.* **66**, 1061.

Gerbner, G., Gross, L., Morgan, M., and Signorelli, N. (1981). Health and medicine on television. *N. Engl. J. Med.* **305**, 901.

Gordon, T. (1964). *Blood pressure of adults by age and sex, United States, 1960–1962.* National Center for Health Statistics, Public Health Service Publication No. 1000 – Series 11-No. 4. Washington, DC.

Gray, N. and Daube, M. (eds.) (1980). *Guidelines for smoking control.* UICC Tech. Rep. Ser., Vol. 52. International Union Against Cancer, Geneva.

Green, D.E. (1975). Teenage cigarette smoking in the United States 1968, 1970, 1972 and 1974. In *Smoking and health,* p. 375. DHEW, PHS, NIH, Washington, DC.

Hammond, E.C. and Selikoff, L.J. (1981). Passive smoking and lung cancer with comments on two new papers. *Environ. Res.* **24**, 444.

Harris, L. *et al.* (1973). *The public and high blood pressure: a survey conducted for the National Heart and Lung Institute.* No. (NIH) 74:356. US Department of Health, Education and Welfare, Washington, DC.

Haynes, R.B. (1976). A critical review of the 'determinants' of patient compliance with therapeutic regimens. In *Compliance with therapeutic regimens* (ed. D.L. Sackett and R.B. Haynes) p. 16. Johns Hopkins University Press, Baltimore.

Hirayama, T. (1981). Non-smoking wives of heavy smokers have a higher risk of lung cancer. A study from Japan. *Br. Med. J.* **282**, 113.

Horn, D. (1960). Modifying smoking habits in high school students. In *Children* **7**, 63.

Hulka, B.S., Cassel, J.C., and Kupper, I. (1976). Disparities between medications prescribed and consumed among chronic disease patients. In *Patient compliance* (ed. L. Lasagna). Futura, Mt. Kisco, NY.

Hunt, W.A. and Matarazzo, J.D. (1973). Three years later: recent developments in the experimental modification of smoking behaviour. *J. Abnormal Psych.* **81**, 107.

Hypertension Detection and Follow-Up Program Cooperative Group (1977). Blood pressure studies in 14 communities: a two-stage screen for hypertension. *JAMA* **237**, 2385.

Johnston, L.D., Bachman, J.G., and O'Malley, P.M. (1980). *Student drug use in America 1975–1980.* Department of Health and Human Services, Washington, DC.

Kasl, S.V. (1975). Social-psychological characteristics associated with behaviours which reduce cardiovascular risk. In *Applying behavioural science to cardiovascular risk* (ed. A.J. Enelow and J.B. Henderson), American Heart Association, New York.

Kirscht, J.P. and Rosenstock, I.M. (1977). Patient adherence to anti-hypertensive medical regimens. *J. Community Health* **3**, 115.

Kirscht, J.P. and Rosenstock, I.M. (1979). Patients' problems in following recommendations of health experts. In *Health psychology: a handbook* (ed. G.C. Stone *et al.*) p. 189. Jossey-Bass, San Francisco.

Kozlowski, L.T. (1979). Psychological influences on cigarette smoking. In *Smoking and health,* p. 5. DHEW, PHS, NIH, Washington, DC.

Leventhal, H. and Cleary, P.D. (1980). The smoking problem: a review of the research and theory in behavioural risk modification. *Psychol. Bull.* **88**, 370.

McGuiness, T. and Cowling, K. (1975). Advertising and the aggregate demand for cigarettes. *Eur. Econ. Rev.* **6**, 311.

National Clearinghouse for Smoking and Health (1976). *Adults' use of tobacco 1975.* DHEW. Bureau of Disease Prevention and Environmental Control, NIH, Washington, DC.

Paul, O. (1978). Complications of mild hypertension. In *Mild hypertension: to treat or not to treat.* (ed. H.M. Perry and W.M. Smith) p. 56. New York Academy of Sciences.

Pechacek, T.F. (1979). Modification of smoking behavior. In *Smoking and health*, p. 50. DHEW, PHS, NIH, Washington, DC.

Promoting Health/Preventing Disease (1980). US Health Human Serv., PHS, NIH, Washington, DC.

Roberts, J. (1975). *Blood pressure at persons 18–74 years, United States, 1971–1972.* National Center for Health Statistics. DHEW Publication No. 75-1632. Rockville, Maryland.

Sackett, D.I. (1976). The magnitude of compliance and non-compliance. In *Compliance with therapeutic regimens.* (ed. D.L. Sackett and R.B. Haynes) p. 9. Johns Hopkins University Press, Baltimore.

Sackett, D.L., Haynes, R.B., Gibson, E.S. *et al.* (1975). Randomized clinical trials for strategies for improving medication compliance in primary hypertension. *Lancet* **i**, 1205.

Schoenberger, J.A., Stamler, J., Shekelle, R.B. *et al.* (1972). Current status of hypertension control in an industrial population. *JAMA* **222**, 559.

Schuman, L.M. (1979). Introduction and summary. In *Smoking and health*. p. 1. DHEW, PHS, NIH, Washington, DC.

Schwartz, J.L. (1969). A critical review and evaluation of smoking control methods. *Public Heatlh Reports* **84**, 483.

Schwartz, J.L. and Dubitzky, M. (1968). Requisites for success in smoking withdrawal. In *Smoking, health and behavior* (ed. E.F. Borgatta and R.R. Evans). Aldine, Chicago.

Schwartz, J.L. and Rider, G. (1975). Smoking cessation methods i the United States and Canada, 1969–1974. In *Smoking an health.* DHEW, PHS, NIH, Washington, DC.

Smith, W.M. (1978). Mild essential hypertension: benefit of treat ment. In *Mild hypertension: to treat or not to treat* (ed. H.M Perry and W.M. Smith) p. 74. New York Academy of Sciences.

Syme, S.L. and Alcalay, R. (1982). Control of cigarette smokin from a social perspective. *Ann. Rev. Public Health* **3**, 179.

Syme, S.L. and Torfs, C.P. (1978). Epidemiologic research i hypertension: a critical appraisal. *J. Human Stress* **4**, 43.

Tagliacozzo, D. and Ima, K. (1970). Knowledge of illness as a pre dictor of patient behavior. *J. Chronic Dis.* **22**, 765.

Trichopoulos, D., Dalandidi, A., Sparros, L., and MacMahon, B (1981). Lung cancer and passive smoking. *Int. J. Cancer* **27**, 1.

US Department of Health, Education and Welfare (1982). *Th health consequences of smoking: cancer*, p. 255. US Departmen of Health, Education and Welfare, Public Health Service, Offic of Smoking and Health, Washington, DC.

West, D.W., Graham, S., Swanson, M., and Wilkinson, G. (1977) Five year follow-up of a smoking withdrawal clinic population *Am. J. Public Health* **67**, 536.

Whiteside, T. (1974). Smoking still. *New Yorker* **50**, 121.

Wilber, J.A. (1967). Detection and control of hypertensive diseas in Georgia, USA. In *The epidemiology of hypertension* (ed J. Stamler, R. Stamler, and Pullman R.N.) Grune and Stratton New York.

Williams, D.C. and Shor, R.E. (1979). The Social support system of smoking. Paper presented at 87th Ann. Conv. Am. Psychol Assoc., New York.

Wilson, R.W. (1979). Morbidity. In *Smoking and health*, p. 3 DHEW, PHS, NIH, Washington, DC.

Global strategies

9 Deterrents to health in developing countries

James Gallagher

HE NATURE OF UNDERDEVELOPMENT

ocio-economic underdevelopment is exemplified in its xtreme form by the 31 countries designated by the United Iations Organization (UN) as least developed countries for urposes of a new programme of action to mobilize resources ɔ accelerate their development. Twenty-one are in Africa, ight in Asia and one each in the Pacific and the Caribbean. ogether they contain some 280 million people of whom bout 200 million are destitute. These countries illustrate vividly ɔoth the part that disease plays in underdevelopment, and how, s a composite phenomenon, underdevelopment, compounded ɔf poverty, ignorance, malnutrition, and disease, constitutes ʰe principal deterrent to health and to measures to improve ⁱealth. It is measured conventionally and roughly by Gross ᵛational Product (GNP) – which in some cases is less than JS$150 per caput – and manifested by such health and socio-conomic indicators as infant mortality rates which can exceed 00 per 1000 live births, maternal mortality rates that in some ɔlaces exceed 1000 per 100 000 births, a life expectancy at birth ɔf 45 years, an adult literacy rate of 28 per cent, a manufactur-ng component of GNP of less than 10 per cent, and an annual ɔublic expenditure on health of less than US$2 per head.

To the interrelated biological and socio-economic forces, ₋nd their magnitude and pervasiveness, that constitute under-devopment are added in many instances, harsh climatic or ₋eological features, scarcity of water, recurring natural and ᵃan-made disasters, and spreading environmental degradation ʳrom the pressures of population on limited farmland and ɔther resources. Associated factors in this degradation are an ₋nrelenting demand for firewood, which is causing, on a large ₋cale in the poorest African countries, the destruction of forests, ₋nd contributing to an accelerating encroachment of desert on ɔreviously arable land, and an apparent lack of political will to ₋pply the technology to combat the process. A high proportion ɔf the world's refugees originate or are sheltered in the least ₋evoped countries.

Most people in the least developed countries depend on ₋ubsistence farming, and there is consequently little surplus to ₋nvest in improving agriculture, building up industry, or expanding such government services as health care and education. Reduced physical and mental capacity consequent ɔn malnutrition and disease also depress productivity. Revenue is so low that public expenditure on health averages ɔnly US$1.70 per person, compared with US$6.50 for other ₋evoping countries and US$244 for developed countries.

Scattered communities spread over vast rural areas and, often, arid land are poorly served by transport and communi-cations, and typically are remote from even elementary health care. They are politically powerless. They remain badly nourished, uneducated, and in poor health as long as they remain destitute, and their destitution continues as long as they continue to be hungry, uneducated, and disease-ridden.

These countries have very restricted internal markets, with no leverage over the supplies of goods or services, have extreme difficulty in securing access to outside markets, and have no basis for export growth. Their economies, based mainly on agriculture, have stagnated and in recent years even declined. They have no control over the prices of their agricultural products, which fluctuate erratically, thus preventing orderly budgeting; their mainly agricultural exports can pay for little more than half of their essential imports. They lack skilled manpower of all kinds, even to make the best use of the aid they receive from rich countries.

This degree of underdevelopment shows strikingly the close interlinkage of socio-economic and health problems, and justifies the formal acceptance by the UN General Assembly in 1979 of health development as an integral dimension of socio-economic development.

The 89 countries at present designated as developing coun-tries present a heterogeneous picture. Latin American countries, compared with those in Africa and Asia have, in general, a longer tradition of political independence and a relatively high level of income per caput; most of their peoples share much common history and similar development experience and problems. The poor countries of Africa and Asia are diverse in culture, economic conditions, and social and political structure.

A few of the developing countries have made substantial progress towards the social objectives of development but in many cases advance has been slow and uneven, and much ground has been lost owing to the oil-price rises of 1973 and 1979 and the economic recession of recent years. A rising GNP as an indicator of economic growth can conceal falling living standards for large rural and peri-urban populations, an increasing incidence of absolute poverty, and widening inequalities in income and wealth. Often the benefits of economic growth apply only to a relatively few who have been able to invest or obtain employment in the modern sectors of industry and agriculture and to senior professionals or public sector officials. Some countries have pockets of affluence, generally in large cities, with living standards comparable to those of the most favoured classes in developed countries and correspondingly strong political leverage. They influence national policies on investment allocation, public expenditure, and trading patterns and they often provide favourable conditions for the special interests of foreign industrial and commercial enterprises. Their diseases are those typical of industrialized countries, and an undue concentration of medical services, public and private, meets their demands for health care and consumes resources that could be applied to reducing the gap in health status between urban and rural populations. This element of social injustice is reinforced by medical education systems which produce graduates whose training has equipped them to serve the demands of this urban elite rather than the needs of peri-urban and rural populations.

POVERTY

The great mass of the people are poor and, according to a World Bank estimate, about 40 per cent – or nearly 800 million, in 1978 – live in absolute poverty (World Bank 1978). Their greatest concentration is in South Asia and Indonesia but it is in Sub-Saharan Africa, which has a much smaller population, that the highest proportion of absolute poor is found. Most live in rural areas, where only 22 per cent of the population have an adequate water supply and 15 per cent satisfactory sanitation services (WHO 1980). A growing number live in the slums and shantytowns of the rapidly growing cities of the Third World, with an almost total lack of basic services such as water, sanitation and electricity. Health services are thinly spread and, for large proportions of rural population, not within walking distance. Their children are often kept away from school, where there are primary schools, because they are needed for work. In cities children may be sent to work in factories at pittance wages and in conditions that contravene the most basic codes of industrial hygiene or occupational health. Families are preoccupied with survival and elementary needs, and live in permanent insecurity, unrelieved by social welfare in the event of unemployment or the sickness or death of a wage-earner. Most of the extreme poverty is associated with a low national output and income, combined with maldistribution of the income that is available.

Besides those in absolute poverty – defined as inability to obtain basic services – many other people have inadequate access to public services. In 1975 about 1200 million people lived in low-income countries in Asia and Africa – which almost by definition means inadequate access to public services – with a median per caput income of US$150; 87 per cent lived in rural areas, 77 per cent of adults were illiterate, 48 per cent of children were not enrolled in primary school, and 75 per cent of the population were without safe water. In middle-income countries, with a population of 900 million in 1975 and median per caput incomes of US$750, 57 per cent were rural, 37 per cent of adults were illiterate, and 48 per cent of the population had no access to safe water (WHO 1980).

According to the Brandt Commission (Independent Com-

mission on International Development Issues 1980) the poorest people in the world will remain, for some time to come, outside the reach of normal trade and communications. The combination of malnutrition, illiteracy, disease, high birth rates, underemployment, and low income closes off the avenues of escape; and while other groups are increasingly vocal, the poor and illiterate are usually and conveniently silent. Their numbers are not expected to diminish substantially in the next decade; World Bank projections indicate that there will still be 600 million absolute poor in the developing countries by the year 2000.

The seeming failure of most developing countries to distribute wealth occurs because, according to the Brandt Commission, their total resources, even if they were equally divided, are insufficient to support their populations. Even countries where a considerable amount of industrialization has taken place have two-thirds or more of their workers in agriculture, and all rely heavily on exporting raw material rather than processed products; the markets of industrial countries are in many cases highly protected against imports of processed products. Developing countries are often highly dependent on the export of a very limited number of commodities whose prices fluctuate erratically in response to factors outside the control of their primary producers.

It is an accepted tenet of socio-economic and health development that the eradication of the mass poverty of the developing countries is a prerequisite for health, as for other dimensions of development in those countries; but in view of the interrelationships of poverty, hunger, ignorance, and disease, and of the scarcity of resources in the developing countries for tackling the composite problem that they constitute, these different elements have to be attacked in co-ordinated and concerted ways which complement and reinforce one another. This demands levels of managerial and administrative competence which are particularly scarce in developing and developed countries alike, and the lack of which has bedevilled much international development effort.

A vast amount of effort and resources has been expended on development in the last three decades. Although with hindsight much of it can be criticized on various grounds, it should be remembered that the concept and the technology of development aid are new to mankind and that earlier experience in respect of some of today's industrialized countries provided no valid precedents for dealing with the nature, magnitude and complexity of current problems. Much has been learned, even if very expensively, and a great deal has been accomplished. The Pearson Commission, set up by the World Bank in 1968, in assessing the results of twenty years of aid, reported that the developing countries had progressed far better than was generally realized and that the richer countries had contributed much aid. The gap between the richest and the poorest countries was still widening, however, and the population explosion, which had not been foreseen, was not subsiding. Also, too much aid had been directed at industry and too little at agriculture (Commission on International Development 1969). The imbalance between development efforts directed at agriculture and rural development, on the one hand, and industrialization and urban improvement, on the other, has persisted (Galbraith 1979).

here is conflict between agriculture and urban industry, and the latter wins. The rural sector contains most of the poverty and most of the low-cost sources of potential advance; but the urban sector contains most of the articulateness, organization and power (Lipton 1977). Not only are sufficiently high levels of managerial and administrative competence in scarce supply but also, apparently, political commitment to redressing this imbalance in favour of agriculture and rural development.

MALNUTRITION AND FOOD PRODUCTION

Malnutrition is a leading cause of illness and death among young children in developing countries but it affects all age-groups. Of 800 millions estimated to be destitute in the Third World most, by definition, cannot afford an adequate diet. In children under 5 years of age the problem is mainly one of protein-energy malnutrition precipitated by diarrhoeal and other infectious diseases and by too frequent births. A UNICEF estimate in 1978 put the number of deaths from hunger of children in this age-group at more than 12 million; among those children who survive, malnutrition brings about chronic debility and impairment of biological, intellectual, and physical functions, contributing in turn to further loss of productivity, consequent low income, and continuing malnutrition.

Of an estimated 22 million births of low-birth-weight babies each year, due mainly to maternal malnutrition, 21 million are born in the developing countries, with a mortality risk up to 20 times higher than that of other babies (WHO 1980). Extremely high rates of maternal mortality among young women in the least developed countries are attributed in part to cephalo-pelvic disproportion caused by pelvic deformation consequent upon malnutrition in childhood.

In its fifth report on the world health situation the WHO draw attention to a reversal of the trend towards nutritional improvement in the developing countries, associated with a general decline in the quality of life; and in its sixth report to the apparent increasing extent of malnutrition in spite of a large number of measures taken by different sectors of government to end it (WHO 1975, 1980).

Improved agricultural technologies, practices and policies enabled the world's farmers to produce twice as much food in 1980 as in 1950 and the potential for further increase is still substantial (Barr 1981). In the developing countries, however, despite a continuous increase in their total food production, per caput food production has increased little in the past decade and in some of the poorest countries it has even declined; and the combination of population growth and rising incomes is limiting the availability of food for their own poor as well as for the least developed countries.

To enable people to buy food rural poverty has to be greatly reduced. This implies that every family must have a reliable livelihood, which means much greater gainful employment in both agriculture and manufacturing (Independent Commission on International Development Issues 1980). However, it is difficult to envisage any substantial reduction in current levels of unemployment and underemployment in the Third World in the face of its projected population increase of 1800 million over the next two decades.

There is at the same time a rising dependence of Third World countries on food imports from the industrialized countries. On current trends, they could be importing 145 million tons of food by 1990, compared with 20 million in 1960 and nearly 80 million in 1978; the Brandt report points out that they are unlikely to be in a position to finance such massive imports from their own export earnings or from additional aid, and that even if they could do so it is doubtful if the major grain producers could supply the amount needed. Moreover, there may well be less food available from the developed countries as their consumption of grain is set to increase in proportion to that of the Third World. Projections indicate that by 1990, barring an unprecedented degree of international co-operation and flexibility, the developed countries, with 24 per cent of the world's population and 85 per cent of its economic activity, will account for 50 per cent of the world's production and consumption of grain, or more than three times as much grain per head as the other three-fourths of the world's population (Barr 1981).

As to prospects for increased food production in the three to four decades before the population of the Third World is expected to stabilize, it must be borne in mind that the great increase in production in the last three decades has taken place under generally favourable conditions of soil and climate, and sufficient water for irrigation. While production is expected to continue to grow in those areas, much of the increase needed will depend on a greater cultivation of infertile land, in places where water is generally scarce and droughts recur regularly, the risk of pest damage is high, expensive pesticides and fertilizers have to be imported, and access to markets is difficult. Adequate and sustained yields of food crops will depend greatly on the ability of chemists and other scientists, in both industrialized and Third World countries, to provide new varieties of crops, improved fertilizer technologies, and integrated pest-management techniques (Brady 1982).

There are also structural deterrents to the eradication of rural poverty and to self-sufficiency in food production. In many poor countries, there are sharp disparities in the ownership of land. A minority of landlords and large farmers, often 5–10 per cent of rural households, may own 40–60 per cent of arable land. The rest of the rural population is crowded on small, often fragmented, pieces of land and many own no land. In many cases, a high proportion of rural land is held on a tenant or sharecropping basis with the landlord appropriating large shares of the total crop (Independent Commission on International Development Issues 1980). A priority role for agriculture in socio-economic development must be accompanied by agrarian reform and land redistribution, which is liable to be opposed by powerful vested interests and which at best cannot provide adequately for the large proportion of landless labourers in many developing countries' populations (WHO 1980). It must be accompanied also therefore by a promotion of small-scale enterprises, as well as by considerable improvement in the organization and delivery of public services.

Clearly, direct health action cannot affect socio-economic

deprivation, the basic cause of undernutrition. But the health sector can prevent and treat the poverty-related factors that generate malnutrition – infections and parasitic infestations, unregulated fertility, and poor environmental sanitation – and substantially improve population coverage. To this extent it can alleviate the problem and contribute to the maintenance of a balance, however precarious, between the nutritional needs of the groups who are most at risk and the supply of food. In addition to direct nutritional health measures, this depends on such indirect means of preventing malnutrition as the widespread use of oral rehydration for diarrhoea in young children, effective measures of birth-spacing, and immunization of the great majority of children against the common infections of childhood. It depends too on supporting women and developing their capacity to promote nutrition in feeding and caring for children, as well as on recognizing their major role in agricultural production: in many places it is women who work in the fields, often for low wages and in poor conditions.

Health action against malnutrition has to be co-ordinated with the activities of various other sectors. This demands a high degree of administrative skill, as well as political commitment, to co-ordinate national food and nutrition strategies with the other components of national development. These national strategies now being adopted in different countries are geared to improving the pattern of income distribution and agricultural productivity; to many other concurrent measures relating to food conservation, processing, marketing, pricing, and distribution; and to environmental measures to reduce the level of the intestinal infections and infestations that are impeding the normal absorption of food by many people (WHO 1980). Increased food aid is essential also but can be only a stop-gap measure which does not fundamentally change underlying longer-term trends. The low-income countries need a massive infusion of capital investment to build infrastructures and give them the capacity to produce, distribute, and market grain. This will require the investment of significant capital in all sectors of a country's economy including grain handling, chemical inputs, and irrigation systems, as well as increased research support and education to implement existing technology in areas such as multiple cropping and higher-yielding varieties (Barr 1981).

DISEASE AND CONSTRAINTS TO ITS CONTROL

The principal diseases of developing countries fall into two basic categories: communicable, i.e. infectious and parasitic diseases, and nutritional deficiency diseases. They reflect well the interrelationships of infection, malnutrition, and an unhealthy environment that characterize those countries.

Nutritional deficiences lower resistance to communicable diseases and increase their severity. Recurrent attacks of diarrhoea, for instance, especially associated with dehydration and lack of early rehydration, exacerbate underlying malnutrition. When combined with malnutrition, the infectious diseases of childhood such as measles, pertussis, and pneumonia have high case-fatality rates. Parasitic diseases

can damage the intestines to the extent that the little food th is consumed is not absorbed.

Three specific nutritional deficiences are of particul importance in developing countries, not only as heal problems but also because of their very serious soci economic effects. These are: vitamin A deficiency and xerop thalmia, causing about 100 000 new cases of blindness young children each year; endemic goitre and cretinisr caused by iodine deficiency and associated with ment retardation, and highly prevalent in various African, Asia and Latin American countries; and nutritional anaem caused by iron or folate deficiency, and affecting lar; numbers of pregnant and lactating women and you children (WHO 1980).

The communicable and nutritional deficiency diseases, a their associated physical, mental, and social disabilitie which affect hundreds of millions of people in the Thi World constitute a massive deterrent to health and to soci economic development; at the same time there are formidab deterrents to their control or eradication. Contrary common belief, many of the diseases of underdevelopme are not necessarily bound up with tropical conditions. T same diseases were common in the industrializing countries Europe and North America in the nineteenth century b have largely disappeared as a result of improvements in san tation, education, and a general rise in living standard Doyal (1979) describes the part played by the slave trade an colonialist expansion in Africa in the spread of infectiou disease and malnutrition, and the influences of monopo capitalism and of development aid tied to the interests donor countries in maintaining disease patterns and deterrir the implementation of effective health policies. Howeve given these causes and deterrents, there have been spectacul successes in controlling these diseases in developing countrie and there are effective technologies to do so. There a deterrents or constraints, however, to their application an adaptation.

The *Sixth Report of the World Health Situation* lists th constraints to applying and adapting effective technology i the control of communicable diseases in the developin countries as: inadequate national commitment; inadequat community understanding and involvement; weakness in th health infrastructure and supporting services; shortcoming in epidemiological surveillance; and lack of managerial capa bility to identify problems and develop the most suitab solutions at all levels of the national health services.

The resurgence of malaria, to become again a major publi health problem in some 70 countries, after the substantia success of the anti-malaria efforts of the fifties exemplifie well the operation of those constraints. Governments wer glad of the opportunity, as they saw it, to apply to othe purposes the funds and other resources that were needed t maintain control over an apparently disappearing disease Many countries did not apply the eradication measures wit the needed epidemiological insight and the required efficienc (Farid 1980). Anti-malaria activities were seriously affecte by the economic and energy crises, by the higher cost o insecticides and drugs, and by the shortage of experience

rofessional and other field personnel. In addition, in the mid-
970s, vectors had become resistant to insecticides, and
lasmodium falciparum to drugs, in 20 per cent or more of
nalarious areas as against 1.5 per cent 10 years earlier.

The effects of those constraints are seen also in the
ncreasing global prevalence and severity of schistosomiasis.
: is endemic in 71 countries, and spreading owing to the
ramatic increase in the developing world's peri-urban
hantytown population, the substitution of perennial for
:asonal irrigation, and the creation of man-made lakes
Chernin 1978). Other intestinal helminthic and protozoal
nfections which affect hundreds of millions of people in
Africa, Asia, and Latin America are generally associated with
oil pollution and contamination of water by faeces and
ncontrolled disposal of solid wastes. Garbage dumps
arbour insects and rodents, which are vectors for a wide
ange of infectious and parasitic diseases. A pandemic of
holera is continuing to spread because of slow progress in
he improvement of water supply and excreta disposal.
)iarrhoea, associated with contaminated water supplies and
oupled with poor nutrition, malaria, or lack of
mmunization, is causing five million deaths a year among
hildren under five years old.

A further five million deaths annually in the same age-
roup, with permanent disabling of an additional five
nillion, are caused by a group of six common diseases –
iphtheria, pertussis, tetanus, measles, poliomyelitis, and
uberculosis; fewer than 10 per cent of the 80 million children
orn annually in developing countries are being fully immun-
zed (WHO 1980). The WHO's Expanded Programme of
mmunization, aimed at immunizing against these diseases
very child in the world by 1990, depends largely for its success
n countries overcoming the constraints mentioned above.

Those constraints may be expressed in other terms. Thus,
he report of the Alma-Ata International Conference on
'rimary Health Care (WHO 1978) states that the technical
nowledge available for health care is not being put to the
est use for the greatest number. Health resources are
llocated mainly to sophisticated medical institutions in urban
reas, and disadvantaged groups have no access to any
ermanent form of health care. Health systems are too often
utside the mainstream of social and economic development,
nd frequently restrict themselves to medical care although
ndustrialization and deliberate alteration of the environment
re creating health problems whose proper control lies far
eyond the scope of medical care. Most conventional health-
are systems are becoming increasingly complex and costly
nd have doubtful social relevance. They have been distorted
y the dictates of medical technology and by the misguided
fforts of a medical industry providing medical consumer
oods to society.

HEALTH HAZARDS OF DEVELOPMENT AND
INDUSTRIALIZATION

t is now well recognized that development and industrializa-
ion carry serious hazards to physical, mental, and social well-
eing. The most dramatic examples are provided by civil

engineering enterprises, particularly the construction of large
water impoundments and artificial lakes constructed for
hydroelectric production and irrigation purposes, which have
provided favourable breeding conditions for the vectors of
schistosomiasis, onchocerciasis, and other intestinal
helminthic and protozoal infections. These and other adverse
environmental consequences of developmental activities often
extend beyond national boundaries. Successful large-scale
control measures have been shown to be feasible but require a
firm commitment on the part of government, and finance
and manpower to a degree that many countries cannot
afford. Yet irrigation and the production of energy are
necessary for economic development, and water is a basic
need for humans and livestock and for the cultivation of
crops.

Accelerated urbanization is associated with the unplanned
growth and spread of large cities and with a continuous
deterioration of the human environment. Industrial pollution, traffic problems, noise, lack of sanitary facilities, and a
reduction in the quality of urban air and water resources have
become very serious problems in many large cities (WHO
1980).

Occupational health hazards are increasing in the
developing countries and control measures are generally
lacking. Their effects are likely to be more serious in the
Third World than in the developed countries for such reasons
as the poor nutrition of workers, high rates of debilitating
disease, and less official concern about pollution and
occupational health hazards (Elling 1977). There has been a
selective transfer of industrial production from the developed
to the developing countries, largely to take advantage of their
flexible and cheap labour supply, and apparently also to
avoid the controls that industrialized countries are imposing
on dangerous or polluting processes. Much of it involves
health and safety hazards, either to workers or to the population at large (Doyal 1979). Developing countries often
welcome even the most hazardous new industries, given their
economic aspirations, but these industries add new environmental hazards to those of rapid urbanization while the basic
sanitation problems have still to be solved.

Developing countries are increasing their use of agricultural
chemicals to raise crop yields and it appears from the scanty
data that can be obtained that up to 40 per cent of spray-men
exposed to such chemicals suffer from poisoning. With a
greater use of agricultural machinery there are more
occupational injuries, and in small industries, in which almost
70 per cent of the world's work force in manufacturing,
mining and related trades is employed, occupational diseases
and injuries are common.

Systematic data on occupational health problems, essential
to assess needs and identify priorities in regard to workers'
health, are limited in developing countries owing to the
weakness of occupational health units at places of work and a
widespread shortage of trained occupational health staff,
epidemiologists and statisticians. The greatest difficulty in
obtaining data, however, is that most workers are outside the
immediate range of occupational health care.

Another health hazard of development is a rapid increase

in tobacco production (FAO 1978). Since tobacco is a major cash crop many governments promote its expanded production. Six of the world's top 10 tobacco-producing countries are in the developing world (Brazil, China, India, Indonesia, Republic of Korea, and Turkey). Besides, multinational tobacco companies are taking advantage of the lack of restrictions on the promotion of cigarettes and on manufacturing standards in developing countries not only to promote aggressively the sale of cigarettes but also to sell cigarettes with a much higher tar content than is permitted in many developed countries.

The smoking habit has spread like an epidemic. Although the developing countries have not yet had time to experience the grim increase in smoking-related mortality that has taken place in the industrialized countries, they must expect it unless they halt and reverse the increase in cigarette consumption. In many less developed countries, the epidemic of smoking-related diseases is already of such magnitude as to rival even infectious diseases or malnutrition as a public health problem (WHO 1980).

It is highly probable, the WHO report points out, that as a result of commercial enterprise and governmental inactivity a major public health problem will have been inflicted on the countries least able to withstand it, and that smoking-related diseases will spread before communicable diseases and malnutrition have been controlled, thus widening the gap between rich and poor countries.

Alcohol consumption is increasing in developing, as it is in developed, countries. Those undergoing rapid socio-economic development and socio-cultural change appear to be particularly vulnerable to alcohol-related problems (WHO 1980). Industrialization of liquor production and the enterprise of multinational companies have resulted in the supplanting of traditional brewing and distilling methods and in a vast increase in supply. Young people, alienated from traditional values, are at particular risk and there is evidence of increasing delinquency and road-traffic accidents related to drinking. Fatality rates from traffic accidents are increasing in rapidly industrializing countries (WHO 1980). Excessive drinking has a special impact where nutritional standards are marginal, not only in causing physical damage but also in precipitating organic psychoses.

Industrialization and urbanization are associated with new forms of malnutrition which are directly related to the export of western commodities and patterns of consumption to the developing countries (Doyal 1979). Those who move to cities no longer have access to traditional vegetables and methods of preparing food, and must purchase food as a commodity. This entails the consumption of processed foods, even highly refined forms of basic grains, and as incomes rise a growing proportion of urban diets consist of such items as white bread, polished rice, refined sugar, soft drinks, snacks, and sweets. The international food industry with its marketing monopoly ensures every inducement to purchase processed foods, especially those with a high sugar content. The decline of breast-feeding and the replacement of breast milk by processed infant-food among urban populations in developing countries is a new health hazard of industrialization.

POPULATION GROWTH AND DEMOGRAPHIC CHANGE

No strategy to improve the health of developing countries ca ignore the expected increase in their population in the ne two decades by about 1800 million; though the populatio explosion of recent decades appears to be abating, the world population by the year 2000 is projected to reach 6000 t 6500 million, of which almost 80 per cent will be in today developing and least developed countries. Some of their citi will have 30 million inhabitants. Projections show stabilization of the world's population in about 40 years between 8000 and 15 000 million. The Brandt report refers t a sense of helplessness at these prospects. The expecte doubling of the world's population in 25 to 35 years:

compounds the task of providing food, jobs, shelter, education ar health services, of mitigating absolute poverty, and of meeting t colossal financial and administrative needs of rapid urbanization. is also difficult to avoid the conclusion that a world of 15 billic people would be racked by a host of potentially devastatir economic, social and political conflicts (Independent Commissic on International Development Issues 1980).

A sharp decrease in early childhood mortality rates considered to be a prerequisite for lowering fertility rates. Th scope for such a decrease is immense. About 17 millio children under five years of age died in 1978. If all th countries of the world had the same early childhood mortalit rates as those of northern Europe, there would have bee only two million such deaths (WHO 1980). When peopl become more confident that their existing children wi survive, they tend to have fewer births. That is the principa reason why no nation has ever seen a significant an sustained fall in its birth rate without first seeing a fall in it child death rate (UNICEF 1982). Family planning service depend for effect on such high survival rates as well as o community development, education, higher status fo women, and other measures that reduce poverty, ill-health and hunger.

For developing countries, where at present about 45 pe cent of people reach the age of 65 years, it is estimated that 7 per cent will do so by the year 2000, and that one person i three will live beyond 80 years; almost 60 per cent of th world's elderly will then be living in the developing countrie (WHO 1980). Thus, before these countries have brough under control their infectious and parasitic diseases an malnutrition they will be faced with the health and welfar needs of their aged, especially where development i associated with the disintegration of traditional supportiv family systems. In addition, they can expect a risin prevalence of the chronic diseases and disabilities typical o today's developed countries, and of the environmental healt problems of industrialization and rapid urbanization.

THE ORGANIZATIONAL CHALLENGE OF 'HEALTH FOR ALL'

When, in 1977, the Thirtieth World Health Assembly decide that the main social target of governments and of the WHC should be the attainment by all the people of the world by th year 2000 of a level of health that will permit them to lead a ocially and economically productive life (popularly known as health for all by the year 2000'), its members were setting hemselves, particularly their health sectors, a formidable rganizational challenge. Since that time the member states of VHO acting collectively have made, in the words of WHO's Director-General, 'remarkable conceptual progress' in the ourse on which the Assembly set out in 1977 (WHO Chronicle 1982b). This progress is indicated particularly in he elaboration by the International Conference on Primary Health Care, at Alma-Ata in 1978, of the concept of primary ealth care as the key to attaining health for all (WHO 1978), nd in the World Health Assembly's adoption in 1981 of the global strategy for health for all by the year 2000 (WHO 981); WHO's Regional Committees have adopted corresponding regional strategies and a growing number of countries re formulating national strategies. Countries now face the ask of putting into practice the concepts enshrined in those trategies, with the support of WHO's Seventh General Programme of Work covering the period 1984–89 which the Health Assembly approved in 1982.

In reviewing the constraints – political, economic, and ocial – faced by countries, the Director-General in his report o the Thirty-fifth World Health Assembly referred to the major organizational constraint represented by the political weakness of many countries' ministries of health for carrying out the responsibilities the Global Strategy assigns to them WHO Chronicle 1982a).

Evans et al. (1981) point to other deterrents presented by he health sector in most developing countries. The administrative chain that the organization of a complex system of services demands depends critically on institutions at district and local levels, which are usually poorly staffed, have nadequate authority or control of resources, and are unable o provide the necessary support and supervision of field staff. The epidemiological perspective, necessary to establish priorities and allocate resources according to a population's health needs, is missing from the training of many in positions of responsibility; and their managerial competence is generally inadequate to the task of gaining the co-operation of highly independent professionals and specialists who have their own constituencies and political support. In the developing as in the developed countries the medical profession, which is often in a position of great political influence, can steer demands for the consumption of very limited resources towards expensive facilities for diagnosis and treatment; and medical education does not concern itself with training in the management of health resources so as to benefit the mass of the people.

Howard (1981) in discussing the possibility of accelerating the flow of external health-development resources refers to two problems. First there is the lack, on the part of most ministries of health, of the professional capability to identify needs, and to design proposals for external funding and defend them before national planning commissions in competition with the needs of sectors other than the health sector. Second, recipient governments have significant managerial difficulties in disbursing and utilizing external resources effectively.

Weak management capability is widely acknowledged as one of the most serious impediments to development in all sectors. Institutional weaknesses, according to Evans (1981), are a key barrier to progress, the limiting factor in absorptive capacity for development assistance, and in local capability for decentralization of management. The management of health services is faced with the special difficulties inherent in that of social sectors in general, viz., weak institutions, susceptibility to social, cultural, and political factors, and dependence for success on the extremely difficult task of changing human behaviour. Yet, as Howard (1981) points out, success in reaching the goal of health for all by the year 2000 will depend on technical objectives and strategies not yet fully determined, on the mobilization of financial and professional resources not yet committed, and on mutually-agreed-upon systems for multilateral and bilateral co-ordination which have not yet been established. These conditions for success pose an unprecedented challenge, particularly in view of the uncertain world economic outlook, and the size and complexity of the managerial and administrative effort involved in recipient countries.

Among significant advances made by WHO is the setting in motion of mechanisms to rationalize the international transfer of resources, technical or financial, for health (WHO Chronicle 1980). At present, over 50 official donor agencies and about 3000 non-governmental organizations transfer annually for health purposes approximately US$3000 million, out of a total annual amount of US$30 000 million in official development aid. Allocations from the latter sum to agriculture, food aid, and support to general development contribute also to health improvement. Besides these sums, which represent mainly grants or concessional loans, recipient countries obtain a much larger amount (US$50 000 million in 1979) in non-concessional flows, a significant proportion of which can be expected to have potential for health development. In addition, these countries are estimated to expend already on health care, mostly private and traditional, up to US$14 000 million annually, much of which would in principle be available for directed health services.

The significance of these figures may be appreciated by comparing them with an estimated US$5000 million required annually to bring about 'vast improvements' in people's health in all the countries of the WHO African Region, as against a current expenditure of US$1500 million on health in the public sector in the same countries (WHO Chronicle 1982b). The former figure is based on a per caput sum of about US$15 per year, compared with an average expenditure in 1978 of US$244 in the world's developed countries.

Despite current and expected economic difficulties the present considerable flow of international health resources is expected to continue and even to increase over the next two decades, although not on the scale proposed by the Brandt Commission. The challenge to the health sector in the developing countries is to provide leadership which will be capable of managing and directing health development as part of social and economic development, using to best advantage these considerable external and internal resources. Not only has the health sector's effort to be harnessed to health for all but also the efforts of other sectors, such as water supply and sanitation, education, agriculture, housing and community development, have to be co-ordinated in an attack on the predisposing causes of ill-health and on the difficult problems associated with socio-economic development and industrialization. This must become a prime function of ministries of health, which at present do not have the co-ordinating authority that this function demands. The least that must be expected of the health ministries in this context is that they specify their health requirements from other sectors, rather than merely attempt to convince the other sectors of the need for multisectoral action for health; also they must be ready to support other sectors through health action whenever this is required of the health sector (WHO Chronicle 1980).

The kind of leadership needed for health development is in extremely short supply in all countries, a deficiency to which universities, schools of public health, and other schools of health sciences must be expected to direct their attention. In this respect the Director-General of WHO refers to a constraint 'that must be converted into an opportunity', viz. the nature of the relationships between ministries of health, on the one hand, and universities, medical schools, and schools of health sciences, on the other hand (WHO Chronicle 1982*a*). With regard to the dialogue between ministries of health and medical schools 'there is too much suspicion on the part of the ministries and too much disdain on the part of the schools . . . social relevance and academic interests are in conflict'. The medical profession has not grasped the seriousness of the world health situation, nor has it realized how inappropriate society's response to this situation is, no matter at what level of social and economic development (WHO Chronicle 1982*b*). It is a striking characteristic of the health scene in developing countries that the leaders of the medical profession and the medical education establishment do not identify themselves with public health action, and that they are preoccupied instead with a medical technology that is wholly inappropriate to any effort to solve their societies' health problems. Many people find it inconceivable that health for all can be attained without the exercise by the profession of its leadership role in health. The risk is real that organized medicine, even if only by default, will be a crucial deterrent to the attainment by the people of the developing countries of a level of health that will permit them to lead socially and economically productive lives.

REFERENCES

Barr, T.N. (1981). The world food situation and global grain prospects. *Science* **214**, 1087.

Brady, N.C. (1982). Chemistry and world food supplies. *Science* **218**, 847.

Chernin, E. (1978). Bilharz's 'splendid distomum': Schistosomiasis 1950–1977. In *Tropical medicine: From romance to reality* (ed. C. Wood). Academic Press, London.

Commission on International Development (Pearson Commission) (1969). *Partners in development*. Prager, New York.

Doyal, L. (1979). *The political economy of health*. Pluto Press London.

Elling, R. (1977). Industrialization and occupational health in underdeveloped countries. *Int. J. Health Serv.* **7**, 219.

Evans, J.R. (1981). *Measurement and management in medicine and health services*. Rockefeller Foundation, New York.

Evans, J.R., Hall, K.L., and Warford, J. (1981). Shattuck lecture – Health care in the developing world: problems of scarcity and choice. *N. Engl. J. Med.* **305**, 1117.

Farid, M.A. (1980). The malaria programme – from euphoria to anarchy. *World Health Forum* **1**, 8.

FAO (1978). *1977 FAO production yearbook*, **31**, Rome.

Galbraith, J.K. (1979). *The nature of mass poverty*. Harvard University Press, Cambridge, Mass.

Howard, L. (1981). *A new look at development cooperation for health*. WHO, Geneva.

Independent Commission on International Development Issues (Brandt Commission) (1980). *North–South: a programme for survival*. Pan, London.

Lipton, M. (1977). *Why people stay poor: urban bias in world development*. Harvard University Press, Cambridge, Mass.

United Nations Children's Fund (1982). *The state of the world's children*. Oxford University Press.

World Bank (1978). *World development report*. Oxford University Press, New York.

WHO Chronicle (1980). Thirty-third World Health Assembly *WHO Chron.* **34**, 251.

WHO Chronicle (1982*a*). Seventh General Programme of Work is approved by World Health Assembly. *WHO Chron.* **36**, 131.

WHO Chronicle (1982*b*). Eighteen years to go to health for all *WHO Chron.* **36**, 215.

WHO (1975). *Fifth report on the world health situation*. Geneva.

WHO (1978). *Alma-Ata 1978. Primary health care* ('Health for all' Series No. 1). Geneva.

WHO (1980). *Sixth report on the world health situation*. Geneva.

WHO (1981). *Global strategy for health for all by the year 2000* ('Health for All' Series, No. 3). Geneva.

20 Deterrents to health in developed countries

Leo A. Kaprio and James Gallagher

INTRODUCTION

The student of public health soon learns that, in the case of many health problems and diseases that can in principle be prevented or brought under substantial control by enlightened public or individual behaviour, or by health action or other means, there are many forces that operate against their prevention or control, which often are not amenable to orthodox public health action. These forces deter individuals or the public from action that could prevent certain diseases or promote or enhance personal and public health. The compulsions of physical or psychological addiction, the pressures that stimulate biological and social appetites and the market forces and peer-value systems that press for their gratification, are instances of such deterrents.

Similar forces undermine or negate the realization of man's potential for physical, mental, and social well-being. If optimal health can be equated with the full and balanced development of man's intellectual and psychosocial faculties, forces that act against the attainment of such development, or that lead it to be over-valued in comparison with other valid means of self-fulfilment, may be considered also as deterrents to health. An educational system that overvalues academic achievement at the expense of craftsmanship or psychosocial 'competence' may be regarded in this light. A mass entertainment medium pitched at a level of mediocrity that demands no intellectual effort and promotes shoddy values can be seen as a deterrent in this context. Any kind of manipulation by special interests of the public or of groups who have not been educated to discern the spurious from the genuine can have a limiting effect on psychosocial maturation.

THE CHALLENGE TO PUBLIC HEALTH

Students or practitioners of public health who see health in the broad terms stated in the Constitution of the World Health Organization (WHO) will find many deterrents to health in the everyday life of developed countries and will share common ground with their counterparts in other fields of endeavour in their perception of human ills and in the contributions they can make to progress towards the betterment of the human condition. The removal or modification of factors that hinder the attainment of optimal health is not the responsibility or the prerogative of the health professions alone, but the multiplicity of such deterrents and of their modes of action pose endless challenges to the public health profession and makes continuous demands on the imaginativeness, ingenuity and creativeness of its members and systems. The broad view of health is essential if these qualities are to be brought into play not only to counter those factors that bring about disease, disability and premature death, but also to foster the conditions that will permit human beings to achieve optimal physical, mental and social well-being. A broad concept of public health is needed to accommodate the kind of professional action that these same qualities imply; conventionality can in itself be a deterrent to effective public health action.

Health not the highest priority

It would be misleading, of course, to imply that formal public health action, even at its most enlightened, will ever have the scope or a mandate to counter in very effective or comprehensive ways many of the social and environmental forces that hinder the attainment of optimal health or give rise to the misuse by man of substances that cause disease and premature death. If freedom from disease and positive health were social values that transcended all others, the picture of disease in modern societies could be radically and fairly rapidly transformed. But no society is likely to accord health a supreme or overriding value; for the human species survival is more important and individual lives may be given up in the process. Similarly, man accords freedom in personal decisions and action higher value than health, including the freedom to make decisions that bear upon health and to behave in ways that may damage health or even lead to death.

Constraints to applying new public-health tools

The 'second public health revolution', which has taken place in the developed countries in the decades following the Second World War, has been fuelled by a great extension and refinement of epidemiological methods and techniques – a 'second epidemiologic revolution' (Terris 1980) – which have forged effective weapons for the control of the main physical diseases of industrialized societies. However, a logical consequence in public health action has not always followed, or such action is circumscribed by restrictions and impeded by barriers imposed in interests other than those of health, and the public health 'revolution' is in many respects frustrated. Governments are loath to follow epidemiology as a guide to health policy. Terris (1980) refers to three factors that singly or together act to restrict the influence of epidemiology in the formulation of health policy: (i) the failure of the health professions and of society to understand the primacy of prevention; (ii) the unwillingness to accept the validity of epidemiological discoveries; and (iii) the power of private interests.

Changes difficult and often slow

Even when in today's developed countries, the killing and disabling diseases were mainly infectious, with their less complex aetiology than the modern, chronic, non-infectious diseases, there were formidable deterrents to public health action. The pioneers of the nineteenth century sanitary revolution and social reform had to contend with powerful political, economical, and industrial interests which were ranged against improvements in the living and working conditions especially of industrial and agricultural workers.

In some respects the potential for countering the noxious influences that give rise to today's common diseases is greater than in the past because of the greater political power of an articulate and more enlightened public. The more educated among the population of developed countries are aware that their own and their children's health, at least their physical health, can be cultivated and protected, and they know how to exercise responsibility for health. The existence of a social gradient of disease, which reflects the ability of the better educated to fashion their living and working conditions, sometimes with smaller incomes than the less educated, and consequently to have lower morbidity and mortality rates for a number of the important causes of disability and early death, indicates the potential of whole societies to achieve better health. In other respects, however, today's deterrents to public health are even more formidable than those that eventually gave way to the first public health revolution. First, their noxious influences can be pleasant, gratifying to biological and social appetites, and generally only very slowly producing disease and disability. Secondly, the interests that promote these noxious influences are often rich, exceedingly powerful and influential, and so complex, as in the case of large multinational industrial concerns, for example, that they cannot 'change course' with regard to the production of hazardous materials or harmful processes without economic and other repercussions that affect whole industrial and commercial systems. Furthermore, the provision of healthy conditions in industry or in urban development, for example, or the elimination of the hazards associated with chemical and nuclear industrial processes and their waste products, at standards that would satisfy proponents of health action, would often incur costs which governments are not prepared to impose or industry to incur.

Governments concerned to ensure an adequate energy supply for their countries, for both present and future needs, are faced with difficult choices with regard to energy policies, all of which carry certain risks to the environment and to human health. Some of these risks are immediate; others are prospective, with implications of possible genetic damage to populations decades or centuries hence. In this case the responsibility of governments with regard to energy conflicts with their responsibilities to avoid harmful health effects on present and future generations.

ECONOMIC AND FISCAL DETERRENTS RELATED TO THE USE OF TOBACCO, ALCOHOL, AND ILLICIT DRUGS

Two of the most pervasive of the noxious influences on health in industrialized countries are smoking and alcohol abuse. A WHO Expert Committee on Smoking and its Effects on Health, which met in 1974, confirmed the conclusion of a report to the Twenty-third World Health Assembly (WHO 1970) that 'smoking-related diseases are such important causes of disability and premature death in developed countries that the control of cigarette smoking could do more to improve health and prolong life in these countries than any other single action in the whole field of preventive medicine' (WHO 1974).

Soon, when mathematical and economical models have been constructed which will predict how tobacco consumption and mortality from smoking-related diseases would change with different kinds of governmental action, governments of developed countries will 'be able to decide how many people they want to die from lung cancer'. Projections of current data show that 10 million Europeans may die prematurely because of smoking during the last two decades of this century. If to Europe are added North America, Australia, and New Zealand, the number reaches 20 million. Almost all of these are already in the 'condemned cell' and are mostly young adults, under 40 years of age, female and male, addicted to nicotine. The Europeans are much less likely to be living in the Nordic countries or in France than in eastern Europe or in the Federal Republic of Germany, the UK, or Italy because the governments of Norway, Finland, Sweden, and France have taken more effective action than others to curb smoking, while in the eastern European countries smoking is still on the increase. Those who smoke heavily are at higher risk than non-smokers of premature death or chronic ill health also from other causes – alcohol abuse, obesity, occupational hazards, traffic accidents, to name the more likely causes.

While there is little that governments or organized social groups can do to save those who are 'condemned' to death or growing disability before the end of the present decade, it is not too much to say that people through their governments and by means of other organized action can decide now to reduce very substantially the number who will die of these diseases or suffer from serious physical, mental or social disability from the same causes during the closing years of this century and the first two decades of the next. One country, Sweden, is already in the fifth year of a 25-year programme to produce a 'smoke-free generation'. In Norway and Finland legislation in the mid-seventies, and other anti-smoking measures, have produced a substantial fall in cigarette smoking. That smoking is now the main preventable cause of death in developed countries – and probably that of the growing numbers of deaths from non-communicable disease in developing countries – is well known to all governments, particularly to health authorities. Students and practitioners of preventive medicine or public health need to understand well the forces that deter all governments from taking the kind of action that a relatively few have taken to curb such an obviously avoidable pathogenic practice.

For public health or community action to be effective against smoking-related diseases it is not enough to direct it exclusively at smoking as the 'cause' of lung cancer and other diseases, because attempts to change the smoker's behaviour while they ignore the pressures to which the smoker – as well as the potential smoker – is subjected will very often have little effect. Smokers also have strong deterrents to giving up the habit.

The sure way of preventing smoking would be to stop the cultivation of tobacco. Less sure ways would be to prevent it being commercially processed or to penalize by taxation the distribution and sale of the finished products to the point that it would be no longer economical to grow tobacco. The steps that are actually taken range from legislation to discourage individual consumption, which is more or less enforced, to voluntary agreements between governments and tobacco companies aimed at limiting the promotion of cigarette sales, which are readily circumvented, to anti-smoking policy statements without commitment or enforcement. The forces that deter governments from taking effective steps are examples of deterrents to public health. They are mainly, in relation to smoking, the interests of tobacco growers, who usually are strongly represented at the political level, and of the other sectors of the tobacco industry – shipping, marketing, distribution, and manufacturing – with large numbers of employees at every stage, not to mention private tobacconists and their assistants in the tobacco kiosk.

Common to all these stages, from production to the retail of the final product, is the fiscal interest of governments. No argument that attempts to base the case for tobacco prohibition or control on the financial costs to the community of medical care for the victims of smoking, and of associated welfare payments and services, and loss of productivity, is tenable in the face of the vastly greater sums collected relatively easily as revenue.

Smoking has been considered at some length because of the public-health importance of smoking-related diseases and since it illustrates well the nature and the mode of action of certain kinds of socio-economic deterrents to public health. Alcohol consumption is the other main cause, comparable to cigarette smoking, in developed countries of ill-health and disability, of death and injuries from traffic and other accidents, and of high cost in terms of medical and psychiatric care, associated welfare costs, and loss of productivity. The Thirty-second World Health Assembly, in 1979, declared that 'problems related to alcohol, and particularly to its excessive consumption, rank among the world's major public health problems' and 'constitute serious hazards for human health, welfare and life'. Alcohol also has its associated agricultural, distributional, processing, marketing, and other interests, and its value to governments as a source of revenue comparable to that of tobacco.

The deterrent effects of these vested interests are reinforced by inconsistencies between alcohol control policies and the evidence that should inform such policies. Often such evidence is imperfect, but countries are slow to seek or act on evaluative evidence of the effectiveness of different kinds of strategies, a strategy of controlling the availability of alcohol, for example, compared with one of treating and rehabilitating problem drinkers while not disturbing the interests of alcohol producers and distributors. 'In many places, the control system has become primarily a means of maintaining the orderliness of the alcoholic beverage industry and protecting its various vested interests. Alcoholic beverage taxes have become essentially an instrument of fiscal policy. The original motivations of the control laws and the situations which brought them about have often been forgotten' (Finnish Foundation for Alcohol Studies 1975).

Serious health problems arise also from the non-medical use of psychotropic drugs other than ethyl alcohol. The promotion of illicit use of narcotic drugs by powerful international crime syndicates constitutes a deterrent to public health action, which no national public health system can, unaided, overcome. Also, some developing countries derive considerable revenue from the production of, and traffic in, drugs the use of which is illicit in developed countries. Opium and coca, like the grape-vine in other countries, have for centuries been staple crops in many rural communities, and regarded as essential to social intercourse and well-being as well as for the treatment of common ailments. Few of the governments of those countries have the resources to replace them by comparably lucrative or useful alternative crops, or are even convinced that the way of life of peasant cultivators should be so seriously disrupted because people in other countries use these products illicitly.

IATROGENESIS

There are public health problems associated also with the medical and other licit uses of drugs. Psychotropic drugs are the most frequently prescribed and used of all drugs. They are often prescribed indiscriminately and continued indefinitely, giving rise to national epidemics of drug dependence. A deterrent to health in this instance may be said to be the predominantly biomedical view of the medical profession which sees the locus of all problems for which doctors are consulted as being within the individual and hence requiring only biological solutions, mainly in the form of pharmacotherapy.

It [the medical profession] tends to see all disease as accounted for by deviation from a measurable biological norm, leaving no room within its framework for the social and psychological dimensions of illness. The benzodiazepines were developed at a time when increasing numbers of patients were presenting symptoms of anxiety and tension related to chronic illness and social and interpersonal problems. The medical profession accepted these symptoms as being legitimately within its domain for treatment. Although the symptoms, which are both vague and immeasurable, are seldom amenable to biochemical solutions, and the underlying problems never, the benzodiazepines were developed to deal with them (Cooperstock 1980).

The powerful pharmaceutical industry reinforces the medical profession's, and the general public's, biomedical view of the psychosocial problems for which psychotropic drugs are prescribed and consumed, and the combination of medical, industrial, and public attitudes constitutes a formidable deterrent to public health.

Dependence on medically prescribed psychotropic drugs is only one instance of a wide range of iatrogenic problems which lay certain kinds of medical practice open to charges of constituting deterrents to public health. Another is the misuse of antibiotics, contributing to bacterial resistance. Adverse drug reactions are not uncommon in hospitals and constitute also an important reason for hospital admission. In the US it has been estimated that two million hospital-acquired infections occur annually, resulting in 150 000 deaths and costing over one billion dollars (Bennett 1978).

Medical diagnoses are often incomplete, and important elements of health care consequently omitted, because doctors find security in simple diagnoses that discount important but not easily classifiable or manageable dimensions of health problems. Much of medical practice consists of unproven procedures and therapies. Medical practice would, no doubt, be radically changed were its most common procedures and treatments to be subjected to randomized controlled trials and the findings universally applied (Cochrane (1972). Unnecessary hospitalization, unnecessary surgery, excessive diagnostic testing, and other instances of undue reliance on expensive technology, are common forms of misuse of resources. Besides their directly damaging effects on the health of individuals, they can, in some countries at least, affect health indirectly because of their serious economic effects on both individuals and societies. Poverty, it has been said, may be a side-effect of medical care in certain countries.

The monitoring and minimization of iatrogenesis, of wrong and dangerous as well as wasteful use of resources in health care, is an important modern challenge to public health.

STRUCTURAL AND ORGANIZATIONAL ASPECTS OF HEALTH SERVICES AS DETERRENTS TO PUBLIC HEALTH

Most of the industrialized countries of the world, even some of the richest, can still be said to be only relatively developed as far as their peoples' health is concerned; for certain segments of their populations they are even poorly developed. Health services as they are at present structured and distributed, and in their modes of functioning, are not producing the results in terms of acceptable levels of health for whole societies that might be expected from their consumption of resources. The accumulation of evidence of the persistence of gross inequalities in health among social and occupational classes more than justifies the adoption by the governments of even the most advanced countries of strategies to attain an acceptable level of health for all their citizens by the year 2000 and of primary health care as the main component of these strategies. Primary health care, as set out in the Declaration of Alma-Ata and as the concept is elaborated in the report of the Alma-Ata Conference (WHO 1978), and in the strategies for 'health for all' adopted formally by the member states of WHO, is designed to harness efforts of other sectors besides the health sector, and of communities and families, to the attainment of acceptable levels of health, especially by the segments of populations who are vulnerable to ill health. It is directed

specifically at deterrents to health, or failings of health services, that are more or less inherent in all our existing health services and, as has been documented in the UK for instance, contribute to the maintenance of a consistent differential between the state of health of 'privileged' and that of 'underprivileged' population groups (DHSS 1980). Conventional health services cannot overcome the inequalities in income, education, nutrition, housing and working conditions, and cultural differences within societies, which together are responsible for this effect.

The need for community participation

Since health is an outcome of many bio-social forces and conditions besides health care services, no conceivable kind of health care system will be capable of overcoming these inequalities without the participation of communities in exercising responsibility for their own health, and the co-operation of other public sectors with the health sector in removing obstacles to health and providing conditions to assure health. Besides the forces that deter existing health care systems from being restructured and from functioning so as to provide the kinds of services that the new primary-health-care strategy implies, there are powerful forces, of which examples have been given earlier in this chapter, which will act as deterrents to other sectors and to communities from realizing their potential for improving and protecting health.

High-technology medicine

Current deterrents within health services include the prominantly individual and clinical orientation of medical care, and its preoccupation with the treatment of established disease or with the relief of symptoms whose origins are ignored or inadequately understood, to the virtually complete lack of concern with primary prevention and with the well established social and physical environmental causes of disease. Typical primary medical care passively satisfies wants; in general, apart from routine immunization, it does not actively seek to prevent, in the sense of dealing with problems before they are expressed. This orientation is reinforced by secondary and tertiary medical care. Particularly in hospital medicine, certain services are based on the use of sophisticated technology to investigate and treat certain symptom-complexes, for no better reason than that such high technology is available in the form of highly trained staff and the equipment, procedures and therapies that permit the practice of super-specialized medicine. Sophisticated equipment is attractive to doctors and technicians, and even to administrators; and it has a particular appeal to an uncritical public, mainly evidenced by the preponderance of hospital services over primary care and preventive medicine. High medical technology has other, more tangible, attractions: it provides employment and produces wealth in its manufacture, marketing, maintenance, and operation; and it can be an important item in a developed country's exports to other developed, and to developing, countries.

Even though the unnecessary use of sophisticated technology represents a wasteful use of resources, it may have little adverse effect on health where manpower and other resources are plentiful, but where they are scarce it diverts resources from health-care problem areas for which, on epidemiological evidence, they could be more effectively used (Kaprio 1979, p. 15). The indifference of the medical and many of its allied professions to epidemiology and public health, which is one indication as well as an effect of the attraction of high technology, is shared by the general public and by health authorities, which are conditioned to, and fascinated by, the super-specialized medicine made possible by high technology. These deterrents are institutionalized in the structures of primary-medical-care services, in conventional modes of practice, both public and private, and in methods of payment for medical services, and they are reinforced by conventional undergraduate, postgraduate, and continuing medical education.

Educational deterrents

Educational systems for health professionals tend to reflect and reinforce dominant modes of health care practice. The role of undergraduate medical education in socializing students to the ideology of the medical profession is considered a strong deterrent of change. Postgraduate or specialty training, with its highly clinical orientation and its lack of concern with prevention or control, strongly reinforces the undergraduate experience. Continuing education for primary-care practitioners further reinforces the clinical emphasis. It is provided almost exclusively for the medical profession, by specialists usually unfamiliar or not concerned with the medico-social and psychosocial problems about which people consult doctors; it thus reinforces the tendency of doctors to medicalize such problems. To the extent that all phases of medical education give inadequate attention to primary health care, they contribute to a devaluation of primary care on the part of the public and to the attraction which hospital and specialist medicine holds for the public.

Inadequate care for the long-term disabled

The principal challenge that faces today's health services in industrialized countries, and which calls for comprehensive action across different sectors, is that presented by the large and growing numbers of the chronic sick and disabled. They represent the successes of medical technology and public health in combating and preventing acute illnesses and injuries. Patients who in the past would have died from their primary defects and illnesses, from injuries, or from secondary infections, are surviving for many years in a more or less disabled state, and at the same time the rising proportion of older people is associated with more long-term disease and disability. Society has still to make a substantial response to this challenge – in new or modified forms of health care and social welfare, for example, or in applying industrial technology to improving the quality of the daily lives of disabled people. The ethos of most industrialized societies accords the elderly and the disabled little political or economical weight, which is an important deterrent to the provision of services and goods to assure them acceptable standards of daily living.

Constraints to environmental health

The environmental dimension of public health in industrialized countries presents various kinds of deterrents (Kaprio 1979, pp. 19–21). Besides the continued existence of pockets of underdevelopment with inadequate basic sanitation, unsatisfactory housing, and low standards of food hygiene, there are serious health problems associated with the effects of toxic materials reaching man through air, water, and food, and in industrial processes. Organizational deterrents to environmental health include a lack of integration between environmental and other public health control measures, and the division of legal and administrative responsibilities for environmental protection between different ministries and authorities. The application of control legislation is often uneven and unsatisfactory. Decisions concerning environmental health are made without due consultation with consumer groups or the general public, which results in misunderstanding and lack of commitment at the community level, where the decisions are to be implemented.

Another class of deterrents in respect of environmental problems is related to the massive increase in the production of new chemicals. Society is slow to realize the need for protective measures and to insist that certain products should not be used or produced before safe and universally acceptable ways are devised to eliminate toxic waste-products. Periodic accidents in nuclear-energy plants and during the disposal of chemical wastes show that the research that leads to technological advances is not always matched by research into the corresponding safety measures.

CONCLUSION: THE CHALLENGE TO EDUCATION

Those who are entering the public health professions in the eighties must expect to have to contend with these institutionalized and other deterrents to public health and to the radical reorientation that is needed in medical care. It cannot be assumed that public health administrations and services, or professional associations, will in all cases be ready to adopt or promote essential features of primary health care, such as community participation and multisectoral co-operation for health, and the innovations in administration, organization, management, and training that the new strategies imply. Public health has its own bureaucracies which may well resist the threatened erosion of the conventional assumptions and standard practices that they embody; new professional and lay roles in health care, and community participation, may well be disturbing and threatening to many officials who function securely within the limits of laws and formal regulations. Professional associations may consider that the concept of primary health care demands an unacceptable erosion of professional authority.

The challenge to organized public health is to convert primary medical care, which is now the norm in developed countries, to the broader, more comprehensive health care that the new strategies demand, and continuously to support and promote it while at the same time conserving the high standards of medical care that the citizens of the developed world have come to expect. This challenge is already being taken up in different ways by pathfinding ventures in countries and localities in Europe, North America, and Australia; a 'primary health care technology' is slowly being forged, and structural and organizational features of primary health care, such as health centres and health care teams, are being tested. Different groups of workers are demonstrating the feasibility of intersectoral collaboration and community participation in health action. Health services research is accepted as an important support measure to primary health care.

However, there can be little doubt that the prime area for action to oppose the deterrents to health which have been illustrated in this chapter must be education: of the public and of all those concerned professionally with protecting and promoting health in its widest sense. Without the pressure of an informed and aroused public, and its support to public health action, it will not be possible to counter the opposition of vested interests that thrive on harmful and pathogenic life-styles and habits, or the inertia of many social institutions, especially health-care and educational systems, which follow standard practices rather than lead the way in finding and applying new solutions to health and health-related social problems. The opportunities, and the responsibilities, of schools and other academic departments of public health, are very challenging. In this context it should be remembered that these educational bodies consist of teachers and students: often it is for the students to take the lead in discarding the conventional and being progressively innovative.

REFERENCES

Bennett, J.V. (1978). Human infections: economic implications o prevention. *Ann. Intern. Med.* **89(2)**, 761.

Cochrane, A.L. (1972). *Effectiveness and efficiency*. The Nuffield Provincial Hospitals Trust, London.

Cooperstock, R. (1980). Psychotropics as a world problem: benzo diazepines and prescribing patterns as a focus of concern. In *Drug problems in the sociocultural context* (ed. G. Edwards and A. Arif) p. 178. WHO Public Health Papers, No 73. Geneva.

Department of Health and Social Security (1980). *Inequalities in health*. HMSO, London.

Finnish Foundation for Alcohol Studies (1975). *Alcohol contro policies in public health perspective*, p. 66. Addiction Research Foundation, Toronto.

Kaprio, L.A. (1979). *Primary health care in Europe*. EURO Reports and Studies 14. Regional Office for Europe of the World Health Organization, Copenhagen.

Terris, M. (1980). Epidemiology as a guide to health policy. In *Annual review of public health*, Vol. 1 (ed. L. Breslow, J.E. Fielding, and L.B. Lave) p. 323. Annual Reviews, Palo Alto, CA.

World Health Organization (1974). *Smoking and its effect on health*. WHO Technical Report Series No. 568. Geneva.

World Health Organization (1978). *Alma-Ata 1978. Primary Health Care*. WHO, Geneva.

21 Global strategies – developing a unified strategy

K.W. Newell

INTRODUCTION

All societies have their own peculiar and special difficulties in making health care decisions. This is partly because health care frequently behaves more as a 'product' than as a 'service'. Health care is clearly 'needed' and 'demanded' as is food, a house, a police force, or a transport system to get to work. But once certain requirements have been met the form, size, and manner of functioning of health care services are less related to a generally accepted set of health objectives or standards than to particular peculiarities of individuals and groups who have their own goals. In their turn these goals may be conditioned by wealth, status, comfort, or a consciousness and concern for the individual's relatives. It is patently absurd to justify spending a large amount of money upon food in a restaurant for purely nutritional reasons, or to demand the use of a Rolls Royce rather than a bus to get to work on the grounds that this is a more appropriate transport solution. Similarly, some patients' demands from general practitioners (GPs) for pharmaceuticals which may be discarded rather than used, the use of a private room in a hospital rather than a four-bedded ward, or a waiting time for elective surgery of one week rather than one month, cannot often be justified using conventional health status objectives. If these 'product' like qualities are combined with the wide spectrum of individual and societal goals which may abut upon health, the conceptual and practical difficulties of designing a standard health care system are even more apparent. A personal decision not to drive racing cars or to take up hang-gliding as a hobby can influence an individual's health, but these are not primarily health decisions. Such extremes may seem of little moment to many, but any individual's ordinary day contains the need to consider both the satisfactions and the risks of such things as smoking or drinking, travelling at high speed or more slowly, or a manner of responding to a family crisis. Societies have similar conflicts ranging from deciding speed limits on the roads to the choice of buying a fighter plane or a warship rather than a hospital.

Despite these difficulties, it is widely agreed that all persons in need should have access to appropriate health care as a human right. This right is justified on the grounds that if an individual does not have this access it is likely to be to his or her disadvantage in terms of 'health' expressed as life expectancy, liability to illness and disease, to the prevalence of and compensation for disability, and to the comfort of caring services for the ill and dying. Where such 'rights' begin and end, at what level, and what forms both the 'essential' and the additional 'product' services should take, is open to question, and it is therefore difficult for a health care system to give as its only objectives a standard set of health status goals, It is equally difficult to formulate a perfect model for the structure of a health care system, both for the reasons given above and also because the risks to health and the resources available vary from country to country. Thus any consideration of a unified health care strategy must include the study of the processes by which decisions are made and the ways in which these decisions are judged to be appropriate and acceptable.

A good health care system could be considered as one which has a mechanism for reaching an acceptable health care solution for that place, at that time, taking existing health and other priorities into account, and conditioning the distribution of possible interventions by the resources available and the demographic and social variables of that society. Decisions taken on these grounds can never be perfect as they attempt to balance the advantages for some against the disadvantages to others. It can never lead to the ultimate solution as the solving of some problems often emphasizes others. Only rarely will the decisions be comparable to those resulting from even similar forces taking place in another situation. If there can be no perfection and no final success a ranking of health systems can be misleading. It can be said that a health system which uses 70 per cent or 80 per cent of its resources for institutional, rather than primary or preventive care, but arranges access for all those persons in need has an unusual pattern. But it cannot be said that it is wrong. Yet a health system which uses 80 per cent of its resources for its teaching hospital in the capital which serves less than 10 per cent of the country's population is unlikely to be providing the basic health care requirements to the majority and may be open to criticism.

Because there is no perfect model and differing health care solutions are possible and necessary between countries and within countries at different times, there is a constant ferment to suggest changes and to adjust the balance one way or another. Some of these innovations and experiments are the product of local events or political forces, or reflections of apparent successes elsewhere, but others are truly international. There are waves of concern relating to one or other facet of health care which sweep the world like a fashion and after a period of prominence are then replaced by others even though the original problem may have been only partially resolved. This chapter considers some of these questions of our time. Neither singly nor together do the possible solutions add up to a unified strategy and the selection of questions to emphasize is very much an individual choice. However, someone looking back at some future time may typify our health era by examining which questions have been our concern, the manner in which they have been approached, and the final outcomes arrived at.

SOME HEALTH STRATEGY ISSUES BETWEEN DEVELOPED AND DEVELOPING COUNTRIES

Any shared strategy between what are now described as 'developed' and 'developing' countries is complicated by some important differences which cannot be glossed over by assuming that all countries are really alike even if they may happen to be at different stages of economic development at any one time. Developing countries as we now know them are largely rural as well as being poor and have few natural resources. They have not historically shared the Greek philosophical traditions, and their objectives, including their health objectives, may be quite different from those of the industrial world. They are not homogeneous as a class and they include the largest and smallest political units in the world. Despite such underlying differences the penetration of western-type medicine into the developing world is as complete as the penetration of the internal combustion engine for transport or electricity for power. Western health technology has conceptually complemented or supplanted indigenous health care systems in the developing world and while western-type medicine may be limited in its application there to but a few problems or distributed to but a selected part of their populations, the degree of spread and dependency upon it is beyond the point where developing countries can stand apart and not be influenced by industrial-world health care developments.

While this spread of western health technology to the developing world has resulted in some visible and important health status advantages it has also led to conflicts and distortions which are continuing and which must be resolved in our time. The World Health Organization (WHO) as the only presently accepted world health forum has highlighted a series of wider eventual common goals such as 'Health for All by the Year 2000' (WHO 1979). It has suggested some likely approaches such as primary health care (WHO/UNICEF 1978) but has been able to make few suggestions as to the way in which some of the primary conflicts can be resolved. These conflicts include the following:

Poverty and health

There is a wide acceptance that the major influence upon the health status of the industrial world in the past century has been the improvement of social and economic conditions and the alleviation of poverty (McKeown 1979). However, this has not been reflected in the health-care thinking and action of most developing countries with a large proportion of their populations in absolute or relative poverty. What evidence is available (World Bank 1975) supports the view that absolute and relative poverty is widespread in the developing world, and that it is largely rural and closely linked with a wide range of mortality, morbidity, and human development outcomes which are largely independent of western-type health-care preventive or curative interventions.

It is unlikely that there will ever be a completely convincing series of separate assessments of the influences upon health of lack of water or sanitation, malnutrition or partial or periodic starvation, lack of education, plus that lack of initiative and hopelessness which make up the poverty syndrome. Whatever the relationships and synergisms of this complex it is now evident that most conventional health care interventions which may be applied to a population experiencing the poverty syndrome are ineffective and may even act as excuses for inaction in dealing with poverty's primary causes. These include overpopulation, the distribution of land, unemployment or underemployment, and the manner of distribution and consumption patterns of certain key things such as food. Planned changes in some countries such as China in recent years have shown that the level of resources required to bring a population above the absolute poverty level is very low and that even many 'poor' countries or areas with a limited productive capacity can reach this level if appropriate distribution mechanisms and consumption patterns are developed. For such events to occur there must be an awareness of the political, economical and social, as well as the health implications of continuing poverty, and political action at both central and local levels.

Many health workers do not consider poverty to be a health 'problem'. Poverty itself may be thought to be outside the boundaries of health and the actions needed to influence it unrelated to the mandate and the competence of health care systems. Others reject this view. While an attack upon poverty does require the orchestrated support of many sectors, the appreciation of the health effects of the poverty syndrome can act as the trigger mechanism which leads to action. In addition, health workers at many levels have been able to play unique roles in anti-poverty programmes when they have kept poverty rather than a limited health status as their primary objective (Newell 1975).

Any syndrome such as poverty which is related to such devastating health outcomes and which affects more than 20 per cent of the world's population must be considered within a world health strategy. If its occurrence and its relationship with health is accepted by health workers, then even if they reject an active role in anti-poverty programmes this knowledge must influence their own programmes and the use of their health resources. At present this is not the case. There are many examples (Newell 1982), some of them extreme, where in poverty situations up to $1000 per caput per year is being expended on conventional health care programmes as ineffective substitutes for anti-poverty programmes which should be justifiable in their own right. Any unified strategy of health care or public health has to accept that the starting point for most health care action starts above the poverty line. Below this line the health services' role must be to advocate and participate in steps aimed directly at the poverty syndrome. Without the humility to accept this reality it is likely that a large part of the world's population will show little improvement in health status terms and their public health programmes may be viewed as either an irrelevance or a negative force decreasing the likelihood of change.

Transfers from developing to developed countries (migration)

Historically the tropical developing countries have been viewed as the continuing reservoirs of a wide range of communicable diseases and therefore a threat to the industrial world. It is less appreciated that disease transfers occur in both directions and epidemics of some temperate communicable diseases have been as devastating to the developing world as were cholera, smallpox, plague, and yellow fever to the temperate countries. This is typified by the Fijian measles epidemic of 1975 where more than a third of the population died from this one cause in one year, or the more gradual effects of pulmonary tuberculosis which have been responsible for the near extinction of some societies.

But disease agents have not been the only transfers between the two worlds: pharmaceuticals have travelled in both directions and it seems probable that more drugs from traditional medical systems will join morphine, quinine and other unique and important substances in the flow to the developed world. However, few transfers of health ideologies have moved in this direction and the developing world still continues to be considered in health terms largely as a disease threat and as a recipient of western health technology. Neither of these flows are now considered to be major issues in the developed world but in recent times there has been a greater concern expressed about the problems presented by the migration of health service manpower.

Prior to the end of the colonial era steps were taken to set up, in some of the colonies, local training institutions to produce doctors, nurses and other health workers. This move towards local self-sufficiency in health service manpower preceded similar moves by other disciplines and resulted not only in a decrease in the number of medical and other expatriates required but also, at independence, in a large proportion of the new leaders having a health service background. As colonialism ended, more training institutions were founded or expanded, supported by governments, bilateral aid programmes, church groups, and international agencies. For the most part these institutions were modelled on those of the industrial world, had similar academic standards, and were planned to produce graduates able to function within a western-type health care system.

By the 1950s the production of developing-world health workers was at such a level that the manpower transfer from the developed to the developing countries was reversed and the industrial world became a recipient in health manpower terms. This change has not been fully documented, but a recent inter-country study (Mejia *et al.* 1979) has attempted to describe some of the flows. Such flows can be viewed as an expression of market forces and a useful safety valve to allow short-term manpower pressures to be relieved. However, in the 1970s the flow became a flood, and the countermeasures which have been taken to limit it may be to the disadvantage of both donor and recipient countries.

The extent of the flow from donor countries may not be fully appreciated. For example, up to 80 per cent of the medical graduates from some high-prestige training institutions in India, Sri Lanka, Thailand, Indonesia, Philippines, and Korea migrate to the developed world within two years of graduation. The advantages of migration to graduates appeared to be so great that private medical schools were formed in some countries to train graduates for migration and some of these graduates did not fulfil the requirements for registration in their home country. A Minister of Health from Colombia stated that even if the cost of medical training in Colombia was said to be one half of that in the US, the cost to Colombia of the medical graduates migrating to the US was greater than the aid transfers of the Alliance for Progress in the reverse direction.

The migrant flow to the developed world in the 1960s and 1970s was to its advantage as it helped to overcome the shortages of doctors and nurses in their expanding health services. The same flow may have also been to the advantage of the donor countries of the developing world as some of these countries did not have the resources to employ all the graduates they produced or the countries discovered that these types of health service workers were sometimes unsuitable or inappropriate to the type of health problems that were present in their largely rural populations. At that time the main question was whether it would be just, and whether a mechanism could be found to reimburse the donor countries for their training investment.

Before this could be resolved the position changed. The openings in the developed world for such health service personnel began to disappear in the 1980s as the health services ceased to expand and as their own training institutions increased their output. Country after country began to limit immigration by immigrant quotas or professional bars. But production of health workers has continued in the donor countries at similar levels leading to a new crisis which has not been resolved.

On the other hand, the health professions continue to emphasize a common background in thought, techniques, and skills directed at mankind as a whole. They advocate a similar type of training everywhere and pride themselves upon the free and uninterrupted exchange of information and ideas. In non-communist countries they also place great store by the idea of the doctor as a free agent and as a person who can accept or alter his role in response to his inclination, or to market or other forces. On the other hand the free flow of even equivalently trained people across national boundaries threatens to over-supply to the richer countries, a lowering of economic and professional standing, or possibly to a dual class system with the immigrants being expected to take those positions which are less popular, less well paid, or the most isolated.

The implication for donor countries is not that now there will be an increased pool of trained manpower which can be used to the national advantage. The reverse may be the case. The presence of an expanded pool of highly trained professionals may act as a force towards moves to provide a high cost health service option mirrored on that of the developed world, even though their resources may be limited and such a service may be inappropriate in such situations. It may also result in waste and dissatisfaction such as is already present in Latin America where trained health professionals are unemployed or forced to retrain in other skills.

The obvious solution of limiting intake and training in the developing countries presents its own difficulties. Few countries have been successful in matching their health training intake with their manpower needs. It is likely that this will rarely be successful if it is dependent solely upon a market orientated health care system. Because of this, the implications of the manpower migration crisis of this time may be a rapid change towards nationally funded and controlled health systems for manpower rather than for need, equity, or other reasons. This may be coupled with the production of health workers in each country with unique qualities which will allow them to practice only in that particular health service. The migration problem will then be solved as health workers would be unemployable outside their own countries, but it will be the end of the universality of the health professions. It is not yet clear whether this is a big or a small price to pay for a solution.

Transfers from developed to developing countries

Transfers of health technology between the developed and developing worlds occur in both directions but the major flow has been towards the developing world. All countries have possessed a health care system of some kind at all periods of their history and the total or partial replacement of indigenous sysems by western medical technology and ideology is the result of a major investment by the developed world's professions, governments, and voluntary associations such as churches. No major replacement of any system can be wholly good and the penetration of western medicine into many societies has led to some losses which are only beginning to be appreciated. While western medicine may be typified by a largely biological view of health and disease, its application to individuals and groups has associated with it some built in assumptions such as that the main health care objective is to increase life expectancy, or that all persons of different ages have equal health care rights, or that services should be provided, or resources allocated, equitably according to need. There may be no fundamental reasons to link such ideas with the application of the interventions developed by the western-type scientific method and yet it is difficult to separate them, and some products are a direct response to these ideas considered as objectives. In many developing countries some of these assumptions are not accepted and can be in direct conflict with their views upon health and disease or man and society. This results in many misunderstandings and an increasing awareness that some western medical solutions are unsuitable or ineffective for them. These differences are not the result of geographical variations, or of wealth and poverty but are more fundamental, as they relate to convictions about the qualities of life, the place of man in his world, and the structure of societies. They result in problems or apparent failures which cannot be explained away be classing them as technical misunderstandings or as irrational actions.

Two examples of unresolved problems relating to transfers from the developed to the developing world are in the ways in which health resources are transferred, and in the manner in which specific items of health technology are developed, transferred, and used.

Recent reviews (King 1976) of transfers of health resources from the developed to the developing world have emphasized that while the international agencies such as WHO, UNDP, UNICEF, and IBRD have played and continue to play an important role, their contributions may be dwarfed by the transfers carried out bilaterally and the amounts used by voluntary and charitable agencies, the foundations, and the churches. No overall total can be given as existing inventories of these transfers take no account of the amounts used for education or fellowships or the sometimes handsome direct or indirect subsidies paid by some developed countries with continuing colonial or trusteeship roles. Despite these unknowns, it is likely that the amount of resources which continue to be transferred are of such magnitude that if they were applied in an organized and sensible manner many developing countries might have sufficient development resources to either make a significant contribution to the resolution of the poverty syndrome or to assist in the evolution of an improved and more effective health care system for a greater proportion of their populations.

This is not the pattern now. Many of the health resource transfers from the developed world are neither given nor received in a way which can have the maximum effect. Indeed, much health care 'aid' is given with such limiting or distorting conditions that some programmes are not only useless and wasted but can be described as harmful. Some bilateral aid programmes may make gifts of what the donor country produces rather than what the recipient needs. Others may subsidize expressions of their own health systems even if these are inappropriate. Contributions may be made on an annual basis because this is how funds are voted in the donor country and yet no change is possible in the recipient country without a five or ten year continuing commitment. Aid may be restricted to the provision of capital equipment or to buildings but a low capital and high recurrent cost solution may be the only one which is useful to the recipient country. A voluntary body may raise money for a highly specific problem such as leprosy, but this may be a low national priority. A country, or the world's conscience, may be stirred by the presence of a disaster such as an earthquake, an epidemic, or a famine, but the resource transfer is restricted to the amount of resources collected rather than to the solution of the problem.

It may seem reasonable to suggest that such problems of giving and receiving should be solved by a firmness of purpose of the recipient governments and a proper dialogue between the two parties but a poor country in an economic, political, and health care crisis can find it difficult to refuse a gift which may appear to help. There are multiple examples where the gift of the capital cost of a new hospital, a specialist unit, or a piece of expensive equipment has resulted in a distortion of national priorities or to the escalation of subsequent recurrent costs so that other wider based priority programmes have had to be limited or cancelled. It takes a special kind of will and maturity for a poor country such as Tanzania to refuse a World Bank loan to rebuild its teaching hospital in the capital because this does not coincide with its priorities.

The transfer of health resources from the rich to the poor, from the developed to the developing world, is a praiseworthy and useful action which has a high political visibility and wide individual support. However, the way in which resources are collected and assigned, the political motives linked with the manner in which some international, bilateral, and voluntary programmes are administered, and insensitivity to the particular needs of the recipients of some professional advisers to the donor groups, sours an otherwise important world endeavour.

The WHO places within its mandate the orchestration of health-related aid programmes, but it finds that it has neither the authority nor the competence to influence anything but a small proportion of the total. It attempts to encourage the development of national infrastructures to cope with aid offers but in many countries these have failed, the methods do not work, or the mechanisms can be sidetracked. Health resources will continue to be transferred, but the ways in which the damage and distortions can be minimized and the advantages maximized while preserving the dignity of the donors and recipients has yet to be evolved. Some programmes have been more successful than others, but no appraisal of the reasons why has been generally accepted.

The transfer of individual items of health technology to the developing world present quite different problems. One concern relates to the manner in which large industrial multi-national companies promote, distribute, and price pharmaceutical and other health care products in the developing world. Even though many of the developing countries are poor the market is large and the mechanisms for regulating importation, distribution and quality control can be less formalized and more loosely monitored than in the industrial world. Recent debates at the World Health Assembly of WHO have highlighted the need for codes of practice to be agreed upon and applied to producers and distributors of such things as substitute breast-milk products (WHO 1981) and for pharmaceuticals. Such actions are the response to a suspicion that the dumping of some products, differential pricing policies, and the encouragement of the substitution of some indigenous products by more expensive imported equivalents still continues, is largely uncontrolled, and is not in the best interests of the developing countries. It seems unlikely that the introduction of international codes of practice will ever stop such trade aggressions completely and national actions will be required in each individual country to limit the reverse transfer of resources, excessive profits, or questionable marketing practices. But this is only one part of a wider problem.

Many western health care products are essential, life saving, developed for a specific need, and have few or no substitutes. Yet many are not directed towards the health problems, such as the parasitic diseases, of the developing countries, or are not suited for the type of developing world health systems where they may need to be applied. For example, in the industrial world, public sponsored research or private industry may develop a new drug which is 10 per cent more effective in treating a specific condition but which has the disadvantages that it is more expensive to produce and has inherent dangers which need to be monitored or countered in a sophisticated way. The benefits in health status terms may be considered to be great enough to produce and use the new substance despite the extra expense of producing it, ascertaining the persons with this particular need, and adapting the health system to allow it to be used with safety. It may become so well accepted and marketed that the previous treatment methods may be completely replaced and the 'old' drugs may no longer be produced. Such an 'advance' or substitution may not be to the advantage of the developing world. The new method may be too expensive for widespread use there and the methods of ascertaining those persons with this special need may be inapplicable in their different types of health systems. The disappearance of the old drug with a lower effectiveness and a smaller complication rate may make the new developing-country solution to this particular health problem less workable than that used in the past.

Such an example is not an argument against research and the search for more specific health-care intervention. Instead it is given to emphasize that increased effectiveness is not the only objective of new advances and that risks, complication rates, costs, the form of delivery systems required, and multiple other variables are also relevant and the significance of these may differ markedly between the developed and the developing worlds. If many of the health care interventions are under-standably developed in the industrial world to help solve *their* problems and fulfil *their* objectives and to fit in with *their* health systems, if the major production resources are geared to western markets, and if the problems in the developing world and other relevant variables are different, then either conflict is likely to occur or the developing world will be at a continuing disadvantage.

Such a problem may have only two possible solutions. One is to increase the pressure on the developing world to develop health care systems similar to those of the developed world even if they appear to have different objectives, to be inappropriate, and to be wasteful. The other is to continue to encourage everywhere the search for global solutions to global problems, but to develop in parallel health research and production enterprises in the developing world which give proper emphasis to the objectives, specific problems, and special needs of these particular countries. Neither solution is comfortable to live with. The first is an arrogant proposal which is in direct conflict with the unique development of the majority of the world's population. The second requires a change in outlook by research workers and industry plus the massive expenditure of resources in countries which have the least to invest. The issue is still unresolved.

SOME WORLD STRATEGY ISSUES

Consideration of differences between developed and developing countries, the rich and the poor, the capitalist or the communist states, or between different eras of health technology, should not be allowed to distract attention from a wide range of unresolved health care issues which are important to all health care systems. Some are clouded biological problems such as our present lack of understanding of cancer, the process of ageing, or of mental illness. Others are technical, including the development and application of methods which are acceptable and objective ways of measuring the effectiveness of new and existing interventions which are also quick and cheap and can be applied to large populations. Still others could be labelled as philosophical questions of direction and include how questions of fertility and population size can be resolved, or how the rights of both individuals and society can be protected in the grossly malformed. All of these types of unresolved questions influence health care strategies but they are expected to be considered elsewhere. In this section some issues have been selected which are *primarily strategic*, and while research and experiment are urgently required to assist in their solution, major decisions have to be made about them in many countries, now, on the basis of our present knowledge. There are many questions in this class and two groups have been selected as examples.

Preventive strategies

Popular sayings such as 'prevention is better than cure' can be an embarrassment rather than a support to a practitioner of public health considering a strategy directed towards a specific health problem. A preventive approach may be both unreasonably costly and inappropriate. It is questionable to disturb millions by a total immunization campaign if the illness to which it is directed is but a minor one experienced by only a few hundreds and if it can be easily and cheaply treated. It is doubtful that a sport such as motor racing should be banned because it involves excessive risks to the trained participants who are involved but none to society as a whole. While curative care is expensive to the individual and to the state, a preventive programme to protect all those at risk may be many times more expensive and may not warrant the use of an unreasonable amount of health care resources. Some preventive actions such as immunization or contraception have their own inherent risks and even though these may be small the *transfer* of risks from one group to another presents ethical issues which cannot be ignored. While emotionally it seems best to stop a health problem from occurring, there are few examples where such a decision can be made without question and without a very detailed balancing of the advantages and disadvantages.

There are four classes of preventive strategies, of which the first is eradication or the abolition of a problem completely. The most dramatic example of eradication in our time has been that of smallpox. National and international endeavours, orchestrated by WHO in a few years and at minor cost, led to the eradication of the agent, so that smallpox does not now have to be considered as a health problem. Some consider this to be the only example of eradication and any future extension of this strategy to be restricted to but a few communicable diseases where man is the sole reservoir of the agent. This is an extremist view. In large parts of the world, many diseases do not occur or are locally eradicated because transmission is not possible or because the agent, or cause, is excluded by quarantine or other measures. The use of the term 'eradication' should not be restricted to the communicable diseases. In many toxic diseases the banning of production and imports, and the use of substitutes for some chemical compounds are forms of an eradication preventive strategy. If the distinction between eradication and control is that eradication removes *all* of a

specific health risk and control *limits* the risk, then eradication can properly be an option of choice where the risk can be identified and is so limited that it can be eliminated. It seems probable that this strategy will become widely used in respect of many new and unique chemical health-hazards as well as for some communicable diseases in many countries.

The second preventive strategy can be labelled collective measures of disease prevention or public health engineering. If the supreme example of eradication is smallpox, the equivalent collective one is the success of the nineteenth century sanitary revolution where the improvement in the supply of water, sanitation, housing, and education, coupled with socio-economic advances, is credited with the major decreases in mortality and morbidity in the industrial world in the twentieth century (McKeown 1979). Many of these prevention actions took place for non-health reasons and included a changed political climate and the need to evolve a tolerable urban society. The measures that were taken could rarely be said to be to the obvious advantage of a specific individual and the benefits, while not being evenly distributed to all, decreased the health risks to the population as a whole. In retrospect it would appear that many of these sanitary and engineering advances could have been justified on purely health grounds and the fact that they were not may be significant.

It is sometimes easier to advocate change, because what is there is 'bad' and what is to come is 'good', than to take part in a visible accounting of who will contribute and who will benefit from a collective action. For example, an immunization programme for rubella including males and females may lead to the control of rubella and to a health advantage for pregnant women, their babies, and society as a whole. But it is of questionable advantage to the males concerned. The addition of nutritional additives to bread may be viewed as an imposition by the well nourished and acceptable in wartime but not in peace. Fluoridation of water supplies changes caries prevalence dramatically in communities with low fluoride intakes, but may be viewed as an aggression by the edentulous or a threat to those who consider all additives to be harmful. Even where such collective measures have no known counter-risks associated with them, they take away the individual's right to choose and can be actively resented. Rejection is common if the measures are restricted to health reasoning and to be successful the justification has to be real, the risks large and frightening, the contributors placed at a minimum disadvantage, and the beneficiaries worthy. Even with such prior conditions, it is sobering to be aware that our expectations of making a proper case are so low that any country which has a water fluoridation programme covering more than 50 per cent of its population is thought to have a successful programme.

But there are many other decisions influencing collective health risks which do not result in such disturbances and negative responses. For example, national decisions are made upon the design of cars and aeroplanes which try to balance safety risks against costs, industrial practicality, and price. Few designs can place the avoidance of death or injury as the dominating issue as it is said that a safe plane would be so heavy that it could not fly. Motor vehicle accidents are closely associated with vehicle speeds and yet reduced speed limits began to be strictly applied in many countries only in response to the oil crisis rather than to accident mortality.

The negative reaction of many groups towards collective health measures may be an expression of a fear of a real or possible threat to personal freedom imposed by an enveloping and dominating state machine, or it may be a lack of feeling of community responsibility among present-day adults. But in reverse a failure to limit or control some risks would be considered to show a lack of responsibility by the same state.

Most collective preventive action or public health engineering seems rational and just, and to the advantage of many. Yet all measures are not the same and negative actions such as limiting toxic substances in food or the air may have a greater acceptability than positive measures such as immunization or the use of additives. Both types of actions are more likely to be acceptable and applied if their primary motivation is not that of health or there are visible associated non-health advantages.

The third preventive strategy is to attempt to change health risks by persuading individuals to undertake a positive or a negative action, e.g. stop smoking, moderate alcohol consumption, do not be promiscuous, change your diet, use your seat belt, or take more exercise. These are examples of pleas to individuals to either decrease their exposures to specific health hazards or to take countermeasures to promote their own health or decrease their individual liability to illness. Many programmes designed to encourage these sorts of behavioural changes start with the assumption that the wide distribution of the evidence linking these actions to a health hazard, plus possibly the use of supporting methods such as anti-smoking clinics or alcoholics anonymous groups, should be sufficient to alter behaviour and therefore health status. While there have been some impressive programmes which do appear to have been at least partially successful, especially to particular groups (Farquhar 1980), the results have been largely disappointing. A spreading awareness of the way certain factors affect health is insufficient to explain either the failure of a family planning programme even when contraceptives are readily available, or its success after a period of lowered infant mortality.

Unassailable arguments can be made to insist that each individual should know and understand the way health relates to all his or her day-to-day actions and decisions. An equal case can be made for the health system and society as a whole to advocate behaviour patterns which would decrease these risks and to build supportive structures to encourage and assist people to change their behaviour. The danger is in the assumption that this alone will be effective.

Such thinking leads to the fourth preventive strategy, which can be labelled as changing the balance. Every action that anyone takes is the product of a complex collection of forces which include the past experience of the person, the availability of products, costs, satisfactions, images of oneself or one's peers, and a wide variety of other things including an understanding of health risks. Alcoholism is not a problem in Java as alcohol is but rarely available. The decrease in the use of hard drugs in some teenage groups may be partly the result of high prices. Obesity in young women may be less common because the peer image of a beauty may be that of a slim person in a summer dress, in a bikini, or in tight jeans. Some may be only marginal while others may be negative. A preventive strategy of changing the balance is designed to support the positive factors and decrease the negative factors in an orchestrated way and in a single direction. It accepts that some parts are hard to change and others are easy, but it also accepts that synergism may occur and the total change may be greater than the influence of the individual parts.

It seems improbable that cigarette consumption will be markedly decreased by anti-smoking warnings on cigarette packets or health-linked education alone. A preventive strategy aimed at causing a change of balance uses these methods but also explores the possibilities of such things as increasing the real price of cigarettes to the consumer, decreasing the places where people can smoke, changing the peer image in the media, decreasing or abolishing advertising, or developing non-risk smoking alternatives.

The difference between the individual and the change of balance approaches is not just one of degree. The individual approach may take general forms but its basis is that if a particular individual or group (such as those with myocardial infarction, pregnant women, or schoolchildren) changes its behaviour then certain health status effects will be less likely to happen. The collective approach may also be particularly directed to certain subgroups of the population, but its message is that a certain type of behaviour is bad, dangerous, and antisocial, and should be discouraged. In the smoking context the individual approach might be evaluated by changes in the incidence of cancer of the lung or some other health status outcome, and the balance approach by the amount of cigarettes smoked or a shift in consumption from high-tar to low-tar cigarette brands.

The strategy of prevention over recent decades has not become a single advised series of actions which can be applied everywhere with comparable chances of success. Rather, recent experiences of success and failure have led to a greater understanding that prevention is but one possibility among a series of choices which must properly be considered. If it is agreed that for a particular health problem prevention is the option of choice then a second series of decisions has to be taken as to which one, or, combination, of preventive strategies is likely to be most effective, acceptable, and at what cost. The answers to these questions are unlikely to be standard and the same in all societies or all health systems. If many of the communicable disease problems of the industrial world were largely solved by collective and eradication actions prior to the discovery of ways of increasing immunity or the production of specific drugs, this does not mean that a different society facing similar problems, now, should necessarily take the same path. Preventive strategies are still in their infancy both because the research which can link many risks to health outcomes and describe their relationships has not yet been done. Also the choice of methods and strategies for prevention are not clear because few have been adequately evaluated. Even when this knowledge becomes available, a unified preventive strategy is likely to take the form of an agreement upon how to choose the appropriate approach and not upon a standard set of actions.

Who should control health and the health services?

The use of the term 'control' worries professionals in any system as it is related to power. If it is a cause of concern in persons working in education, transport or even the armed forces, it results in even greater sensitivities when used in relation to health and health services which deal so largely with individual intimacies and where one-to-one relationships between patient and doctor or nurse are understandably so important. Despite this, there have always been controls, and even in a completely private health care system decisions must be taken that influence the structure and functioning of the system which in their turn are conditioned by political considerations, resource allocation methods, manpower and training questions, medical audit, or the boundaries of professional responsibility. The resolution of all such questions requires decision mechanisms and these are controls whether they are the responsibility of the professions themselves, the consumers, or the government. If controls are required in a private system, of which there is no recent example, it certainly applies to mixed or national systems where there has to be some accountability for the use of public funds. As controls are required in all health systems a consideration of some of the issues involved does not have to be restricted to a comparison of different health systems under different political banners but can use general questions which apply to them all. Three examples are given here.

The first one is to review the mechanisms which can be used to decide health rather than health service questions. In the preceding section on prevention, examples were given of certain risks which influence health but which are not generally considered to be directly within the responsibilities of the health care system. These include such things as housing, education, unemployment, speed limits or seat belts in motor vehicles, or the limitation of the production of noxious substances. Although some decisions upon these matters may be taken on health grounds alone, most decisions are some sort of compromise between the alleged individual or societal needs and the health implications. The problem of motor vehicle accidents can be completely solved by the abolition of motor vehicles, but if it is agreed that society must have them, then a decision has to be made about an acceptable balance between the controls which need to be imposed and the accidents which will result as a consequence of having them at the agreed level. This is quite an easy issue to resolve because most of the controls used come within a single sector and include such things as safety standards, road design, speed limits, seat belts, or the licensing of drivers. But other health issues such as heart disease have risks which involve many different sectors. Some health professionals deny that they have a role in influencing decisions on such risks. They state that their responsibilities are limited to describing the health consequences of the risks and dealing with the victims of the risks which continue. This restricted view of the professional's role is not widely held and many health workers feel that they should play a greater part in influencing decisions which, while not being directly within the responsibilities of the health care system, may be the dominating factors in deciding health or illness and the sort of patients who require assistance.

Involvement in such decisions can take different forms and indirect methods such as the collection and distribution of information, the mounting of public campaigns, the attachment of professional advisers to decision bodies in other sectors, or other lobbying mechanisms have all been used and appear acceptable. But this is not enough, as there may be no single body to lobby to make decisions upon health questions which have multiple risk factors under the control of a number of different sectors. Various solutions have been proposed and they include the formation of single bodies with responsibility for specific health questions, such as national committees on smoking, or multipurpose mechanisms such as national health councils which may be chaired by a senior cabinet minister, or the head of state, and involve decision-makers from all relevant sectors. At provincial and regional levels the health council idea has had remarkable success and the heart disease and stroke programme in Finland is a good example (National Public Health Laboratory of Finland 1981).

There is no accepted model for such health-, rather than health-service-controlling mechanisms and the qualities of success have not been systematically studied. However, it is generally held that such bodies need to be visibly separated from the health system so that there is no question of any conflict of interest, that the decision body should include more than token consumer participation, and that there must be prior acceptance by all the different sectors involved to use their own resources to implement the decisions which are made. Such new types of controlling mechanisms are at the stage of exploration and experiment.

A second control example revolves around the unknowns relating to the presence of or the relationships between public and private health care systems within a single country. Both capitalist and communist health service systems face two apparently opposing sets of principles or qualities. There is the view that a certain level of health care is a human right and if this is to be expressed equitably then there has to be a method by which resources can be collected so that they can be distributed in the form of health care to those with a health care need. It is difficult to do this without some form of public system. In parallel with this is the view that any person should have the right to spend his own resources in any way he wishes as long as this is not anti-social. He can decide to use some of them upon lavish personal living, his family, or such things as health care even if this is at a level which is above that which others say that he needs, or at a level of comfort which he decides that he wants. Superficially these two qualities or rights do not appear to be in conflict and it would seem that a country could comfortably have a health care system that included a public collection and allocation system for all and a parallel complementary private system for those who wish to use their own resources to obtain the additional services that they think they need or want. In practice, two such parallel systems cannot function completely independently of each other and they interact at many levels.

Some, for example, consider that any country has a finite amount of health care resources and that the very existence of a private system therefore takes resources away from the public system to the disadvantage of the public good (WHO/UNICEF 1981). Others state that if a person spends his vn resources on a private health care solution this allows the ıblic system to assign the resources which would otherwise be ed for him to other people, and this is thus a type of extra conıbution to the public sector. Still another view is that many ıvate health care systems are partly financed by tax missions on income or other forms of public subsidy and that these sums are added up, the result is two health systems with e private system being an excessive and inequitable charge ıon the public purse. Such reasoned possibilities are ıdependent of the more emotional responses of some who ıpress their suspicions that health professionals who were ısisted in their training by public subsidies, and who may ıactise in dual public–private roles, are finding it to be to their ırsonal advantage to enlarge their involvement in the private ıctor and to increase the difficulties of the public sector.

Politically, these and similar questions are not presented as ı matter of conflict between the state and the consumer, but ıther as one between doctors and the state. While the ıguments put forward by both sides are often based upon ıknowns, of which many are measurable, there is a proper ıubt whether measurement will help to resolve the issues. ıther methods may need to be found to address the two ıimary issues and resolve them.

A third example is the manner in which public health care ısources are controlled or 'rationed'. There is an increasing ıreement that there is no upper limit to the amount of ısources a health care system *could* use if it was given the ıportunity (Cooper 1975). National bodies such as parliaents properly decide what the actual public expenditure ıon health care will be, but a comparison of expenditures by fferent countries gives no indication of what a 'reasonable' ınount is either as a percentage of GDP or in per caput ıpenditure terms. One country can spend twice as much as ıother and this can bear no relationship to either need or ıccess as judged by the conventional health status indicators. ıstead health care expenditures may be directly related to the ıverall wealth of each country (Office of Health Economics ı79). There is, therefore, one level of 'rationing' directed ıwards the total size of the national public resource cake but ıis is a political control with but little input, or direct ırticipation, from the health care system itself.

A second level of 'rationing' is in the manner of distribution ı public health care resources within countries. Many ıuntries show great variations in their resource allocation ıtterns between different geographical areas. Some of these ıfferences are the result of historical accident, population ıovements, or past political or other pressures and have ıecome frozen or increased as a result of an incremental ıpproach to budgeting. Where this has been adjusted, methods ıch as the central planning processes in the USSR or the use of ı weighted population based formula in the UK (DHSS 1976) ıave tried to make some compromise between equity and ıquality. This form of control is often the responsibility of the ıinistry of Health or the equivalent although it has political ıvertones. There are few direct health service or consumer ıputs at this level.

The third level of 'rationing' or control is at regional level ınd here decisions relate to the distribution of a fixed amount ı resources between different services or competing needs. It is here that issues such as the resource allocations for institutional or domiciliary care or the relative needs of the old or the young are decided. The elected or appointed decision makers may be restricted in their decisions by national policies or guidelines, but it is at this level where the submissions by the services themselves begin to exert a major influence. While the manner of arriving at a decision or the nature of the decisions themselves may be affected by the structure of the controlling body, the outcomes may be even more influenced by factors such as whether the region's independence has been reinforced by access to local as well as central resources.

The last level of control is in the actual assignment of resources within a service. The way in which a waiting list is constructed and functions, the form of agreement upon what patients with what conditions have emergency or nonemergency status, or the appointment system for out-patients are all expressions of a rationing system. An extreme form could be the criteria for the selection of priority candidates for renal dialysis, a transplant, or for cardiac surgery. While the size of the resource cake for each service may have been decided at other levels and by other persons, the actual selection of who will receive care and who will not, is decided largely by professional groups using professional reasoning which may not be overt.

The presentation of a multi-tiered description of control makes each level appear as independent and yet the relationships between each level may be close. A national health budget may be increased in response to long waiting lists and a professional judgement of how to rank individuals for a particular service may be influenced by national guidelines. The point of emphasis here is that *despite* these links the *types* of decisions made are very different, made in response to quite different types of responsibility. It seems reasonable for this to be structured and implemented by different groups, but because the reasoning influencing the different levels of decisions may be very different, and because one level can at last partly counter another one, such a process of control can create suspicion and mistrust and result in real conflict or disorder.

The development of solutions to an acceptable control or rationing mechanism is beset by the same difficulty as that of so many health care decisions – there are no real measures of success or failure. It cannot be said that a country which spends 10 per cent of GDP on health care has made a better or worse decision than one which has spent 6 per cent. Similarly, a renal dialysis service which limits acceptances to persons under 50 years is no better or worse than one which makes the cut off at 55 years. All one can say is that a well functioning health service is one where the criteria of assigning resources and the manner in which they are administered reflect the views of most citizens and the health service workers involved.

Few health services have even partially reached this level of success. Some consumers and administrators feel that nearly all health service decisions are dominated by proposals put forward by doctors and that most doctors speak with a single voice tinged with self-interest because of a collegiate type of relationship between them. They also feel that many national or other decisions at different levels can be blocked or distorted by the manner in which doctors and other health service workers express a growing irritation with what they consider are bureaucratic and nonsensical decisions which are inhuman and quite at variance with what they judge to be the needs and aspirations of their patients and society as a whole. This real annoyance is compounded by their conviction that some of these decisions have been taken without any chance being given for their views to be considered.

Both of these purposeful distortions of the extremes are likely to contain elements of truth and are only likely to be overcome if members of the health services have a greater formal voice at the upper levels of the decision and control tree in some sort of exchange for a greater consumer participation in true decision making at the periphery. This in itself has its own difficulties and progress will probably be slow.

The answer to the question of who should control health and the health services cannot be a simple one like the doctors, the government, the patients, or the Ministry of Health. So many of the decisions must be compromises and the proper answer will vary in different groups, different countries, and at different stages of history. For this reason any overall strategy for health services has to concentrate on processes as much as upon outcomes at the risk of moving into a position which may be thought of as partly irrelevant or insensitive to real health needs.

Conclusion

The arguments presented and the examples given in this chapter may appear to be destructive, as they may seem to attack the case that a unified health care strategy is either possible or useful. If many health care expenditures are 'product' responses but little related to health care needs, if few health benefits do not have also some risks and disadvantages, if there are few specific objectives which can be linked to judgements of success or failure, and if some decisions must be made upon issues where equally valid arguments can be made for quite opposing courses of action, then it might be thought that to propose any unified strategy is nonsensical or just an attempt to cover up an irrational process. The consideration of some of the relationships between developing and developed countries may appear to add to the confusion rather than to emphasize that the differences between such countries are but extreme expressions of the similar sorts of conflicts which are present within countries.

It is unreasonable to come to such a negative conclusion. There is no reason to confuse the need for different countries, regions, or groups to come to different conclusions about their health and health care problems with an acceptance that the overall ways in which these decisions can be taken can have so much in common that they can be described as a unified strategy. A unified strategy for health and health service development might have to state that *because* there is no single objective, *because* populations differ, *because* people live under different political systems, and *because* the components of any decision have to be differently weighted under different circumstances, then the end products must vary.

The acceptance of a strategy, not just of diversity, but of decision choices made at different levels and with decision structures suited to the consideration of different sorts of questions, plus an awareness of possibly unique objectives and philosophies, is not a cowardly acceptance of failure to reach a global agreement. It can be the basis of a practical positive strategy with merit if it has its own internal discipline and is not just a cover for an acceptance of the status quo. Few countries now have health systems which possess these qualities and many existing decision processes and the decisions taken can be described as unjust, inefficient, and ineffective. The start of any movement towards other systems which will work better probably has to be a fuller understanding of the absurdity of looking at health, disease and health systems in isolation from other societal goals and decisions.

There are dangers in proceeding along such a strategic path. There will be resentment among health service workers in appearing to lose more of their authority. There will be the inevitable comparisons between regions and countries when health status indexes are compared without taking the decision choices into account. There will be the pressures by the health care workers, political figures and citizens, properly concerned about their own or their family's health, to try to chase the possibly false advantages of the most elitist high technology solutions that some other country may have decided to have.

All these and other arguments can be foreseen, but the complexities of many of the issues involved and the gaps in many aspects of our present knowledge should not be used as a justification for passivity. There is a sufficiently strong case already made for persons in medicine, nursing, economics, sociology, social administration, political science, and other disciplines to become involved and to assist in implementing such a strategy at the international, national, regional, and other levels. Such persons have the responsibility to experiment, observe, and to describe the possibilities and implications of such a strategy. The needs and opportunities for these disciplines within such a strategy are already apparent in some health systems. They will have to become more intense and organized if they are going to result in a second leap forward in health comparable to the successes of the nineteenth century.

REFERENCES

Cooper, M.H. (1975). *Rationing health care.* Croom Helm, London.

Department of Health and Social Security (1976). *Sharing resources for health in England. Report of the resource allocation working party.* HMSO, London.

Farquhar, J.W. (1980). Changing cardiovascular risk factors in entire communities: the Stanford three community project. In *Childhood prevention of atherosclerosis and hypertension* (ed. R.M. Lauer and R.M. Skekelle) p. 435. Raven Press, New York.

King, S.C. (1976). *Health sector aid from voluntary agencies. The British case study.* Institute of Development Studies D4.85, University of Sussex.

McKeown, T. (1979). *The role of medicine—dream, mirage or nemesis.* Blackwell, Oxford.

Mejia, A., Pizurki, H., and Royston, E. (1979). *Physician and nurse migration. Analysis and policy implications.* WHO, Geneva.

National Public Health Laboratory of Finland (1981). *Community control of cardiovascular disease. The North Karelia Project.* WHO, Copenhagen.

Newell, K.W. (ed.) (1975). *Health by the people.* WHO, Geneva.

Newell, K.W. (1984). Primary health care in the Pacific. *Soc. Sci. Med.* In press.

Office of Health Economics, London (1979). Scarce resources in health care. In *Issues in health care policy, Milbank Reader 3.* (ed. J.B. McKinlay). MIT Press, Cambridge, MA.

World Bank (1975). *The assault on world poverty. Problems of rural development, education and health.* World Bank Series, Johns Hopkins University Press, Baltimore.

World Health Organization (1979). *Formulating strategies for health for all by the year 2000.* WHO, Geneva.

World Health Organization (1981). *International code of marketing of breast milk substitutes.* WHO, Geneva.

WHO/UNICEF (1978). *Primary health care. Report of the international conference on primary health care,* Alma Ata, USSR, 6–12 September 1978. WHO, Geneva.

WHO/UNICEF (1981). *National decision making for primary health care.* WHO, Geneva.

ndex